Lectures On the Diseases of Infancy and Childhood: By Charles West

Charles West

LECTURES

ON THE

DISEASES OF INFANCY

AND

CHILDHOOD.

BY

CHARLES WEST, M.D.,

FELLOW OF THE ROYAL COLLEGE OF PHYSICIANS; PHYSICIAN TO THE HOSPITAL FOR SICK CHILDREN.

FIFTH AMERICAN

FROM THE SIXTH REVISED AND ENLARGED ENGLISH EDITION.

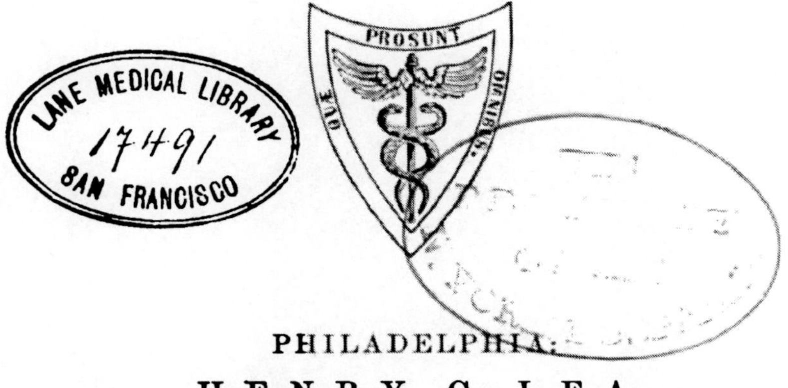

PHILADELPHIA:
HENRY C. LEA.
1874.

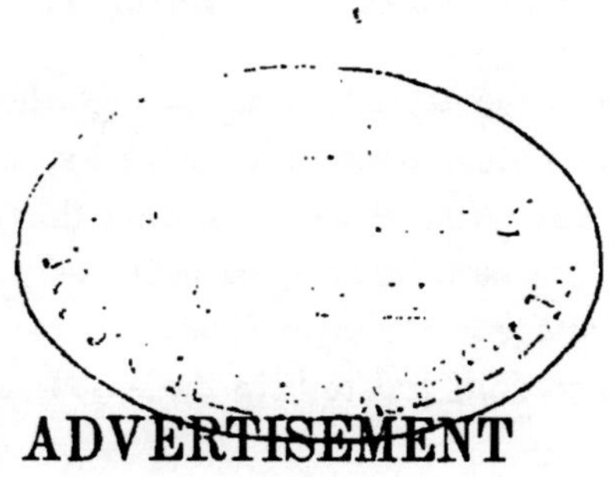

ADVERTISEMENT

TO

THE SIXTH EDITION.

THERE remains but little to add to the Preface to the former edition. Seven years more of clinical observation, and the records of 743 more cases, and of 181 more post-mortem examinations, making in all nearly 2000 cases, and nearly 600 post-mortem examinations, have, it may be hoped, enabled me to add something to the value of the work. I have striven not to increase its bulk, and have omitted much that seemed to me less important, in order to obtain space for the introduction of additional matter which appeared to me of greater moment. In spite, however, of all my pains, this volume is bigger than its predecessor by more than thirty pages.

An Italian translation, accompanied with notes, was published by Dr. Blasi of Rome in the year 1869; a second edition is now in preparation. Causes which it is not worth while to mention having interfered with the publication of the French translation of the former edition, the present is in the most competent hands of Dr. Archambault, Physician to the Hôpital des Enfants Malades.

Any one in his fifty-eighth year must feel it very doubtful whether his life will be so prolonged as to allow him to take part in the publication of another edition of a book which first appeared more than twenty-five years ago; or whether some better, completer work will not before long occupy its place.

But be this as it may, to me it is no small satisfaction to feel that future laborers will have their tasks lightened by my endeavors; that while thirty years ago there was not a single hospital for children in the whole British dominions or in America, the Hospital for Sick Children in Great Ormond Street and its thirty daughters will now tell, if my name should be at all remembered, that it was permitted me to live not altogether to myself, but in some small degree at least to serve my generation, and to help those little ones whom I so much love.

CHARLES WEST.

61 WIMPOLE STREET,
December 1, 1873.

PREFACE

TO

THE FIFTH EDITION.

TWENTY-SIX YEARS AGO the kindness of DR. ROBERT WILLIS threw open to me the field of observation afforded by the Children's Dispensary in Lambeth, and in 1842, I succeeded him there in the office of Physician.

In 1847 I gave a series of Lectures on the Diseases of Children, based on observations made at the Children's Dispensary, to the Pupils of the Middlesex Hospital; and these Lectures appeared in the "Medical Gazette" during the summer and autumn of the same year.

In 1848 these Lectures were published as a distinct book; founded on the notes of 600 cases, and 180 post-mortem examinations, which I had observed at the dwellings of the poor in the district where I labored.

The establishment of the Children's Hospital, in Great Ormond Street, brought me readier means of more careful observation, and the appointment within the past four years of different gentlemen to the office of Registrar, has provided for the record of cases of which want of leisure would have otherwise prevented me from preserving an account.

I have thus been enabled in each successive edition to add to the preceding one, and I trust to improve upon it. The present edition embodies the result of 1200 recorded cases, and of nearly 400 mortem examinations, collected from between 30,000 a children who, during the past twenty-six years, have come under my care, either in public or private practice.

While improving, as far as I could, the substance of this book, I have not attempted to alter its form; for the fact that it has passed through three editions in America, and through four in Germany, while it has also been translated into Danish, Dutch, and Russian, and that the French translation is now in the press, may be taken as good proof that it has to a great extent met the wants of the Profession both here and abroad.

A moment's satisfaction may be pardoned me in thankfully acknowledging these evidences that my toil has not been fruitless. But it is with no feeling of flattered vanity that I now lay down my pen. The revision in mature age of the labors of one's youth must, with most persons, minister to self-reproach rather than to self-satisfaction. The same unsolved problems meet one's eye now as met it years ago; one's deficiencies are felt more deeply; they seem graver and less excusable, as the time for remedying them passes by; one longs for the leisure gone, for the energies of former years, which one fancies, coupled with the soberness of advancing life, might help to add something more and better to the common store of knowledge.

I can for my part say most honestly, that nothing will give me greater pleasure than to see some younger man, better furnished for the task than I was, devote himself to the cultivation of that field where I have labored. No one would greet the skilled husbandman more heartily than I, nor rejoice more sincerely to see him reap, as he cannot fail to do, a most abundant harvest.

CHARLES WEST.

61 WIMPOLE STREET,
June 1, 1865.

CONTENTS.

LECTURES

ON THE

DISEASES OF INFANCY AND CHILDHOOD.

INTRODUCTORY.

On the Study of Children's Diseases.—Its difficulties, and how to overcome them—Rules for the examination of sick children, and for taking notes of cases—General plan and objects of the Course.

Gentlemen: It is not without hesitation that I have determined on adding another to the already numerous courses of lectures that you are called on to attend while engaged in the study of medicine. My reasons—and I trust my justification—for so doing are furnished partly by the frequency of the diseases of infancy and childhood, partly by their fatality, but still more by their many peculiarities.

Children will form at least a third of all your patients; and so serious are their diseases, that one child in five dies within a year after birth, and one in three before the completion of the fifth year. These facts, indeed, afford conclusive arguments for enforcing on you the importance of closely watching every attack of illness that may invade the body while it is so frail; but they alone would scarcely be adequate reasons for my bringing these diseases under your notice as objects for special study.

The body, however, is not only more frail in infancy than it becomes in after life, but the sympathies between its different parts are more extensive and more delicate. One organ seldom suffers alone, but the effects even of local diseases extend to the whole system, and so disorder its workings that it is often no easy matter to determine the seat of the original mischief. Nor is this all; but many important consequences result from the period of childhood being one of unceasing development. In the adult the structure of the body is complete, and its functions are the same to-day as they were yesterday: but the child learns successively to breathe, to feel, to think; and its body is daily undergoing modifications to fit it for new duties, as well as daily growing in size and strength. Disease, therefore, not merely disturbs the present, but its influence reaches to the future; it not only interrupts the present function of the organ that is affected, but it puts a stop for a time to the completion of the general machinery of the body, or disarranges the due proportion of one part of that machinery to another. Moreover, there are periods, namely, those of the first and second dentition, when very great changes take place in the organism of the child, and when all these dangers are especially to be feared. Disease is then frequent and serious beyond what it is at other times, and every ailment then warrants a double measure of anxiety; while, on the other hand, if these epochs are safely passed, there succeeds a season of comparative immunity from many affections that before were both common and perilous.

But, if this be so, you will at once perceive that something more is essential to the successful treatmennt of children's diseases than to watch their advances carefully, and to adapt the strength and doses of your remedies to the tender years of your patients. It is not mere hyperbole to say that you have to study a new semeiology, to learn a new pathology and new therapeutics. Matters of such importance cannot be properly examined at the end of a course of lectures on midwifery. I have therefore preferred making them the subjects of separate consideration during the summer, when the comparative leisure of the season will, I hope, enable you to devote some of your time to the practical as well as the theoretical study of the diseases of children.

I must warn you, however, of one difficulty which you will encounter at the very outset—a difficulty that disheartens many, and makes them abandon in despair the study of children's diseases. Your old means of investigating disease will here to a great degree fail you, and you will feel almost as if you had to learn your alphabet again, or as if, entering a country whose inhabitants you expected to find speaking the same language and having the same manners as the people in the land you had lately left, you were to hear around you everywhere the sounds of a foreign tongue, and to observe manners and customs such as you had never seen before. You cannot question your patient; or if old enough to speak, still, through fear, or from comprehending you but imperfectly, he will probably give you an incorrect reply. You try to gather information from the expression of his countenance, but the child is fretful, and will not bear to be looked at; you endeavor to feel his pulse, he struggles in alarm; you try to auscultate his chest, and he breaks out into a violent fit of crying.

Some practitioners never surmount these difficulties, and the diseases of children are consequently a sealed book to them. After a time they grow satisfied with their ignorance, and will then with the greatest gravity assure you that the attempt to understand these affections is useless. They have fallen into this unfortunate error from not taking the pains to start aright; they have never learned how to interrogate their little patients, and hence they have never received satisfactory replies. I speak of interrogating them; for though the infant cannot talk, it has yet a language of its own, and this language it must be your first object to learn, if you mean ever to acquire the character of successful practitioners in the diseases of children. But, if you have not cultivated your faculties of observation, you cannot learn it, for it is a language of signs, and these signs are such as will escape the notice of the careless; if you are not fond of little children, you cannot learn it, for they soon make up their minds as to who loves them, and when ill they will express their real feelings, whether by words or signs, to no one else.

There is, moreover, a certain tact necessary for successfully investigating the diseases of children. If, when summoned to a sick child, you enter the room abruptly, and going at once to your patient, you begin to look closely at it, while at the same time you question the mother or nurse about its ailments in your ordinary pitch of voice, the child, to whom you are a perfect stranger, will be frightened, and will begin to cry; its pulse and respiration will be hurried, its face will grow flushed, and you will thus have lost the opportunity of acquainting yourself with its real condition in many respects. Besides this, the child's alarm once excited, will not subside so long as you are present; if you want to see its tongue, or auscultate its chest, its terrors will be renewed, and it will scream violently: you will leave the room little wiser than you entered it, and, very likely, fully convinced that it is impossible to make out children's diseases.

Very different would be the result if you conducted this examination properly; and though, I believe, where there is real love for children, the tact necessary for examining into their ailments will not be long in being acquired, still a few hints on this subject may not be out of place in an introductory lecture.

The quiet manner and the gentle voice which all who have been ill know how to value in their attendants, are especially needed when the patient is a child. Your first object must be not to alarm it; if you succeed in avoiding this danger, it will not be long before you acquire its confidence. Do not, therefore, on entering the room, go at once close up to the child; but, sitting down sufficiently near to watch it, and yet so far off as not to attract its attention, put a few questions to its attendant. While doing this, you may, without seeming to notice it, acquire a great deal of important information; you may observe the expression of the face, the nature of the respiration, whether slow or frequent, regular or unequal; and if the child utters any sound you may attend to the character of its cry. All your observations must be made without staring the child in the face; little children, especially if ill, seem always disturbed by this, and will be almost sure to cry. If the child is asleep at the time of your visit, your observations may be more minute: the kind of sleep should be noticed, whether quiet or disturbed, whether the eyes are perfectly closed during it, or partly open, as they are in many cases where the nervous system is disordered: you may, too, if the sleep seems sound, venture to count the frequency of the respiration and the beat of the pulse, but in doing this you should be careful not to arouse the child. It should be awakened gently by the nurse or mother, and a strange face should not be the first to meet its eye on awaking. If it were awake when you entered the room, it will probably in a few minutes have grown accustomed to your presence, and will allow you to touch its hand and feel its pulse. This must always be done at as early a period in your visit as possible, in order that you may count it while the child is undisturbed, since the pulsations of the heart vary in young children, as much as twenty in a minute under comparatively slight disturbing causes; and any inferences that you might draw from the pulse of the child, when frightened or excited, would almost certainly be erroneous. Here, as throughout when children are your patients, your difficulties will be great or small exactly in proportion to your tact. If you grasp the hand, however gently, and try to feel the pulse, the little one will struggle to be free. If you place your hand as if accidentally on its arm, and gradually move your fingers downward to the wrist, you will often unobserved and unsuspected count the pulse. Or if the nurse or mother takes the babe's hand in hers it will leave it there with confidence, and will not heed the pressure of your fingers. Besides the pulse, the frequency of the respiration should, if possible, be noticed, since the results obtained by a comparison of the two are always more valuable than those of either taken alone. But if this is your first visit to the child, do not, for the sake of ascertaining either of these points exactly, persevere in attempts which irritate or frighten it: probably you would, after all, be unsuccessful; and even though you were to succeed, the knowledge would not repay you for the loss of the child's confidence, which it must be your grand object to acquire and to keep.

With management and gentleness, however, you will comparatively seldom fail; and while you are feeling the pulse, or with the hand on the abdomen are counting the frequency of the inspirations, you will also learn the temperature of the body and the condition of the skin. Supposing your examination has thus far been pretty well borne, you may now probably, venture to talk to the child, or to show it something to amuse it—as your watch or stethoscope; and while thus testing the state of its mental powers, you may pass your hand over the head, and note the state of the fontanelle, and the presence or absence of heat of the scalp.

Often, though not always, it is important to ascertain the temperature with greater exactness than is possible without the aid of the thermometer; and its neglect would then be at least as culpable as the omission of auscultation, and would lead to just as grave mistakes. When practicable it is best to take the temperature in the axilla, but where the restlessness of the patient, as is often the case with infants and very young children, renders this impossible, the thermometer can almost always be placed in the fold of the groin without exciting resistance, and the results thus obtained are very little less accurate.

The examination of the state of the abdomen, though too important to allow of its ever being omitted, will often lead to no satisfactory result unless carefully managed. If you allow the nurse to change the child's posture and to lay it back in her lap, in order that you may pass your hand over its stomach, the child will often be alarmed, and begin to cry. Its abdomen then becomes perfectly tense, and you cannot tell whether pressure on it causes pain, or whether the cries are not altogether the consequence of fear. It is therefore the best plan to pass your hand beneath the child's clothes, and to examine the abdomen without altering its posture, while, at the same time, the nurse talks to it to distract its attention, or holds it opposite the window, or a bright light, which seldom fails to amuse an infant. If there is no tenderness of the abdomen the child will not cry on pressure; or if, during your examination, the presence of flatus in the intestines should occasion pain, gentle friction, instead of increasing suffering, will give relief.

You must next examine the chest: and for this purpose immediate auscultation is always to be preferred, since the pressure of the stethoscope generally annoys the child. If the child is not in its bedgown, it will usually be your best course to have the back of its dress undone, and then, while it is seated in its mother's or nurse's lap, to kneel down behind it, and apply your ear to its chest. In all acute diseases of the lungs in infancy, the condition of their posterior part is a sure index to the extent of the mischief from which they are suffering; for owing to the infant passing so much of its time in the horizontal position, the blood naturally gravitates towards the back of the lungs, and the secretions are much more likely to accumulate in the bronchi in that situation than elsewhere: hence, if air is heard permeating the lungs throughout the whole posterior part of the chest, and unaccompanied with any considerable amount of crepitation, it may fairly be inferred that their front parts are free from serious disease, even though you should be unable to ascertain the fact by actual observation.

When you have listened thoroughly to the back of the chest, you may next percuss it. You must not percuss first and listen afterwards, as you often do in the adult; for, even when practiced with the greatest gentleness, percussion sometimes frets the child, and makes it cry, whereby any subsequent attempt to listen to the breathing will often be rendered unsuccessful. But you must not neglect percussion: it is of peculiar value in childhood, since auscultation is then unavoidably incomplete in many instances, sometimes quite impracticable. In practicing it, however, there are some rules without attention to which you will very likely fail of acquiring any information. You must never, in the child, attempt to percuss the walls of the chest immediately, but should strike on your finger, and even then very gently. The chest of the child is so resonant, that, if you percuss smartly, you will fail to perceive the finer variations of sonority which would be readily appreciable on gentle percussion. Always compare the results obtained by percussing opposite sides of the chest, since otherwise you may overlook a very considerable degree of dulness. It often happens, too, that the lower lobes of both lungs are involved nearly equally; you must therefore notice the resonance of the lower as compared with that of the upper part of the chest. Sometimes you are compelled, by the fretfulness of the child, or by the tenderness of the walls of its chest, to percuss so gently as scarcely to elicit any sound. It is of importance, therefore, to attend to the sensation of solidity communicated to the finger, as well as to the sound of dulness that falls upon the ear, since if your sense of touch is delicate, it will correct or confirm the evidence of hearing.

Having thus examined the back of the chest, you may, if the child is likely to tolerate it, try to listen at its sides, and then in front. You can, however, scarcely auscultate the front of the chest in infancy without a stethoscope, and this you will often be unable to use; for, if the child is not frightened, it will probably be so exceedingly amused at what it regards as specially intended for its own diversion, that it will join in the game, and disconcert you by playing with the instrument. You will encounter this difficulty in cases of phthisis in early childhood, and will sometimes find it no easy matter to ascertain the character of the respiration in the front of the chest. In such cases you will learn all the value of percussion, which may be practiced over the front of the chest as well as the back, while the state of the breathing in the upper and back part of the chest will generally afford a tolerably accurate clue to its condition in front; though, except in instances of great tubercular enlargement of the bronchial glands, the signs of pulmonary consumption are perceived earlier, and in a more marked degree, under the clavicle than in any other situation.

Your examination of the chest will not be complete until you have noticed the character of the breathing, whether the whole of the chest is expanded by it, or whether the respiration is merely abdominal—whether the child breathes as deeply as it should, or whether it makes frequent short inspirations which cannot fill the smaller bronchi. The time for ascertaining these points must vary in each case; but the earlier they are observed the better, since otherwise you run the risk of drawing your inferences, not from the child's ordinary condition, but from its state when excited and alarmed. Some of these points may be noticed though the child be so fretful that you cannot auscultate even the back of its chest satisfactorily. An imperfect auscultation, however, is better than none; for at the very worst, during the deep inspirations that are made at intervals in a fit of crying, you may ascertain how far the lungs are permeable to air, and whether the bronchi are much loaded with mucus. Independently of auscultation, too, much may be learned from the cry. If its two periods are clearly marked—the long loud cry of expiration, and the shorter, less loud, but perfectly distinct sound that attends inspiration—you may feel convinced that there exists no important ailment of the respiratory organs.

It will still remain for you to examine the tongue, and to ascertain the condition of the gums; and it is wise to defer this to the last, since it is usually the most grievous part of your visit to the child. If during any part of your previous examination it had cried, you might seize that opportunity to look at its tongue, and, if necessary, to pass your finger over the gums; thus sparing it any further distress about the matter. If you had not this opportunity, you will generally get a good view of the mouth and throat in young infants by gently touching the lips with your finger; the child opens its mouth instinctively, and then you can run your finger quickly over its tongue, and down towards the pharynx, and thus secure a perfect view of the mouth and throat. With older children a good deal of coaxing is sometimes necessary to persuade them to open their mouth; but, if once you get your finger on the gum, you can usually keep the patient quiet by rubbing it, and, by a little address, will then seldom fail in opening the mouth wide enough to get a view of the tongue.

If little children are very ill, all this minute care in the order of your examination is not so much needed, because they will not notice so quickly; but gentleness of tone and manner will be even more necessary to soothe the pettishness and quiet the alarm of the little sufferer.

Many of the directions that I have just given you refer to the examination of infants, and become less applicable in proportion to the greater age of the patient. Minute rules for your examination of children from three years old and upwards are not needed: but patience the most untiring, and good temper the most unruffled, are indispensable.

The previous history of a patient, the circumstances in which his present illness came on, and the symptoms that at first attended it, often help to remove our doubts with reference to the nature of a disease, and sometimes greatly modify our diagnosis, and influence our plan of treatment. Really trustworthy information on these points, however, is often difficult to be obtained, and the attempt to elicit it is almost sure to be unsuccessful, if the questions put to the patient are proposed at random, and without some previously well-digested plan on the part of the physician. One great object of clinical instruction is to teach the student so to conduct this as well as other parts of his examination of the sick, as to throw from every source the greatest possible amount of light upon the nature of the disease, and thus to fit himself to decide with some approach to certainty on the means most likely to effect its cure. Such instruction has been amply afforded you in the wards of the hospital; but you must allow me to detain you while I point out the subjects towards which your inquiries must be especially directed in the case of children, since they differ in many respects from the questions that you would propose if your patient were an adult.

We will suppose, if you please, that a child is brought to you of whose case you wish to preserve a record. Its name, age, sex, and residence will form of course the first entry in your note-book; but your next inquiries should be as to the number of living children that the parents have had, whether any of those children have died, and, if so, at what age, and of what diseases, and as to the health of both parents, and of their immediate relatives. The object of these questions is to ascertain whether there exists any hereditary tendency to disease in the family, since that plays a most important part in many of the affections of childhood, and symptoms that in the child of healthy parents would cause you but little uneasiness, would at once excite serious alarm if you knew that some members of the family had died of hydrocephalus, or of consumption, or had been the subjects of scrofula.

Many of the most serious affections of childhood occur within the period of a few years, and after a certain age are comparatively rare in their occurrence, and generally mild in their character. It is therefore very desirable when any ailment is coming on, the nature of which is not yet quite apparent, to know which of the diseases incidental to childhood have already affected your patient. With this view you would ask whether the child has been vaccinated, or has had the small-pox, and whether it has passed through any other of those affections—such as chicken-pox, hooping-cough, measles, or scarlatina—which generally come on in early life. If the child had suffered from any other disease, you should learn its nature, the age at which it occurred, and any other point of importance connected with it.

In writing out your history of the case, these preliminary matters would naturally be mentioned at the beginning; and, though you would not follow any very strict order in proposing your questions, yet it is always desirable to obtain information on these points at an early stage of your examination, since it may guide you in some of the questions that you afterwards propose, or may lead you to pay particular attention to symptoms which otherwise would not seem to be of much moment. Besides, if you postpone these inquiries till you have nearly completed your examination of the patient, the parents will probably apprehend that they are suggested by some doubt and apprehension in your mind as to the nature of the case, and will distress themselves by causeless fears, or perhaps disconcert you by questions to which you are not prepared to return a positive answer.

There are two other points which bear on the general condition of the child, to one or both of which your inquiries must in many instances be directed. If your patient is an infant at the breast, you must learn whether it lives entirely on its mother's milk, or has other food besides. If it has been weaned, you must ask its age at weaning; whether it was taken from the breast on account of any failure in its own health or its mother's, and on what diet it has since been fed. The process of dentition is the other subject for examination; and in reference to it you must ascertain how many teeth the child has, and which they are; whether they were cut easily or with difficulty, the age at which teething commenced, and the time that has elapsed since any fresh teeth appeared.

You may now endeavor to obtain a clear and connected history of the present illness; and for this purpose it is well to begin with asking, When did the child last seem quite well? since you thus get a fixed starting-point from which you can make the mother or nurse set out in her detail of symptoms. The date thus assigned, indeed, will often be a wrong one, the disease having begun before with some symptom that was not noticed, or its real origin having been considerably subsequent to its supposed commencement. But notwithstanding this possible error, you derive much advantage from thus making sure of the symptoms being told you in something like their chronological order, since otherwise it is very likely that those only would be mentioned which had chanced to strike the mind of the mother or of the nurse, while the others would be passed over in silence. Your object in the examination must not be to curtail the garrulity of the nurse, or to suppress the mother's expression of her sometimes imaginary fears, but to get as clear an account as possible of everything that has been observed. You must be careful not to underrate the value of the information they communicate, or even of the opinions they express. Both are much more likely to be correct when your patients are children, than when they are adults. A mother hanging over her sick infant, or a nurse watching the child she has helped to rear from babyhood, may sometimes see dangers that have no existence, but will generally be the first to perceive the approach of such as are real. You see the child but for a few minutes and at distant intervals, and the excitement or alarm which your presence is so likely to occasion may greatly modify its condition during your visit. They tend the little one by day and night, notice each movement, and seize the most transient variations in its expression.

I need not say much concerning the necessity of inquiring about the appetite and thirst, the state of the bowels, and the appearance of the evacuations; for these are points which you would investigate in patients of every age. I will just mention, however, that the degree of appetite and thirst cannot be so readily determined in the infant as they may be in the adult, or even in the weaned child; for an infant may suck, not because it is hungry, but in order to quench its thirst. That extreme craving for the breast, which is appeased only so long as the child is sucking, while the milk swallowed is speedily vomited, may be taken as a sign of thirst; but it is always better to record the fact than the inference. It is likewise often desirable to let the infant be put to the breast in your presence, not only for the sake of observing the above-mentioned facts, but also in order to notice the vigor with which it sucks, the ease or difficulty with which it swallows, and other similar points, from which very important conclusions may often be drawn.

Before you venture on drawing any inferences from the state of the child at the time of your visit, you should ascertain whether it has just before been taking food, or has been recently excited or fatigued by being washed or dressed; since comparatively trivial causes are sufficient to accelerate the pulse and respiration, and to give rise to changes which might, if unexplained, lead you to very erroneous conclusions. Any such circumstances ought of course to be mentioned in your notes, as should also the fact of the child being asleep at the time of your visit, since that would explain even a very considerable diminution in the frequency of the pulse and respiration.

But if you are carefully to observe all the points which I have mentioned, and to make yourselves thoroughly masters of a case, you must be most lavish of your time; you must be content to turn aside from the direct course of investigation, which you would pursue uninterruptedly in the adult, in order to soothe the waywardness of the child, to quiet its fears, or even to cheat it into good humor by joining in its play; and you must be ready to do this, not the first time only, but every time that you visit the child, and must try to win its affections in order to cure its disease. If you fail in the former, you will often be foiled in your attempts at the latter. Nor is this all: you must visit your patient very often, if the disease is serious in its nature and rapid in its course. New symptoms succeed each other in infancy and childhood with great rapidity; complications occur that call for some change in your treatment, or the vital powers falter suddenly, when you least expect it. The issues of life and death often hang on the immediate adoption of a certain plan of treatment, or on its timely discontinuance. Do not wait, therefore, for symptoms of great urgency before you visit a child three or four times a day; but if the disease is one in which changes are likely to take place rapidly, be frequent in your visits as well as watchful in your observation.

You will naturally think, that before I finish this lecture I should tell you something definite about the subjects that I mean to bring before your notice, and the manner in which I propose to treat them. The title of these lectures can, I should think, scarcely need any explanation, for by the diseases of infancy and childhood you will naturally understand all those affections which are either limited in the time of their occurrence to early life, or which, though incidental to all ages, yet in the child present many peculiarities in their symptoms, and require many important modifications in their treatment. Some of these diseases, indeed, are usually allotted to the care of the surgeon, and on their examination I will not enter, since I could tell you nothing more than has already been better said by others. For the same reason, too, I leave untouched the very important class of cutaneous affections, well worth your study indeed; but that study should be carried on under a more skilful guide than I could prove myself.

In the description of the diseases of children, no practically useful end would be attained by following any elaborate nosological system. I shall therefore adopt the most simple classification possible, and shall treat in succession of the diseases of the nervous system, of the respiratory and circulatory, and of the digestive systems and their appendages. There will still remain one very important class of affections, namely, fevers; and these I propose to consider last of all, because much of their danger arises from their complications, and to treat them judiciously you must be familiar with the diseases of the brain, the lungs, and the bowels. In this plan it will be easy to detect a want, perhaps too great a want, of scientific arrangement; but the one object of my endeavors will be to communicate to you, as clearly as I can, such information as may be most useful to you in the discharge of your daily duties.

With this view I have, while composing these lectures, tried to think over the doubts I felt, the difficulties I met with, and the errors I fell into, when, now many years ago, I entered on the office of physician to a large institution for the treatment of children's diseases. I have presumed that where I had encountered difficulties, there you might meet them too; that where I had made mistakes, there you would need a guide; and, remembering the many anxious hours I passed when I hesitatingly adopted some course which I feared might after all be a mistaken one, it has been my aim to lay down, not only the rules for the diagnosis, but also the indications for the treatment of each disease as minutely as possible.

To the task before me I now apply myself, with a deep conviction of the narrow limits of my own knowledge, but still feeling that I have contracted an obligation to impart to others what I trust experience has taught me. My end will be answered, if you learn it at an easier rate than I did, and if I can be the means of saving you from some of those errors in diagnosis, and some of those mistakes in treatment, which, for want of some one to guide me aright, I committed.

LECTURE II.

INTRODUCTORY.

ON THE TREATMENT OF CHILDREN'S DISEASES.—Influence of remedies modified by the age of the patient—Rules for the practice of depletion, for the use of mercury, antimony, opium, and other sedatives, and for the employment of blisters—Suggestions as to the mode of prescribing for infants and children.

IN the introductory lecture, I tried to point out the main peculiarities which distinguish the diseases of early life, and to furnish you with some general rules for their investigation. It may not be time misspent, if, before we begin the examination of any special class of ailments, I endeavor to give you a few general *directions for their treatment*, though in so doing I must of necessity anticipate some things which will require notice hereafter, and must occasionally presuppose the possession of that knowledge which it is the main object of these lectures to impart.

The importance of great exactness in prescribing for infants and children, and the necessity for regulating the doses of our remedies according to the tender years of our patients, are self-evident. Posological tables, as they are termed, are, however, of very little value for our guidance, since the susceptibility of the young to the action of different remedies varies greatly according to their nature, so that the rule which safely defines the dose of an opiate, would be altogether inapplicable as determining the strength of a purgative or of an emetic.

The abstraction of blood, the use of emetics and purgatives, the employment of antiphlogistics, and the administration of sedatives, are the great weapons with which we endeavor to combat the advances of acute disease. The safe use of each of these in early life implies the observance of certain precautions which I will now attempt to explain, and will then try to furnish you with a few general directions that may be of service in prescribing for infants and children.

The early age of our patients imposes of necessity some restriction on the mode in which *depletion* can be practiced; for venesection in the arm is hardly ever possible before the age of three years, often not till later, in consequence both of the small size of the veins, and of the quantity of fat in which they are imbedded. In cases of extreme urgency the jugular vein may be opened, and I have never found any difficulty in the operation, though I believe the necessity for the proceeding very seldom arises, and the only cases in which I have had recourse to it were either instances of violent convulsions succeeded by profound coma, or else of very acute inflammatory croup.

For almost all purposes of depletion in early life we are dependent on the use of leeches, and by this means, if rightly managed, we may attain nearly all the ends of general bleeding. The great objection to the employment of leeches rests on the difficulty of estimating and of controlling the quantity of blood abstracted by them. This objection, however, applies almost entirely to the common practice of putting on a comparatively small number of leeches, and trusting to the application of a poultice, or the employment of fomentations, for obtaining a sufficient quantity of blood. Instead of adopting this plan, than which nothing can be more uncertain, it is far better to apply a larger number of leeches, and to allow of no subsequent bleeding. It may be calculated that each leech takes about two drachms of blood, and we are thus enabled to estimate the quantity removed with a certainty little less than we are possessed of if we employ venesection, while, further, the blood is removed in the course of fifteen or twenty minutes, instead of draining away, as in the other case, for six or eight hours, weakening the patient, and yet exercising comparatively small influence on the disease.

To insure certainty and safety, however, in the employment of leeches, there are several precautions which must not be neglected. Of these the most important is, that their application should not be left to a nurse, but that, wherever it is at all practicable, the medical attendant should himself superintend it. This is of special moment in all acute diseases in which it is desired to obtain by local bleeding the constitutional effects of general depletion; since, according to the result produced, it may, on the one hand, be desirable to put on a larger number, or, on the other, to remove some before they have completely filled themselves. The effects produced by the loss of blood often influence the character of the subsequent treatment. On this account, therefore, as well as with the view of lessening the risk of hemorrhage going on from the leech-bites unperceived, it is desirable to apply leeches by day, not towards evening, or at bedtime, as is commonly the practice. Attention should further always be paid to apply leeches in situations where they will not alarm the child by being within his sight, and where, also, there is a firm surface beneath against which pressure can be made, so as readily to control the bleeding. Behind the ears, therefore, or on the vertex, are the best situations for applying leeches to the head, and under the scapulæ when it is necessary to deplete from the chest; while, in many abdominal affections, all the advantages of local bleeding may be most safely obtained by the application of leeches to the anus.

The above rules apply to the *mode* of practicing depletion in early life; but, independently of the mere manner of drawing blood, there are some still more important cautions which have reference to the general principles that should govern us in resorting to depletion at all.

1st. It should be remembered that large losses of blood are worse borne by the child than by the adult; that if syncope is produced, its effects do not pass away so speedily, but leave a much more abiding depression.

2d. That the shock consequent on large losses of blood, shows itself, not merely by causing syncope, but also, not very seldom, by producing convulsions; and such convulsions are specially apt to be excited in cases where the previous disorder of the nervous system was considerable, even though that disorder depended on congestion of the brain which called for depletion to relieve it. It seems as if in these cases, just as in some of comparatively slight disease of the heart, if the equilibrium of the circulation is suddenly disturbed it altogether fails to recover itself. A child of ten months old was brought to me many years ago with symptoms of cerebral congestion—a hot head, a raised fontanelle, a burning skin, and twitching of the tendons of the arms and legs. I ordered leeches to the head, which drew freely: but the convulsions which it was hoped they would ward off, occurred while the bleeding was still going on, and the child sank at once into a state of coma, from which it never rallied completely, and died in the course of forty-eight hours. Now, in this case, the abstraction of blood was indicated, and the appearances discovered after death showed that the depletion had not been excessive. It had, however, been too sudden; and probably, had I been present when the leeches were applied, I should have noticed some change in the child's condition which would have warned me to put a stop to further bleeding, and might thus have led to an entirely different result. In proportion, therefore, to the youth of our patient, must be our caution in ordering free depletion, and our care in watching its effects; and these must both be greater when marked disorder of the nervous system forms the indication for our treatment.

3d. Not only are very large losses of blood hazardous, and great shock by its too sudden abstraction also attended with danger in early infancy, but repeated bleedings are also inexpedient. The system rallies from them with proportionately far greater difficulty than in the adult, and that peculiar class of symptoms, by which exhaustion is apt to simulate congestion of the brain, is specially likely to be induced. It may be added that, to a considerable degree, the same caution holds good with reference to all other antiphlogistic remedies; that free purgation, spare diet, and depressing measures of all kinds, though often requisite, yet require most heedful watching, and generally need to be soon discontinued.

Changes in medical opinion, such as have taken place within the past twenty years, influence one's conduct by slow and almost imperceptible degrees, and I find that my practice now differs much from what it was a quarter of a century ago; that I deplete less than I did, that I have less faith in mercury, that I employ antimony more rarely, that I have more confidence in nature's powers, less reliance on my own resources. And yet I am unwilling to believe that all my former observations were erroneous and that my old faith was entirely misplaced; but unhappily I have no longer the leisure to test the value of these changes as I could wish; while the peculiarities of consultation practice in a large city, though they may sharpen one's perception, and increase one's promptness in action, are anything but favorable to scientific investigation or to accurate reasoning.

With this explanation, and if need be, apology for my still entertaining views on some subjects opposed to, or as may be said, behind the opinions of the day, I will now proceed to tell you what I think about other great remedies that one employs in the diseases of childhood.

And first, with reference to *mercury*. I still believe that it possesses a peculiar and specific power in controlling acute inflammation of the serous membranes of the chest and abdomen; and that both acute pleurisy and acute peritonitis (the latter, by the by, as rare as the former is frequent in early life), yield to a combination of calomel and opium more speedily than to opium alone. I feel also persuaded that in severe inflammation of the mucous membrane of the large intestines —in other words, in dysentery in childhood—the part borne by mercury in its cure is at least of as much moment as that of the opium with which it is right to combine it; but the latter alone will fail when the two together will save the patient.

In laryngeal inflammation, or true croup, after the first active symptoms have been subdued, mercury often plays an important part in its more chronic stages; and I still hold to the belief that in some forms of chronic non-tuberculous consolidation of the lung, recovery is expedited by the careful employment of mercurials. I do not regard it as of any service in acute affections of the pulmonary tissue, nor in any form of bronchitis, but I still regard mercury as of service in acute pericarditis; and I say this with full consciousness of the sources of fallacy which in this case may readily interfere with the formation of a correct judgment.

In cachectic diseases its utility is far more limited. The earlier symptoms of congenital syphilis yield rapidly to the employment of small doses of mercury; but the tertiary results of the disease are often aggravated, very seldom indeed benefited, by that medicine. In the majority of disorders connected with the tubercular diathesis, mercurials are not beneficial, and in tubercular meningitis in particular, in which they are so often given, I never saw even momentary improvement from them, apart from their occasional action as purgatives. It must, however, be confessed that in their powerlessness to control this disease, they do but stand on the same footing with all other medicines. There is one class of ailments, too, connected with tuberculosis, in which the action of mercury is almost uniformly beneficial, and that is tubercular peritonitis, and those vague disorders of the functions of nutrition so commonly, though so often erroneously, referred to disease of the mesenteric glands.

In administering mercury to infants and young children, it must be borne in mind that evidence of the system being affected by it is seldom afforded, as in the adult, by the occurrence of salivation. So rare, indeed, is mercurial stomatitis in early life, that I have seen but one instance in which it proved fatal, and have very seldom met with it in such a degree as to be troublesome. I should therefore regard the production of gangrene of the mouth by the administration of mercury, as an evidence of some rare idiosyncrasy on the part of the patient rather than of want of due care on that of the doctor. In early life, mercury, instead of affecting the mouth, usually acts very speedily as an irritant on the intestinal canal; and the green stools, which are often looked on with satisfaction as a proof of the system being brought under the influence of the medicine, are far from always having that meaning. They prove its action as a local irritant—a result which may be most undesirable, and which often compels us to diminish its dose, sometimes even completely to suspend its administration. Sometimes, too, calomel acts as an irritant on the mucous membrane of the stomach, producing nausea and vomiting, and giving rise to so great a degree of depression as to necessitate its discontinuance.

Besides its use in those more formidable diseases to which reference has hitherto been made, mercury is also often employed as a purgative and alterative. There is no doubt but that used with either of these objects it is a remedy of great value, and the objection to its employment is, not that it fails to accomplish these ends, but that it answers them at a greater expense of constitutional power than is necessary. Rhubarb, soda, the mineral acids, aloetic preparations, taraxacum, and other remedies, exert an alterative power over the secretions, without any of that depressing influence which attends the use of mercurials. In the same manner, there are many purgatives no less certain, and no less speedy in exciting the action of the bowels; so that, before prescribing calomel or gray powder, both of which ought to be absolutely banished from nursery use, the practitioner ought to be satisfied that there is some special end, in producing an increased secretion of bile, in controlling an excited state of the circulation, or in rapidly modifying the condition of the intestinal mucous membrane, which no other remedy would attain, or at any rate would not attain so certainly or so quickly.

A second remedy of great value in early life is *antimony*, though one which also is not infrequently misapplied. It is not as a simple emetic that antimony ought to be employed, for, unlike ipecacuanha, its influence is not confined to inducing vomiting, but it also exerts a most powerful depressing action on the circulation, and is therefore especially indicated in acute inflammation of the lungs and air-tubes. When the object is merely to empty the stomach, to produce that revulsion which follows the operation of an emetic, and which leads us often to prescribe it at the onset of a febrile attack for the sake of the moist skin and tranquil pulse which seldom fail to succeed its operation; or when we seek simply to free the bronchi from the secretions poured into them in too great abundance, as in catarrh or in simple hooping-cough; every end is answered by the use of ipecacuanha. On the other hand, in the onset of croup, in the early stage of acute pneumonia or of capillary bronchitis, when disease is advancing every hour and when its advance directly threatens life, antimony is the only medicine sufficiently speedy and sufficiently powerful in its action to keep pace with the advances of the disease, and to hold it in check. Even in these cases, however, the administration of antimony needs care, and after tolerance of it has been established we cannot, so safely as in the adult, continue its use. I shall hereafter have to explain to you the liability to collapse of the lung in early life, when feeble inspiratory power is associated with the presence of secretion in the air-tubes. In this state the pulmonary tissue tends by its own elasticity to exclude the air from the air-vesicles; and if the muscular power is reduced below a certain point, the patient's efforts fail to dilate them, and by degrees more and more of the lung becomes dense, unaerated, and as useless for the time, for all purposes of respiration, as if it had been solidified by inflammation or compressed by fluid. This danger is always to be borne in mind in the pulmonary affections of early life, and the vigor of the patient's powers must be the measure of our treatment, as much as the urgency of the disease.

As a mere diaphoretic, antimony, when administered in small doses, is as useful in the case of the child as in that of the adult. I am not fond of its use, however, as an antiphlogistic in ordinary febrile affections; for the nausea which it is apt to produce may obscure the approach of cerebral mischief, or lead to an erroneous interpretation of the symptoms.

A third great remedy in the diseases of early life is *opium* in its various preparations; and with it may be classed, though separated by a wide interval, other sedatives, such as hemlock, henbane, hop, and lettuce. Perhaps no remedies are so often needed in the diseases of early life as sedatives, for at no other age is the nervous system so easily disturbed. At the same time, the susceptibility to the action of narcotics and sedatives is so remarkable, and the evils which result from their unnecessary employment or from their administration in excessive doses are so serious, that some practitioners altogether abstain from their use. To do so, however, is to deprive ourselves of one of the most important classes of remedies, and of one for which no substitute can be devised.

The danger which especially attends the use of opium arises partly from the employment of uncertain preparations, such as the syrup of poppies; partly from the administration of overdoses, or from their too frequent repetition: of which two errors, the latter is more frequently committed. In prescribing for children, preparations of definite strength should always be used, as the compound tincture of camphor, tincture of opium, or Dover's powder. The weaker preparation, the compound tincture of camphor, is often preferable to laudanum, since a slight error in dispensing is of so much less moment. Sometimes the comparative tastelessness of laudanum renders it the more suitable; but if so, even though only a single dose is needed, it is wiser in the case of infants to order a mixture containing two or three doses, in order to lessen the risks of error. But mischief is more frequently done by the frequent repetition of opium, than by the improper prescription of overdoses; and I am always averse to the common practice of giving small quantities of opium at short intervals, for the purpose of checking diarrhœa or of soothing restlessness in young infants; and prefer, unless there be some strong reason to the contrary, to give a larger dose of the remedy once or twice in the twenty-four hours.

In addition to these general precautions with reference to the mode of administering opium, special care is needed in its employment in some conditions. It must be given charily in all cases where the system has been exhausted by the previous disease, or by the previous treatment; and this caution must be particularly borne in mind during convalescence from fever, where yet the patient's restlessness not seldom requires its employment. In all cases of cerebral excitement the use of opium calls for great watchfulness; sometimes it must be given rather as an experiment whereby the real nature of the disease is tested, and when so employed its results must be scrutinized with the most anxious care. In severe diarrhœa, too, the transition from a state of excitability of the nervous system to a condition of coma is often very rapid in its occurrence; an overdose of opium may hasten or induce this catastrophe, or, even though it should not have this result, yet without great care we shall be at a loss to determine how far the disease, and how far the medicine, has induced the symptoms.

The subcutaneous injection of morphia is an exceptional means for obtaining relief from intense pain which once or twice I have had recourse to. It is, however, hazardous in early childhood, and the few instances in which it is likely to be needed will be met with in surgical rather than in medical practice.

In mere restlessness, unattended by severe pain, other sedatives are often preferable to opium: thus, for instance, the feverish disquietude of a child during teething is often soothed by henbane, while that which manifests itself by a disposition to carpopedal contraction and to spasm of the glottis is mitigated by small doses of hydrocyanic acid and chloric ether as effectually as by opiates, and with far greater safety.

Two additional sedatives have of late years been introduced into practice, both of them of great value, and both free from the special risks of opium. The *bromide of potass* and the *hydrate of chloral*, either alone or in combination, seem to exercise special influence in producing sleep in various disorders of the nervous system, such as spasm of the glottis in infancy, or chorea in subsequent childhood. They are of equal service in overcoming the persistent sleeplessness for which in delicate children it sometimes happens that no definite cause can be discovered. In cases where cerebral disease is suspected they may be given with advantage, and without obscuring the symptoms, and also in the restlessness of fever, provided the stimulating power of opium is not indicated. They do not, however, annul pain as opium does, even though they may produce sleep; the sleep is not refreshing if the actual suffering is severe when the patient awakes; and as they both tend to depress the circulation, they must not be given in cases of great exhaustion, nor, I think, when there is serious organic disease of the heart.

The difficulties in the administration of internal remedies in early life have had no small share in leading practitioners to the employment of outward applications with much greater frequency than in the adult. Fomentations, poultices, and liniments of various kinds relieve pain, abate spasm, or serve as useful counter-irritants, in very many cases which I need not now occupy your time in specifying. But, besides these, *blisters* are also much used in different inflammatory affections, more particularly in those of the lungs and air-tubes, though I think their application is more restricted and is resorted to with greater caution now than formerly; and I see far fewer instances of unhealthy ulceration of blistered surfaces among the children of the poor now, than came under my notice twenty years ago.

In applying blisters to infants and young children, it must be borne in mind, not only that they vesicate more speedily that in the adult, but that the vesicated surface is apt, especially in some diseases, to pass into a state of ulceration; and, further, that the amount of constitutional disturbance produced by blisters is considerable in proportion to the youth of the patient.

The ordinary rule, which prescribes four hours as the longest time during which a blister should be allowed to remain on the skin in infancy, is on the whole a good one, but it must be remembered that some parts of the surface are far more sensitive than others. Thus, for instance, the skin on the front of the chest is peculiarly delicate, and a blister applied there for two hours would almost certainly vesicate, while it might not produce the same effect in double the time if applied beneath the scapulæ. On the other hand, the scalp is remarkably deficient in sensitiveness, and a blister may be allowed to remain on it for eight hours without any risk of mischief ensuing. There are, moreover, some diseases which increase the susceptibility of the skin to the action of irritants: thus, for instance, in all the ailments which accompany or succeed to measles, and especially in the pneumonia which often complicates it, a vesicated surface is apt to pass into a state of dangerous ulceration. Nor is this the only hazard that attends their use; but the constitutional disturbance which they produce, the pain while they are drawing, the soreness of the surface while they are being dressed, and the itching and irritation which accompany their healing, often keep up an amount of restlessness, and a state of feverish irritation, that are in every way prejudicial to the child's recovery.

On these accounts, therefore, I have almost entirely abandoned the use of blisters in infancy and early childhood, and am always most careful that no extensively abraded surface shall be left by their application. Partly with this object, and partly in order to avoid the inconvenience of the blister being dislodged by the movements of the child, I make use almost exclusively of the blistering fluid, which is painted once or oftener over the surface, according as it is wished to produce a more or less considerable degree of irritation. If vesication takes place, the serum is let out by pricking with a needle, and a layer of cotton-wool being applied over the surface is allowed to remain there until, healing being completed, it drops off of its own accord. In addition to the avoidance of danger and the lessening of constitutional disturbance by these means, we have the great advantage of being able, if it should be desirable, to repeat the same proceeding in the course of three or four days, while, by the ordinary mode of employing blisters, ten days almost invariably elapse before the sore left by their application is healed. In other cases, such as those of chronic pleurisy, where we are anxious to promote the absorption of the effused fluid, or in cases of consolidation of the lung, associated with signs of tubercular mischief, the application of tincture of iodine once a day over the surface takes the place most advantageously of the blisters which we should employ in the adult.

The whole range of remedies might thus be gone through; and with reference to each it might be pointed out how its employment requires to be more or less modified according to the age of the patient. But to do this would be more tedious than profitable, and the majority of details will find their fittest place when we notice the disease for the cure of which this or the other medicine is specially indicated.

A few general hints may, however, be given with reference to the *art of prescribing* for infants and children of tender age. But first of all I must remind you of the twofold difficulty which you encounter in the treatment of the diseases of children, owing partly to the waywardness of the little patients themselves, partly to the prejudices of their parents, while your success as practitioners will depend on the amount of tact with which you avoid coming into direct collision with either. To prescribe nauseous medicine, when with a little care you could order it in a palatable form; to insist on a particular article of diet being given, or on a particular remedy being employed, which the parents fancy will not suit, unless you believe one or the other to be absolutely indispensable to your patient's cure—is needlessly to weaken that authority which in the graver maladies it is absolutely essential that you should be able to exert. As has been truly said by MM. Rilliet and Barthez, it is in the slighter much more than in the serious diseases of children that waywardness, fretfulness, and obstinate refusal of medicine are met with. In the majority of such cases nature alone suffices for the patient's cure, and, while you watch carefully the approach of any serious symptoms, you will lose nothing in the confidence of the parents, and gain much in the love of your patients, by sparing them the nauseous draught, and the agony of tears and fright and temper which they often undergo before they swallow it. The battle with a child to compel it to take medicine, to force it into a bath, or to give it an emetic, generally does far more harm than the remedy so administered can do good; and the many tears saved by it in the nursery are one of the strongest practical recommendations of homœopathy to the public.

But even the most expectant plan of treatment does not leave you without the power of regulating to a great degree the diet of the child, the temperature of its room, the nature of its amusements, and of excluding bright light and loud sounds from its apartment; and nothing beyond these simple measures is needed to remove many of the minor ailments of the young child. Many medicines, too, can be given without any trouble either to the child or to its attendants. A few drops of ipecacuanha wine will be unperceived in its drink, a little James's powder may be concealed in some arrowroot or on a bit of bread and butter, or a dose of scammony may pass unnoticed in a little hot and sweetened milk; while, if tonics are needed, the saccharine carbonate of iron or the steel wine will seldom be refused by the most spoiled and most wilful inhabitant of the nursery. Your own ingenuity will suggest many other remedies which may be given without exciting suspicion, or at any rate without causing disgust; and, believe me, the doctor who brings smiles rather than tears into the nursery, he whom the children love most, the parents will trust most, and that love and trust will stand him much in stead when he has to combat serious illness.

As far as may be, then, it is well to avoid formal prescriptions in treating the ailments of early life. Often, however, this is not possible; but something may still be done to make physic at any rate supportable. Let its bulk be small: two teaspoonfuls will be swallowed readily by many a child whom no persuasion could induce to take two tablespoonfuls. For the same reason, powders, except when very small, are often worse than useless; and yet one sees powdered bark or powdered calumba, or large doses of rhubarb and soda, prescribed for little children of two or three years old: and they must have been educated with far more than average wisdom, or be possessed of more than average docility, who will be prevailed on to take the nauseous compound.

In the heat and fretfulness of fever, when the child would gladly drink any moderately palatable medicine, the solution of acetate of ammonia is not seldom prescribed, and the return of the time for giving each dose of medicine is but the signal for a fresh combat between the child and its attendant, in which, whoever gains the victory, the patient is sure to suffer. A few moments' thoughtfulness would avoid the trial both to the child and its parents, for nothing would be easier than to prescribe a mixture such as it would take eagerly. A solution of carbonate of potash saturated with citric acid and flavored with syrup of mulberries, or a few grains of nitre dissolved in water and rendered palatable with syrup of lemons, form a febrifuge mixture to which very few children would object. If it is desirable to give antimony, a watery solution of tartar emetic may be substituted for the wine, the unaccustomed taste of which might be disagreeable. If a stimulant is needed, milk well sweetened conceals to a great extent the pungency of ammonia; while the chloric ether, on account of its sweet taste, is almost always taken readily.

Of course it is not possible to make all medicines palatable, and then you must confine yourselves to giving that which is unpleasant in as small a bulk as possible. Still, if you keep this object in view, it is remarkable to how large an extent it is attainable. The compound jalap powder is almost the only aperient powder which children do not very much object to, and the small bulk of jalapin enables us to dispense even with that in the greater number of instances. Scammony, and especially its extract, can be concealed in milk; and even castor oil shaken up in a bottle with hot sweetened milk, in which a piece of cinnamon has been boiled, is so disguised as scarcely to be suspected. The addition of a little chloric ether to the infusion of senna covers its nauseous taste almost completely, and an extra quantity of licorice makes even the decoction of aloes palatable, while powdered aloes, occupying a small space, can often be given in brown sugar. Rhubarb is the one medicine which nothing effectually disguises, though a little spirit of nutmeg mitigates the nauseous flavor of the infusion. Even the difficulty of administering rhubarb may often be surmounted, if we employ the extract, which is thrice as strong as the powder. Each grain of the extract may be divided into four or six tiny pills, and these, if silvered, may be given unsuspected, or at any rate quite untasted, in a little arrowroot or currant jelly. We seldom, however, need be at a loss in selecting some of the milder laxatives; for the senna electuary, the various syrups and essences of senna, the nursery infusion of senna and prunes, fluid magnesia, the saccharine carbonate of magnesia, or the very palatable Limonade Purgative of French chemists, may each in turn be employed.

It is not in general difficult to prescribe a tonic which shall both be suitable for a child, and at the same time not very unpalatable. The ordinary bitter infusion, as gentian, cascarilla, and calumba, are out of the question with young children; but the mineral acids can always be made tolerable, and the infusions of roses, cloves, and orange-peel, though perhaps of little value except as vehicles for some other remedy, are by no means unpleasant. The decoction of logwood is very valuable as a tonic and astringent, and a little sugar and a teaspoonful of port wine generally render the dose popular. In spite of its bitter flavor, the small bulk of quinine often enables us to give it without much difficulty; while the Vin de Quinquina is rarely objected to by any but very young children; and the most rebellious little ones generally grow fond of the Vin de Bugeaud—a compound of bark, cacao, and Burgundy. Cod-liver oil, disgusting as it seems to be, is comparatively seldom objected to, and orange syrup or orange wine usually conceals its taste very effectually. It happens frequently, indeed, that children grow very fond of the oil; and I have known quarrels to take place in the nursery over the spoon which had contained it. The steel wine, the saccharine carbonate of iron, and the syrup of the phosphates, which goes by the name of Parrish's chemical food, are the best and most digestible chalybeates for children; but if iron is needed in stronger forms, the syrup of orange-peel covers the taste of the muriated tincture of iron, and even the compound iron mixture of the London Pharmacopœia is taken readily if sufficiently diluted with almond emulsion.

But enough has probably been said on these preliminary subjects. Your own experience will every year deepen the conviction that in dealing with the diseases of early life nothing can be considered trivial. The object of my first lecture was to show you how it is only by attention to little things that you will learn rightly to discriminate their nature; the purpose of this has been to teach you how necessary the same attention is to their successful treatment.

LECTURE III.

DISEASES OF THE BRAIN AND NERVOUS SYSTEM.—Their extreme frequency in early life favored by the rapid development of the brain, and the wide variations in the cerebral circulation during childhood—Peculiar difficulties of their study—The Ophthalmoscope—Symptoms of cerebral disease in the child—Convulsions, symptomatic value very various—Their frequency in great measure due to the predominance of the spinal system in childhood—May be excited by many causes—Hence attention should always be paid to the precursors of an attack—Description of a fit of convulsions.

IT can scarcely be necessary to assign many reasons for beginning this course of lectures with the study of the *diseases of the nervous system.* The subject, although beset with many difficulties, has always engaged much attention; partly, no doubt, from the natural tendency of the human mind to inquire most curiously into those truths that seem most hidden; but still more from the alarming nature of many of the symptoms that betoken disturbance of the nervous system, and from the frequently fatal issue of its diseases. But besides the general interest and importance of these affections, at whatever age they may occur, *their extreme frequency in early life* gives them an additional claim on our notice.

It appears from the Reports of the Registrar-General, that 16,258 out of 91,225 persons who died in the metropolis during the years 1842 and 1845, of ascertained causes, were destroyed by the various diseases of the nervous system. But 9350 of these 16,258 deaths took place during the first five years of existence; or, in other words, 57 per cent. of the fatal disorders of the nervous system occurred within that period.[1] Even after making a very large allowance for the possible errors of statistical data, this predominance of the diseases of the nervous system in early life is far too remarkable to be overlooked; though some persons, not being able to account for the fact, have affected to doubt its reality.

The fact is one which cannot be gainsaid; and though we do not pretend thoroughly to account for it, yet *two considerations may help in some degree to explain it.*

The *first* is derived from our knowledge of the fact, that in an organ whose development is rapidly advancing, many diseased processes also, if once set up, will go on with proportionate activity. Now there is no organ in the body, with the exception of the pregnant womb, which undergoes such rapid development as the brain in early child-

[1] These numbers, which yield results differing but very little from those given in the first edition, are deduced from the returns furnished in the Fifth and Eighth Reports. The returns for 1846, which are also given in the Eighth Report, are not included, since, owing to the epidemic prevalence of diarrhœa in the autumn of 1846, they would not yield average results.

hood. It doubles its weight during the first two years of life, and though it does not absolutely cease to grow, even after adult age has been attained, its growth is slow and comparatively inconsiderable after the end of the seventh year. This same active state of the nutritive or vegetative processes in the brain of the child renders the organ liable to have disease set up in it by causes which would produce little or no injurious effect on the brain of the adult.

In the *second* place, the brain in infancy is much more exposed to disorder than that of the adult, owing to the far wider variations of which the cerebral circulation is susceptible in early life than subsequently. Nor is the cause of this difficult to discover. The cranium of the adult is a complete bony case, and the firm substance of the brain affords a comparatively unyielding support to the vessels by which it is nourished. It has been proved, indeed, by Dr. Burrows,[1] that the quantity of blood which these vessels contain is not always the same, as some have erroneously supposed; still its variations must needs be circumscribed within far narrower limits than in the child, whose cranium, with its membranous fontanelles and unossified sutures, opposes no such obstacle to the admission of an increased quantity of blood, while the soft brain keeps up a much lighter counter-pressure on the vessels than is exerted by the comparatively firm parenchyma of the organ in the adult. If the circulation in the child is disturbed, whether from difficulty in the return of venous blood as during a paroxysm of hooping-cough, or from increased arterial action as at the onset of a fever, or during the acute inflammation of some important organ, the brain becomes congested, and convulsions often announce the severity of the consequent disturbance of its functions. The same causes too, which expose the brain to be overfilled with blood, render it possible for it to be drained of that fluid more completely than in the adult. This fact, which you should always bear in mind when treating the diseases of infants, is one reason why excessive depletion induces a far more serious train of symptoms in young children than succeed to it in the grown person.

It happens, unfortunately, that while there are special reasons for studying the diseases of the nervous system in childhood, *their study is beset with special difficulties* which we do not meet with in the adult. Disordered intellect, altered sensation, impaired motion, are the three great classes to which the symptoms of disease of the nervous system may be referred. If our patient is an adult, he tells us of his altered feelings; he perhaps experiences some disorder of his intellectual powers even before it has become observable to others, and, thus timely warned, we can often take measures to prevent the advance of

---

[1] In his Lumleian Lectures, published in the Medical Gazette, April 28 and May 6, 1842, and subsequently in his work on Disorders of the Cerebral Circulation, &c., 8vo., Lond., 1846 The general accuracy of Dr. Burrows's conclusions, though called in question by the late Dr. John Reid, in the London and Edinburgh Monthly Journal for August, 1846, and more recently by Dr. Hamernjk, of Prague, in the Vierteljahrschrift für die praktische Heilkunde, vol. xvi, p. 38, seems to be placed beyond doubt by the very careful experiments of Dr. Berlin, published in the Nederlandsche Lancet, February, 1850, and in Schmidt's Jahrbücher for 1851, No. 1, p. 14-16.

disease, and to ward off that impairment of the motor powers, which, in his case, we know usually indicates the occurrence of some grave organic lesion. In the child, things follow a very different course. At first it cannot express its sensations at all, while, long after it has acquired the power of speech, it knows too little how to shape its ideas into words to give a correct account of what it feels; and we cannot expect to learn much from the disturbance of an intellect which as yet has scarcely asserted its claim to be anything higher than the instinct of the animal. The value of the symptoms, too, is different; for disturbance of the motor power, which is comparatively rare in the adult, except as the consequence of some serious disease of the brain, takes place in the child in cases of the mildest as well as of the most serious ailments; and we may even observe convulsions recurring several times a day for many days together, apparently without adequate cause, and not leading to any serious impairment of the child's health.

How, then, are we to attain in the child to anything beyond the merest guesswork in our diagnosis of diseases of the nervous system, when we are deprived to so great an extent of that information which the state of his intellect and the description of his sensations afford us in the adult? What meaning are we to attach to that symptom, the impairment of the motor power, which in the adult we look on as of such grave import, but which we meet with in the child under such varying conditions and in by far the greater number of cases? The task, indeed, is attended with difficulty, and the solution of these inquiries will need that you should devote to it some time and some careful observation; but if you do this, you need not despair of learning much about an infant's sensations and the state of its mind, and will at length become able rightly to interpret the meaning even of a fit of convulsions.

And here will, perhaps, be the fittest place for saying a few words about the Ophthalmoscope—an instrument by which we may be said to see into the brain, and to gain that kind of knowledge of its state with which the stethoscope furnishes us in the case of the heart and the respiratory organs.

Unfortunately I have no skill in its use; but I do not, therefore, underestimate its value. On the contrary, I counsel you most earnestly to make yourselves familiar with its employment, in order that you may start in practice furnished with the amplest resources possible for the solution of the difficult problems which we have to encounter. I shall, hereafter, try to give you some account of the special information which, in different circumstances, it conveys to the instructed observer; but must beg leave now to give you in better words than my own an estimate of its value, and a caution as to its use. The words are those of M. Roger,[1] physician to the Hôpital des Enfans Malades at Paris, my much-valued friend, and one of the ablest physicians of our time; whose only fault is that he plans his works as though he reckoned on

[1] Recherches cliniques sur les Maladies de l'Enfance, 8vo., Paris, 1872, vol. i, pp. 156, 157.

an antediluvian length of days, and that he forgets the "vita brevis" for whose span all our undertakings should be calculated.

"The use of the ophthalmoscope," says he, "is by no means as easy in the child as in the adult, especially when we have to do with any acute affection of the brain, as, for instance, with meningitis in its early stages. It often happens either that the indications which it yields are scarcely marked, and have no definite value; or that if they are more distinct, they have become so only at a time when the disease is already advanced, and has declared itself by unmistakable symptoms. Be this as it may, however, to be furnished in doubtful cases with even one new sign to guide us is well worth having; and if the ophthalmoscope did no more than confirm a diagnosis already arrived at on other grounds, its importance would be very real, and skill in its use well worth acquiring.

"Do not imagine, however, that by this instrument you can read as it were in the eye the diseases of the brain; and can even, with much practice in its use, read them readily. Our diagnosis of these affections must be based on a complete view of all their signs and symptoms, and not upon one solitary sign, whether it be the *tache méningitique* which Trousseau made so much of, or the *souffle cérébral* to which I myself paid so much attention, or whether it be the changes in the optic disk. It is not the corporeal eye, it is the eye of the mind which alone can see and recognize the different diseases of the brain; whose diagnosis will always continue most obscure in spite of the ophthalmoscope, as it used to be before its invention."

I need then make no apology for asking you to study well now, with just as much attention as I should have bespoken twenty years ago, *the symptoms* by which disease of the nervous centres, and especially of the brain, manifests itself in infancy and early childhood.

The painful sensations which the infant experiences soon show themselves in the haggard, anxious, or oppressed look, which takes the place of the naturally tranquil expression of its countenance. It often puts its hand to its head, or beats or rubs it, or, while lying in its cot, bores with its occiput in the pillow; owing to which, in children who have suffered for any time from uneasy sensations in the head, you will often find the hair worn quite off the occiput. It turns its head away from the light, and lies much with its eyes half closed, in a state of apparent drowsiness, from which it often arouses with a start, and cries. The cry, especially in inflammatory disease, is peculiar; it is generally a low, almost constant moan, very sad to hear—interrupted occasionally by a sharp, piercing, lamentable cry, almost a shriek. If the child is young, it will often seem relieved by being carried about in its nurse's arms, and while she is moving will cease its wail for a time, but begin it again the moment she stands still. You will sometimes observe, too, that if moved from one person's arms to those of another, or even if its position is but slightly altered, a sudden expression of alarm will pass across its features; the child is dizzy, and afraid of falling.

You see, then, that even in the infant there is a language of signs by which we learn with certainty the existence of pain in the head, and the connection of this pain with dizziness and intolerance of light.

You must beware, however, of concluding from any one set of symptoms that the head is the seat of real disease. The child, as well as the adult, may have sick headache; and the degree of febrile disturbance, of heat of surface, and of heat of head, together with the state of the digestive organs, are all to be taken into account in forming your diagnosis.

Something may be learned of the state of the mental powers and of the feelings even in early infancy. Have you never watched an infant on its mother's lap, and noticed the look of happy recognition with which its eye meets that of its mother? An early result of cerebral disease is to interrupt this intercourse: the child now never seems to catch its mother's eye, but lies sad and listless, as if all persons were alike indifferent to it; or at other times even familiar faces cause alarm, the child apparently not recognizing those who yet have always tended it. This disturbance, however, is but momentary, and the child subsides into its former condition, and allows itself to be taken by those at whom a minute before it seemed frightened.

But these symptoms are to be interpreted by the light thrown on them from other sources, and by the information, both positive and negative, thus obtained. You fear that disease is going on in the brain; but is the skin hot?—is there heat of head?—are there frequent flushings of the face, and does the accession of each flush seem connected with an increase of agitation and distress, or followed by a deepening of the drowsiness? Is the fontanelle prominent and tense, or are the pulsations of the brain to be felt with unusual force through it?—are the veins of the scalp full, or do the carotids beat with unusual force? What is the character of the pulse?—is it not merely increased in rapidity; but even when examined under exactly similar conditions, does it afford a different result each time? Do you find it irregular in frequency, or unequal in the force of its beats, or even distinctly intermittent? Again, what is the state of the pupil?—is it generally contracted, as if to exclude light as much as possible from the oversensitive retina? or is it usually dilated, and does it act slowly, as though disease had deadened the sensibility of the nervous system? or do the pupils of the two eyes not act simultaneously, but one more readily than the other? Do the pupils oscillate under the light, at first contracting, then dilating, and either remaining dilated or continuing to oscillate, though within narrower limits, and with a tendency to remain more dilated than at first? Or, lastly, do you find, when the child is roused, this oscillation of the pupil going on under the ordinary amount of light that enters the chamber? Now all of these are indications of disordered function of the brain, and many of them point to disorder of a very serious kind.

But there are yet other sources from which we must not neglect to seek for information. Much may be learned from the state of the digestive functions. The bowels are almost always disturbed; usually, though not invariably, constipated; while nausea and vomiting are seldom absent. I am not acquainted with any one symptom which should so immediately direct your attention to the brain, as the occurrence of causeless vomiting, and especially its continuance. At first, perhaps, the child vomits only when it has taken food; but before long the stomach will reject even the blandest fluid, and then the efforts at vomiting will come on when the stomach is empty, a little greenish mucus being rejected with no relief, the retching and vomiting soon returning. I shall have occasion to dwell again upon the importance of this symptom, which I have known continue for several days before any other indication of cerebral disease could be discovered. In children of three or four years old this occurrence would scarcely be overlooked; but the case is different with infants, who so often vomit the milk when ill, that the mother or nurse might fail to mention it to you, if you did not make special inquiries with reference to that point.

The manner in which the functions of the respiratory organs are performed is also not to be overlooked. That peculiar, unequal, irregular breathing, to which the name of cerebral respiration has been applied, though of considerable value when present, is sometimes not observed, or not until the disease of the brain is already so far advanced that all questions of diagnosis have long been set at rest. There is, moreover, a short, hard, hacking cough, which you may sometimes hear, and the import of which you ought to be acquainted with, since it betokens disease of the brain, not of the lungs. There are peculiar sounds, too, which sometimes attend respiration, and are known as indicating disturbance of the nervous system. To these, however, I shall have to return hereafter, since they betoken a disease of a serious nature, known by the name of spasmodic croup, and which I must in the course of these lectures describe in full.

I have purposely delayed till now speaking of the indications of cerebral disease afforded by the occurrence of *convulsions*. The symptom is one undoubtedly of great importance, since it is observed in almost every case of serious disease of the brain, at some stage or other of its progress. The very frequency of the phenomenon, however, and the great variety of the circumstances in which it occurs, render it difficult for us rightly to interpret its meaning. Perhaps it will help us to understand it, if we bear in mind that in a large proportion of cases convulsions in the infant answer to delirium in the adult. In early life the superintendence of the motor power is the chief function of the brain, which has not yet attained to its highest office as the organ of the intellect. Hence the convulsions which you may observe to come on in infancy in the course of some acute diseases, such as inflammation of the lungs, do not import that any new malady has invaded the brain, but simply that the disease is so serious as to disturb the due performance of all the functions of the organism, and of those of the brain in common with the rest. Convulsions at other times take place in infancy not as the result of any abiding disease of the brain, but simply in consequence of those anatomical peculiarities which allow of a much more sudden and more considerable congestion of the cerebral vessels than can occur in the adult. Of this kind are frequently the convulsions that come on during a paroxysm of hooping-cough, which are induced by the impediment to the return of blood from the head, and which often cease so soon as that impediment is removed by the child taking a deep inspiration. But these two considerations are, it must be owned, by no means adequate to explain the very great frequency of convulsions in children, though they account for much that otherwise would be inexplicable.

The grand reason of their frequency is no doubt to be found in the *predominance of the spinal over the cerebral system in early life.* In the adult, the controlling power of the brain checks the display of those reflex movements which become at once evident if disease highten the excitability of the spinal cord, or cut off the influence of the brain from the paralyzed limb, or even if sleep suspend that influence for a season. When the child is born the brain is but imperfectly developed, its functions are most humble, and convulsions are then so frequent, that they are computed to occasion 73.3 per cent. of all deaths which take place during the first year of existence from diseases of the nervous system. In the next two years the brain more than doubles its weight, and deaths from convulsions sink to just a third of their former frequency. In proportion as the brain increases in size, and its structure acquires perfection, and its higher functions become displayed, convulsions grow less and less frequent, until from the 10th to the 15th year they cause less than 3 per cent., and above 15 less than 1 per cent., of the deaths from diseases of the nervous system.[1]

But a little observation will show you, that though convulsions are often the immediate cause of death, yet this fatal event is rare during childhood in comparison with those instances in which they pass off without any serious result; and that in proportion to their frequency they less often betoken grave disease of the brain in the child than in the adult, while any cause which greatly excites the spinal system may be attended by them. The disturbance of the spinal system which ushers in fever in the adult, shows itself by shivering; while in the child the same disturbance often manifests itself, not by shivering but by convulsions. Convulsions may be induced in early life by a constipated state of the bowels, by the presence of worms in the intestinal canal, or of a calculus in the kidney, or by the pressure of a tooth upon the swollen gum,—causes wholly inadequate to occasion so serious an occurrence in the grown person. Hence your first duty is, in every case, to ascertain where is the seat of the irritation which excited the nervous system to this tumultuous reaction. If the fits come on in an advanced stage of some serious disease, they are probably only the

[1] The first line in the accompanying table shows the proportion per cent. of deaths from diseases of the nervous system at different ages, to the deaths from all causes at the same ages, in the metropolis; and the second line, the proportion borne by deaths from convulsions to deaths from diseases of the nervous system in general.

Under 1 year.	From 1 to 3 years.	From 3 to 5 years.	Total under 5 years.	From 5 to 10 years.	From 10 to 15 years.	Total above 15 years.
30.5	18.5	17 6	24.3	15.1	10.6	10.4
73.3	24.9	17.8	54 3	9.9	2.4	.8

Deduced from the Fifth and Eighth Reports of the Registrar-General.

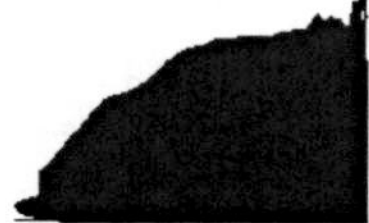

indications that death is busy at the centres of vitality; if they occur during hooping-cough, they point to a congested state of the brain, the consequence of the impeded circulation through the lungs; if they attack a child apparently in perfect health, they probably indicate that the stomach has been overloaded, or that some indigestible article of food has been taken; or, if this be certainly not the case, one of the eruptive fevers is perhaps about to come on; most likely either small-pox or scarlatina.

To determine the *cause of convulsions*, you must acquaint yourself with the history of the child's health for some time before any threatening of them had appeared; you must learn whether the child has ever suffered from worms, whether its digestive functions have long been out of order, or whether the process of dentition, which is now perhaps going on, has been attended with much constitutional disturbance. But, besides all these points, your inquiries must be still more carefully directed to ascertain whether any cerebral symptoms preceded the attack, and if so, what was their nature, since it is seldom that acute disease of the brain sets in with convulsions. You will sometimes, indeed, be told that the child was well until a convulsive seizure suddenly came on; but on inquiring minutely it will usually be found that some indications of cerebral disease had been present for days, though not sufficiently severe to attract much attention. In cases of apoplexy, of intense cerebral congestion, and of phrenitis, convulsions occur at a very early period; but even then, extreme drowsiness, great pain in the head, and vomiting, usually precede for a few hours the convulsive seizure. When the brain is thus seriously involved, the recovery from the convulsions is very imperfect; coma perhaps succeeds to them, or other evidences of cerebral disease are so marked as to leave no doubt of the brain being affected. Tubercle sometimes remains for a long time after its deposition in the brain, without giving rise to any well-marked symptoms, till its presence is at length announced by a fit of convulsions. These convulsions are seldom at first very severe, but you will learn to dread them more than those which assume a more formidable appearance, from noticing either that one side of the body is exclusively affected, or, at least, that there is a marked preponderance of the affection on one side. It is well to bear in mind, too, that convulsions may occur from a want of blood in the brain as well as from its excess, and that the convulsions which come on in some ill-nourished infants may indicate a state of atrophy of the brain.

I must, however, have said enough already to impress upon you the importance of narrowly scrutinizing the meaning of every attack of convulsions. But though so important, there are few tasks more difficult. You have to maintain your own self-composure at a time when all around you have lost theirs; to extract truth as you best may from the imperfect, often exaggerated, accounts of anxious relatives; to observe not only minutely but quickly, and to come to a speedy decision: since while in those cases which require active treatment delay is almost synonymous with death, there is at least as great danger of destroying your patient by that "*nimia diligentia*" to which the prejudices of the nurse and the fears of the friends will often conspire to urge you.

It is well to watch closely the *first indications* of that disturbance of the nervous system which will be likely to issue in *convulsions*. And here let me recommend you not to listen with too incredulous an ear to old nurses, who may tell you that a child has been much convulsed, while you find upon inquiry that it has not had any fit. When they say that a child has been much convulsed, they mean usually that it has shown many of the symptoms which forebode an attack of general convulsions. These forebodings are often induced by dyspepsia or by disorder of the bowels in young infants, and have been described by writers under the name of "inward fits." A child thus affected lies as though asleep, winks its imperfectly closed eyes, and gently twitches the muscles of its face—a movement especially observable about the lips, which are drawn as though into a smile. Sometimes, too, this movement of the mouth is seen during sleep, and poets have told us that it is the "angel's whisper" which makes the babe to smile—a pretty conceit of which we can scarcely forgive science for robbing us. If this condition increase, the child breathes with difficulty, its respiration sometimes seems for a moment almost stopped, and a livid ring surrounds the mouth. At every little noise the child wakes up; it makes a gentle moaning, brings up the milk while sleeping, or often passes a great quantity of wind, especially if the abdomen be gently rubbed. When the intestinal disorder is relieved, these symptoms speedily subside; nor have we much reason to fear general convulsions so long as no more serious forebodings show themselves. There is more cause for apprehension, however, when we see the thumbs drawn into the palm either habitually, or during sleep; when the eyes are never more than half-closed during sleep; when the twitching of the muscles is no longer confined to the angles of the mouth, but affects the face and extremities; when the child awakes with a sudden start, its face growing flushed or livid, its eyes turning up under the upper eyelid, or the pupils suddenly dilating, while the countenance wears an expression of great anxiety or alarm, and the child either utters a shriek or sometimes begins to cry.

When a *fit* comes on, the muscles of the face twitch, the body is stiff, immovable, and then in a short time, in a state of twitching motion, the head and neck are drawn backwards, and the limbs violently flexed and extended. Sometimes these movements are confined to certain muscles, or are limited to one side. At the same time neither consciousness nor sensation is present. The eye is fixed and does not see; the finger may be passed over it without winking; the pupil is immovably contracted or dilated; the ear is insensible even to loud sounds; the pulse is small, very frequent, often too small and too frequent to be counted; the breathing hurried, labored, and irregular; the skin bathed in abundant perspiration.

After this condition has lasted for a minute, or ten minutes, or an hour or more, the convulsions cease; and the child either falls asleep, or lies for a short time as if it were bewildered, or bursts into crying, and then returns to its senses, or sinks into a state of coma in which it may either be perfectly motionless, or twitching of some muscles may still continue; or, lastly, it may die in the fit. This, however, is not usual except when the convulsions have come on in subjects exhausted by previous disease, or when they are the result of apoplexy or of intense cerebral congestion, such as takes place occasionally in hooping-cough, or when they are associated with that closed state of the larynx which occurs sometimes in spasmodic croup.

This preliminary examination of the symptoms of disturbance of the nervous system has placed us in a position to commence our investigation of the different forms of cerebral disease; on which we will enter at the next lecture.

LECTURE IV.

CONGESTION OF THE BRAIN.—Often supposed to be present when the symptoms are not really due to it—Active congestion—Its causes, symptoms, and treatment—Notice of conditions once supposed to be due to congestion, as sunstroke, and head symptoms preceding eruptive fevers—Passive congestion, its causes, symptoms, and treatment.

IN my last lecture I endeavored to point out to you some of the reasons for the greater frequency of affections of the nervous system in infancy and childhood than at other periods of life. I dwelt especially upon certain structural peculiarities of the brain, and of its bony case, which render the cerebral vessels liable to become overloaded with blood, under the influence of causes that would be wholly inadequate to produce such an effect in the adult. With the advance of the ossification of the skull, and the closure of its fontanelles and sutures, these peculiarities are rendered fewer and less important; but still a remarkable liability to congestion of its vessels continues to characterize the brain through all the years of early childhood. A late distinguished German physician, Dr. Mauthner, of Vienna,[1] on examining the bodies of 229 children who had died at different ages and of various diseases, found a congested state of the vessels of the brain in 186 of the number. In some of these cases it is probable that this condition had come on only a short time before the patient's death, since in them no symptoms of cerebral disturbance had appeared during the progress of their illness; but in many it was not so; and I shall have occasion to warn you over and over again to be on the watch against *congestion of the brain*, as a condition which is very likely to come on in the course of affections even of distant organs. Nor is it merely as a serious complication of many other diseases that this cerebral congestion deserves

---

[1] Die Krankhei en des Gehirns und Rückenmarks bei Kindern. 8vo., Wien, 1844, p. 12. See, however, the cautions given by Niemeyer as to the sources of error with reference to this very point in post-mortem examinations of the brain, in his Lehrbuch der speciellen Pathologie. 8th ed., Berlin, 1871, vol. ii, p. 163.

your notice; its importance depends still more on its constituting the first and curable stage of many diseases of the brain, which, unless arrested at the outset, soon pass beyond the resources of our art. Neither, indeed, must it be forgotten, that although inflammation, hemorrhage, and the effusion of serum are the three results to one or other of which congestion of the cerebral vessels tends, yet the exceptions to their occurrence are by no means few, even when that congestion has been very considerable or of long continuance; and that not only may the functions of the brain be seriously disordered, but the life of the patient may be destroyed, without the anatomist being able to discover any one of these results, or indeed anything more than a general repletion of the vessels of the organ.[1]

Any cause which greatly increases the flow of blood to the head, or which greatly impedes its reflux, may give rise to a congested state of the brain; and according as this state is induced by the one or the other cause, it is said to be *active* or *passive*. The active form of cerebral congestion is associated with and in measure dependent on excitement of the heart's action, and is therefore observed in connection with various forms of febrile disturbance; while the passive form receives its best illustrations in cases of hooping-cough, and of spasm of the glottis, in which violent and fruitless expiratory efforts are made. The brain may become actively congested at the time of teething, or from a blow on the head, or the state may come on independently of any definite exciting cause; or a state of passive congestion may be induced by some mechanical impediment to the return of blood from the organ—such as the pressure of a hypertrophied thymus, or of enlarged and tuberculated bronchial glands upon the jugular veins; or it may be merely the result of a languid circulation from the want of pure air, or of nourishing and sufficient food.

I have been used, in common with other physicians, to believe and to teach that the symptoms of violent cerebral disturbance which sometimes usher in the eruptive fevers, and even prove fatal before the rash has had time to show itself, were among the most striking illustrations of active cerebral congestion.[2] It seems, however, more than doubtful whether this opinion is correct, and some of the best authorities assure us that they are positively erroneous. These symptoms, it is said, do not in any sense depend on an increased flow of blood towards the brain produced by the excited action of the heart, but partly on the high temperature of the blood circulating in the cerebral vessels, partly on its altered composition due to the greatly intensified metamorphosis of tissues which the fever produces. The so-called asthenic fevers are a remarkable example of the truth of this opinion, since in

[1] Dietl's Anatomische Klinik der Gehirnkrankheiten, 8vo., Wien, 1846, contains, at pp. 58–78, a very able exposition and defence of views concerning cerebral congestion in many respects similar to those expressed in this lecture.

[2] See Armstrong's notice of these suddenly fatal accidents at the outset of scarlatina, at p. 30 of his work on Scarlet Fever, &c., 2d edit., London, 1817; and Von Ammon's mention of it in his description of the epidemic of malignant scarlatina at Dresden in 1831–2, in the Analekten über Kinderkrankheiten, 11tes Heft, p. 42. Stuttgart, 1836.

them we have an extremely high temperature associated with enfeebled though accelerated action of the heart, but with no determination of the blood to the brain, while yet we meet in them with most marked delirium, and with the gravest disturbance of the brain functions.[1]

The same explanation is given of the nature and cause of the symptoms of sunstroke, which the late unhappy Franco-German war afforded so many opportunities of observing. A remarkable support is given to this view by the fact that in the infant and young child all the symptoms of sunstroke may result from lengthened exposure to a very high temperature even though the day is cloudy, or the child sheltered completely from direct action of the sun's rays.

But, even though we separate these two classes of cases from their supposed connection with cerebral congestion, there yet remain many others in which the symptoms may still with propriety be referred to that cause. Such, for instance, are many of the disorders of the nervous system, and especially of the cerebral functions, which occur during teething. Febrile disturbance almost always attends upon the process of dentition, and it is not difficult to understand how, when the circulation is in a state of permanent excitement, a very slight cause may suffice to overturn its equilibrium, and occasion a greater flow of blood to the brain than the organ is able to bear. Sometimes too, and that by no means rarely, symptoms of cerebral congestion come on for which it is not possible to assign a distinct exciting cause, and for the explanation of which we have to fall back on the well-known fact that all periods of development such as childhood, are periods during which the growing organs are most apt to become disordered.

Let us now then pass to an examination of its *symptoms*. In the great majority of cases they come on slowly; and for the most part, general uneasiness, a disordered state of the bowels, which are usually though not invariably constipated, and feverishness, precede for a few days the more serious attack. The head by degrees becomes hot, the child grows restless and fretful, and seems distressed by light or by noise or by sudden motion, and children who are old enough sometimes complain of their head. One little boy, nearly three years old, who died of congestion of the brain, had seemed to suffer for some days before any alarming symptom came on, from severe pain in the head. He sometimes awoke crying from his sleep, or when awake would suddenly put his hands to his ears, exclaiming, "Oh, hurt! hurt!" Usually, too, vomiting occurs repeatedly; a symptom on the importance of which I have already insisted, since it is not only confirmatory of others, but also may exist before there is any well-marked indication of the head being affected, and when, though the child seems ailing, there is nothing definite about its illness. The degree of fever which attends this condition varies much, and its accessions are irregular; but the pulse is usually much and permanently quickened; and if the skull is unossified, the anterior fontanelle is either tense and prominent, or the brain is felt and seen to pulsate forcibly through it. The sleep is disturbed, the child often waking with a start, while there

[1] Niemeyer, Op. cit., vol. ii, p. 165–6.

is occasional twitching of the muscles of its face or of the tendons of its wrist.

The child may continue in this condition for many days, and then recover its health without any medical interference; but a slight cause will generally suffice to bring back the former indisposition. You will sometimes see striking instances of this in children while teething; the fever subsiding, the head growing cool, and the little patient appearing quite well, so soon as the tooth has cut through the gum, but the approach of each tooth to the surface being attended by the recurrence of the same symptoms.

But though the disturbance of the brain may pass away of its own accord, yet we cannot reckon on such a favorable result occurring, for symptoms such as I have mentioned are often the indications of the organism generally having begun to suffer from mischief which has been going on for months unnoticed, and which is now about to break out with all the formidable characters of acute hydrocephalus. Or should they have no such grave import, yet congestion of the brain is itself a serious, sometimes a fatal malady. Even though no treatment should be adopted indeed, the heat of head may diminish, and the flush of the face grow slighter and less constant; but the countenance becomes very heavy and anxious, the indifference to surrounding objects increases, and the child lies in a state of torpor or drowsiness, from which, however, it can at first be roused to complete consciousness. The manner on being roused is always fretful, but if old enough to talk the child's answers are rational, though generally very short; and murmuring, "I am so sleepy, so sleepy," it subsides into its former drowsiness. The bowels generally continue constipated and the vomiting seldom ceases, though it is sometimes less frequent than before. The pulse is usually smaller than in the other stage and it is often irregular in its frequency, though not actually intermittent. An attack of convulsions sometimes marks the transition from the first to the second stage; or the child passes without any apparent cause from its previous torpor into a state of convulsion, which subsiding, leaves the torpor deeper than before. The fits return and death may take place in one of them, or the torpor growing more profound after each convulsive seizure, the child at length dies comatose.

This second stage, if so it may be called, is usually of short duration; and if relief is not afforded by appropriate treatment, death is seldom delayed beyond forty-eight hours from the first fit, though no graver lesion may be discovered afterwards than a gorged state of the large vessels of the membranes of the brain, and perhaps a little clear fluid in the ventricles and beneath the arachnoid; together with a generally white color of the cerebral substance, due to an œdema of its tissue which has succeeded to the previous congestion of its capillaries.

Occasionally, indeed, death does not so speedily follow these symptoms; but they continue slightly modified for days, or even weeks, and contrary to all expectation recovery now and then takes place. This protracted course of the affection is I believe met with only in the case of very young children, in whom, the congestion having relieved itself by a copious effusion of serum into the ventricles, the yielding skull accommodates itself to its increased contents. The symptoms, though to a great extent the same as before, are now due to the presence of water in the brain—a disease which, though dangerous and often fatal, is yet chronic in its course, and may even admit of cure.

In the *treatment* of congestion of the brain, whatever may be the circumstances in which it has come on, our first and best attention ought always to be paid to just those things which in far too many cases receive it least. The temperature of the room, the amount of light admitted into it, the number of persons present, the position of the child's cot, the material of its pillow (which ought to be horsehair, and not down), and the nature of its food, are matters of the greatest importance. All these things, however, are so simple that their value is frequently underrated; and it is so often said, almost as a matter of course, "*Keep the child quiet and the room cool, and apply cold to the head,*" that it does not strike the parents how much depends upon those directions on which the doctor seems to lay so little weight. You must learn, however, that in the treatment of children's diseases none of these things are trivial, but that on their due performance often hangs the life of your patient. Do not content yourselves then with merely giving directions, but stay to see them attended to; and do not leave the house till the chamber is darkened, the cool air freely admitted, the cold application to the head properly adjusted, nor till all persons who are not actually waiting on the child have left the apartment.

Next in importance in these cases are the arrangements for keeping the head cool. For this purpose it is necessary that the infant should be removed from its nurse's lap: where lying with its head resting on her arm and pressed against her bosom, all attempts to keep it cool are idle. The child should be placed in bed, its head resting on a horsehair pillow, and if it will not (and indeed it seldom will) allow a linen rag soaked in some evaporating lotion to be kept on its head, the following simple plan will usually be found very efficient, and will be readily submitted to in most instances. Let two bladders be half filled with pounded ice, or cold water, and be placed, each wrapped in a napkin, the one under and the other upon the child's head. By pinning the corners of the napkin to the pillow, you can secure them from being displaced, and can also prevent the weight of the upper bladder from resting too heavily on the child's head.

At the outset of the affection the bowels are usually constipated, so that an active *purgative* is in most cases called for. You may give a dose of calomel and jalap, or the calomel may be administered alone, and followed by the infusion of senna, which may be repeated every three or four hours till the bowels act. Should the stomach be very irritable, a larger dose of calomel may be given, and after the lapse of a couple of hours an attempt may be made to quicken its action by administering a purgative enema, or by dissolving some sulphate of magnesia or the less nauseous phosphate of soda in the child's drink, and giving it at short intervals. In many cases the disorder will be speedily removed by this treatment, and the child, whose life had seemed to be hanging by a thread, will, in the course of twenty-four hours, be almost well.

Next in order comes the question of depletion, and I purposely say next, because the simple measures already pointed out not infrequently so relieve the urgency of the symptoms that one passes within twelve hours from a state of great anxiety about the patient to one of comparative tranquillity. If, however, these means are not succeeded by a speedy and marked improvement, if the heat of the head has not sunk down to the same temperature as that of the body, if the fontanelle is tense or strongly pulsating, or the carotids are beating visibly, if the pupils are very contracted and light is ill borne, if the hands twitch, or if sickness continues and there is much distress and fretfulness, with frequent cries and moaning, the abstraction of blood is then plainly indicated, and will give relief which no other measures can procure. This depletion may be accomplished by means of leeches, and should when indicated be effectually done, and once for all. It may be calculated that a good leech will draw ʒij of blood; and the application of one leech for every three months of a child's life, assuming that no bleeding is allowed to take place after the leech falls off, may, I think, be adopted as a fairly safe rule for your guidance in the case of infants and young children. It is truer economy of the child's strength to deplete once sufficiently to produce a decided influence, than by acting with too timorous a hand to be compelled to repeat the abstraction of blood again and again.

Supposing now, that by the employment of these means you have removed the imminent danger and that your patient is going on favorably, still it will be generally desirable to continue treatment for a few days.* Free action of the bowels must be maintained, for which purpose small doses of calomel may be given two or three times a day, and it may be desirable to accompany each powder with a dose of a mixture containing nitre and sulphate of magnesia.[1] Or, if there is no indication for acting on the bowels, but yet a good deal of heat of skin, a rapid pulse, and much cerebral excitement are present, you may employ with advantage the bromide of potass with small doses of aconite.[2] You must, however, bear in mind that you will do less harm by allowing a child to go without medicine than by forcing on it remedies which it dislikes and resists taking. Calomel, indeed, can almost always be given; and even sulphate of magnesia will very often be taken if mixed with the drink, or dissolved in a little veal broth. But how much

---

[1] (No. 1.)

℞. Potassæ Nitratis, gr. xij.
Magnesiæ Sulph., ℥j.
Syr. Limonum, ʒiij.
Aquæ destill., ℥ix. M. ʒij three times a day.
For a child a year old.

[2] (No. 2.)

℞. Potassæ Citratis, gr. xx.
Potassii Bromidi, gr. xv.
Tinct. Aconiti, ♏iij.
Tinct. Chloroformico, ♏xv.
Syrupi Mori, ʒiv.
Aquæ destill., ℥j. M. ʒij every four hours.
For a child a year old.

soever a child may resist medicine, the abstraction of blood, a spare diet, a cool and dark and quiet chamber, are remedies always at command, the value of which you must not underrate.

I need not tell you that all cases do not admit of this treatment. When the disease creeps on with febrile symptoms, occasional vomiting, constipation, loss of appetite, and restless nights, with complaints if the child is old enough to speak, of pain in the head or limbs, or vertigo, and with a quick and variable pulse, you must treat it very gently, and must trust much to quiet and the careful regulation of the diet. In such cases you will often find a tepid bath night and morning soothe the child and tranquillize the circulation far more than you might have expected from so simple a remedy. Drastic purgatives must be avoided; but small doses of mercury and chalk, or of calomel, either alone or combined with rhubarb, may be given with advantage once or twice a day. Half a grain of calomel, or two grains of the Hydr. c. Creta, with three of rhubarb, or one of the powdered extract, would be a proper dose for a child a year old. If there is much feverishness and restlessness during the day, you may give a mixture of bicarbonate of potash not quite saturated with citric acid, and containing small doses of ipecacuanha wine, if the stomach is not extremely irritable, and of the tincture of hyoscyamus, the value of which last medicine as a sedative in the diseases of children can scarcely be too highly estimated. The addition of a little syrup of mulberries will render the above mixture extremely palatable.[1]

I have already referred to various conditions, once assumed to be due to intense cerebral congestion, by which the correcter pathological knowledge of the present day has proved to depend on other causes. It is hard to know where to classify them, for there are many points still uncertain with reference to their mode of production; and therefore, as a mere matter of convenience I notice them here, on the ground of the similarity of their symptoms in many respects to those which congestion of the brain occasions. It is true that pathological anatomy lays the only ground on which we can securely tread; but when that fails us, or is insufficient, we must be guided by symptoms in our arrangement, not forgetting how lifelike are the portraitures of disease which Hippocrates and Aretæus have drawn, although morbid anatomy was a sealed book to them.

The great peculiarity of these cases, whether they occur as the result of blood-poisoning in the incubation period of a fever, or from sunstroke, or from the irritation produced by unwholesome or undigested food, is the suddenness of the onset of their symptoms, and their violence. A child who went to bed well, is seized in the night with

---

[1] (No. 3.)

℞. Potassæ Bicarbonatis,
Acidi Citrici, āā gr. xx.
Vin. Ipecac, ♏xij.
Træ. Hyosc., ♏xviij.
Syr. Mori, ℥iij.
Aquæ destill., ℥ix. M. ℥ij every six hours.
For a child a year old.

vomiting, followed by convulsions of extreme severity, which leaves it comatose, with burning skin, rapid pulse, twitching of the limbs, and stertorous breathing—a state that may continue for some hours, and then slowly pass away: or which may be interrupted by renewed convulsions, to end in still more profound coma, and at last in death; or the appearance of the rash of one of the eruptive fevers may indicate the cause of the attack, and at the same time dissipate it: or abundant action of the bowels may remove the cause of disorder, and leave the child quite well; or the functions of the nervous system disordered by intense heat may but slowly return to their regular performance; and heat of skin, and hurried pulse, and disturbed brain may continue for days—really a brain fever; but the term must not be used, as it might lead to misconstruction.

Whenever any symptoms such as these come on, you must endeavor to make out what has been the antecedent of the attack. Inquire whether your patient has had the eruptive fevers, especially scarlatina or small-pox, or whether he has been recently exposed to their contagion, and examine the arm to see whether there are good cicatrices as evidences of successful vaccination. Learn what the child has eaten during the previous twenty-four hours; or if the attack comes on during the summer, ascertain at what time of the day the child was taken out, where it was taken, and what covering it had on its head. Learn, too, whether the child appeared quite well, or whether it was hot, and seemed languid or drowsy when it came home.

An emetic, followed by an active purge, will often remove the symptoms which were due to an overloaded stomach, but it must be remembered that be their cause what it may, these attacks inflict a shock upon the brain (I use popular language, for scientific terms are to be avoided where our ideas are not definite), the effects of which may last for weeks in disorder of its functions, and that sometimes such attacks appear to be the exciting cause of organic disease, especially in children who inherit a predisposition to tuberculosis.

In the case of the formidable symptoms which usher in the exanthemata, one's first impulse is to deplete, and to deplete largely, and I have certainly seen good results follow from this treatment. I have, however, of late years tried the use of the wet sheet in these cases, and with results all the more satisfactory, since they are obtained without any of that depression of the vital powers inseparable from the free abstraction of blood. I have seen the packing in the wet sheet followed, in the course of one or two hours, by an abatement of temperature, a cessation of convulsions, and a return of consciousness, as remarkable as I have ever observed follow from even a copious bleeding, while the action of the skin has certainly been more speedily established, and the appearance of the eruption has been brought about [illegible] and more satisfactorily, than by any other means with which I [illegible]. While, therefore, I would not say that depletion [illegible] be practiced, and while, if hydropathy failed, I should [illegible] to it, I no longer employ, nor should I advise that [illegible] which, in ignorance of these other means, I was ac-[illegible] recourse.

The effects of sunstroke in our climate are, in general, less formidable than those which are sometimes produced by the fever-poison. Alarm, restlessness, and fretfulness, alternating with drowsiness, hurried irregular breathing, intense heat of skin, violent pulsation of the anterior fontanelle if still unossified, a pulse almost too rapid to be counted, twitching of the limbs, and starting of the tendons of the wrists, such are the usual symptoms of its severer forms. Sickness is generally present, the stomach rejecting immediately even the simplest fluid, the bowels are usually relaxed, while sometimes there is severe diarrhœa; and occasionally, though not I think usually, the disorder of the nervous system is so severe as to give rise to convulsions. Occasionally as the signs of cerebral disturbance abate, the diarrhœa increases, and in young infants I have even known fatal dysentery succeed to the other symptoms of sunstroke. In other instances, while the first urgent symptoms abate, the general feverish condition continues, accompanied with signs very similar to those I have already enumerated as characterizing cerebral congestion, while the bowels are irregular, though acting with undue frequency, and the evacuations are almost always destitute of bile. My experience of these cases is that, unless the first shock proves fatal, or the dysenteric symptoms carry off the patient, recovery is tolerably certain to take place.

These cases require very gentle treatment, and especially the observance of all those minor precautions which I dwelt on as of so much moment in the treatment of cerebral congestion. The tepid bath often soothes remarkably, and may be repeated two or three times in the twenty-four hours. The diarrhœa which is so often present is not to be checked by astringents; but ¼ grain of calomel and 1 grain of Dover's powder, given every 8 hours to an infant of a year old for one or two days, will generally improve the state of the secretions, and check the irritability of the bowels; while the simple soothing febrifuge medicines which have already been suggested, will favor the action of the skin, and abate the excitement of the circulation. The difficulty in these cases is to read them aright, to discover the nature of the possible danger, and to avoid in treatment the too little or too much, each of which has its own danger.

Thus much may suffice for these conditions; but we must now briefly notice those cases in which congestion of the brain exists in what may be called the *passive state*. In the paroxysms of hooping-cough the brain becomes congested by the impediment to the return of the blood from the head; and cerebral congestion is induced in a similar manner when the larynx becomes spasmodically closed in the disease known by the name of Laryngismus Stridulus. But we likewise meet with cases where the passive succeeds to the active form of cerebral congestion, or becomes more or less gradually developed out of some disorder of the abdominal viscera; or, lastly, where it supervenes towards the close of life in weakly children, whose vital powers have at length become too feeble to propel the blood.

In children who have suffered long and severely from hooping-cough, you often notice a general lividity of the face and lips, a puffed and anxious countenance, and the child makes grievous complaints about its head, while the skin is moist and cool, and the pulse soft, though frequent. Many of these symptoms indicate an overloaded state of the cerebral vessels; and if a paroxysm of coughing occurs, and the circulation is thus further disturbed, the child may die in a fit, or may sink after some convulsive seizure into a state of coma, which sooner or later proves fatal. In such a case you will find the vessels of the brain and its membranes universally gorged with black blood, the choroid plexuses of a deep purple color, and more bloody points than natural will present themselves on a section of the brain being made.[1] Both the symptoms during life, and the appearances after death, are only a rather exaggerated illustration of what occurs in all cases of passive congestion of the brain. It is not, however, always easy to explain why this condition comes on. Among the poor you often find it connected with general disorder of the digestive organs, and occurring as one of a long train of ills induced by destitution and neglect. It was so in the case of a little boy four months old, whom I saw some years ago. His parents were young and healthy people, but they had already lost three children, apparently in consequence of their inhabiting one of those narrow courts so numerous in London, into which the sun never shines, and where young children pine and fade like tender plants shut up in a cellar. When ten weeks old, this little boy was taken with pain in his bowels and diarrhœa, and at three months old he began to suffer from fits, which came on daily, sometimes several times a day. No efficient treatment had been adopted when he was brought to me. He was then as large as most children of his age, and by no means emaciated; but his flesh was flabby, his face unintelligent, puffed, and livid, his head hot, the veins of the scalp and eyelids were turgid, the eyes prominent, lustreless, covered by mucus, and the pupils scarcely acted under light. He lay on his mother's lap, uttering a constant hoarse moan; his head thrown rather back, and in incessant rotatory motion; his mouth was open, his tongue red and parched, and the papillæ on its surface were very prominent; his abdomen was rather full, and his legs were constantly drawn up towards it. He vomited much; his bowels were open three or four times a day, the motions being green and offensive; his pulse was frequent, but without power. In this, as in many instances of passive congestion of the brain, local depletion was resorted to at first, and, benefit resulting from it, was repeated more than once. It is not, however, every case that will admit even of local depletion, which whenever employed, must be practiced only with the view of affording relief to the gorged cerebral vessels, not with the idea of curing the patient by bleeding; for repeated congestion is often associated with atrophy of the brain-substance, as well as with marked dilatation of its vessels. The greatest attention must in every case be paid to diet and to the state of the bowels, and you will find no means of inducing their healthy action better than the employment of small doses of mercury

[1] Niemeyer's caution must not be forgotten as to the dependence of the number of bloody points apparent on a section of the brain, on the degree of fluidity of the blood rather than on the distension of the vessels. Op. cit., vol. ii, p. 164.

and chalk two or three times daily for a couple of days. If the child is not weaned, you may find it desirable, if there is constant sickness, to take it almost or entirely from the breast for a day or two, and to substitute barley-water, sugar and water, or a weak solution of isinglass, with the addition of one-third of milk, which should be given in quantities of one or two tablespoonfuls at a time till the stomach becomes more settled. A stimulating bath, as a hot salt-water bath, or a bath into which a handful of mustard has been put, and in which the child is to be kept for four or five minutes, night and morning, will often be found a valuable auxiliary to the general treatment, as well as very useful, if combined with the application of cold to the head, in cutting short the convulsive seizures.

If the case is associated with much diarrhœa and general impairment of nutrition, the extract of bark with a few drops of sal volatile, or of the compound tincture of bark, should be given two or three times a day, and you should not let the head symptoms lead you to keep the child on a low diet.[1] Remember, too, that when nutrition is much impaired, farinaceous food is not usually well digested; you must, therefore, be sparing of arrowroot, and give milk and water, or milk and water with isinglass, or with the white of egg beaten up with it; or veal tea; or some concentrated meat essence, as Brand's or Gillon's, in very small quantities. If all animal broths or meat essences should purge, as they sometimes do, the white decoction of Sydenham[2] will for a time be a useful substitute for them. As the child improves, the ferrocitrate of quinine will be one of the best remedies you can give,[3] and throughout the whole progress of the case you will remember the tonic influence of pure air; and may even find the removal to a healthier spot and a purer atmosphere absolutely necessary to the recovery of your patient.

Lastly, I will just allude to the head symptoms that sometimes for a few days precede death in children who have been long ill. You may in such cases find the vessels of the brain turgid, and be disposed to reproach yourselves for not having adopted active treatment. Such self-reproach would be unmerited; the streams have stagnated, because the vital powers were all too feeble to keep them in motion.

---

[1] (No. 4.)

℞. Extr. Cinchonæ. ʒj.
Træ. Cinch. Co., ʒij.
Aquæ Carui, ℥ij. ʒvj. M. ʒij three times a day in milk.

For a child a year old. The taste of the above mixture is best concealed by sweetening it, and mixing it with twice the quantity of milk.

[2] This, the Décoction Blanche of the French Pharmacopœia, is made by boiling half an ounce of hartshorn shavings, and the inside of one French roll, in three pints of water, till reduced to two; when it may be sweetened, and given either alone or with the addition of one pint of milk.

[3] (No. 5.)

℞. Syrupi Quinæ et Ferri Citratis, ʒiss.
Syrupi Aurantii, ʒijss.
Aquæ Flor. Aurantii, ℥j. M. ʒj three times a day.
For a child a year old.

LECTURE V.

CEREBRAL HEMORRHAGE.—The rupture of any large vessel in childhood very rare, but effusion of blood into arachnoid frequent—Reasons for its especial frequency in new-born infants—Its association with infantile asphyxia—Blood sometimes effused external to the skull in new-born infants—Cephalhæmatoma, its characters, changes in the effused blood, and process of cure—Its treatment—Hemorrhage into arachnoid in childhood—Changes in the effused blood—Obscurity of the symptoms—Occurs sometimes in very feeble children, or in connection with changes in the blood—Illustrative cases—Hemorrhage into cerebral substance in childhood extremely rare—Cases in illustration of its causes and symptoms—Capillary hemorrhage in connection with tubercle in the brain.

WHEN we last met, I called your attention to the very important consequences that may result from the vessels of the brain becoming overloaded with blood. I pointed out to you a train of symptoms, rising in severity, from mere pain or heaviness of the head, to convulsions or coma, according to the degree of the cerebral congestion; and told you that death itself might take place, without any mischief being discoverable afterwards, more serious than a general turgescence of the vessels of the brain and its membranes. *Simple apoplexy*, indeed, is by no means rare in childhood, and the knowledge of this fact may furnish encouragement to us in cases where the symptoms of present danger are most alarming. We may hope, that if the instant peril can be averted, the blood, which has not burst its vessels, will flow again tranquilly through them, and the functions of life once more go on in their wonted course. In the adult we could scarcely indulge such an expectation, for the import of apoplectic symptoms is generally far more serious. If the patient die, we look for, and seldom fail to find, blood poured out into the brain, compressing its substance, and lacerating the delicate fibres along which the nervous influence travels. Or, even should he survive, it often is to pass through a tedious convalescence, with palsy, and weakened senses, and impaired mental powers—the sad and standing evidence of the grievous injury which the brain has sustained.

You may naturally inquire how it happens that in the child, the very structure of whose skull favors the occurrence of cerebral congestion, hemorrhage into the brain is comparatively so rare; while in the adult, whose unyielding cranium and firmer brain tend to check congestion, the extravasation of blood into its substance takes place so often? The changes which advancing age induces in the structure of the cerebral vessels are probably the chief cause of this difference. In early life, the arteries are yielding, and admit of being greatly distended without giving way; but in the course of years they lose their elasticity, their calibre becomes diminished and unequal, and their coats grow brittle by the deposit of fatty or earthy matter in their tissue.

But though the larger arterial trunks withstand the constantly recurring variations in the cerebral circulation during infancy and childhood, the smaller and more delicate vessels of the brain are very liable to give way, and *capillary hemorrhage*, or hemorrhage by exhalation, as it has been often though incorrectly termed, takes place with greater frequency than in adult age.

All periods of childhood are not equally exposed to this accident, but it is oftenest met with immediately after birth; and no circumstances can be imagined more favorable to its occurrence than those which then concur to produce it. The head of the infant has been subjected to severe and long-continued pressure during its progress through the mother's pelvis; immediately on its birth, the course of the circulation is altogether changed, and, should any difficulty occur in the establishment of the new function of respiration, a long time will elapse before the blood flows freely through its unaccustomed channels. No one will wonder that death should frequently take place during this transition to a new kind of existence. The tumid scalp and livid face of some stillborn children point to one of its most important causes, since they are but the measure of that extreme congestion of the vessels within the skull that has at length ended in the effusion of blood upon the surface or at the base of the brain.

There would be reason to fear that this occurrence had taken place, if an infant, when born, were to present great lividity of the surface, and especially of the face; and if the heart were to beat feebly, and at long intervals, although the pulsations of the cord were slow and faint, or had altogether ceased. In these circumstances, death sometimes takes place without any effort at respiration being made, the beatings of the heart growing feebler and fewer till they entirely cease; but at other times the child breathes irregularly, imperfectly, and at long intervals. The hands are generally clenched, and spasmodic twitchings are of frequent occurrence about the face, or these twitchings are more general and more severe, and amount almost to an attack of convulsions. The symptoms, however, are by no means uniform, for it sometimes happens that the breathing is not much disturbed, and that after living for a few hours in a state of weakness and torpor, with chilliness of the whole surface, the child dies without any signs of convulsion.

In these cases it must not be supposed that the stillbirth of the infant is due solely or directly to the congestion of the brain, or to the effusion of blood interfering with respiration, as cerebral apoplexy does in the adult. The violent uterine action which has compressed the head has at the same time interfered with the placental circulation, and the child is born asphyxiated from the hindrance to fœtal respiration before the influence of the medulla oblongata is called into play, as it is after birth in the establishment and continuance of pulmonary respiration. Cerebral congestion, or actual effusion of blood, may complicate the asphyxia, or render the carrying on of breathing difficult or even impossible, but apnœa is the cause of stillbirth; and the establishment of respiration as speedily as possible is its great remedy.[1]

[1] Schultze, Der Scheintod Neugeborner, 8vo., Jena, 1871, pp. 97–150.

I shall hereafter return to this subject when we come to speak of affections of the respiratory organs. At present, however, it may suffice to say that we do sometimes meet with instances in which, notwithstanding most persevering attempts at inducing respiration, these attempts fail owing to the injuries received in birth, either from instruments or from the mother's passages, having issued in such an extravasation of blood as to paralyse the functions of the medulla oblongata. In such cases the extravasation is sometimes limited to the neighborhood of the cerebellum, but at other times it covers a considerable part of the convex surface of the brain, and even occupies the spinal canal; as you see in this by no means exaggerated representation of a case of infantile apoplexy in Cruveilhier's great work on Morbid Anatomy.[1]

It fortunately happens that the overcharged vessels of the head in the new-born infant do not always relieve themselves by pouring out blood within the skull, but sometimes the capillaries of the scalp give way, and blood is extravasated into its tissue; or, at other times, the effusion of blood takes place between the bone and pericranium. When this last accident occurs, it often gives rise to the formation of a tumor upon the head, that presents peculiarities sufficient to call for some notice.

This tumor (*cephalhæmatoma*, as it has been called, from κεφαλή, head, and αἱματῶμα, from αἷμα, blood) makes its appearance within forty-eight hours after birth—often much sooner—on one or other parietal bone, most frequently on the right, as a circumscribed, soft, elastic, slightly fluctuating, painless swelling, beneath the unchanged integument. On a careful examination, it is generally felt to be bounded by a firm, apparently osseous ridge, which usually encircles it completely, though more distinct at one part than another. On passing the finger over the summit of this ridge, and down towards the base of the tumor, the impression is at once conveyed of the parietes of the skull being deficient at this point, and of the ridge being the edge of a hole in the bone. When first discovered, the tumor is usually small, but increases in the course of two or three days, from the size of a marble to that of a chestnut, or of half a hen's egg. As it grows larger, it generally becomes tenser, but still seems to cause no pain, and the child's health continues good. After it has attained its full size, it often remains stationary for a few days, and during this time a gradual increase in the distinctness of the ring which surrounds it is the only change that it undergoes. A slight diminution in the size of the tumor at length becomes perceptible, and then it slowly disappears, though its removal occupies a month, six weeks, or more; and a slight elevation of the skull at the point where it was situated sometimes remains even longer. The centre of the tumor generally retains its soft and fluctuating character nearly to the last, but occasionally it loses this, and communicates to the finger a sensation of crackling, such as we should experience if we pressed on a piece of tinsel.

Although once the subject of much difference of opinion, the mode

[1] Anatomie Pathologique, liv. xv, pl. 1.

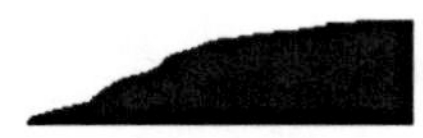

of formation of these tumors, and the nature of the changes they undergo, are now tolerably well understood. The edges of the os uteri, compressing the fœtal skull during labor, just as in this engraving[1] the hands are represented compressing it, often produce an effect similar to that which you see depicted here, and occasion an oozing of blood from its surface; or the same result may follow from undue pressure of the fœtal head against the pelvic walls. The quantity of blood thus poured out is usually small, and is then speedily absorbed, without having at any time produced a perceptible swelling. If, however, it is more considerable, a tumor is formed on the exterior of the skull, and this tumor may continue to enlarge for some time after birth, owing, possibly, to the influence of causes calculated to keep up a congested state of the brain, and to favor the effusion of blood.[2]

The blood thus effused coagulates after very various intervals (often, however, remaining fluid for a considerable time), and the edge of the coagulum sometimes conveys to the finger an indistinct sensation of a raised border surrounding the tumor. The elevated ring that is afterwards plainly felt circumscribing it, is however the result of a reparative process, in the course of which new bone material is poured out from the inner surface of the detached pericranium, and is heaped up in especial abundance just where the bone and its investing membrane come into apposition. This is proved to be its real source, by the fact that the ring becomes much more evident after the absorption of the blood has commenced than it is at first; while in those cases where the effusion of blood has been very considerable, no ring is perceptible during life, and it is found after death that scarcely any attempt at reparation has been made, and that the fibrinous exudation is very scanty, or altogether absent.

This exudation is generally absorbed in course of time, but sometimes a process of ossification is set up in it; the fibrinous ring becomes converted into an osseous ridge, and that part of the cranium over which the blood had been poured out is roughened by the formation of new bone upon its surface. The meaning of the appearances thus produced was long misunderstood, and they were thought to be owing to a process of destruction, not to one of cure. The roughened surface

---

[1] In Valleix's Clinique des Maladies des Enfants Nouveaux-nés, Paris, 1839, planche i, fig. 2.

[2] The various questions relating to the mode of formation of these tumors are fully discussed by Feist, Ueber die Kopfblutgeschwulst der Neugebornen, 4to., Mainz, 1839; and by Burchard, De Tumore Cranii recens natorum sanguineo, 4to., Vratislaviæ, 1837; where are likewise mentioned various exceptional cases in which the swelling formed on the parietal bone that had been directed towards the sacrum, and not, as is usual, on the bone which had presented during labor. The investigations of Professor Levi, of Copenhagen, published in the Journal für Kinderkrankheiten, March, 1852, show fresh exceptions to this, which had been supposed to be the general rule, and prove that sudden pressure, however exerted, is quite adequate to occasion this accident. M. Seux's laborious essay on the subject, which forms the second number of his Recherches sur les Maladies des Enfants Nouveaux-nés, 8vo., Paris, 1863, and the remarks of Virchow in his great work (Die Krankhaften Geschwülste, vol. i, p. 128–135, Berlin, 1863), in which, however, he states the fact of the blood remaining fluid for a long time, much more absolutely than either my own experience or the statements of other observers bear out, do but confirm in all other points the results arrived at by previous observers.

of the skull was looked on as the result of ulceration by which its outer table had at one part been destroyed, and the bony ridge around it was supposed to be the edge of that part of the outer table to which the disease had not yet extended. The real nature of these changes was extremely well exemplified in a very remarkable case that came under my notice, in which blood was effused between the skull and dura mater, as well as between it and the pericranium.[1] This drawing shows the processes of cure in progress. First, however, you may notice the perfect smoothness of the inner surface of the bone, in order to display which the edge of the clot is raised. Its outer as well as its inner investment had been detached from this portion of the skull by the effusion of blood beneath them, and the bone continues unroughened, because an attempt at reparation was impossible here. At the edge of the clot, the dura mater and the bone come again into contact, and nature has here begun the cure. New bone has been deposited, and an osseous ridge has been formed precisely similar to that which in so many instances surrounds the external effusion. Nor is this all; but bony plates are beginning to be deposited between the layers of the dura mater, exemplifying the manner in which, when blood has been poured out beneath the pericranium, that membrane sometimes becomes ossified, and accounting for the crackling sensation that in these cases is felt on pressing the tumor.

The characteristics of these tumors are so well marked, that they are not likely to be confounded with swellings of the scalp produced by any other cause. A hernia of the brain, indeed, may present some resemblance to them, since it forms a soft painless tumor, unattended by discoloration of the integuments, and the edges of the aperture in the bone through which the brain protrudes may easily be taken for the ring surrounding an effusion of blood beneath the pericranium. Independently, however, of the pulsating character of the swelling formed by hernia of the brain, its situation at one of the fontanelles, probably the posterior, or in the course of one of the sutures, will generally distinguish it sufficiently from these sanguineous tumors, which are almost always seated on the parietal bone, and near to its protuberance.

While the nature of this affection was ill understood, many practitioners regarded it as of very serious import, and thought that *its cure* could be effected only by making a free incision into the tumor, and emptying it of the effused blood, or else by applying caustic to its surface, with the view of exciting suppuration within it. There is, however, no real necessity for these severe measures, which appear in not a few instances to have caused the death of the child; for the blood will in the course of a few weeks be absorbed, and the tumor diminish and disappear of its own accord. I have even seen a tumor of larger size than my fist, which was seated on the right parietal bone, but extended considerably beyond the mesial line, disappear completely of its own accord in the course of four months. The great difficulty, indeed,

---

[1] A description of this case will be found at p. 397 of vol. xxviii of the Medico-Chirurgical Transactions.

that you will encounter will consist in persuading the parents to let the swelling alone, and to wait till time effects its removal. While, however, the affection requires no treatment, and is generally not attended by any danger, it is yet right to bear in mind the possibility of internal as well as external effusion having taken place. In this case, as happened in an instance that came under my notice, the sudden increase of the internal effusion may be followed by apoplectic symptoms, and death; or, as in the other instance which I have just mentioned of the very large effusion, the injury inflicted on the brain may be so considerable, that the child may survive only to present every sign of hopeless idiocy.

Perhaps I may be pardoned if I digress for a moment to notice the occasional *pouring out of blood beneath the occipito-frontalis* or temporal muscle in children as the result of a blow on the head. Unlike a bruise, this effusion does not always take place at the precise spot where the injury was inflicted, but the greater size of the vessels that traverse the skull at the side seems to be the reason why a shock, such as a fall on the occiput, is sometimes succeeded by the formation of a tumor of this kind at the side of the head, and not at the part which received the blow. It has twice come under my notice in these circumstances. The tumor thus formed is soft, painless, and fluctuating, and its size at first increases very rapidly, but the integuments covering it are neither hot nor discolored. It is not surrounded by so well-defined a ring as circumscribes the swelling formed by the effusion of blood beneath the pericranium; the ridge is imperfect, its edge is much less sharp, and it is often to be felt nowhere except near to the insertion of the temporal muscle.

In this as in the other case nature herself is usually fully equal to the removal of the blood, and the consequent dispersion of the swelling.

Cerebral hemorrhage, though at no other time so frequent as immediately after birth, may occur at any period of subsequent childhood, under the influence of causes that favor congestion of the brain, or even independently of any cause that we can discover. The *hemorrhage* still takes place almost invariably *into the arachnoid cavity*, and blood is sometimes poured out there in very large quantity; but the accident is neither so invariably nor so speedily fatal as in the new-born infant.

If death should follow very soon after the occurrence of the effusion, the blood is found unchanged, forming a more or less extensive layer upon the convex surface of the brain, and extending downwards and backwards towards the base of the organ, but seldom situated at its anterior part unless the hemorrhage have been unusually profuse. If life is prolonged, the clot speedily separates into serum and crassamentum, and a series of changes commences in the latter, the effect of which is to deprive it of its coloring matter, and to convert it, in course of time, into a delicate false membrane, which lies in close apposition with the parietal arachnoid. This transformation may sometimes be observed while in course of progress, and a central clot may then be seen gradually losing itself in a membrane that grows more and more delicate towards its periphery. If, as occasionally happens, successive effusions of blood take place at somewhat distant intervals, this membrane may become thick and firm, and may even present a pearly lustre; changes which have led some observers into the error of attributing the appearance to alteration and thickening of the dura mater. The amount of the original effusion has much to do with the rapidity of the changes in the clot. If the effusion were but inconsiderable, the serum of the blood soon becomes absorbed, and no other trace of the occurrence remains than the false membrane lining a portion of the arachnoid. If the hemorrhage were at all abundant, the reddish serum will, even after the lapse of a considerable time, be very evident on opening the sac of the arachnoid, and some of it will probably be found entangled in the substance of the clot. By degrees the serum loses its color, but its quantity may still continue for a long time undiminished, or the efforts of nature may even entirely fail to accomplish its absorption. The fluid in such cases is either simply contained within the arachnoid cavity, or, having remained inclosed within the clot during the changes which it underwent, appears at length to be situated within a delicate cyst or shut sac. If the hemorrhage, in the first instance, were very considerable, or if it were to recur two or three times, the yielding cranium of the child will enlarge, the head will alter in form, and the case will assume many of the characters of chronic hydrocephalus.[1]

All writers, even those who, like MM. Rilliet and Barthez, have thrown the most light on the anatomy and pathology of cerebral hemorrhage in the child, concur in representing its *symptoms* as extremely obscure. Paralysis, which, in the grown person, is one of the most frequent results of the escape of blood from the cerebral vessels, is so rare in the child that it was observed by M. Legendre[2] only in one out of nine cases, and by MM. Rilliet and Barthez[3] in one out of seventeen cases. This peculiarity is doubtless in great measure accounted for by the circumstance of the blood being almost always poured out into the cavity of the arachnoid, so that the pressure which it exerts on the brain is generally diffused over the surface of the organ, and is nowhere very considerable.

The absence of paralytic symptoms, however, is not the sole cause of the obscurity of these cases, but the indications of cerebral dis-

[1] Not having had the opportunity of observing the whole series of changes said to take place in blood effused into the sac of the arachnoid, I have chiefly followed the account given by MM. Rilliet and Barthez, in their Traité des Maladies des Enfans, 2e éd., Paris, 1853, vol. ii, pp. 247-255. I am not, however, prepared to say how far this, which was the generally received opinion as to the source of the hemorrhage and the mode of formation of the false membrane associated with it, is still to be regarded as correct. The observations of recent writers, as, for instance, Virchow, in his work Die Krankhaften Geschwülste, 8vo., Berlin, 1863, p. 140; and Lancereaux, in the Archives de Médecine, 1862, vol. ii, p. 526-679, and 1863, vol. i, p. 38, tend to prove the formation of inflammatory false membranes to be the first step in the morbid process, the occurrence of hemorrhage the second. I can, however, scarcely imagine that accidents which seem so sudden as hemorrhages into the arachnoid in children can really be due to a long train of previous morbid phenomena. The observations which have led to this conclusion were all made in the adult and in the aged. The subject seems to me to require further investigation in infancy and early childhood.

[2] Recherches Anatomo-Pathologiques sur quelques Maladies de l'Enfance, 8vo., Paris, 1846, p. 130.

[3] Lib. cit., p. 257.

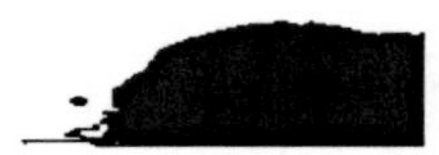

turbance by which they are attended vary greatly in kind as well as in degree. The sudden occurrence of violent convulsions, and their frequent return, alternating with spasmodic contraction of the fingers and toes in the intervals, appear to be the most frequent indications of the effusion of blood upon the surface of the brain. I need not say, however, that such symptoms taken alone would by no means justify you in inferring that effusion of blood had taken place. Many circumstances having reference to the previous history of the child, as well as to its present condition, must be taken into account in forming a diagnosis. Hemorrhage into the arachnoid cavity is most frequent in early childhood—symptoms such as have been enumerated would therefore acquire additional diagnostic importance in proportion to the tender age of the child in whom they occurred. The probability of their betokening this accident would be still further strengthened if the child who experienced them had previously suffered from frequent attacks of cerebral congestion, or had been recently exposed to the sun without proper covering for the head; or had been placed in other circumstances calculated to favor determination of blood to the head.

The popular notion that associates the idea of rude health and general plethora with the occurrence of apoplexy in the adult, is in many instances altogether fallacious. In the case of the child it has still less foundation, since the effusion of blood upon the brain occurs much more frequently in weakly children than in such as are robust. There seems to be reason, indeed, for supposing that the hemorrhage is sometimes of a purely passive character, and dependent on an altered state of the blood. I will relate to you a case or two as illustrations of this *cachectic form of cerebral hemorrhage.*

Some years ago, I saw a little boy, five weeks old, the child of healthy parents, and who had been perfectly well for the first fortnight after his birth: he then, without any evident cause, grew drowsy, and vomited often, and his skin became quite jaundiced. His abdomen at this time was large and hard, and he cried when pressure was made on the right hypochondrium: these symptoms still continued when he was brought to me. A leech now applied on the right side drew a good deal of blood, and the hemorrhage was stopped with difficulty; the bowels, previously constipated, were acted on by small doses of calomel and castor oil, and in three days the child lost the yellow tinge of his skin, became cheerful, and seemed much better. He was now, however, on July 18, suddenly seized with hurried respiration and great depression, soon followed by violent convulsions, during which he screamed aloud. At the same time it was observed that his left hand had begun to swell, and to put on a livid hue, and on the 20th, the right hand also became œdematous. His whole surface grew quite sallow, and, on the day before he died, the œdema of the left hand had much increased; the liver had become considerably deeper, and there were small spots of extravasated blood over each knuckle. The right elbow was slightly livid; the right hand much swollen, but of its natural color; and a small black spot had appeared under the chin corresponding to the knot of the cap-string. The fits recurred very frequently, the child in the intervals lying quite still; the pupils were contracted, and the condition seemed to be one of extreme exhaustion rather than of coma. On the 20th, the power of deglutition was lost; and after several returns of less violent convulsions the child died at 9 A.M., on July 21; about sixty hours after the occurrence of the first fit.

The sinuses of the brain were full of fluid blood; a black coagulum, three or four lines thick, covered the whole posterior part of both hemispheres, extending from the posterior third of the parietal bones, occupying the whole concha of the occipital bone, and reaching along the base of the skull to the foramen magnum. A little blood was likewise effused about the anterior part of the base of the brain, though the quantity was very small in comparison with what was found at its posterior part. The substance of the brain was very pale, and all the organs of the body were anæmic, except the liver, which was gorged with fluid blood, while the heart was quite empty. The ductus arteriosus was closed, the foramen ovale admitted a probe with ease; the ductus venosus admitted one with difficulty.

Another instance has since then come under my notice, in which passive hemorrhage took place into the arachnoid in a child exhausted by long-continued illness, the effects of which were aggravated by poverty and want. From the age of two to that of five months the child had been under my care in consequence of frequent attacks of hæmatemesis and purging of blood, and though his health afterwards improved, yet he never became strong, and his evacuations were almost always white, and deficient in bile. After he was weaned, the coarse food which his indigent parents gave him did not nourish him; he lost flesh and strength, and when almost three years old was puny and emaciated. Three days before his death an attack of diarrhœa came on, which induced great exhaustion; and while suffering from this affection, he suddenly grew comatose, cold, and almost pulseless, and his breathing became so slow that he inspired only four or five times in a minute. In this state he lay for twenty-four hours, and then died quietly. Nearly six ounces of dark coagulated blood were found in the sac of the arachnoid over the right hemisphere of the brain; a little blood was likewise effused beneath the arachnoid, and there was a very small clot in the lower and front part of the right middle lobe of the brain, but no ruptured vessels could be perceived. Great anæmia of every organ, and a state of extreme attenuation of the walls of the heart, were the only other remarkable appearances.

Hemorrhage into the substance of the brain, though extremely rare in infancy and childhood, does sometimes occur, and then gives rise to appearances similar to those with which we are familiar in the adult. Death, however, usually takes place too speedily in these cases for any of those changes to occur in the apoplectic effusion which are often observed in the adult, and which betoken the advance that nature has made in her efforts to repair the injury of the brain.

I have only twice met with distinct extravasation of blood into the substance of the brain in children. In the first case, that of a little girl eleven months old, the occurrence was evidently due to the impediment to the circulation through the brain produced by the formation, of a thrombus in the longitudinal sinus, and consequent inflammation of the sinuses of the dura mater. In addition to other appearances, which I shall describe in a future lecture,[1] there was great venous congestion of the membranes covering the middle lobe of the left hemisphere of the brain, the cerebral veins were distended with coagula, and their coats were thickened. At the anterior part of the lower surface of the left middle lobe of the brain there were four apoplectic effusions, in all of which the blood still retained its natural color, and each effusion was situated close to an obliterated and distended vein. The largest clot extended for an inch into the substance of the brain, and the others were of smaller dimensions. Head symptoms, as might be expected, had existed in this little child for a long time before her death. The occurrence of the effusion was probably synchronous with a sudden attack of extreme faintness that came on forty-eight hours before she died, and from which she never completely rallied.

The other instance of hemorrhage into the substance of the brain occurred in a girl eleven years old, the child of healthy parents, and whose own health had been quite good until she was six years of age. At that time the extraction of a molar tooth was followed by necrosis of a large portion of the lower jaw, and by the formation of abscesses in the face and head, from which bone escaped. An abscess, attended with similar exfoliation of bone, formed likewise on the right foot, and it was three years before the child had recovered completely. Though much disfigured by the disease, her health ever after continued good until April 12, 1846. She was then suddenly and causelessly attacked by vomiting and pain in the head, for which no other treatment was adopted during ten days than the occasional administration of an aperient. During this time, however, a condition of stupor gradually stole over the child, for which, on April 21, a blister was applied to the back of her neck with great relief. On April 23 she had two attacks of convulsions, with an interval of four hours between each. She struggled much during their continuance, especially with the right side; when the convulsions subsided partial palsy of the left side remained; the child complained much of her head, and sank from time to time into a state of stupor, from which, however, she could always be roused. Very free purgation on April 24, and the application of another blister to the back of the neck, were followed by some amendment. On the evening of the 25th another fit occurred, with symptoms similar to those that had been observed on the previous occasions; but it was not followed by any increase in the palsy of the left side, nor was the degree of stupor so considerable as on the former occasion. Mercurials, which had been employed from the commencement of the attack, had now produced a decided influence on the mouth, and the abundant action of the bowels was again succeeded by much improvement in the child's condition. The pulse, which had varied from 60 to 70, now continued about 70, and was natural in character, and the child improved daily, though taking no other medicines than occasional aperients. The headache returned occasionally, though

[1] See Lecture VIII.

each time it was less severe than the time before; but on the evening of May 15, this amendment was suddenly interrupted by an attack of violent pain in the abdomen, which was soon followed by convulsions and coma, and the child died convulsed in sixteen hours; on the 36th day from the first attack of pain in the head.

On making an examination of the head, blood was found to be effused into the subarachnoid tissue over a great part of the right hemisphere of the brain. The quantity of blood, however, was nowhere very considerable, but merely occupied the sulci between the convolutions. The brain presented no remarkable appearance, except that, on a level with and just exterior to the right lateral ventricle, there was a large clot of blood, rather larger than a hen's egg, but of more irregular shape, around which the brain was softened. This effusion was perfectly black throughout, the coloring particles of the blood being equally diffused through it, and no appearance betokened that hemorrhage had previously taken place in this situation. The anterior cerebral artery ran for a considerable distance just outside the clot, but it could not be ascertained that it had given way at any point.

Cerebral hemorrhage is one of the few affections of early life concerning the *treatment* of which but little can be said; for where the symptoms of a disease are so obscure, it would be idle laying down elaborate rules for its cure. The general principles, according to which you would manage a case of congestion of the brain, would still guide you if hemorrhage had taken place. It cannot, however, be necessary for me to repeat to-day the observations on that point to which I yesterday directed your attention.

Before concluding, I must for a moment refer to a form of cerebral hemorrhage, which, though of no great importance, yet forms an exception to what has been stated as to the rarity of the accident in early life. In children who have been affected with tubercular disease of the brain, it is by no means unusual to observe very small effusions of blood in the midst of the softened cerebral matter that surrounds the deposit. This *capillary apoplexy*, produced by some of the minute vessels of the brain giving way, is, however, seldom extensive, and probably has but little share even in accelerating the fatal event.

When next we meet, we shall pass from this subject, which, it must be owned, has more of a pathological than of a practical interest, and shall enter on the study of the inflammatory affections of the brain in childhood.

LECTURE VI.

Inflammatory Affections of the Brain.—Frequent in childhood, but overlooked by early writers—First noticed about a century ago—Their most common form described under the name of acute hydrocephalus by Dr. Whytt—Progress of knowledge with reference to these diseases—Gradual recognition of importance of affection of the membranes—Its two varieties—The simple and the tubercular—Reasons for rejecting old nomenclature, and treating of Simple and Tubercular Meningitis—The latter name restricted in these lectures to scrofulous inflammation of the brain, which is much more frequent than its simple inflammation in childhood.

Tubercular Meningitis.—Morbid appearances in it—Due either to inflammation or to tubercular deposit—Alterations more apparent in the membranes at the base of the brain than in those of its convexity—Increase of fluid in the ventricles almost invariable—Central softening of the brain not a post-mortem alteration—Frequently connected with changes in the lining of the ventricles—Inferences to which these facts lead.

Symptoms of the three stages of the disease.

Few of the diseases of childhood are more serious than those *inflammatory affections of the brain* on the examination of which we are now about to enter. They occasion 9.8 per cent. of all deaths under five years of age in this metropolis, while they are so especially the diseases of early life, that 81.1 per cent. of all cases of fatal inflammation of the brain occur in children under five years of age, 90.2 per cent. before the age of ten, and 92.4 per cent. before the age of fifteen.[1]

But though the frequency of these affections in the young is a matter of such popular notoriety that most of you were familiar with the fact long before you were engaged in your present profession, yet if you turn to the writings of any of the old physicians, you will find in them no mention of inflammation of the brain in childhood. At first this may surprise you, but a few moments' consideration will explain the seeming oversight. Convulsions, which form a prominent symptom in most cases of inflammation of the brain, occur, as I need not remind you, in the course of many other affections of the nervous system. An accident so alarming as a fit of convulsions is sure to attract attention, but much careful examination is often needed to distinguish those minor differences between the symptoms that precede or accompany it, which alone would indicate its cause. It cannot, then, be surprising, that in the absence of this minute care, many diseases, though differing in most important particulars, should have long been classed together under the head of convulsions, and that inflammation of the brain should not have been recognized as a distinct affection. The importance of some of those less obvious structural changes which we know to be most significant of the nature of previous diseases, was not then understood, so that an alteration in the consistence of the brain, or a

[1] Deduced from 5th and 8th Reports of Registrar-General for 1842–5.

diminution in the transparency of its membranes, often passed unnoticed; and anatomical research was not exact enough to make up for the deficiencies in clinical observation.

But just as the physician's attention was fixed on the convulsive seizures which in so many cases affected his patients, so the eye of the anatomist was often arrested by the discovery of a large quantity of fluid in the interior of the brain. Sometimes this fluid had been secreted in such quantity, as not only to distend the ventricles of the brain, but to occasion a manifest enlargement of the skull. In such cases the disease was essentially chronic in its course, and was called, from its most striking characters, dropsy of the brain, or chronic hydrocephalus.

Speculation, however, was set afloat by the occasional notice of cases in which, though fluid was found in large quantity within the brain, yet the previous disease had been of short duration, its symptoms had been acute, and the fever, drowsiness, and cerebral disturbance which attend it had run a very rapid course to their fatal termination. Dr. Whytt was the first[1] who, in the year 1768, clearly pointed out the connection between these symptoms and the accumulation of fluid in the ventricles. His attention, like that of previous observers, was mainly fixed on this point, to the exclusion of other morbid appearances, and he was thus led to regard the disease as an acute dropsy of the brain. Little can even now be added to his description of the malady; but further observation has shown that the presence of an increased quantity of fluid in the brain, on which he laid so much stress, is not of invariable occurrence; that there is no certain relation between the amount of the fluid and the intensity of the symptoms, or the rapidity of their course; and that it is always associated with other very important lesions, some of which are the evident results of inflammation. Many years were occupied in the investigations which led to this conclusion; so that long before Whytt's theory had been ascertained to be erroneous, people had grown familiar with the name of acute hydrocephalus which he proposed for the disease, and continued to employ it as a convenient term long after it was known that it expressed a part only, and that not the most important part, of the truth with reference to its nature.

The first great step towards a knowledge of the true pathology of the affection, was the discovery that the fluid poured out into the ventricles is not a mere dropsical effusion, but that it is the result of previous inflammatory action. Next came the observation, that the effects of inflammation are as remarkable in the membranes of the brain as in its substance; or in other words, that the meningitis is as important as the cerebritis. A further advance was made when it was ascertained that the occurrence of Whytt's disease was associated during life with more or less marked evidences of the tubercular diathesis, and that deposits of tubercle were invariably found after death in various organs of the body of patients who had died from it; and last of all came the discovery, which we owe to the acuteness of French anatomists, that

[1] In his Observations on the Dropsy in the Brain, 8vo., Edin., 1768.

in these cases the inflamed membranes of the brain themselves have been the previous seat of inflamed deposit—that the disease is not a *simple* but a *tubercular* meningitis.

One difficulty still remained in the occasional occurrence of cases similar to, but yet not altogether identical with Whytt's disease, either in their symptoms or their course, the former being usually more violent, the latter more rapid, in which meningitis was discovered, after death, associated with more or less fluid in the ventricles, and more or less softening of the brain-substance; but in which no trace of tubercle is to be found, either in the membranes of the brain or in any organ of the body.

Careful observation brought to light the curious fact, with reference to the two classes of cases, that the membranes covering the upper surface of the brain were mainly affected in simple meningitis, those of the base in the tubercular form. So constantly, indeed, does this rule hold good, that some writers of great authority employ the terms *meningitis of the convexity* and *basilar meningitis* as synonymous with *simple* and *tubercular meningitis* respectively.

To one or the other of these classes may be referred almost all cases of what used to be called acute hydrocephalus on the one hand, and encephalitis, or simple inflammation of the brain, on the other. I propose therefore to discard phraseology which no longer represents the state of pathological knowledge, and to speak first of *Tubercular Meningitis*, which is vastly the more frequent form, then of *Simple Meningitis*, and afterwards to notice the rare instances of inflammation of the brain-substance—*Encephalitis*, or still more properly *Cerebritis*.

We will commence this investigation with an inquiry into the nature of *the appearances found after death* in cases of Tubercular Meningitis. These may be divided into two classes, according as they are the result of inflammation or of the deposit of tubercle; and changes due to both of these causes are often found in the membranes of the brain as well as in its substance.

The appearances which present themselves on the skull being opened are seldom very striking, for the dura mater is usually healthy, and the changes in the arachnoid are not in general of a kind at once to attract attention. Sometimes, indeed, the eye is struck by an excessive vascularity of the membranes, but this appearance often depends on the overfilling of the large vessels, as the result of position. Attentive examination will enable us to distinguish between this, and that increase of vascularity which is produced by a uniform injection of the minuter vessels; and moderate pressure, while it causes the disappearance of the apparent vascularity in the former case, will produce no effect on the true congestion in the latter.

The secretion that naturally moistens the sac of the arachnoid is altered, increased, or suppressed; but the last of these changes is the most frequent, while the first is seldom observed. The preternatural dryness of the membrane is usually connected with some diminution of its natural transparency; it looks dull and lustreless, and feels sticky—a state to which the French have applied the term "*poisseux*." The dulness of the arachnoid is sometimes more considerable, and it then presents an opaline appearance, which is very evident at those parts where the membrane passes from one convolution to another. This opalescence is not often general, but is usually most marked about the upper part of the hemispheres, and in the neighborhood of the longitudinal fissure.

When any considerable degree of vascularity of the membranes is evident, this is, of course, chiefly due to the injection of the minute vessels of the pia mater. Such intense injection of the pia mater is, however, far less frequent than the effusion of fluid between it and the arachnoid, and it is still less common to find the two appearances in the same subject. The effused fluid is for the most part colorless and transparent, and if present in any considerable quantity, the surface of the convolutions appears as if covered by a layer of transparent jelly, though on puncturing the membrane a drop of clear serum will exude. The effusion of lymph or pus into the pia mater covering any considerable extent of the convexity of the brain is very seldom met with, but deposits of a yellow puriform lymph are not unfrequently seen occupying the depressions between the convolutions, or following the course of the vessels along the sides, or at the upper surface of the hemispheres.

But though the alterations presented by the membranes at the convexity of the brain are usually comparatively trivial, the membranes at the base of the organ almost always show unequivocal traces of inflammatory action. The predominance of the affection of the membranes at the base of the brain may indeed, as I have already stated, be regarded as pathognomonic of scrofulous inflammation of the organ;[1] for even if the rule is not absolutely without exception, it yet holds good in the vast majority of cases. In 75 out of 80 cases under my care, in which the symptoms during life were those of acute hydrocephalus, the membranes at the base of the brain were found to be the seat of disease more or less extensive, and always more considerable than that which existed at the vertex. I hesitate to draw any conclusion from the five remaining cases, since they were recorded many years ago, and I am more disposed to believe that my observation was inaccurate than that a pathological law which seems so well established should have so many exceptions.

The least considerable of the morbid changes in the membranes at the base of the brain consists in a milky or opaline condition of the arachnoid and pia mater, but chiefly of the former, sometimes extending over the whole lower surface of the cerebrum, but seldom being equally apparent in that part of the membrane which invests the cerebellum. But, besides this opacity, we usually observe much more distinct evidences of inflammatory action in the effusion of yellow lymph beneath the arachnoid. This is generally found about the olfactory nerves, which are often completely imbedded in it, while a similar effusion extending across the longitudinal fissure unites the two hemi-

[1] On which subject, the valuable essay of M. Rilliet, De l'Inflammation franche des Méninges chez les Enfants, in the Archives de Médecine for December, January, and February, 1846–7, may be consulted with advantage.

spheres of the brain together. A deposit of the same kind likewise reaches up the fissure of Sylvius in many cases, and connects the anterior and middle lobes of the brain with each other; or if poured out in less abundance, it may be seen running up in narrow yellow lines by the side of the vessels as they pass from the base of the brain towards its convexity. It is in the neighborhood of the pons Varolii, however, and about the optic nerves, that the most remarkable alterations are met with. The opacity of the arachnoid is here particularly evident, while the subjacent pia mater is opaque, much thickened, and often infiltrated with a peculiar semi-transparent gelatinous matter, sometimes of a dirty yellowish-green color. This matter is occasionally so abundant as perfectly to conceal the third and fourth nerves, and at the same time to invest the optic nerves with a coating two or three lines in thickness; though, on being dissected off, the substance of the nerves beneath appears quite healthy. When this morbid condition exists in any very considerable degree it extends beyond the pons, and involves the membranes covering the medulla oblongata, especially at its anterior surface.

It is little more than forty years since attention was first drawn to the importance of *another element, besides mere inflammation*, in the production of tubercular meningitis. The peculiar granular appearances which various parts of the membranes of the brain almost invariably present in this disease, though noticed many years before, began then to engage the special attention of several French physicians.[1] The conclusion to which we are led by their careful investigation of the subject is, that this appearance is not due to inflammation, as was once supposed, but that it is occasioned by the presence of tubercular deposits. These deposits often assume the form of minute, flattened, spherical bodies of the size of a small pin's head, or smaller, and either of a yellowish color, and rather friable under pressure, or grayish, semi-transparent, and resistant, almost exactly resembling the gray granulations which are sometimes seen in the lungs or pleuræ of phthisical subjects, and, whatever appearance they ultimately assume, they all originally begin in the form of gray granulations. They are likewise sometimes met with in what would seem to be an earlier stage, when they appear like small opaque spots of a dead white color, much smaller than a pin's head, and communicating no perceptible roughness to the membrane. This appearance is often observed in the arachnoid covering the cerebellum, and those parts of the base of the brain where the arachnoid is stretched across from one part of the organ to another. The flattened yellowish bodies are most frequently seen at the convexity of the brain, and on either side of the hemispheres. They generally follow the course of the vessels that ramify in the pia mater, and accordingly occupy the sulci between the convolutions much oftener than their summit. The firm gray bodies are mostly seen about the pons, or imbedded in the pia mater in the neighborhood of the optic

[1] M. Papavoine appears to have been the first who, in the Journal Hebdomadaire for 1830, vol. vi, p. 113, clearly established the tubercular nature of these granulations of the membranes of the brain.

nerves, or projecting from the surface of the membranes that cover the medulla oblongata. They are also often deposited in the arachnoid lining the occipital bone, and are then sometimes collected in considerable numbers around the foramen magnum. These bodies, sometimes of a gray, at other times of a yellow color, are likewise met with, though less frequently, in the substance of the velum interpositum, or imbedded in the choroid plexuses, and in both of these situations they are sometimes very abundant.

These bodies, however, do not always retain the appearance of distinct granules, but sometimes on separating two folds of the arachnoid which had seemed to be glued together by an effusion of yellow lymph or concrete pus, we find that the matter which forms these adhesions is not homogeneous, but that it consists of an aggregation of minute granular bodies connected together by the lymph or pus in which they are imbedded. This appearance is often met with at the convexity of the brain, and close to the longitudinal fissure, and rather more towards its posterior than its anterior part: a strip of this yellow matter, half an inch long by two or three lines broad, connecting together the two hemispheres of the brain or the two surfaces of the arachnoid. Sometimes two or three deposits of this kind are observed at the convex surface of the brain, but they are generally more extensive at the base of the organ, where they occupy the longitudinal fissure and the fissure of Sylvius, and frequently connect opposite surfaces of the brain so closely together as to render their separation impossible without injury to its substance.

The nature of these granular bodies was for a long time much debated, and I was accustomed once to state fully the reasons which led to the conclusion that they are really tubercular deposits, and not the products of inflammation. It would, however, be needless to do so now, for on this point all morbid anatomists without exception are agreed; and all too are agreed in regarding their presence as essentially characteristic of this form of cerebral disease. We may now, therefore, with great propriety discard the long-used but incorrect term of Acute Hydrocephalus, and speak as I have already done only of *Tubercular Meningitis*.[1]

---

[1] It is perhaps scarcely necessary to give a caution against confounding with these tubercular granulations those small corpuscles, the Pacchionian bodies as they are termed, which are met with either singly or in groups upon the upper surface of the hemispheres near the falx cerebri in the early years of childhood. They are minute round excrescences of the arachnoid, either semi-transparent or of a white color, made up of dense fibrous tissue like that of lowly organized cellular tissue. The arachnoid around them is not infrequently somewhat thickened; but they are in no other respect to be regarded as pathological conditions, than that there appears to be some connection between their development and the previous frequent occurrence of cerebral congestion. In the course of time they sometimes perforate the dura mater, and form little depressions in the bone, in which they become imbedded. They not seldom undergo conversion into the carbonate and phosphate of lime, and yield also slight traces of silex; and are in all respects different from the bodies referred to in the text. See Luschka, in Müller's Archiv, 1852, p. 101; a review of a thesis by M. Faivre, in Arch. Gén. de Méd., Avril, 1854; and Rokitansky, Pathol. Anat., Wien, 1856, vol. ii, p. 407. The laborious investigations of Dr. Meyer, of Hamburg, published in Virchow's Archiv, 1860, vol. xix, pp. 171–288, support the view that the development of these bodies is associated with fre-

Notwithstanding the important nature of the changes presented by the membranes of the brain, it was long before they attracted as much attention as the *alterations in the substance of the brain* itself, and especially as that *distension of its cavities with fluid* from which the malady derived its name of acute hydrocephalus. The surface of the brain, indeed, generally presents but few traces of disease, though sometimes the convolutions are greatly flattened, and the sulci between them almost obliterated by the pressure of the fluid from within. The cerebral substance is often healthy as low down as the centre of Vieussens, or presents no change more important than the presence of an unusual number of bloody points, the divided cerebral vessels. But, though unaltered to the eye, a diminution of consistence is often perceptible as the ventricles are approached. Sometimes the whole brain seems softer than natural, while at other times, though not actually softened, it is infiltrated with fluid, as though it had soaked up the serum from the ventricles.

The presence of a larger quantity of fluid than natural in the lateral ventricles is of almost constant occurrence. In 78 out of 80 cases in which death had taken place under the symptoms of tubercular meningitis, I found an appreciable quantity of fluid in the ventricles; and in 65 of these cases the quantity was considerable, amounting to several ounces. The fluid is in general a perfectly transparent serum, resembling passive effusions poured out from other serous membranes; and such it doubtless is in many cases in which it is found distending the lateral ventricles. But, in a large proportion of instances, the increased secretion in the ventricles is associated with a very notable change in the surrounding cerebral substance. This change consists in a loss of the natural firmness of the central parts of the brain; varying in degree from a slight diminution of consistence to a state of perfect diffluence, in which the cerebral substance forms a pulpy mass that is easily washed away by a stream of water; or the softening may be even more considerable, and the cerebral matter may become semifluid, and closely resemble thick cream. The parts thus affected are perfectly pale and bloodless, and the adjacent substance of the brain is usually rather anæmic. The fornix, septum lucidum, corpus callosum, and posterior horn of the lateral ventricles, are the parts most frequently affected; the optic thalami, corpora striata, and lower parts of the middle and posterior lobes of the brain, rank next in this respect, while the anterior lobes are but seldom softened. In a few instances the cerebellum is involved in the softening, and now and then the whole brain is found to have lost much of its natural firmness—a change, however, which is usually much more marked on one side than the other. Closely allied to this softening is the state to which I have already referred, wherein the whole brain appears perfectly infiltrated with

---

quent and long-standing variations in the cerebral circulation; and my own impression is that they are discovered in children who have died of hydrocephalus with much greater frequency than Meyer's statement of their extreme rarity before the sixth year would lead one to anticipate, though I do not know that I could state the fact numerically. It gives, however, to these appearances that position on the border land between physiological and pathological products which is, I apprehend, their proper place.

serum, as though it had been long soaked in it, and had imbibed it like a sponge.

A mechanical explanation has been frequently suggested to account both for this appearance and for the central softening of the brain, which you will observe is most marked in those very parts to which the fluid in the ventricles would naturally gravitate after death. Many facts, however, are opposed to this view of the cause of softening of the brain. If it were a change induced by the imbibition of fluid after death, we should expect to find it as constant as is hypostatic congestion of the lungs; but instead of this being the case, fluid is found in many instances in the ventricles without the consistence of the brain being in the least diminished. In a German work on Acute Hydrocephalus, which embodies the results of a very large number of dissections, it is stated that central softening of the brain existed only in 47 out of 71 instances, in which the ventricles contained a quantity of serum varying from 3 to 11 ounces.[1] In my records of the examination of the brain in hydrocephalus, I have preserved an accurate account of the condition of the cerebral substance in 78 cases, and find that in 35 instances there was not the least central softening, although the ventricles contained fluid in every case but one, and the quantity amounted on 21 occasions to several ounces. M. Louis, too, mentions in his work on Phthisis,[2] that in 75 out of 101 tubercular subjects, each ventricle contained a quantity of fluid varying from half an ounce to two or three ounces, but yet in only 6 of these 101 cases were the central parts of the brain at all softened. And not to dwell on any other arguments which might be adduced, it may be added that M. Rokitansky has subjected the supposed hygroscopic property of the brain to the test of experiment, and found that no change whatever was produced in slices of cerebral matter by soaking them for hours in serum.

But if we reject the theory of this change in the brain being a mere post-mortem occurrence, the question still remains, to what is it due? M. Rokitansky regards it as a condition of acute œdema of the brain, often, though not invariably, associated with inflammation, since its products, pus and exudation corpuscles, are usually found in the broken-down or infiltrated nervous matter.

One very strong proof of the close *connection* that subsists *between softening of the brain and an inflammatory process* going on in the organ, is furnished by the changes which in many of these cases may be observed in the *lining membrane of the ventricles*.

My own observation would lead me to believe that in at least two-thirds of the cases these changes exist to such a degree as to be readily appreciable by the naked eye, and the microscope would, I have no doubt, ascertain their almost invariable existence. The first alteration that takes place in the membrane is the loss of its transparency, which is often, though not always, associated with a turgid state of its vessels.

[1] Beobachtungen und Bemerkungen über den rasch verlaufenden Wasserkopf. von K. Herrich. 8vo., Regensburg, 1847, p. 161, § 126.

[2] Recherches sur la Phthisie; 2d éd., 8vo., Paris, 1843, p. 160, § 161.

At the same time it loses its polish, and next acquires an unnatural toughness, so that it can be raised by the point of the scalpel; and sometimes it is not merely opaque and tough, but greatly thickened, forming a dense firm membrane; and sometimes it presents a granular appearance, which is usually most marked over the optic thalami and corpora striata. This granular condition is sometimes so slight as to be perceptible only when the membrane is looked at in certain lights; sometimes so extreme as to present a distinct roughness to the finger. It is due to the presence[1] of small new-formed papillary outgrowths, consisting of an accumulation of roundish cells with transparent nucleoli, which spring from an unevenly deposited layer of cells superimposed on the lining of the ventricle itself.

These changes, though observed in cases of tubercular meningitis, are present in their most characteristic degrees in chronic internal hydrocephalus, and are the evidence of inflammatory action which dates back in some instances even to the time of fœtal life. Now and then, indeed, the lining of the ventricles, instead of presenting the above described changes, is thickened, pulpy, and softened, so as to fray with the slightest touch; or participates in the general diffluence of the central parts of the brain. This, however, is a decidedly exceptional occurrence, and opacity, loss of polish, thickening, toughening, and granular deposit on its surface, are the changes almost invariably presented by the lining membrane of the ventricles. I have not been able to satisfy myself that these changes bear any certain relation to the quantity of fluid, or to the degree of central softening, though it is rare to find an extreme degree of change in the lining of the ventricles without a considerable quantity of fluid in their cavity, and great softening of the brain around them.

It is clear that in cases of tubercular meningitis there are two distinct elements, which have no constant relation to each other, which even are not invariably associated. The one of them manifests itself in the affection of the membranes at the base of the brain, and is characterized by the deposit of tubercle there, as well as of the exudation-products of inflammation. The other displays itself in the affection of the lining of the ventricles, in the changes which that undergoes, and in the alteration of the adjacent brain-substance.

It were well worth the inquiry to determine the exact connection of the two; to make out which is the earlier occurrence, which predisposes to the other, which contributes most to bring about the fatal event, to ascertain what symptoms betoken the one order of changes, what the other; and so to arrive, if possible, at some means of distinguishing cases which admit of remedy from those in which treatment is vain and hope has no place.

One sometimes hears the complaint that the field of science has been reaped so thoroughly by previous laborers as to leave but scanty gleaning for those who come after. But surely this is an idle lamentation while problems such as these remain unsolved, to which it so much

---

[1] See the minute researches of Dr. Löschner on this subject in his Aus dem Franz Joseph-Kinder-Spitale, I Theil, 8vo., Prag, 1860, pp. 48–85.

imports the practical physician as well as the pathologist to be able to return a correct answer.

It happens sometimes that we find large patches of tubercular matter deposited beneath the membranes on the convex surface of the brain, and extending to the depth of about a line into its tissue, in children who have died of tubercular meningitis. Now and then, also, masses of tubercle, of a spheroidal shape, and of various sizes, are found imbedded in the cerebral substance. This latter appearance, however, is not frequent: it existed only in 8 out of the 80 cases on which I have founded my remarks on the morbid anatomy of the disease, and even in these cases peculiar symptoms existed which during the lifetime of the patient led to the suspicion of the disease being something else than an ordinary attack of water on the brain.

The *complications* of tubercular meningitis consist almost entirely in the deposit of tubercle in many organs of the body, and in the various results to which that tubercular deposit may have given rise. The lungs and the bronchial glands are the parts most frequently and most seriously invaded by the tubercular deposit; the spleen, liver, mesenteric glands, and intestines, rank next in frequency as the seat of tubercle. The association of meningitis with tuberculous ulceration of the intestines is an accident which, though not very frequent, must not be lost sight of, since its existence may give rise to diarrhœa, and thus lead to an error of diagnosis on your part, if you look for constipation of the bowels as an invariable symptom of water on the brain.

But let us now pass to the examination of the *symptoms* of tubercular meningitis. We cannot, however, do more to-day than familiarize ourselves with the main features of the disease, and must leave all attempts at filling up the outline to our next meeting.

The *first* or *premonitory stage* of the affection is attended by many indications of cerebral congestion, coupled with general febrile disturbance, and presenting exacerbations and remissions at irregular periods. The child becomes gloomy, pettish, and slow in its movements, and is little pleased by its usual amusements. Or, at other times, its spirits are very variable; it will sometimes cease suddenly in the midst of its play, and run to hide its head in its mother's lap, putting its hand to its head, and complaining of headache, or saying merely that it is tired and sleepy, and wants to go to bed. Sometimes, too, it turns giddy, as you will know, not so much from its complaint of dizziness, as from its suddenly standing still, gazing around for a moment as if lost, and then either beginning to cry at the strange sensation, or seeming to awake from a reverie, and at once returning to its play. The infant in its nurse's arms betrays the same sensation by a sudden look of alarm, a momentary cry, and a hasty clinging to its nurse. If the child can walk, it may be observed to drag one leg, halting in its gait, though but slightly, and seldom as much at one time as at another, so that both the parents and the medical attendant may be disposed to attribute it to an ungainly habit which the child has contracted. The appetite is usually bad, though sometimes very variable; and the child, when apparently busy at play, may all at once throw down its toys and beg for food; then refuse what is offered, or taking a hasty bite, may seem to nauseate the half-tasted morsel, may open its mouth, stretch out its tongue, and heave as if about to vomit. The thirst is seldom considerable, and sometimes there is an actual aversion to drink as well as to food, apparently from its exciting or increasing the sickness. The stomach, however, seldom rejects everything; but the same food as occasions sickness at one time is retained at another. Sometimes the child vomits only after taking food; at other times, even when the stomach is empty, it brings up some greenish phlegm without much effort and with no relief. These attacks of vomiting seldom occur oftener than two or three times a day; but they may return for several days together, the child's head probably growing heavier, and its headache more severe. The bowels during this time are disordered, generally constipated from the very first, though their condition in this respect sometimes varies at the commencement of the disease. The evacuations are usually scanty, sometimes pale, often of different colors, almost always deficient in bile, frequently mud-colored, and very offensive. The tongue is not dry, generally rather red at the tip and edges, coated with white fur in the centre, which becomes yellowish towards the root. Occasionally I have seen it very moist, and uniformly coated with a thin white fur. The skin is harsh, but there is no great heat of surface; the nares are dry, the eyes lustreless, the pulse accelerated, but seldom exceeding 120 in children of four years old and upwards; not full nor strong, but often unequal in the force and duration of its beats. The child is drowsy, and will sometimes want to be put to bed two or three times in the day; but it is restless, sleeps ill, grinds its teeth in sleep, lies with its eyes partially open, awakes with the slightest noise, or even starts up in alarm without any apparent cause. At night, too, the existence of intolerance of light is often first noticed in consequence of the child's complaints about the presence of the candle in the room.

I need scarcely say that you must not expect to find all these symptoms in every case, neither, indeed, when present, are they persistent, but the child's condition varies greatly in the course of a few minutes; cheerfulness alternating with depression, and sound sleep being now and then enjoyed in the midst of the unrefreshing dozes of the night. It will not be by a hurried visit of a few minutes that you will learn these things; you must not grudge your time if you hope ever to attain to excellence in the management of children's diseases.

This precursory stage is of very variable duration, but on the average does not exceed four or five days. If the disease is not recognized, or if the treatment adopted is unsuccessful, it will pass into *the second stage*, in which the nature of the affection is very apparent, though unhappily the prospect of its cure is almost lost. The child no longer has intervals of cheerfulness, nor attempts to sit up, but wishes to be left quiet in bed, and the face assumes a permanent expression of anxiety and suffering. The eyes are often kept closed, and the eyebrows are knit, the child endeavoring to shut out the light from its morbidly sensitive retina. The skin continues dry, the face is sometimes flushed, and the head often hot; and though these two symptoms vary much in their duration, coming and going without any evident cause, yet there is a permanently increased pulsation of the carotids, and if the skull is not ossified the brain may be felt and seen forcibly beating through the anterior fontanelle. The child is now very averse to being disturbed, and often lies in a drowsy condition, unless spoken to, when, if old enough to answer, it usually complains of its head, or of weariness or sleepiness. Its replies are generally rational, but very short; and if it needs anything, it asks in as few words as possible, in a quick pettish manner, and shows much irritability if not at once attended to. At other times it lies with its face turned from the light, either quite quiet, or moaning in a low tone of voice, and now and then uttering a short, sharp, lamentable cry, which M. Coindet, of Geneva, regarded as characteristic of the disease, and hence termed it *cri hydrencéphalique;* but making no other complaint than the low moan and the occasional plaintive cry. To this, however, there are exceptions, and children sometimes scream with the intensity of the pain, or cry out, "My head! my head!" most piteously. As night comes on there is almost always a distinct exacerbation of the symptoms, and the quiet of the day is frequently succeeded by a noisy and excited state, in which vociferous cries about the head alternate with delirium. This, however, is not by any means a constant occurrence; an increase of restlessness being often the only difference from the state of stupor in which the child lay during the day. At the commencement of this stage the pulse is quickened, sometimes very much so, and is in many cases unequal in the force and quickness of the beats. Irregularity of its rhythm, or distinct intermission in its beat, is the next change, and is usually perceived at the same time with a great diminution in its frequency, which often falls in a few hours from 120 to 90 or 80. At the same time that these changes take place in the general characters of the pulse, its power becomes manifestly diminished, while the slightest exertion, such as attends any alteration in the child's position in the bed, will often suffice to increase its frequency twenty beats or more in the minute. The child sometimes keeps its eyes so firmly closed that we can scarcely see the state of its pupils. Usually they are not much affected, but sometimes one is more dilated and acts more sluggishly than the other, or, in other cases, strabismus exists, though perhaps in a very slight degree, or confined to one eye. It is seldom that vomiting continues beyond the commencement of this stage, but its cessation is not followed by any desire either for food or drink. The bowels usually become even more constipated than they were before, and the evacuations continue quite as unnatural, while all flatus disappears from the intestines, and the abdomen thus acquires that shrunken form on which much stress has been laid by some writers as characteristic of the disease.

The transition from this to the *third* stage is sometimes effected very gradually by the deepening of the state of drowsiness, till it amounts to a stupor, from which it is impossible to arouse the child. At other times, however, this stupor comes on very suddenly, succeeding immediately to an attack of convulsions. The convulsions usually affect one side much more than the other, and after the fit has passed off, one side is generally found partially or completely paralyzed, while the child makes constant automatic movements with the other, carrying the hand to the head, and alternately flexing and extending the leg. The side which is the most affected during the fit is generally, though not invariably, the most palsied afterwards. When the third stage is fully established, the child lies upon its back in a state of complete insensibility, with one leg stretched out, the other drawn up towards the abdomen. The tremulous hands are either employed in picking the lips or nose till the blood comes, or one hand is kept on the genitals while the other is rubbing the face or head. The head is at one moment hot, and the face flushed, and then the heat disappears and the flush fades, though usually there is a permanent increase in temperature about the occiput. Sometimes the skin is dry, and then, though the extremities are cold, a profuse sweat breaks out on some parts of the body or on the head. The pulse often loses its irregularity, but at the same time it grows smaller and more rapid, till at length it can be counted only at the heart. The eyelids now close only very partially, and in most cases there is some degree of strabismus. Light is no longer unpleasant, for the dilated pupils are either altogether motionless, or they act very sluggishly, frequently oscillating under the stimulus of a bright light, alternately contracting and dilating, till at length they subside into their former dilated condition. The child now often makes automatic movements with its mouth, as though chewing, or as though endeavoring to swallow something. It generally happens that, although sensibility is quite extinguished, the child will still swallow anything that is put into its mouth, and the power of deglutition is in most cases one of the very last to be abolished.

An attack of convulsions now sometimes puts an end to the painful scene; but often the child lives on for days, though wasted to a skeleton, and its features so changed by suffering, that those persons who had seen it but a short time before would now scarcely recognize it. The head often becomes somewhat retracted, and the child bores with the occiput in the pillow: the eyelids are wide open, and the eyes turned upwards so as to conceal three-fourths of the iris beneath the upper lid, while the countenance is still further disfigured by a horrible squint, or by a constant rolling of the eyes. The pupils are now fixed and glassy, the white of the eyes is extremely bloodshot, and their surface is besmeared with a copious secretion from the Meibomian glands, which collects in their corners. One leg and arm are stiff and motionless, the other in constant spasmodic movement, while the hands are often clenched and the wrists bent upon the forearm. At the same time there is frequently so much subsultus as to render it impossible to count the pulse, and the muscles of the face are thrown from time to time into a state of spasmodic twitching. Cold clammy sweats break out abundantly about the head, the breathing is labored, deglutition becomes difficult, and the child almost chokes with the effort to swallow, or lets the fluid run out at the corners of its mouth. It is uncertain how long this condition may endure: the recurrence of convulsions usually hastens the end, but sometimes many days will pass, during which death is hourly expected, and earnestly prayed for, to put an end to the patient's sufferings.

LECTURE VII.

TUBERCULAR MENINGITIS, continued.—Diversities in its course and in its modes of attack—Insidious approach in phthisical subjects—Resemblance of its symptoms to those of typhoid fever—of simple gastric disorder—Serious import of continued sickness in cases of gastric disorder.

Prognosis.—Disease almost always fatal—Appearances of improvement often delusive—Cautions against being misled by them.

Duration of the disease.

Treatment.—Prophylaxis.—Treatment of the disease—Rules for depletion, for use of purgatives, mercurials, application of cold—Diet of patients—Circumstances in which opiates may be useful—When blisters are to be applied—Alleged efficacy of tartar-emetic ointment as a counter-irritant—Conclusions about treatment.

It can scarcely be necessary to observe that tubercular meningitis does not always run precisely that course which I described to you at our last meeting. Almost every case, indeed, presents some slight peculiarity, either in the comparative severity of the different symptoms, in the date of their occurrence, or in the order in which they succeed each other. Convulsions, for instance, though hardly ever absent, occur earlier in one case than in another—affect in one the whole body, in another are limited to one side—are succeeded in one instance by paralysis, in another by a stiff and contracted state of the limbs. Again, coma sometimes comes on gradually, at other times takes place suddenly; in one instance it continues long, in another is speedily followed by death. The pupils sometimes become early insensible to light; at other times they continue to act, though slowly, almost to the time of death; and in like manner strabismus may exist in various forms, or there may be constant rotation of the eyeball, or neither of these symptoms may be present; and yet we cannot couple these diversities in the signs of the disease with any certain differences in the morbid appearances. But, how much soever one case of tubercular meningitis may differ from another in these respects, such differences are of comparatively but little moment, since, whether these symptoms occur early or late—whether they are slight or severe—short in their duration, or of long continuance—the appearance of any one of them stamps the character of the disease too plainly for it to be mistaken, and indicates not the incipient but the fully developed evil. The *deviations from the ordinary mode of its attack* are far more important, since they may lead you to mistake the nature of the disease during the only time when treatment is likely to be of much avail.

The healthy and robust are comparatively seldom attacked by tubercular meningitis, and in many instances the indications of declining health precede for weeks or months the real premonitory symptoms of the disease. You may, however, be so much taken up with watching the former as to overlook the latter, or to misinterpret their meaning. Your solicitude is excited by the gradual decacy of a child's strength, and the wasting of his flesh. You observe that he becomes subject to irregular febrile attacks—that he coughs a little—that he loses his appetite—that his bowels are almost always disordered, and generally constipated—and that he makes frequent vague complaints of pains in his limbs, or of weariness or headache. These symptoms, which depend upon that general deposit of tubercle in the different organs of the body which almost every dissection of fatal cases of the disease reveals, make you apprehensive lest phthisis should be about to come on, and you often auscultate the chest in the expectation of discovering some signs of disease in the lungs. At length, the child seems worse —he coughs more, and is more feverish—grows heavier and more dull, but does not complain more about his head—or, at most, says that the cough makes his head ache. The parents think the child must have caught cold, and you do not see the indication of any new disorder; for, though listless and moody, he still moves about the house, and sometimes plays, though in a spiritless manner. Simple treatment seems to do a little good, and you not unnaturally hope that the aggravation of the symptoms will prove only temporary; but, after an unusually restless night, a fit of convulsions comes on, or the listlessness deepens in the course of a few hours, and without any evident cause, into profound coma, and a very few days terminate the patient's life.

A little girl, nearly eight years old, was brought to the Children's Hospital one December. She was very pale, very languid, and so emaciated that she looked as if far advanced in consumption. Her mother stated that from birth the child's health had been delicate, but that she had had no disease until the previous July, when hooping-cough came on, which in a few days was complicated by the occurrence of measles, attended with diarrhœa. She recovered from these ailments, though they left her very thin and very weak, and the hooping-cough did not completely cease until late in the autumn.

From the time of the hooping-cough ceasing, the child's health improved, but her appetite was never very good, and she seemed by degrees to become more and more unable to eat the coarse food of poverty. She next was sick sometimes after taking food, and then complained occasionally of headache; and after these fresh symptoms had continued for a few days, her mother brought her to the hospital. She attended as an out-patient for nearly a fortnight, during which time no new symptom appeared; but the child grew daily weaker, and, accordingly, was received into the house on December 16. The fact that the auscultatory signs of phthisis which were present, consisted merely in slight impairment of resonance on the left side posteriorly, with coarse breathing and loud expiratory sounds, led to the hope that the mischief in the lungs was not very considerable. She was ordered beef tea, with a little wine, and a mixture containing the nitro-muriatic and hydrocyanic acids.

For a few hours, the comforts of the hospital made a change in her for the better; but, on the night of the 17th, she slept badly, complained of headache on the following morning, and was sick after her breakfast. A single dose of calomel freely relieved her bowels, blisters behind the ears removed the headache, and the sickness was quite stopped by the prussic acid given in an effervescing mixture. This improvement, however, lasted only for twenty-four hours. On December 20, after a restless night, she became very drowsy, refused her beef tea, asked for nothing, complained of nothing, but, if much pressed, said that her head ached. A blister was put on the shaven scalp; the wine, which flushed her, was discontinued, while an attempt was made to nourish her with beef tea enemata. The drowsiness, in spite of the blister, deepened on the next day into coma; and thus she lay, in a state of unconsciousness, with occasional convulsive twitchings of the muscles of the face for the last two days of her life, till she died quietly on the morning of December 25.

On examining the body after death, there was found advanced tuberculous disease of the bronchial glands at the left side of the trachea, but the lungs were quite free from tubercle. The ventricles of the brain contained some fluid; the arachnoid at the base was less transparent than natural; while a thin layer of toughish yellow lymph extended over the pons Varolii, being rather more considerable at the right than the left side. The two hemispheres of the brain were united by old adhesions along the longitudinal fissure, and the anterior and middle lobes were connected along the fissure of Sylvius; but there was scarcely any effusion of hyaline matter or any granular appearance between the pons and the optic commissure, where usually it is so marked.

There were but few symptoms of the coming disease; for the same reason, I imagine, as that which will account for the comparatively slight appearances after death: namely, that it takes but little to extinguish life, when long standing ailments have so enfeebled all the vital powers.

In cases such as this, you will, it is true, most likely be able to do little or nothing, even if you recognize the approach of the disease from the earliest indication of its coming. But you will save your patient's friends some sorrow, and yourself some reproach, if you discover the danger at a distance. Now, whenever any child, especially if it is of a consumptive family, has been failing in health for some weeks or months, without evident cause, I advise you to look with much suspicion on the supervention of unusual drowsiness or listlessness, or on any aggravation of the cough, for which you cannot find adequate reason in the information afforded by auscultation. A frequent, short, dry cough is not infrequent at the commencement of tubercular meningitis: but in cases where cough has existed for some time, you are very likely to refer its aggravation to mischief in the chest, and to lose sight of its possible connection with affection of the brain. Inquire, therefore, in every doubtful case, whether there has been any vomiting—for sometimes it is but slight, and occurs only after food has been taken, and then only occasionally, so that it may seem to the parents to be a symptom of little importance. Ascertain the condition of the bowels; watch the pulse most carefully; it may not be irregular nor intermittent, but you will probably find a little inequality in the force and duration of its beats: if so, you may be sure that the head is suffering, and if the head suffers in such a patient, it is in ninety-nine cases out of a hundred from the approach of tubercular meningitis. Do not content yourselves with seeing your patient once a day; visit him at least morning and evening—stay some time with him, watch him closely, and see how far he is capable of being amused: but if you are still strangers to that freemasonry which assures a little child that you love it, you will very likely fail of arriving at the truth.

But it may happen that a child, though not robust, had yet been tolerably well till a week or two before you visited it, and that it was then attacked by febrile symptoms, with a little headache, and perhaps with vomiting and constipation. You learn that these two symptoms were but of short duration, but that the fever has continued ever since, and that the child has been very taciturn, rather drowsy, and averse to being disturbed, though giving rational answers when spoken to. You regard the case as one of what you call remittent fever, and treat it without either improvement or deterioration, till the appearance of convulsions or of coma corrects your diagnosis, though unfortunately too late.

This error would indeed be avoided three times out of four if you would once for all recognize the fact that apart from ague and from the eruptive fevers,[1] typhoid is the only essential fever with which we have to do; that all other fevers are but indications of the constitution sympathizing with local mischief somewhere. But still it must be confessed that it is not always easy to distinguish between the milder forms of typhoid fever and the early symptoms of tubercular meningitis. It may help you, however, to bear in mind that typhoid fever is very rare before five years of age, and is hardly ever met with in children under three; while at least half of all cases of tubercular meningitis occur in children who have not completed their fifth year. Still this is not the kind of evidence on which you can place much reliance in a doubtful case, but there are differences in the symptoms, which will generally enable you to discriminate between them, if you have acquired the habit of minute and careful observation. The vomiting, on which I have laid so much stress as a symptom of approaching tubercular meningitis, is generally absent even at the onset of typhoid fever; it soon ceases, and is not followed by that abiding nausea which is frequent in meningitis. In typhoid fever the bowels are often relaxed from the very outset, or speedily become so, and the evacuations present no resemblance to the scanty, dark, or mud-colored motions which are voided in tubercular meningitis; but are usually watery, fecal, and of a lightish yellow color. Tenderness of the abdomen is nearly constant in typhoid fever, and is greater in the iliac regions than elsewhere, and wind can always be felt in the intestines. The tongue is not moist as in meningitis, and is seldom much loaded, but has in general only a thin coating of yellow fur at the centre and towards the root, while it is very red at the tip and edges, and becomes dry at an early stage of the disease. In tubercular meningitis there is

[1] Typhus fever, in London, at least, is of such rare occurrence in childhood, that I have not thought I am wrong in passing it over here without notice.

frequently a great distaste for drink as well as for food, while although the appetite is lost in cases of typhoid fever, yet the patients have great desire for drink, especially for cold drink, to quench the urgent thirst. The heat of the skin in typhoid fever is extremely pungent, it is usually greater than in tubercular meningitis, and more abiding, in which, although there is great dryness of the surface, yet the temperature is either not much increased, or else fluctuates independently of corresponding changes in the disease. It is in such doubtful cases that the full value of the thermometer as an aid to diagnosis becomes apparent. Not only is the temperature in typhoid fever higher as a rule than in tubercular meningitis, but it follows laws with reference to its increase and diminution, a knowledge of which ought to save us from error. It increases slowly day by day during the first stage of the disease, and this independently of corresponding acceleration of the pulse, the evening temperature being constantly from half a degree to a degree and a half higher than that of the preceding morning. So invariably is this the case that Wunderlich and Griesinger[1] on the one hand deny that any acute disease on the second evening of which the temperature is 104° Fahr. can be typhoid, and on the other hand they equally deny its being typhoid if the evening temperature on the fourth day does not reach 103.1°; or if between the eighth and eleventh day it remains permanently below this point. On the other hand, in tubercular meningitis the variations of temperature seem to obey no law, to bear no relation to the frequency of the pulse, but to vary much, being sometimes very high quite early in the disease, at other times continuing low long after the temperature of typhoid would have reached its maximum, while of all the fluctuations which it presents, the most remarkable is the sudden decline of heat for a few hours or a day, and its equally sudden subsequent rise without any corresponding change in the symptoms or course of the disease.

The pulse in typhoid fever is much quicker than in tubercular meningitis; it continues quick throughout, and never becomes unequal or irregular, while its frequency is in direct proportion to the elevation of the temperature of the surface. In typhoid fever the child makes few complaints about its head, but delirium is of early occurrence, especially at night; in tubercular meningitis, on the contrary, true delirium hardly ever occurs till an advanced period of the disease, and is sometimes absent altogether. In typhoid fever, there are distinct remissions and exacerbations of the symptoms, the patient getting better towards morning when the temperature falls, and worse again as night approaches and the temperature rises; while, though there are many fluctuations in the course of tubercular meningitis, yet we observe no *definite* periods at which the symptoms invariably remit or are increased in severity.

With due caution you will scarcely take a case of incipient tubercular meningitis for one of simple gastric disorder, though there are many points of resemblance between the two. Vomiting and consti-

[1] Roger, Op. cit., pp. 275 and 320–328.

pation occur in both, and there is usually some degree of headache in the latter affection, though seldom severe or lasting. Mere gastric disorder is not attended with much febrile disturbance; the face, though heavy, is not distressed nor anxious, while the tongue is usually much more coated than at the onset of an attack of tubercular meningitis. The relief that follows the use of remedies in the less dangerous affection is complete as well as speedy; the sickness will cease after the operation of an emetic, the bowels will act copiously after the administration of a brisk purgative, and in a day or two your patient will be quite well. The persistence of vomiting, however, in any case, which you had thought to be one merely of gastric disorder, must be looked upon by you with great suspicion, and this, even though the bowels have acted freely from medicine, and though there should be no obvious indication of mischief in the head. I once saw a case in which the continuance of intractable vomiting for more than six weeks after the cessation of a short but severe attack of diarrhœa, was the only symptom of illness in a boy five years of age. At length he became a little drowsy, and once or twice when closely questioned, said that his head ached. Not quite two days after the first complaint of headache, the child had a violent fit of convulsions, and in the course of the succeeding week he died, having suffered during that time from all the symptoms of tubercular meningitis, and his body presenting after death its characteristic lesions.

Before taking leave of the diagnosis of tubercular meningitis, we must consider for a moment the question of how far the ophthalmoscope may serve our purpose. At present I believe the ophthalmoscope occupies somewhat the position as an aid to diagnosis which auscultation did some fifty years ago, and I anticipate that in the course of time it will yield us much more help than it does at present; so I beg that my opinion may be taken as referring to the present, and to the present only; and further as being the opinion of one unskilled in its employment. My impression is that in the acute disorders of the brain in childhood it adds but little to the knowledge which we derive from other sources. Its use, never very easy in the case of children, is rendered still more difficult by the fretfulness, restlessness, and intolerance of light which characterize all cases either of meningitis or of disorders resembling it; while next, the signs of optic neuritis, which in some cases it discloses to us, are neither sufficiently constant in their presence, nor uniform in their import to justify us in drawing any very definite conclusion either from the discovery of them in one case, or from our inability to detect them in another. I do not think, therefore, that at present we can afford to neglect any of the ordinary means for arriving at a diagnosis, since all that at present we can safely expect from the ophthalmoscope is the confirmation of an opinion arrived at on other grounds than those with which it can furnish us.[1]

---

[1] With the sincerest respect for the researches of Dr. Clifford Allbutt, I am not at present prepared to subscribe to his opinion as to the not infrequent recovery from tubercular meningitis; and the cases of assumed meningitis in the appendix

An inquiry of little less importance than that concerning the means of distinguishing between one disease and another, respects the *prognosis* that we are to form, the inferences that we may draw, from the course of the malady, either to encourage hope or to excite anxiety. Unfortunately the prognosis in tubercular meningitis is so unfavorable that we can scarcely speak of the circumstances which regulate it: for under almost every variety of condition, of symptoms, and of treatment, the patients die. The cases are but very few in which I have seen any other than a fatal issue follow on even the premonitory symptoms of water on the brain. Once I saw recovery take place after the second stage of tubercular meningitis had commenced, and once I watched with surprise the gradual subsidence of the disease, though convulsions had already taken place, and had been followed by coma. In that instance the child, three and a half years old, was a member of a phthisical family, and her younger brother had died a year before of hydrocephalus. The disease in her case ran its ordinary course, unchecked by the customary treatment. Convulsions took place, coma succeeded them, deglutition was very difficult, the pupils were dilated and almost motionless, the pulse was very feeble and very frequent, and everything portended the speedy death which one looks for as the usual termination of such symptoms. Food was still given, as the power of swallowing was not entirely lost, and ammonia and ether were administered, which after a time were exchanged for quinine. For days unconsciousness continued, and the first return of voluntary effort was shown by the child raising her hand to steady the cup that was put to her lips. She next recovered the power of vision, but still could not move her legs, nor utter any articulate sound. The power of speech was not regained for some weeks, nor that of walking for many months; the gait long continued tottering and uncertain, and the child's manner half-idiotic. When last I saw her three years had elapsed, and recovery was then as perfect as probably it ever will be; but the child, though not deficient in intelligence, had never regained flesh, nor recovered the look of health, nor the manners of a child, but walked about unsteadily, with a weird cast of countenance, and a vacant smile, and I felt surprise that the disease, evidently still latent, had not yet returned. I do not know what eventually became of her.

I am aware that other practitioners have arrived at results far more favorable than those to which my own experience has led me; but while I would gladly, if it were possible, modify my statements, I feel sure that a careful perusal of the cases of alleged recovery recorded by different writers must satisfy every one that the disease in almost every instance was not tubercular meningitis at all; and that often it was some ailment bearing to it but a very slight resemblance. It is remarka-

---

to his work appear to me to be most inconclusive, and as far as I can judge from the brief account of symptoms were not meningitis at all.

His treatise on the "Use of the Ophthalmoscope," London, 8vo., 1871, is, however, deserving of the highest praise for careful and patient research, and lucid statement. It is by far the most valuable contribution to our knowledge of this new means of diagnosis of which we are at present possessed.

ble, indeed, as M. Rilliet[1] well observed in a very valuable paper on this subject, that almost all the instances in which recovery is stated to have taken place, occurred before the real nature of the disease was understood, while, since its tubercular nature has been recognized, not a single authenticated case of the kind has been published by any French physician.

M. Guersant, of Paris, who probably had seen more than any man now living of children's diseases, gives the following statement as the result of his experience:

"Tubercular meningitis," says he, "may sometimes terminate by recovery in the first stage, though the nature of such cases is always more or less doubtful; in the second stage I have not seen one child recover out of a hundred, and even those who seem to have recovered have either sunk afterwards under a return of the same disease in its acute form, or have died of phthisis. As to patients in whom the disease has reached the third stage, I have never seen them improve even for a moment."[2]

The minuteness with which M. Rilliet records the history of his patient's recovery, leaves little room for doubt that the case was one of tubercular hydrocephalus in the third stage; and the bare possibility of error is removed by the circumstance that the child died five years afterwards under a recurrence of the former symptoms; and that on a post-mortem examination the old mischief at the base of the brain was clearly distinguishable from the effects of the recent disease under which the child had sunk. This case, however, and the few others which are scattered through the annals of medicine, can be regarded only as the exceptions which prove the rule that hydrocephalus following the law of tubercular disease in general is almost incurable, while it proves mortal all the more frequently owing to the importance of the organ which is its seat.

Since, then, the fatality of the disease is almost invariable, it may seem to you superfluous for me to say anything more with reference to the prognosis; but I am desirous of guarding you against being deceived by certain *delusive appearances of improvement* which are by no means unusual even in cases where the real nature of the disease has for some two or three days been clearly manifest. Many years ago, a little girl, three years old, was brought to me in a state of profound coma, and presenting the symptoms of the third stage of acute hydrocephalus, of which she died forty-eight hours afterwards, without having had any return of consciousness. I learned from her mother, that, fourteen days previously, the child had been attacked by vomiting, attended by fever and great drowsiness; but that these symptoms abated in three days, and that the child improved and was regaining her cheerfulness until the morning of the day before she was brought to me, when her mother found her comatose, and in just the condition in which she was when I saw her. A more acute observer than this

---

[1] Archives Gén. de Médecine, Dec. 1853.

[2] Dict. Méd., t. xix, p. 403; quoted by MM. Rilliet and Barthez, op. cit., 1st edition, t. iii, p. 531.

child's mother would probably have seen something to make her distrust the apparent improvement; but it is evident that the change was great from fever and drowsiness, and frequent vomiting, to a cessation of the sickness, diminution of the fever, and a return of cheerfulness; and yet during all this time disease was going on, and producing the very extensive softening of the central and posterior parts of the brain which was discovered after death. The cases in which you are likely to fall into error are for the most part such as have come on insidiously, unattended by very violent symptoms, and about which you perhaps hesitated some little time before you became convinced that so grave a malady could wear so mild a form. Treatment for some days produces no effect, the disease remaining stationary; but at length your hopes are raised by finding that the vomiting has ceased, and that the constipated condition of the bowels has been overcome. The heat of head has disappeared, the pulse presents much less irregularity than before, or may even have lost it altogether; the child's restlessness has subsided, and its manner is almost natural. Perhaps the child seems rather drowsy, or it may be sleeping at the time of your visit; but the account you hear of it seems satisfactory; its repose is quiet, and the mother rejoices: her little one has had no sound sleep for many days, and will, she thinks—and you may think so too—be much better when it wakes. It does not wake up, but it swallows well when some drink is given in a spoon, and the mother is still content. Presently slight twitchings of the face and hands are seen, but the child does not wake —you cannot rouse it; the sleep has passed into coma, and the coma will end in death. Always suspect the sleep which follows continued restlessness in a case of affection of the brain.

In other instances, although the disease did not come on so insidiously, and although it has reached a stage at which all its characters are well marked, you may yet be led for a few hours to entertain, and perhaps to express, ill-founded hopes, in consequence of the symptoms having somewhat abated, of the child having had some hours of quiet sleep, or having ceased to vomit, or no longer complaining of its head, or being visited by a short gleam of cheerfulness. You must not forget, however, that it is characteristic of tubercular meningitis to present *irregular* remissions, that they last but for a few hours, and that at your next visit you may find every bad symptom returned, and, possibly, some fresh one superadded. Usually, too, you may be guarded from error by observing the suddenness of the change, and that the condition which has now come on is the very opposite of that which before existed, preternatural excitement having been succeeded by an equally unnatural apathy, or great talkativeness having taken the place of obstinate silence, or the pulse, which before was above 130, having sunk all at once to 90 in the minute. At other times, though there is a general abatement in all the previous symptoms, yet some new one may have appeared; not more formidable, perhaps, than the occurrence of a slight degree of strabismus, which had not existed before, but still enough to indicate that the mischief is still going on, and that you must not dare to hope.

A still more remarkable temporary improvement is sometimes ob-

served, that "lightening before death," which seems, contrary to all expectation, to warrant a hope of recovery even when dissolution is impending. The only instance of it which has come under my notice occurred in a girl, aged seven years, who died on the fifteenth day of an attack of acute hydrocephalus. She had been in a state of stupor for six days, and profoundly comatose for two days, when she became conscious, swallowed some drink, spoke sensibly, and said she knew her father. She became worse again, however, in the course of an hour and a half, though she did not sink into the same deep coma as before, and in another hour she died.

A few points still remain on which I must touch before passing to the consideration of the treatment of hydrocephalus. One of these is the question of its *duration*. The exact determination of this is not always easy, owing to the insidious manner in which the disease comes on; but, on the whole, there is less discrepancy than might have been expected between the statements of different writers. Of 117 cases observed or collected by Dr. Hennis Green, 80 terminated within 14 days, and 31 more within 20 days. Of 28 cases recorded by Gölis,[1] 18 terminated within 14 days, and only 2 exceeded 20 days. MM. Rilliet and Barthez[2] state the average duration of 28 cases that came under their observation to have been 22 days; and the average duration of 73 fatal cases of which I have a complete record, was about 20 days. Of these 73 cases, that which ran the most rapid course terminated fatally in 48 hours, and 3 in five days; death took place in 24 more before the fourteenth day; in 25 others during the third week, and in 18 during the fourth week. In the remaining 8 cases indications of cerebral disturbance had existed for four, six, or eight weeks; but death took place in every instance but two in less than 21 days after the appearance of well-marked symptoms of hydrocephalus, and in one on the eighth day from their becoming clearly manifest. We are, then, warranted in stating that the disease usually runs its course in from two to three weeks.

In describing this disease I divided it into three stages, but did so simply for convenience. Many physicians, however, have attached much greater importance to this division, regarding the first as the stage of turgescence; the second as that of inflammation; the third, that of effusion. Again, the first has been characterized as the stage of increased sensibility; the second, of diminished sensibility; the third, of palsy. Lastly, Dr. Whytt proposed a division that has been much followed, based on the variations of the pulse, which is usually quick and regular in the first stage, slow and irregular in the second, and quick in the third. There are too many exceptions, however, to the order of these changes, for it to be right to make them the foundation of any division of the disease into different stages; and the same remark may be made with reference to any arrangement founded on the variations in the sensibility of the patient.

I have said that the phenomena of the pulse are not constant; I need

---

[1] Praktische Abhandlungen, &c. 8vo., Wien, 1820, vol. i.
[2] Op. cit., vol. iii, p. 497.

scarcely add, that the slow irregular pulse is no proof of the occurrence of effusion; neither is the dilated pupil a proof of it: it is a proof of great mischief having been inflicted on the brain; so are the strabismus and the rolling of the eyes which frequently accompany it; but you cannot connect these symptoms with injuries of a special kind, or involving particular parts of the brain.

Although a disease of childhood, tubercular meningitis is by no means most frequent in early infancy. In only 5 of 79 fatal cases in which the diagnosis was confirmed by a post-mortem examination, were my patients under a year old; 19 were between 1 and 3 years of age; 38 between 3 and 6; 13 between 6 and 9; 2 between 9 and 10; 1 between 10 and 11; and 1 between 12 and 13 years old.[1]

From all that I have told you about this disease, you have, I doubt not, already deduced the practical inference, that the only *treatment* likely to avail much is the prophylactic; and that, if you would hope ever to save a patient, you must treat the mere threatenings of his malady, and not remain inactive until you see it fully developed before you.

The *prophylactic treatment* of tubercular meningitis must be in the main the prophylactic treatment of consumption, since not only is tubercle invariably present in the various organs of children who have died of tubercular meningitis, but the disease itself often supervenes on more or less definite phthisical symptoms, as is shown by the fact that the previous health of the children was indifferent in more than two-thirds of the cases that came under my notice. The influence of hereditary predisposition to phthisis, in favoring its development, on which almost all writers have insisted, is illustrated by the fact, that in 27 out of 42 instances, in which the health of the relatives was made the subject of special inquiry, it was ascertained that either the father, mother, aunt, or uncle had died of phthisis.

In any case where several children of the same family have already died of tubercular meningitis, or have shown a marked tendency to the disease, the mother should for the future abstain from suckling her infants, and they should be brought up by a healthy wet-nurse. In such circumstances, too, it is desirable that a child should always live in the country; should be warmly clad, and should wear flannel next its skin. Its diet should be simple and any change in it should be made with the greatest caution, while milk should for a long time form one of its chief aliments; and it would be desirable not to wean it until after it had cut four molar teeth, as well as all the incisiors. As it grows up, overexertion, either of mind or body, must be most carefully avoided: and on this account, though free exercise in the air is highly

[1] This statement as to the time of life at which hydrocephalus is most frequent is fully borne out by the Fifth and Eighth Reports of the Registrar-General, from which it appears that while only 7 per cent. of the total deaths under one year old in this metropolis resulted from cephalitis and hydrocephalus, these diseases caused 12.5 per cent. of the deaths between 1 and 3; 12 5 per cent. of those between 3 and 5; 11.1 per cent of those between 5 and 10; and 5 9 per cent. of those between 10 and 15. I must, however, add that, since at the Children's Hospital only few and exceptional cases are admitted under two years of age, the figures given above understate the frequency of hydrocephalus in early infancy.

beneficial, gymnastic exercises are by no means to be recommended. The child must be watched carefully during the whole period of dentition, and every precaution must be taken to shield it from the contagion of measles, hooping-cough, or scarlatina; since these diseases, which tend to excite the tuberculous cachexy, would be likely greatly to aggravate the disposition to hydrocephalus, or even to bring on an attack of the disease. The condition of the bowels must be most carefully watched; constipation must not be allowed to exist even for a day, and the least indication of gastric disorder must be regarded as a serious matter. It is not desirable that calomel should be used as a domestic remedy; but if the simplest aperients do not act, the child should be immediately placed under proper medical care. If at any time there should be heat of head, and the child appear squeamish, you must be at hand with your remedies, and those well chosen. Any bulky remedy would probably be rejected; but the stomach is almost sure to bear a grain or two of calomel with sugar, and you may follow this up with small quantities of the sulphate of magnesia[1] every hour until the bowels act freely. A small dose of mercury and chalk, or of calomel, may be continued every night for two or three times; and if any feverishness remains, or if the bowels are disposed to be constipated, the sulphate of magnesia may still be given twice or thrice a day. Leeches should not be applied to the head without very obvious necessity, nor then in large numbers, for strumous children do not bear the loss of blood well; and your endeavor should therefore always be, not simply to cure, but to cure at the smallest possible expense to the constitution. After attacks of this kind, children sometimes recover their health very slowly, and much good may then be effected by a judicious use of tonics. The infusion of calumba,[2] with small doses of rhubarb, is a very suitable medicine, and one which children generally take tolerably well. Or you may give the ferro-citrate of quinine in orange-flower water, and sweetened with the syrup of orange-peel,[3] while you secure the healthy action of the bowels by a grain or two of Hyd. c. Cretâ, combined with five or six of rhubarb, administered every night, or every other night.

If threatenings of head affection have frequently occurred, it has been recommended that an issue should be inserted in the back of the neck. I have no personal experience of its utility, but I can readily believe that it may be of service; though one's natural repugnance to

---

[1] (No. 6.)

℞. Magnes. Sulphat., ʒij.
Syr. Aurantii, ʒij.
Aquæ Carui, ʒvj. M. ʒij every hour till the bowels act.
For a child three years old.

[2] (No. 7.)

℞. Inf. Calumbæ, ℥ij. ʒij.
Inf. Rhei, ʒivss.
Træ. Aurantii, ʒiss. M. ʒiij twice a day.
For a child three years old.

[3] See Formula No. 5, p. 57; or the Vin de Quinquina, or the Vin de Bugeaud of French pharmaceutists, which both have the recommendation of being nice.

cause constant annoyance to children has prevented my giving it a trial. A most remarkable instance of its value is recorded by Dr. Cheyne, who mentions that all the children in a numerous family were carried off by water on the brain, with the exception of one, in whose case the precaution was adopted of putting a seton in the back of his neck.

But the opportunity may not be afforded you of adopting any prophylactic treatment; and when you first see your patient, the existence of headache, vomiting, constipation, and a quickened pulse, with perhaps a very slight inequality in its beat, may leave you but little doubt as to the formidable nature of the disease with which you have to contend. In doing this, there are three remedies on which practitioners commonly rely, namely depletion, purging, and the administration of mercury.

With reference to *depletion*, you must not forget that the disease in which you are about to employ it, although of inflammatory nature, is inflammation in a scrofulous subject, and is in many cases grafted on previous organic disease; such as those tubercular deposits in the membranes of the brain which I have already described to you. You cannot, therefore, hope to cut short the affection by a large bleeding, but your object must be to take blood enough to relieve the congested brain, and no more than is necessary for that purpose. Avoid precipitancy in what you do, and do not let your apprehensions betray you into that overactivity which is sometimes more fatal to a patient than his disease. If you feel any doubt as to the necessity of depletion, visit your patient again before determining on it, but do not delay that visit long. Order a dose of calomel, to be followed by some sulphate of magnesia, if, as is most probable, the bowels are confined, and return again in three or four hours. You may then find that the bowels have acted, and the sickness has ceased; that the head is cooler, and aches less; and that depletion is, for the present at any rate, unnecessary. Or the child's state may be the same, and you may still feel uncertain as to the right course. In that case, at once obtain the assistance of some other practitioner. This is the season when advice may be really useful, for it is only at the outset of the disease that its cure is possible; when convulsions have occurred, or coma is coming on, your treatment matters but comparatively little, for the season for hope and the opportunity for action have then fled.

Though you may have determined on the propriety of depletion, it will seldom be found, even at the outset of the disease, that the character of the pulse is such as to warrant venesection. Local bleeding will generally answer every purpose, and, indeed, the application of leeches may, as I have already mentioned to you,[1] be so managed in the case of infants or young children, as to answer every purpose of general depletion. One caution may not be out of place with reference to the part of the head on which leeches should be put; since, though the reasons for it are obvious, it nevertheless is often forgotten. They should be applied to the vertex, because, if put on the temples, they

[1] See Lecture II, p. 28.

hang down over the eyes and terrify the child ; if behind the ears, they are very likely to be rubbed off as it rolls its head from side to side. I will not say that this depletion is never to be repeated, but I believe that in by far the greater number of cases you will do no good whatever by its repetition, and the exceptional cases will generally be those in which, very marked relief having followed the first bleeding, the same symptoms appear to be returning twenty-four or thirty-six hours afterwards. If you do not see the child until the second stage of the disease is far advanced—till general convulsions have occurred, or till twitchings of the limbs, or of the muscles of the face, an appearance of extreme alarm, or a state of alternate contraction and dilatation of the pupils, show them to be impending—you must be exceedingly careful in abstracting blood. In such circumstances, I have seen convulsions, to all appearances induced, and the fatal course of the disease accelerated, by a rather free, though by no means immoderate loss of blood.

The value of *purgatives* in the treatment of tubercular meningitis can scarcely be overrated; but they must be given so as not merely to obtain free action of the bowels, but to maintain it for some days. After having once overcome the constipation, you will secure this end best by giving small doses of a purgative every four or six hours. The administration of a strong cathartic every morning will not answer this end nearly so well; for, independently of the chance of its being rejected by the stomach, you will find that the dose which sufficed the first time will not be large enough the second, and that there will be a constantly increasing difficulty in obtaining an evacuation. The nausea and vomiting which at first stood in the way of your administering any medicine, are often so much relieved by depletion, that the stomach will almost immediately afterwards bear a dose of calomel and jalap, or calomel and scammony, which may be repeated every three hours, until it acts, while you at the same time endeavor to quicken its operation by the administration of a purgative enema. There is no use, however, in persevering with these medicines if they excite sickness, and it is then better to give a single large dose of calomel in some loaf sugar, and to follow it up by a solution of sulphate of magnesia, which should be repeated at short intervals. When a free evacuation has been obtained, the same salt, in combination with the nitrate of potash, will often keep up a free action of the bowels as well as stimulate the kidneys to increased activity. These remedies may be either mixed with the child's drink, or be dissolved in water flavored with syrup of lemon or of orange-peel.[1]

Mercurial preparations, and especially *calomel*, have long had a high reputation in all the cerebral diseases of early life. Unhappily my own experience does not bear out the common practice, and I put no faith in calomel, nor in the production of salivation, as a means of curing tubercular meningitis. I have seen children die whose mouths had been made sore by mercury, without any influence appearing to have been thereby exerted on the disease; and I recollect two who, at the

[1] See Formula No. 1, p. 52.

time of their death, were in a state of most profuse salivation. Whatever good I have seen in these cases from calomel has been when it was given in combination with purgatives, or when it produced a purgative effect.

Let me, however, again remind you that you may have meningitis combined with tubercular ulceration of the intestines, and that in such a case diarrhœa may exist from the outset, or may come on after a mild dose of some aperient. Now and then, too, without such a cause, constipation is absent, while diarrhœa comes on occasionally in the advanced disease. You must not, therefore, draw inferences as to the state of the patient too exclusively from the condition of the bowels.

There is still one remedy, the iodide of potassium, to which some practitioners cling with a sort of half faith in its specific virtues; and its proved utility in various forms of scrofulous disease furnishes without doubt an argument in its favor. I myself give it likewise, and think that I have seen good from its employment, while in one instance of what seemed to be advanced tubercular meningitis under the care of my former colleague, Sir W. Jenner, recovery took place under its employment. No other case of equal success has come under my own notice, and I can therefore by no means indorse all that has been said in its favor, though I have seen symptoms of a very threatening kind subside under its continued use; and this especially in those cases which were the least active in their character. After the bowels have been freely relieved, and with due care still to keep them daily acting, I give about two grains of the iodide of potass every four hours to a child three years old; either alone, or if the child seems feeble, and the case is one whose symptoms seem to occupy the boundary line between true and spurious hydrocephalus, in combination with a third of a grain of the sulphate of quinine; and I can recommend this practice as yielding results, on the whole, more encouraging than any other with which I am acquainted.

I insisted much on the *local employment of cold* when speaking about the management of cases of cerebral congestion. It is likewise a very valuable agent in the treatment of tubercular meningitis, but its application requires to be judiciously regulated. You will generally find it of service after depletion, for you have abstracted blood on account of the febrile disturbance, and heat of head, and other indications of congestion of the brain, all of which cold will be a powerful auxiliary in subduing. So long as the signs of active congestion of the brain are present, cold will be of service; but it should not be employed independently of the symptoms which betoken the existence of that condition; nor can you hope to see any benefit result from cold applications to the head in the advanced stages of the disease. I need scarcely say that the application of cold with a shock, or the pouring cold water from a height upon the head, though a very valuable means of arousing the child from the state of coma into which it sinks in some cases of intense cerebral congestion, is wholly inapplicable in the coma of tubercular meningitis. The functions of the brain are here not merely interrupted by the excess of blood in the organ, but they are abolished by the disorganization of its tissue, or the compression of its substance by the effusion of fluid.

In the management of children attacked by tubercular meningitis you must not forget that for the most part they are of feeble constitution, and that they will not bear too rigorous a *diet*. Just at first, indeed, while the febrile symptoms run high, and the bowels are unrelieved, or the sickness is urgent, the less the patient takes the better. Afterwards, however, it is desirable that he should be supplied with as much light and unstimulating nutriment as he will take; such, for instance, as arrowroot, or veal or beef tea, either of which will often remain on the stomach when most other articles of food or drink would be rejected.

In the treatment of many diseases you see physicians destroy the sense of pain by *narcotics*, and the question naturally suggests itself to you whether you may not sometimes venture, in the management of hydrocephalus, to mitigate by their means your patient's sufferings. The inquiry is one not very easy to reply to satisfactorily. I think, however, that there are two conditions in which you will be justified in trying the experiment of giving them. Sometimes the disease sets in with great excitement, and a condition closely resembling mania in the adult, symptoms which may have been ushered in by convulsions. In such a case, although the heat of head and the flush of the face may have disappeared after free depletion and the copious action of purgative medicine, and though the pulse is feeble as well as frequent, yet the excitement may be scarcely if at all diminished. Here an opiate will sometimes give the relief which nothing else will procure; your patient will fall asleep, and wake tranquillized in the course of two or three hours. In other cases, which did not set in thus violently, restlessness, talkativeness, and a kind of half-delirious consciousness of pain in the head, become very distressing as the disease advances, being always aggravated at night, so that the patient's condition seems one of constant suffering. But he is not able to bear any more active treatment, and, indeed, you have already emptied your quiver of such weapons. In these circumstances I have sometimes given a full dose of morphia, and have continued it every night for several nights together with manifest relief.

There are two or three remedies comparatively recently introduced into practice, from whose employment I have seen relief in cases of cerebral excitement, whether dependent on tubercular meningitis, or on some less grave cause. One of these is the aconite, from which in cases of general febrile disturbance accompanied with excitement of the brain from whatever cause, I have seen much good result. I have never given it in any large dose; but half a minim every four hours to an infant of a year old, in conjunction with any simple febrifuge medicine, and to older children in proportionately increased doses.

The hydrate of chloral is another remedy of comparatively recent introduction, and one which in these cases appears usually to act as a sedative, better even than any preparation of opium, obtaining sleep especially in those cases where wakefulness is due to restlessness rather than to pain. The bromide of potass, while powerless to retard the progress of the disease, still sometimes does much to mitigate distress, especially by restraining those convulsions which are, perhaps, more grievous to the bystanders than to the patient. For this purpose, however, it must be given in large and frequently repeated doses, such as 10 grains to a child of 3 years old, every two or three hours till the convulsions cease; but when this end has been attained, I have seen no further influence exercised by it on the progress of the disease. It still, however, given in a single large dose at night, sometimes procures quiet, and even sleep, especially if combined for this purpose with the hydrate of chloral.

Another inquiry that you may put is, when are you to employ *blisters?* Certainly not at the beginning of the disease, when they would increase the general irritation, and do more harm than good. At a later period they may be of service, when the excitement is about to yield to that stupor which usually precedes the state of complete coma. They should then be applied to the nape of the neck or to the vertex; and I am disposed to think the latter the better place, since, when applied to the nape of the neck, they often become displaced by that boring movement of the head which the child in many instances keeps up unconsciously. It is well, too, to remember that the skin in this disease is very inapt to vesicate, so that a blister will require to be kept on for ten or twelve hours; contrary to what ought to be your usual practice with children. Cases enough are on record proving the utility of blisters thus applied, to render it your duty not to neglect this means.

I have made a few trials of a very energetic counter-irritant which has been strongly recommended by a German physician,[1] but my experience does not induce me to recommend its adoption. Dr. Hahn employs an ointment composed of one part of tartar emetic and two parts of lard; of which a portion, the size of a hazelnut, is to be rubbed on the shaven scalp over a surface some two and a half inches in circumference, every two hours, till an abundant pustular eruption is produced. The sores which follow this inunction are remarkably intractable, requiring sometimes many months for their cure; but Dr. Hahn asserts, and gives some cases in proof of the assertion, that even in an advanced stage, and after the supervention of coma, recovery has often taken place under the use of this remedy. Many of the cases that he relates, however, are clearly not instances of tubercular meningitis at all, while the theory which he propounds of the existence of a sort of antagonism between it and certain pustular eruptions of the skin, and on which he founds the assumption of a sort of specific virtue in the tartar-emetic ointment, is a mere hypothesis, of the correctness of which, as a general law, we have no sort of evidence. In the cases in which I tried it, it produced most formidable ulcerations of the scalp: it did what a very energetic counter-irritant might be expected to do, but nothing more, and it was difficult to convince bystanders that a large black-looking wound did not increase the suffering of patients whose disease it certainly failed to arrest.

Need I say that you must not think of treating a case of tubercular

---

[1] De la Méningite Tuberculeuse, &c., par H. Hahn. 8vo., Paris, 1835.

meningitis throughout just in the same way as you did at its commencement? There is, if the disease does not run a very rapid course, a stage of weakness and exhaustion, often associated with a half-comatose condition, though sometimes attended with a considerable degree of suffering, which frequently precedes the signs of approaching death. The bowels are now sometimes relaxed, though oftener they continue constipated, because the nervous energy which kept up the peristaltic movements of the intestines is worn out. The powers of organic as well as those of animal life are palsied. This is the time for the administration of quinine, for the employment of nutritious broths and jellies, and even of wine.

You may perhaps be disposed to ask me what I think of this remedy or the other, which has at different times been boasted of, as having done good when other means had failed. Now you must not infer from my silence that I do not believe that other medicines besides those which I have spoken of have been of service; but to attempt to canvass the respective merits of each would, I fear, be a tedious task, and one from which you would derive but little profit.

Besides, let me remind you of what Sydenham says: . . . "In eo præcipuè stat Medicina Practica, ut genuinas Indicationes expiscari valeamus, non ut remedia excogitemus quibus illis satisfieri possit; quod qui minus observabant, Empericos armis instruxere, quibus Medicorum opera imitari queant."

Looking over, at the end of nearly thirty years, what I wrote, and have but little altered, as to the treatment of tubercular meningitis, I cannot but ask myself what more I have learned since then, whether I have gained the use of new weapons, or whether I wield the old ones with greater skill than heretofore? I fear that I cannot profess to do either. With the advance of life, one's private practice becomes more and more that of a consultant, and one sees less of slight ailments, and of the beginning of disease; while further, one loses much when one no longer has the leisure to attend the out-patients of a Children's Hospital. One gains in diagnostic skill, one sees the danger further off, and foretells the inevitable sorrow earlier and more surely than in former years, but that is all.

I leave what I wrote but little changed, because I believe that on the whole the rules laid down procure by their observance the greatest relief to the symptoms; because, in that large class of cases which occupy, as it were, the border land between the curable and the irremediable, they hold out the best prospect of doing good, and because, if the ophthalmoscope should confirm the, I fear too sanguine, views of some as to the curability, of tubercular meningitis, it is by such and such like means that I believe its cure will be most probably effected.

LECTURE VIII.

SIMPLE MENINGITIS.—Its differences from tubercular meningitis—Occasional extreme rapidity of its course—Cases in illustration.—Morbid appearances—Frequent connection with meningitis of the cord—Extreme rarity as an idiopathic affection—Treatment.

INFLAMMATION OF THE BRAIN-SUBSTANCE SUCCEEDING TO DISEASE OF THE EAR.—Digression concerning otitis—Its symptoms—Distinctions between it and inflammation of the brain—Treatment—Chronic otorrhœa with disease of the temporal bone—Case.

THROMBOSIS OF THE SINUSES OF THE DURA MATER.—Circumstances in which it occurs—It sometimes succeeds to large collections of pus in distant organs—Case in illustration.

WE have been engaged at our last two meetings with the study of one form of inflammation of the brain in the young subject. We found tubercular meningitis to be an affection almost exclusively confined to children whose previous health had been indifferent, who had shown some indications of phthisis, or in whose family phthisical disease existed. We observed its development to be gradual, its progress often tardy and attended with irregular remissions, but its issue almost always fatal. The alterations of structure discovered after death were seen to be slight at the convexity of the brain, but very obvious at its base, where, in addition to the effects of inflammation, the membranes often present a peculiar granular appearance, due to the deposit of tubercle. The fluid contained in the ventricles of the brain is almost always transparent, and tubercle is discovered in some, often in many, of the viscera.

But we sometimes meet with cases in which *inflammation of the membranes of the brain* has given rise to changes that contrast remarkably with those which true hydrocephalus produces. We find the cerebral membranes intensely injected, the effusion of lymph or pus abundant, especially about the convex surface of the brain, where it sometimes forms a layer concealing the convolutions from view. Moreover, the fluid that occupies the cavity of the arachnoid, as well as that within the ventricles, is turbid and mixed with lymph, while the membranes present no trace of that granular appearance so remarkable in tubercular meningitis, and the various organs of the body are usually free from tubercle; or if not, its deposit is comparatively small and unimportant.

If we inquire as to the symptoms by which this disease was attended during the lifetime of the patient, we shall most likely find that they present fresh reasons for distinguishing between it and tubercular hydrocephalus. We shall learn that the attack came on in a previously healthy child, that it was either ushered in by convulsions, or that they soon recurred; that they returned often, and probably that they continued with but little intermission until death took place. We shall be told, moreover, that the disease set in with violent vomiting and intense febrile excitement; and that having commenced thus severely, it advanced rapidly, and without remission, to its fatal termination, which may have arrived in the course of a few hours, and is seldom delayed beyond the first week.

Some cases of this *simple encephalitis*, or more correctly of *simple meningitis*, are recorded by Gölis,[1] under the name of Water-stroke: I will select one of them, as affording a good specimen of the most acute form of the disease.

"A little girl, 14 months old, who was healthy and strong and fat, was suddenly seized at 5 o'clock in the morning, after a restless night, with violent fever and frightful general convulsions. Medical assistance was at once obtained, and in less than thirty minutes from the commencement of the attack four leeches were applied behind the ears, which drew three ounces of blood: calomel and other remedies were administered internally, and mustard poultices were applied to the soles of the feet. These measures soon alleviated the symptoms, but the relief lasted for but a very short time; the fever returned as intensely as before, convulsions came on again, attended with opisthotonos, and the child became comatose. Hemiplegia succeeded; the pupils became extremely contracted; complete loss of vision, and spasmodic twitchings of the muscles of the face soon followed, and, thirteen hours after the first convulsive seizure, in spite of most appropriate and energetic treatment, the little child died.

"The vessels of the scalp were loaded with blood, and the skull was so intensely congested as to appear of a deep blue color. The sinuses were full of coagulated blood mixed with lymph, and all the vessels of the brain and its membranes were enlarged and turgid with blood.

"A large quantity of coagulated lymph covered the convolutions of the brain and the corpus callosum like a false membrane, and furnished a delicate lining to the lateral ventricles, whose walls were softened and in part broken down. The ventricles contained about three ounces of turbid serum, and there was a considerable quantity of lymph at the base of the brain."

As I have never seen an instance of this most rapid form of meningitis, I will draw for another illustration of it upon that valuable storehouse of facts, Dr. Abercrombie's work on Diseases of the Brain.[2]

"A child, aged two years, 21st May, 1826, was suddenly seized in the morning with severe and long-continued convulsion. It left her in a dull and torpid state, in which she did not seem to recognize the persons about her. She had lain in this state for several hours, when the convulsion returned, and during the following night it recurred a third time, and was very severe and of long continuance. I saw her on the morning of the 23d, and while I was sitting by her she was again attacked with severe and long-continued convulsion, which affected every part of the body, the face and the eyes in particular being frightfully distorted. The countenance was pale, and expressive of exhaustion; the pulse frequent. Her bowels had been freely opened

---

[1] Praktische Abhandlungen, &c., vol. i, Case 2. [2] Case 10, p. 52.

by medicine previously prescribed by Dr. Beilby, and the motions were dark and unhealthy. Farther purging was employed, with topical bleeding, cold applications to the head, and blistering. After this attack she continued free from convulsion till the afternoon of the 23d; in the interval she had remained in a partially comatose state, with frequent starting; pulse frequent but feeble; pupils rather dilated; she took some food. In the afternoon of the 23d the convulsion returned with greater severity; and on the 24th there was a constant succession of paroxysms during the whole day, with sinking of the vital powers; and she died early in the evening.

"On removing the dura mater, the surface of the brain appeared in many places covered by a deposition of adventitious membrane betwixt the arachnoid and pia mater. It was chiefly found above the openings between the convolutions, and in some places appeared to dip a little way between them. The arachnoid membrane when detached appeared to be healthy, but the pia mater was throughout in the highest state of vascularity, especially between the convolutions: and when the brain was cut vertically, the spaces between the convolutions were most strikingly marked by a bright line of vivid redness, produced by the inflamed membrane. There was no effusion in the ventricles, and no other morbid appearance."

It would not answer any useful purpose to multiply the recital of cases, since though there are great varieties in the duration of the disease, yet its general features are the same in almost every instance, and will, I think, readily be recognized by you as betokening an affection very different from tubercular meningitis.

The morbid appearances are sometimes found to vary both in their degree and in their extent, without any corresponding difference being observed in the symptoms. With the exception of its course being more rapid, Gölis's case differed but little from that recorded by Dr. Abercrombie. I believe that in the majority of instances the lining of the ventricles is affected; and it is certainly more common for the membranes at the base of the brain to be involved in the disease, than for it to be entirely limited to those at the convexity. My own experience, which, however, unfortunately extends only to six complete post-mortem examinations, would lead me to believe that the inflammatory mischief extends in general to the membranes of the spinal cord; and the symptoms observed during life, even when no opportunity was afforded for a post-mortem examination, confirm this opinion.

Acute inflammation of the membranes of the brain is fortunately of very rare occurrence except as the result of fracture of the skull, or of injury to the head or neck, and hence comes more frequently under the observation of the surgeon than of the physician. In the nine cases which came under my own notice, I was unable to discover any adequate exciting cause for the attack, though I was not in all as alive to the probable extension of inflammation from the cavity of the tympanum as I ought to have been; for there can be no doubt but that long-continued otorrhœa, and extension of disease to the temporal bone, are by no means essential to the production of serious disease of the brain or its membranes. This fact serves to give increased importance to every attack of earache in childhood; and will keep you from looking on it as a trivial ailment, painful indeed, but calling for no remedies beyond what the nursery furnishes.

Exposure to the heat of the sun, cold, damp, and overfatigue, are all alleged causes of meningitis probable enough, though I can say nothing concerning them, while as a secondary occurrence and in a somewhat masked form it occasionally complicates the eruptive fevers, especially scarlatina and typhoid fever.

In the *treatment* of this affection in its idiopathic form, our remedies must be, in the main, the same as we should employ to combat the acute inflammation of any other vital organ. Bleeding, purgatives, mercurials, and the application of cold, are the grand means on which we must rely; and these must be used with an unsparing hand if we would have any chance of saving our patient. Our prospect of success, however, depends almost entirely upon our seeing the patient at the very outset. The case which I quoted from Gölis showed you what extensive mischief may occur in thirteen hours, and instances are on record in which a greater amount of injury has been discovered after a still shorter train of symptoms. Even in those cases which do not run this extremely rapid course, and in which the mischief found after death is not so considerable, there is little less need for speedy as well as active interference, for if life be prolonged for a day or two without the disease being overcome, the patient often sinks into an exhausted condition, in which active treatment can no longer be ventured on.

But besides these cases in which the membranes of the brain are alone affected, others are occasionally met with in which the gradual extension of disease beginning without the skull involves not the membranes only but also in many instances the *substance of the brain,* producing extensive softening, or even giving rise to the formation of a distinct abscess. Instances of this are occasionally furnished by children who have suffered from scrofulous disease of the cervical vertebræ, when a life of suffering is terminated by a most painful death; or inflammation of the brain, proving very quickly fatal, may come on in a child who has long had discharge from the ear, with occasional attacks of earache. Vague threatenings of mischief in the head may perhaps have existed for some time, just sufficient to excite your apprehension, but not so serious nor so definite as to call for decided interference; and yet, when death takes place, you will find it almost impossible to reconcile the existence of lesions so extensive and of such long standing as a post-mortem examination discovers, with the long-continued absence of definite cerebral symptoms.

In Dr. Abercrombie's work on Diseases of the Brain,[1] an account is given of a boy, aged 14 years, who had been affected for two months with headache and discharge of matter from the right ear. A week before his death the pain increased, and was accompanied by great debility, giddiness, and some vomiting. He continued in this state, without stupor or any other remarkable symptom, until the day of his

[1] Page 87; quoted from Mr. Parkinson, in London Med. Repository, March, 1817.

death, when he was suddenly seized with convulsions, and died. An abscess was found in the middle lobe of the right hemisphere of the brain, and another in the cerebellum, and there was extensive caries of the pars petrosa, with effusion of three ounces of fluid in the ventricles.

I have quoted this case in order to impress upon your minds that every, even the slightest, indication of cerebral disturbance is to be looked on with the greatest anxiety in children who have suffered from chronic otorrhœa. Your solicitude must be redoubled if the discharge from the meatus had ever been attended with the formation of abscesses at the back of the ear, or burrowing between the cartilage and the bone, since they would render it extremely probable that caries of the bone had existed, and that the membranes of the brain had been reached by the advance of the disease.

Nor indeed is this the only caution which you will do well to bear in mind. Another scarcely less important is, that even very great improvement must not lead you to look upon the danger as really at an end in any case where head symptoms have succeeded to disease of the internal ear. A boy between 8 and 9 years old had suffered for 2 years from attacks of earache, which had been followed about a month before his admission into the Children's Hospital by the formation of an abscess behind the right ear. For four days he had been sick, and had had much frontal headache; and when admitted there was ptosis of the right eyelid, the pulse was irregular, the pupils were dilated, and the boy was so drowsy as to be almost unconscious. From August 14 to September 15, his condition may be said to have seemed hopeless, but then improvement began; and in a month he seemed almost well. He had gained much flesh, was cheerful, his appetite was good, and his pulse was regular. The grasp of his hands was good and there was no difference between the power of the two, and the only remarkable thing about him was that he walked with effort, his body erect, his elbows out as though like a rope-dancer trying to balance himself. He was sent to the seaside, and there for six weeks he improved; he then for a day or two complained of his head; and next violent convulsions came on, in which at the end of 36 hours he died.

In addition to a large quantity of fluid in the lateral ventricles there were two abscesses in the right lobe of the cerebellum. The larger of these was egg-shaped; of about the size of a bantam's egg, perfectly encysted, with cretaceous substance covering the whole of its inner surface, and containing very thick pus. Behind this was another smaller more recent abscess, containing similar pus, but not furnished with a lining. There was no affection of the membranes of the brain except slight thickening on the inner surface of the carious mastoid process of the right temporal bone.

The possibility of inflammation either of the brain or of its membranes following upon attacks of *Otitis* gives as you have seen its chief importance to that affection. But even independently of that grave consequence, the ailment deserves attention on account of the severe suffering by which it is accompanied. In many instances, too, needless alarm is excited by the symptoms of inflammation of the ear being supposed to betoken that the brain is the seat of mischief. The one indeed may follow on the other, but on this account it is all the more necessary to become familiar with the diagnostic marks that distinguish the less from the more dangerous affection.

The name of *Otitis* has been applied to inflammation of very different parts of the organ of hearing, and in common speaking no adequate distinction has been drawn between the affection of the external auditory canal, and that of the more deeply seated parts of the ear, posterior to the membrana tympani. The earache of infants and children is sometimes due to inflammation of one, sometimes of all of these structures. It is more frequent in all its forms in early life than in adult age, and it is the more deserving of mention since the amount of suffering by which it is attended is by no means a certain criterion by which to judge of its importance. When limited to the external auditory canal, the inflammation, though apt to recur from slight causes, and though very painful, seldom leads either to permanent discharge from the ear, or to permanent impairment of hearing. Inflammation of the mucous membrane lining the cavity of the tympanum, when occurring as an acute idiopathic affection, is usually associated with affection of the external auditory canal, and then often greatly aggravates the child's sufferings. It does, however, often run a comparatively chronic course attended with uneasiness rather than with severe pain, but which betokens the progress of mischief within the ear such as is likely to lead to abiding dulness of hearing. The deafness that follows measles and scarlatina is due to inflammation, which terminates in secretion of pus within the cavity of the tympanum, whence it escapes through the membrana tympani; a mischief either repaired as the inflammation declines by the closure of the opening, or rendered altogether incurable by the detachment of the bones of the ear. In strumous subjects, too, the evil which thus originated may become chronic, may involve the petrous portion of the temporal bone, and may thence eventually extend to the brain. The same result may also follow on long-standing purulent discharge from the ear dependent on chronic inflammation of the external meatus; and it is this circumstance which gives to otorrhœa in childhood its most grave significance.

The full detail of the symptoms and management of these various affections comes rather within the province of the aural surgeon[1] than within mine. I must not, however, pass them entirely without mention. Attacks of earache are most frequent before the completion of the first dentition, and are by no means rare in young children who are perfectly unable to point out the seat of their sufferings. The attack sometimes comes on quite suddenly, but usually the child is fretful and languid for a period varying from a few hours to one or two days before acute pain is experienced. In this premonitory stage, however, it will often cry, if tossed or moved briskly, noise seems un-

[1] Two papers by Mr. Toynbee may be consulted with advantage: the one a pamphlet on Otorrhœa and Otitis, the other in vol. xxxiv of Med.-Chir. Transactions, on "Those Affections of the Ear which produce Disease in the Brain;" and also chap. xiv of his work on "The Diseases of the Ear," 8vo., London, 1860. There are also some good practical remarks on internal Otitis in a paper by Dr. Schwartze, J. f. Kinderkr., vol. xl, p. 305.

pleasant to it, and it does not care to be played with; while children who are still at the breast show a disinclination to suck, though they will take food from a spoon. The infant seeks to rest its head on its mother's shoulder, or, if lying in its cot, moves its head uneasily from side to side, and then buries its face in the pillow. If you watch closely, you will see that it is always the same side of the head which it seeks to bury in the pillow, or to rest on its nurse's arm, and that no other position seems to give any ease except this one, which, after much restlessness, the child will take up, and to which, if disturbed, it will always return. The gentle support to the ear seems to soothe the little patient; it cries itself to sleep, but after a short doze some fresh twinge of pain arouses it, or some accidental movement disturbs it, and it awakes crying aloud, and refusing to be pacified, and may continue so for hours together. Sometimes the external ear is red, and the hand is often applied to the affected side of the head, but neither of these symptoms is constant. The intensity of the pain seldom lasts for more than a few hours, when in many instances a copious discharge of offensive pus takes place from the ear, and the child is well. In some instances, indeed, the subsidence of the disease on one side is followed by a similar attack on the opposite side, and the same acute suffering is once more gone through, and terminates in the same manner. Sometimes, too, this complete cure does not take place, but the earache abates, or altogether ceases, for a day or two, and then returns; no discharge, or but a very scanty discharge, taking place, while for weeks together the child has but few intervals of perfect ease. In infants earache seldom follows this chronic course, though I have occasionally seen it do so in older children; and the disease is in these cases seated within the cavity of the tympanum.

In children who are too young to express their sufferings by words, the violence of their cries, coupled with the absence of all indications of disease in the chest or abdomen, naturally lead to the suspicion of something being wrong in the head. There are three circumstances, however, which may satisfy you that the case is not one of ordinary hydrocephalus: the child does not vomit, the bowels are not constipated, and there is but little febrile disturbance. The loud and passionate cry, the dread of movement, and the evident relief afforded by resting one side of the head, are evidences of the ear being affected; while in many instances the movement of the hand to the head, and the redness of the external ear, with the swelling of the meatus, concur to make the diagnosis easy. Sometimes, when in doubt, you will be able to satisfy yourselves that the cause of suffering is in the ear, by pressing the cartilage of the organ slightly inwards, which will produce very evident pain on the affected side, while if practiced on the other side, it will not occasion any suffering.

The *treatment* of this painful affection is very simple. In many instances the suffering is greatly relieved by warm fomentations, or by applying to the ear a poultice of hot bran or camomile-flowers. A little oil, to which some laudanum has been added, may be dropped into the ear, and repeated from time to time, while if the pain is extremely severe, or has continued for several hours, it may be wise to apply a few leeches to the mastoid process. If the earache returns frequently, a small blister should be applied behind the ear, or slight vesication may be produced by means of the acetum cantharidis. After the cautions I have already given it is scarcely necessary for me to add, that the possible supervention of inflammation of the brain must of course be borne in mind, and any indication of its approach must be immediately combated.

In those cases where offensive puriform discharge from the ear has been of long continuance, and the matter is sometimes tinged or streaked with blood, astringent injections must be used only with the greatest care, while their employment is not at all advisable if exfoliation of bone has taken place, since in such a case not only is the internal ear disorganized, but the dura mater has very probably become exposed. Attention to cleanliness, by frequently syringing out the ear with warm water, or with a solution of gr. j or gr. ij of the acetate of lead in an ounce of water, constitutes all the topical treatment on which it would be safe to venture, while the most sedulous attention must be paid to the general health of the patient.

It still remains for me to notice one singular form of cerebral disease, which, though not confined to children, is seen much oftener among them than among adults; namely, *thrombosis of the sinuses of the dura mater*. In grown persons it usually succeeds to some injury of the head, but in the child it has generally been observed as a consequence of long-continued purulent otorrhœa, combined with disease of the temporal bone, or it has been connected with disease of the frontal sinuses, or has followed an abscess of the scalp. In some instances, also, it has seemed to be excited by the presence of large collections of pus in distant parts of the body. M. Tonnelé, who has written a very valuable paper on inflammation of the sinuses of the dura mater in children,[1] records one instance in which it coincided with a pleuritic effusion; and a somewhat similar case has come under my own notice, which I will relate, partly on account of its rarity, partly because it illustrates exceedingly well the morbid appearances observed in cases of this description.

A healthy little girl was attacked by scarlatina when eight months old. The attack was not severe, but, after it had passed away, she did not regain her previous health, but continued restless and feverish; she was sometimes sick, and her eyelids were often slightly swollen. A fortnight after the rash appeared, she had one or two violent convulsive seizures, but they ceased after her gums were lanced, and did not appear to be in any way connected with her subsequent illness. She continued out of health until she was 10½ months old, when her mother noticed, in addition to the puffiness of the eyelids, a swelling of the legs and abdomen, for which she came under my care when eleven months old. The legs were then very œdematous, and fluctuation was distinctly felt through the parietes of the abdomen, the urine being scanty and high-colored. In the course of about three weeks her condition had improved considerably, the urine having increased much, the anasarca

[1] Journal Hebdomadaire, vol. v, p. 337. 1825.

having greatly diminished, and the abdomen being 1½ inch less in circumference. A fit of convulsions now came on without any apparent cause, but no other symptoms of cerebral mischief followed it, and the convulsions did not return. After the lapse of another week, a discharge of sero-purulent fluid took place from the umbilicus, and continued for several days in quantities of from a quarter to half a pint daily. This discharge was attended with an improvement rather than a deterioration in the child's health; but after it had continued for eleven days, fever and dyspnœa suddenly came on, with dulness on percussion over the right side of the chest, and absence of respiratory murmur in that situation. The discharge ceased for a week during the urgency of the thoracic symptoms, but then reappeared, though scantily. The child now grew thinner and weaker, and sank into a state of hectic. No new symptom came on till she was suddenly seized with extreme faintness, amounting to almost perfect syncope. She rallied, however, under the use of stimulants, but forty-eight hours afterwards the faintness returned, and terminated in death, without any convulsion having preceded it, just five months and a half after the attack of scarlatina, and two months after she came under my care.

On an examination of the body after death, pleurisy of the right side was discovered, with about ℥vj of pus in the right pleura, and peritonitis, with Oiij of pus in the abdomen; the passage being still traceable through which the fluid had escaped at the umbilicus.

The dura mater adhered firmly to the skull along the posterior half of the longitudinal sinus, at the torcular Herophili, and along the left lateral sinus; but elsewhere it was easily detached from the cranium.

The sinuses on the right side were healthy, but the blood within them was almost entirely coagulated. The posterior half of the longitudinal sinus, the torcular, the left lateral and left occipital sinuses, were blocked up with fibrinous coagulum, precisely such as one sees in inflamed veins, and the clot extended into the internal jugular vein. The coats of the longitudinal and of the inner half of the lateral sinus were much thickened, and their lining membrane had lost its polish, was uneven, and presented a dirty appearance.

There was some congestion of the arachnoid, a considerable quantity of fluid in the ventricles, and sections of the brain presented more bloody points than natural, especially on the left side. The base of the brain was perfectly healthy on the right side, but there was great venous congestion beneath the middle lobe of the left hemisphere; the cerebral veins in that situation were distended with coagulum, and their coats were thickened. Towards the anterior part of the left middle lobe were four apoplectic effusions, in all of which the blood retained its natural color. Each of these effusions was connected with an obstructed and distended vein. The largest clot extended an inch into the substance of the brain; the others were of smaller extent.

I cannot speak to you of any symptom as pathognomonic of this occurrence: it usually comes on, as in this instance, in much debilitated children, and though it generally follows some injury or disease in the neighborhood of the brain, you will bear in mind the possibility of its occurrence whenever large collections of pus exist in any part, and will draw a very unfavorable prognosis in the event of head symptoms coming on in such circumstances.

It is now many years since I observed this case, and made with reference to it the above remarks. No other instance has come under my notice in which the thrombosis was so extensive, or in which its results were so characteristic, and I therefore retain mention of it here, though the subject has lost its novelty since the condition has been described by several recent writers, who have brought to bear on it the light which the researches of Virchow have thrown on clot formation in the bloodvessels.

The most elaborate essay on the subject is that of Von Dusch;[1] who divides all cases of "Thrombosis of the Cerebral Sinuses" into two classes, according as they are the result of inflammation in the neighborhood, or as they depend on the indirect influence of general debilitating causes. The effects of local injuries to the skull, and the extension of disease of the internal ear illustrate the former mode of its production; but the latter would seem to be much the more frequent in early life, and in many instances of it, in addition to the influence of general debilitating causes in its production, there was superadded some condition or other obstructing the respiration, and thus preventing the right side of the heart from emptying itself properly, thereby retarding the current of the blood.

Neither the researches of Von Dusch, nor the observations of other writers indicate any symptoms as pathognomonic of this affection, and the only conclusion at which we can arrive with reference to it is, that when head symptoms set in suddenly in previously debilitated subjects, and do not run the course of any ordinary form of cerebral disease, such symptoms will probably be found to be due to the formation of thrombus in the sinuses.

One additional suggestion, which we owe to the acuteness of Dr. Gehrhardt, of Jena, is, that the occurrence of thrombosis may probably explain the sudden tension of the fontanelle and enlargement of the skull, and the hydrocephalic symptoms that sometimes succeed to the depressed fontanelle and sunken sutures which one may observe in the course of the diarrhœa, and some other exhausting diseases of early infancy.

---

[1] The essay of Von Dusch, on Thrombosis of the Cerebral Sinuses, is translated in vol. xi of the publications of the New Sydenham Society, 8vo, London, 1861. Several interesting cases have been contributed by Dr. Löschner, of Prague, in the Prague Vierteljahrsschrift. and in the Jahrbuch für Kinderheilkunde, vol. iv; Analecten, p 49, who dwells especially on the absence of any characteristic symptoms during life; and a case with remarks by Dr. Langenbeck, of Göttingen, will also be found in the Journal für Kinderkrankheiten, vol. xxxvi, 1861, p. 75. In Gehrhardt's Lehrbuch der Kinderkrankheiten, Tübingen, 1871, p. 500, there is also a very able chapter on this affection.

LECTURE IX.

CHRONIC HYDROCEPHALUS.—Various conditions under which fluid collects in the skull—Divided into the external and the internal—Symptoms of both nearly identical—Changes in form and size of the head—And their mode of production—Course of the disease—Termination almost always fatal.

INTERNAL HYDROCEPHALUS.—Important questions involved in its pathology—Frequent connection with malformation of brain—But also follows inflammation of lining of ventricles—Description of post-mortem appearances—Case illustrative of its connection with inflammation—Process of cure usually mere arrest of disease—Effusion occasionally passive—Alleged share of rickets in its production.

EXTERNAL HYDROCEPHALUS.—Circumstances in which it exists—Its relation to hemorrhage into the arachnoid—Treatment of both forms of the disease—Importance, but difficulty, of distinguishing curable and incurable cases—Compression—Puncture—Cases suited for each mode of treatment.

WE have now completed our examination of the acute inflammatory affections of the brain, and with them we may consider that we have dismissed the most important class of diseases of that organ. Before we pass, however, to those in the production of which inflammation bears no part, we must study one malady, which forms a kind of connecting link between the two.

Chronic Hydrocephalus, or dropsy of the brain, is a morbid condition met with in children at various ages, and coming on in a great variety of circumstances. Sometimes it is congenital, and is then often, though by no means invariably, associated with malformation of the brain. In subsequent childhood, an excess of blood in the brain, or its deficiency, or the existence of some impediment to the circulation through the organ, are conditions all of which have been found to give rise to the effusion of fluid into the cavities of the brain, or upon its surface. Instances of chronic hydrocephalus are on record, which have succeeded to hemorrhage into the sac of the arachnoid; others that have been connected with wasting of the brain, in consequence of the supply of blood being inadequate to its due nutrition, or in which obliteration of the sinuses by disease, or the pressure of a morbid growth upon some of the vessels of the brain, has interfered with the due performance of the cerebral circulation. In many cases, however, I believe, as do MM. Rokitansky and Vrolik,[1] that the disease is not merely a passive dropsy, nor simply a consequence of arrested cerebral development, but that it is the result of a slow kind of inflammation of the arachnoid, especially of that lining the ventricles, which may have existed during fœtal life, or may not have attacked the child until after its birth. I may further add that each year leads me to estimate more highly the share of inflammation of the lining of the ventricles in the production of chronic hydrocephalus.

[1] Rokitansky. Pathologische Anatomie, vol. ii, p. 754; Vrolik, Handboek der Ziektedundige Ontleedkunde, Amsterdam, 1840, 8vo., pp. 514–537.

According to the situation in which the fluid collects, a division has been made of chronic hydrocephalus into the *external* and the *internal;* the former term being applied to cases in which the fluid collects in the sac of the arachnoid; the latter to those in which it accumulates in the ventricles of the brain. The two conditions sometimes coexist, but generally they are independent of each other; the internal hydrocephalus being the more frequent and the more important; and to it we will therefore first direct our attention.

The early *symptoms of the disease* vary. When it is congenital, indications of cerebral disturbance are generally apparent from the infant's birth. These are sometimes serious—such, for instance, as convulsions recurring almost daily; at other times they are comparatively slight, and consist in nothing more than strabismus, or a strange rolling of the eyes, unattended by any very definite sign of affection of the brain. The size of the head generally attracts attention before long, and causes importance to be attached to symptoms which otherwise might have given rise to but little anxiety. In some instances, however, the increased size of the head is not very obvious until the child is a few weeks old, although well-marked symptoms of mischief in the brain existed from its birth. Enlargement of the head, indeed, is by no means invariably the first indication of chronic hydrocephalus. In 12 out of 45 cases, fits, returning frequently, had existed for some weeks before the head was observed to increase in size; in 6, the enlargement of the head succeeded to an attack resembling acute hydrocephalus; and in four other instances it had been preceded by some well-marked indication of cerebral disturbance. In the remaining 23 cases no distinct cerebral symptom preceded the enlargement of the head; but in almost every instance the child's health had been noticed to be failing for some time, although the cause of its illness was not apparent.

In whatever way the disease begins, impairment of the process of nutrition is sure to be one among its earliest symptoms. The child may suck well, and, indeed, may seem eager for food, but it loses both flesh and strength; and often, although the head has not yet attained any disproportionate size, the child is unable to support it, either losing the power it had once possessed, or never attaining that which, with its increasing age, it ought to acquire. The bowels are usually, though not invariably constipated. Sometimes diarrhœa comes on for a day or two; but, under either condition, the evacuations are almost always of an unhealthy character. Thus far, indeed, there is but little to distinguish the case from any other in which a young infant is imperfectly nourished; but, even though no well-marked cerebral symptom should be present, occasional attacks of heat of head will be observed, attended with pulsation or tension of the anterior fontanelle, while crying and restlessness often alternate with a drowsy condition, though the child almost always sleeps ill at night. In many instances, too, the open condition of the fontanelles and sutures excites attention long before any enlargement of the head becomes perceptible.

By and by, however, the increased size of the head grows very manifest, and the child's physiognomy soon assumes the distinguishing features of chronic hydrocephalus. As the disease advances, the unossified sutures become wider, the fontanelles increase in size, their angles extend far into the sutures in which they terminate, while the fluid, pressing equally in all directions, tends to impart a globular shape to the receptacle in which it is contained. Some of the casts upon the table afford striking illustrations of this change in the form of the cranium, which would be still more remarkable were it not for the very unequal resistance of different parts of its walls. The bones at the vertex of the skull are much less firmly fixed than the others, and ossification is nowhere so tardy as at the anterior fontanelle, and along the inner edges of the parietal bones. Hence it results that the great increase in the size of the head is effected by enlargement of the anterior fontanelle, and by widening of the saggital suture. The os frontis consequently becomes pushed forwards, the parietal bones are driven backwards and outwards, and the occipital bones downwards and backwards. The displacement of the bones is very obvious in this hydrocephalic skull, but it is still more striking in the two engravings which I here show you.[1] You notice the great prominence of the forehead, and the alteration in the position of the parietal bones, which are driven backwards as well as outwards, so that the natural relations of their protuberances are altogether changed; while in this remarkable case of a man named Cardinal, who though hydrocephalic from his infancy, lived to the age of 29 years, the occipital bone lies almost completely in a horizontal position. You will observe, too, another remarkable alteration produced by the yielding of the orbitar plates of the frontal bone, which are driven by the accumulating fluid from a horizontal into an oblique direction. Sometimes, indeed, they become nearly perpendicular, when, by contracting the orbits, they give to the eyeballs that unnatural prominence, and that peculiar downward direction, which constitute one of the most remarkable features in cases of chronic hydrocephalus.

Few objects are more pitiable than a little child who is the subject of far-advanced chronic hydrocephalus. While the skin hangs in wrinkles on its attenuated limbs, the enlarged head appears full, almost to bursting, owing to the stretching of the scalp; and the scanty growth of hair does not at all conceal the distended veins that run over its whole surface. The size of the skull, too, appears greater than it really is, since the face not only does not partake of the enlargement but retains its infantile dimensions much longer than natural. The eyes are so displaced by the altered direction of the orbitar plates that the white sclerotica projects below the upper lid, and the iris is more than half hidden beneath the lower. Often, too, there is a considerable degree of convergent strabismus, or a constant rolling movement of the eyeballs which the child is unable to control; or the pupils are dilated, and quite insensible to light.

The symptoms of cerebral disturbance that attend the advance of the disease differ much in severity. Sometimes there is little besides a state of uneasiness and restlessness, aggravated at intervals when the

[1] Baillie's Morbid Anatomy, fasc. x, plate iii, fig. 1, and the drawing of Cardinal's skull, in Bright's Reports, vol. ii, part 2, plate xxxv.

head grows hot and the fontanelle becomes tense. In other cases convulsions occur very frequently, being induced by extremely slight causes, or coming on without any. In several instances I have observed spasmodic attacks of difficult breathing, attended with a crowing sound in inspiration, and those symptoms which constitute spasmodic croup, seizures of which sometimes come on even before there is much enlargement of the head. But, whether the cerebral symptoms are slight or severe, almost every case of chronic hydrocephalus has pauses in its course, during which the child seems to enjoy a comparative immunity from suffering, and gains flesh, while its head ceases for a time to enlarge. Nothing, however, can be more variable than the frequency of these pauses, or their duration.[1]

Though almost every case of chronic hydrocephalus is fatal, yet death takes place in very different ways. Children who are the subjects of the disease are almost always very weakly: hence, they frequently give way under the first serious illness that attacks them, and are carried off by maladies totally unconnected with their head affection; while many others sink into that state of atrophy by which the disease of the brain is often accompanied, and die exhausted. Others are carried off suddenly by convulsions, or fall victims to some severe paroxysm of spasmodic croup: and there are other instances in which the disease seems lighted up again after a pause, by the irritation of teething, or by some trivial accident, and death is preceded by the indications of acute cerebral mischief.

The pathology of chronic internal hydrocephalus involves questions not merely of scientific interest, but of great practical moment; for if we come to the conclusion at which some observers of high authority have arrived, that it is almost invariably the effect of arrest of the development of the brain, all therapeutical proceedings must be worse than useless. The early date of the occurrence of its symptoms in the great majority of cases, lends support, indeed, to the opinion that the causes to which it is due must generally have existed before birth; for I find, on examination of the history of 54 cases, 18 of which came under my own observation, that some indications of it were observed in 50 of this number before the child was six months old; that in 14 of these its symptoms existed from birth; and that in 21 more they appeared before the completion of the third month. The knife of the anatomist, too, has discovered evidences of congenital malformation of the brain, in some instances in which no sign of hydrocephalus was apparent until several weeks after the child's birth; a fact which still further deepens the dark colors in which this malady has been portrayed.

Still, large as is the proportion of cases in which symptoms of chronic hydrocephalus have existed from birth, I am disposed to believe

---

[1] I make no reference to the results of cerebral auscultation in this or other affections of the brain in early life. M. Roger's essay, Sur l'Auscultation de la Tête, in vol. xxiv of the Mémoires de l'Académie de Médecine, has completely settled the imaginative character of MM. Fisher and Whitney's discovery. I have myself listened, without success, for the cerebral souffle in several cases of chronic hydrocephalus.

that even in them the condition is by no means constantly due to arrest of development or to malformation of the brain, but rather to a process of inflammation of the lining of the ventricles, such as we know may produce effusion into the cavities of the brain after birth. To this cause is doubtless due that occlusion of the cerebro-spinal openings to which Mr. Hilton was the first to draw attention as one very important pathological element of chronic hydrocephalus.[1]

In seven post-mortem examinations of children affected with chronic internal hydrocephalus, who died at the respective ages of 16 months, 3 years, 8 months, 19 months, 2 years, 3¼ and 3½ years, I found the corpus callosum perfect in every instance. In all, also, the fornix was present; thrice it and the septum lucidum were thickened and tough: twice they were found torn and softened; acute hydrocephalus having supervened on the chronic disease. Once the septum lucidum was absent, and once both it and a large portion of the fornix also were wanting. In one case the state of the membranes lining the ventricles was not noted; in the other six it was thickened, four times very remarkably; and twice it was roughened and granular, presenting an exaggerated degree of that condition which is also so often met with in fatal cases of acute hydrocephalus, and to which I directed your attention when speaking of that disease.

In some cases—as, for instance, in this drawing by Professor Vrolik[2] of the brain of a young man who died of chronic hydrocephalus at the age of 20—a false membrane is found in the interior of one or other ventricle, and may even occlude the foramen of Monro; an accident which, by interrupting the communication between the two sides of the brain, may serve to account for the unequal distension of the two ventricles, and the great want of symmetry occasionally observed in hydrocephalic skulls. The marks of inflammation of the membranes at the base of the brain are, moreover, in many instances, very evident; and there is often an extremely abundant effusion of that hyaline matter in the meshes of the pia mater, to which I called your attention when speaking of acute hydrocephalus.

Lastly, I may remark, that the observation in a large number of instances, that the cerebral substance has been simply unfolded by the accumulation of the fluid in the ventricles, so that even when of extreme tenuity the gray and white matter could still be distinguished, proves not merely that the brain was not melted down by the action of the fluid, but also that its accumulation could not, in these instances, be due to the arrest of cerebral development.

Besides the evidence which post-mortem examinations often furnish of the connection of chronic internal hydrocephalus with previous inflammatory action, the history of the patient's illness sometimes affords distinct proof of its occurrence. A striking instance of this has been

---

[1] See his Lectures on Rest and Pain, 8vo., London, 1863, pp. 34–44, and also "Some Remarks on changes in the Ventricular Lining during Fœtal Life," by Dr. Löschner of Prague, at p 54 of Part I of Aus dem Franz Josef Kinder-Spitale, &c. 8vo., Prague, 1860.

[2] Traité sur la Hydrocéphalie Interne, 4to., plate iii. Amsterdam, 1839.

published by M. Rilliet, of Geneva,[1] in the case of a little girl 10½ years old, in whom the symptoms of acute cerebral inflammation were succeeded by those of chronic disease in the brain, which terminated fatally at the end of four months. Ten ounces of transparent but highly albuminous fluid were contained in the lateral ventricles, the lining membrane of which was nearly half a line thick, having a gelatinous appearance, as if softened, but being in reality so tough that it could be torn away from the cerebral substance in long strips.

Though in the following history the connection between the acute and the chronic evil is far less striking than in M. Rilliet's case, yet I think few will refuse to admit the injury to the head and the subsequent cerebral symptoms as the first steps in the chain of morbid processes which led to the distension of the ventricles of the brain with fluid, and to the development of all the symptoms of chronic hydrocephalus.

A little girl, the child of healthy parents, was healthy when born, and continued so until she was five months old, when she fell out of the arms of the person who was nursing her, and on the same day was taken in a fit, and lay stupid and senseless for some hours. She was leeched and blistered for these and other head symptoms, which the parents were unable to describe very accurately, and to all appearance recovered. When a year old, however, head symptoms returned, and for several weeks convulsions were of extremely frequent occurrence; but at length ceased. About that time, the child being then 15 months old, her mother first noticed that her head was beginning to enlarge, since which time she had no return of fits but the head continued to increase in size down to the time when I first saw her, she being then just three years old.

Her countenance presented all the peculiarities of chronic hydrocephalus in a very marked degree: her head was large, measuring 20 inches in circumference, and 13¼ from one meatus auditorius to the other; her forehead was prominent, and her eyes were directed downwards, while her body was very ill nourished. Her bowels were regular, her bodily functions generally natural, and she was very voracious. She was by no means stupid, but on the contrary showed much shrewdness, though she was noisy and almost constantly chattering.

I had not seen her above once or twice when she was attacked by measles, on the second day of which convulsions came on, and she sank into a comatose state, interrupted only by convulsive twitchings of the limbs, and died in this condition on the fourth day of her illness.

The head was examined 48 hours after death.

The bones of the head were quite firm and hard; the posterior fontanelle was closed, but the anterior was open; its diameter in either direction being about 3½ inches.

There was no fluid in the sac of the arachnoid, nor morbid condition of the membranes either at the vertex or base of the brain.

A very small quantity of fluid was in the subarachnoid tissue, and a pint of perfectly transparent serum in the lateral ventricles.

---

[1] Archives Gén. de Médecine, Dec. 1847.

The convolutions of the brain were quite flattened: its cortical substance was of natural thickness, the white substance very thin, and expanded around the ventricles, which were dilated to four times their natural size.

The white substance of the wall of the ventricles was quite firm, and separable into a thin tough layer, leaving the substance of the brain quite natural beneath. The septum lucidum was tough and membranous and much thickened. The edges of the fornix were firmly adherent to the upper surface of the optic thalamus, and included between them a portion of the choroid plexus.

The membrane lining the ventricles was universally thickened; where it covered the corpora striata, the optic thalami, the commissures, and the floor of the fourth ventricle, it was not only peculiarly tough, but granular, and presented an appearance just like shagreen.

The size of the head in this case had been increasing but slowly, and probably, had the child not been cut off by the intercurrent attack of measles, the effusion of fluid would at length have come to a standstill, and the hydrocephalus would have been cured; at least, as much as hydrocephalus usually is. Strictly speaking, however, there is in general no cure of the affection, but merely an arrest of its progress; no more fluid is poured out, but that already effused is unabsorbed; the sutures and fontanelles become ossified, and the enormous size of the head attracts less attention, not because there is any diminution in its dimensions, but because the disproportion between the cranium and the face becomes less striking, owing to the development of the latter as the child grows older. In some instances, indeed, Professor Otto[1] is of opinion that a real cure is effected by an increased activity of the nutrition of the brain, producing hypertrophy of the organ; the fluid being absorbed, and nerve-matter deposited in its stead. This, however, is, in all probability, a purely exceptional occurrence; and the majority of hydrocephalic patients who survive the advance of the disease still have their lateral ventricles distended with fluid. This was all that occurred in the well-known case of Thomas Cardinal, whose bust I here show you. Having been hydrocephalic from infancy, he yet lived to the age of 29, in the possession of a tolerable amount of bodily and mental activity. On examination of this body after death, between seven and eight pints of fluid were found in his cranium. In the greater number of instances symptoms exist during life which show clearly enough that the arrest of the disease differs widely from its cure, or that the malady of the brain which its produces, or with which it was associated, is irreparable; for the intellectual powers are generally feeble, and the temper very irritable, while the child is often unable to walk, and its sight is very imperfect.

Although inflammation of the ventricular lining is, as I believe, by far the most frequent cause of chronic hydrocephalus, there can be no doubt but that the effusion of fluid is occasionally a purely passive dropsy due to the accidental pressure of some morbid growth upon the Venæ Galeni, or upon the lateral sinus. Such cases, however, are not

[1] Rokitansky's Pathologische Anatomie, 1st ed., vol. ii, pp. 749–769.

only of rare occurrence, but the effusion plays in them a very secondary part, being merely an accidental consequence and complication of the graver disease.

The frequent observation of evidence of rickets in children who are hydrocephalic has also given rise to the suggestion[1] that the diminished pressure of the cranial parietes in consequence of their tardy and imperfect ossification is in very many instances the exciting cause of the effusion, the enlargement of the head being due to diminished resistance, rather than to increased pressure. I cannot subscribe to this opinion, for not only is hydrocephalus present in a very large proportion of cases independent of any sign whatever of rickets, while the most extreme degrees of rickets are not usually associated with hydrocephalus; but the evidences of rickets when present are comparatively slight, and do not precede but follow the enlargement of the skull. Further, the most marked imperfection in the ossification of the skull, as in the so-called craniotabes, is observed independent of effusion of fluid into the ventricles, while lastly the shape of the head associated with rickets, is peculiar, characteristic, and entirely different from that produced by chronic hydrocephalus.

The presence of a large quantity of fluid in the sac of the arachnoid, constituting what is called *external hydrocephalus*, may arise from several causes.

1st. The commissures of the distended brain may yield, and a portion or the whole of the fluid which it contains may escape into the cavity of the cranium. This seems to have taken place in the case of Cardinal, whose skull contained seven or eight pints of fluid, while "the brain lay at its base, with its hemispheres opened outwards like the leaves of a book."[2]

2d. An atrophied condition of the brain may exist, and fluid may be poured out to fill up the vacuum thus produced in the skull; and such cases are generally of a very hopeless kind, the defect of cerebral development being almost always the result of congenital malformation or of intra-uterine disease.

3d. A large quantity of fluid is sometimes found in the sac of the arachnoid, as the result of hemorrhage into its cavity, and of the changes subsequently undergone by the effused blood. MM. Rilliet and Barthez, who have most ably investigated the subject of hemorrhage into the arachnoid, believe that chronic hydrocephalus frequently has this origin. I have seen a few and only a few cases which I suspect were of this nature, but have never had the opportunity of confirming my suspicion by a post-mortem examination; and doubt much whether this cause of chronic hydrocephalus is not rare and exceptional.

In cases of this last kind, more may be expected both from nature's own reparative powers, and from the resources of art, than in any other form of chronic hydrocephalus. Unfortunately, their symptoms so closely resemble those of the other less hopeful varieties of the disease, that their diagnosis is attended by much difficulty and uncertainty, and

[1] Dr. Dickinson, in his lectures on Chronic Hydrocephalus, published in the Lancet for July and August, 1870.

[2] Bright's Reports, vol. i, part 1, p. 433.

must be founded, in great measure, on the previous history of the patient. "It is never congenital, but generally begins about the tenth month; that is to say, about the time when the teeth begin to appear. The head, indeed, enlarges gradually, but does not acquire so large a size as in internal hydrocephalus; while, lastly, it is always preceded by repeated convulsions, or by some other form of active cerebral disturbance, which marks the date of the occurrence of hemorrhage."[1]

The observation has often been made, that the reputed means of cure of any disease are generally numerous in a directly inverse proportion to its curability; and to this rule chronic hydrocephalus certainly forms no exception: "its remedies have been derived," as Gölis says, "from all the kingdoms of nature, and include almost every kind of surgical contrivance and pharmaceutical compound." It would be an almost endless task to attempt estimating the comparative value of them all; and I think it more useful to direct your attention to a few points of real importance.

First of all, I would have you bear in mind that there are some cases in which you can do no permanent good, but in which treatment must fail, not because it is improper, but because the malady does not admit of cure. Such cases are those in which the accumulation of fluid within the brain is associated with extensive congenital disease, or malformation of the organ. If aware of its existence, our treatment would, of course, be simply palliative, and our efforts would be limited to securing euthanasia, since we could not hope to avert death. We should suspect the affection to be incurable, if, though the head were large, and its ossification very imperfect, the forehead were low and shelving; if a considerable degree of paralysis were present, if convulsions occurred daily and causelessly, and especially if these or other indications of serious cerebral disorder had existed almost from birth. Unfortunately, these hopeless cases are by no means invariably characterized by peculiar symptoms, and the amount of functional disturbance often affords but a very incorrect index to the extent of organic lesion: your prognosis, therefore, must always be most guarded, and even when you see every reason to expect success, you must yet be prepared for failure.

On the other hand, you must not regard a case as hopeless, and abstain from remedial measures, merely on account of the head having been larger than natural at birth, or its ossification having been less advanced than usual, since we have evidence of perfect recovery from chronic hydrocephalus in cases where many circumstances had appeared to indicate that the disease was congenital. The state of the cerebral functions must influence your prognosis as much as the size of the head, or even more.

In either form of chronic hydrocephalus, the success of treatment must depend, to a great degree, upon its being adopted early, but in no stage of the disease can good be expected from violent remedies; rough measures would be likely to destroy the patient rather than the malady. I tried for many years the plan of treatment suggested by Gölis of

[1] Legendre, Recherches Anatomo-pathologiques, p. 185. See also Rilliet et Barthez, op. cit., 2d ed., vol. ii, p. 259.

Vienna, consisting in the inunction of mercurial ointment into the head, which was to be covered with a woollen cap, in the constant administration of small doses of calomel, and the occasional employment of counter-irritation. The details of this plan were, however, irksome to carry out and the results which I obtained were not remarkable. I am now therefore accustomed instead of following any specific course to employ salines, with diuretics, and small doses of the bichloride of mercury; with cold or tepid applications to the head whenever the symptoms present any degree of activity, and to give small doses of the iodide of potassium, and the syrup of iodide of iron with cod-liver oil when the state is one of cachexia rather than of active cerebral disorder; and I think I have effected at least as much by these means as by any other.

The observation that in some cases where the spontaneous cure of chronic hydrocephalus takes place, the ossification of the head, previously so imperfect, makes rapid advances, and the bones become early united, led Mr. Barnard,[1] of Bath, to imitate nature's processes, and to bandage the head so as to prevent its yielding to the accumulating fluid. He has related several cases of the successful adoption of this practice, though, like many other persons, he rides his hobby rather too hard, and advocates his mechanical method to the exclusion of all other treatment. It is, however, a valuable adjunct to other treatment in some cases. Unless you apply it well, it will be of little service, and the plasters by which the compression is exerted will come off. You cannot do better than follow M. Trousseau's rules for their application.[2] He uses strips of diachylon plaster about one-third of an inch broad; and applies them—1st, from each mastoid process to the outer part of the orbit of the opposite side; 2d, from the hair at the back of the neck along the longitudinal suture to the root of the nose; 3d, across the whole head, in such a manner that the different strips shall cross each other at the vertex; 4th, a strip is cut long enough to go thrice round the head. Its first turn passes over the eyebrows, above the ears, and a little below the occipital protuberance, so that the ends of all the other strips shall project about one-fourth of an inch below the circular strip. These ends are next to be doubled up on the circular strip, and its remaining two turns are then to be passed over them just in the same direction as the first turn. By these means you secure a firm, and equal, and very powerful pressure on the head. You must watch the results of this proceeding very carefully, and loosen the plasters if symptoms of compression appear, since it once happened to M. Trousseau, from neglect of this precaution, that the fluid acted on the base of the skull, detaching the ethmoid bone from its connections, and thus occasioned the infant's death. The pressure of a broad elastic band around the head, as I have seen it applied by my colleague, Dr. Dickinson, is a safer proceeding, and is more readily manageable than is the use of plaster. Both act on the same principle as tight bandaging in cases of ovarian dropsy. The pressure is in neither instance curative, it merely retards the outpouring of the fluid, but with this special advantage in the case of chronic hydrocephalus, that time brings with

[1] Cases of Chronic Hydrocephalus, &c., by J. H. Barnard, 8vo., London, 1839.
[2] Journal de Medecine, April, 1843.

it increased ossification of the skull, and resistance to the effusion similar to, but more efficient than, the temporary obstacle which the bandage furnished.

You will naturally inquire whether pressure is applicable to every case, and if not, when it should be employed? I regret that I cannot answer these inquiries so satisfactorily as I could wish. It is my belief, however, that cases of external hydrocephalus, which have succeeded to previous hemorrhage into the arachnoid, will be found better adapted than any others to treatment by mechanical means; while I am quite sure, from actual experience, that when there is any appearance of *active* cerebral disease, pressure will not do good.

Puncture of the cranium, and the evacuation of the fluid, is another proceeding which has been ocasionally resorted to from a very early period in the history of medicine, and which is even at the present day strongly advocated by some writers; not merely as a palliative measure, or as an adjunct to other remedies, but as a means of effecting the radical cure of the disease. Opinion, however, is much divided as to the propriety of this practice, the statistics of which certainly do not yield any very encouraging results. Fifty-six cases, the particulars of which I published many years ago,[1] as I found them recorded in various publications, yielded a proportion of fifteen alleged recoveries; but on subjecting these cases to a rigid analysis, it appeared that in only four of this number were the particulars recorded with sufficient accuracy, or had the interval since the performance of the operation been long enough to warrant our admitting them as permanent cures. The very unfavorable conclusions which I then expressed with reference to this operation were afterwards criticized by M. Durand-Fardel,[2] a gentleman whose opinion on any question connected with cerebral disease is entitled to very great weight. He observed, that while it is admitted that in a few cases puncture of the cranium has been followed by complete and permanent cure, its failure on other occasions was often manifestly due to the existence of utterly incurable malformation of the brain; while in many instances, though the operation failed to effect a cure, yet the very frequency with which it was repeated proved that in itself it is not usually attended with any considerable danger. Since, then, it may do good—since, if it should fail, its failure is often due to causes which no remedy could remove—since, even if it should do no good, yet in the majority of instances it will do no harm, while if left to itself the course of the disease is almost invariably to a fatal result, he advocates its performance in cases of chronic hydrocephalus. Though I cannot but fear that this gentleman rather underrates the amount of immediate risk attendant on the operation, yet I think that his authority ought at least to have so much weight with you as to prevent your looking upon its performance as altogether unjustifiable, and the rather since there is good reason for believing that the accumulation of fluid in the ventricles is frequently the result of previous inflammation of their lining membrane, and that puncture of the cranium may therefore

[1] In the Medical Gazette, April, 1842

[2] In the Bulletin Générale de Thérapeutique, vol. xxiii, p. 190.

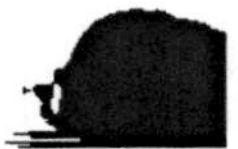

contribute to the cure of dropsy of the brain, just as tapping the abdomen does to the cure of ascites.[1]

I should regard any case as favorable for the operation, which, on the whole, there was good ground for believing to be one of external hydrocephalus, or in which the enlargement of the head had not been attended by indications of active cerebral disease. Though less promising, I should not reject the operation simply because enlargement of the head had been congenital; while I should always be more ready to operate if nutrition were well performed than if the child were emaciated. I would not, however, have you operate simply because the head is large; for it does not appear that diminution in its size has resulted from the puncture, but only arrest of its enlargement: and if the disease is at a standstill, and the cerebral functions are tolerably well performed, you would risk much, with the chance of gaining but very little. The proper situation for the puncture is the coronal suture, about an inch or an inch and a half from the anterior fontanelle. A fine trocar and canula are the best instruments; and care must be taken not merely to withdraw only a very few ounces of fluid at a time, but to keep up pressure both during the escape of the fluid as well as afterwards.

LECTURE X.

Hypertrophy of the Brain.—Usually associated with general disorder of nutrition—Symptoms and course—Seldom directly fatal—Nature of change in brain—Alterations in form of skull, and difference from chronic hydrocephalus—Treatment—Partial hypertrophy.

Atrophy of the Brain.—Case illustrative of its defective development—Wasting of the brain in protracted illness—Temporary retrocession of mental powers in children after long illness—Case of partial atrophy.

The anxiety of parents is sometimes needlessly excited in consequence of an infant's head being larger than common; and even though the child's health be good, the relations are apprehensive lest it should be affected with water on the brain. Now you must not be too ready to take up this cry, which is one often raised by nurses and ignorant persons, or to suppose that every large head is therefore unnatural; for one child may have a bigger head than another, just as it may have a bigger hand or foot. But it may be that the child's head is not only larger than natural, but that well-marked symptoms of cerebral dis-

---

[1] See, moreover, some remarks on this operation, and cases of its successful performance, in the Oesterr. Med. Jahrbücher, vol. xxii. p. 27, by Dr. Schöpf-Merei, late of Manchester, and previously the distinguished director of the Children's Hospital at Pesth.

turbance are present, and you may feel yourself compelled to adopt the opinion that the case is one of incipient chronic hydrocephalus. The subsequent history of the patient may in many respects confirm your original diagnosis, so that great will be your surprise, on examining the body after death, at not finding a drop of serum in the ventricles, although, when you opened the skull, the cerebral convolutions had appeared flattened, as if the brain were greatly distended with fluid.

Individual cases of this kind had been mentioned by medical writers at different times, but Laennec[1] was the first who drew attention to *hypertrophy of the brain* as a condition resembling chronic hydrocephalus in many of its symptoms, and liable to be mistaken for it. It has since then been frequently noticed, and I am not sure that an undue importance has not sometimes been attached to it, as though it were of much more common occurrence than you will really find it to be in practice.

I have placed upon the table a cast taken from the head of a child who was affected with hypertrophy of the brain, and whose very remarkable case is related by Sir Thomas Watson.[2] He came under the care of the late Dr. Sweatman when two years old, and his head, which had been gradually increasing from the age of six months, was then so large as by its weight to prevent the child from continuing long in the upright posture. The boy was active and lively, though thin. He had never any fit or convulsion, but occasionally seemed uneasy, and would then relieve himself by laying his head upon a chair. He had never squinted, nor was he subject to drowsiness or starting during his sleep, and his pupils contracted naturally. His appetite was good, and and all the animal functions were well performed. The case was supposed to be one of chronic hydrocephalus; but no urgent symptoms being present, active remedies were not employed. About six months afterwards the child died of inflammation of the chest, and Dr. Sweatman examined the head. It measured 12 inches from ear to ear over the vertex, 13 inches from the superciliary ridges to the occipital, and 21 inches in circumference. The anterior fontanelle, which was quite flat, measured 2¼ inches by 1½ across its opposite angles; the posterior fontanelle was completely closed, as was the frontal suture. The skull generally was increased in thickness; the morbid appearances in the membranes of the brain were quite trivial; the ventricles were empty, not dilated; the convolutions were perfectly distinct, and retained their proper rounded shape. The medullary matter, however, presented a very unusual vascularity.

It is not merely on account of the great size which the head attained that I have quoted this history, but because it affords an instance of the overgrowth of the brain unconnected with any general disorder of the processes of nutrition. Such an occurrence is very rare, for hypertrophy of the brain is usually only one manifestation of a deepseated disorder of the nutritive process, and is met with, in connection with rickets or scrofula, in the narrow lanes of a crowded city, or in the

[1] Journal de Médecine, Chirurgie, et Pharmacie, 1806, t. xi, p. 669.
[2] Lectures, 5th ed., vol. i, p. 384.

unhealthy valleys of mountainous districts, where goitre and cretinism are endemic.

The majority of cases of hypertrophy of the brain that have come under my notice in London have occurred in infants about six or eight months old. Their history had usually been, that without any definite illness, the children had lost their appetite, and grown by degrees dull and apathetic, though restless and uneasy. Notwithstanding the general apathy, this restlessness is often very considerable, though it does not show itself in cries so much as in a state of general uneasiness, and in frequent startings from sleep. Short gleams of cheerfulness occur when the children are awake, but these are usually very transient. The head seems too heavy to be borne, and even when its size is not much greater than natural it hangs backwards, or to one side, as if the muscles were too weak to support it. If placed in its cot, a child who is thus affected bores with its occiput in the pillow, while its head is almost constantly in a state of profuse perspiration. Convulsions sometimes occur without any evident cause, but threatenings of their attack are much more frequent than their actual occurrence, the child awaking suddenly with a start and a peculiar cry, like that of spasmodic croup, the surface turning livid, and the respiration becoming difficult for a few moments, and the symptoms then subsiding of their own accord. Such attacks may issue in general convulsions, which may terminate fatally, but infants thus affected do not by any means invariably die of the cerebral disorder; but, being weakly, they are often cut off by the first malady which attacks them.

If life be prolonged, it becomes more and more evident that the process of nutrition is imperfectly performed: the child loses flesh and looks out of health, and enlargement of the wrists and ankles shows the connection between this disease and rickets—a connection which becomes more evident in the second and third years of the child's life. When the child survives infancy, or when, as occasionally happens, the symptoms of hypertrophy of the brain do not come on until dentition has been in a great measure accomplished, convulsions are of very rare occurrence. Complaints of headache, however, are frequent and severe; and, though drowsy in the daytime, the child generally rests ill at night, and often awakes crying and alarmed. Besides the symptoms, too, the child has occasional attacks of feverishness, with great increase of the headache and giddiness, which last for a few hours or a day, and then subside of their own accord, while it grows by degrees more and more dull and listless, and its mental powers become obviously impaired.

It happens, in some cases, that as the child grows older, these symptoms become less and less severe; the health improves, the rickety deformity of the limbs gradually disappears, and the infant who had excited so much solicitude, becomes at length a healthy child. There is a termination in complete idiocy, which I have never seen in this country, but some years ago I observed some instances of it in the Hospital for Cretins, which then existed near Interlachen; and I believe that the association of cretinism and idiocy with hypertrophy of the brain is by no means of unusual occurrence. Death is not often the direct result of the affection of the brain, but generally takes place owing to the supervention of some other disease. The affections, however, which prove most fatal are those which favor cerebral congestion—such as hooping-cough, or the eruptive fevers, especially scarlatina.

You must not infer that hypertrophy of the brain has existed in every instance in which the organ may appear to be large, and its convolutions somewhat flattened, although the ventricles are free from fluid. The weight and apparent size of the brain are much influenced by the quantity of blood contained within it, and it may appear too large for the skull simply because the vessels are over full.[1] In true hypertrophy, on the contrary, the brain is generally pale and anæmic, unless death should chance to have taken place as the result of an attack of cerebral congestion. Neither, indeed, is the process one of mere increased growth, but the nutrition of the organ is modified in character as well as increased in activity. The gray matter of the brain is but little involved in it, and, with the exception of its color being somewhat paler than natural, it shows scarcely any alteration. The white matter, on the contrary, is both paler and firmer than in a state of health; and Professor Rokitansky[2] states, as the result of many microscopical examinations, that its augmented bulk is not produced either by the development of new nervous fibrils, or by the enlargement of those already existing, but by an increase in the intermediate granular matter, most probably due to an albuminoid infiltration of that structure.[3] These changes, too, do not affect indifferently all parts of the brain, but are confined to the hemispheres, and do not implicate either the base of the organ or the cerebellum.

Chronic hydrocephalus is the only affection with which hypertrophy of the brain is liable to be confounded: the diagnosis between the two affections is often by no means easy, though it is of much importance with reference both to our prognosis and our treatment, for we should have more hope of the recovery of a child whose brain is merely hypertrophied than of one whose brain is distended with fluid, while the means by which we should endeavor to effect a cure would differ widely in the two cases. The history of the patient would afford some help towards determining this question; for the symptoms of chronic hydrocephalus generally come on earlier, and soon grow much more serious, than those of hypertrophy of the brain, and the cerebral disturbance is throughout much more marked in cases of the former than in those of the latter kind. The form and size of the head, too, present peculiarities by which you may often be enabled to distinguish between the two conditions. Both diseases are attended by enlargement of the head, and in both the ossification of the skull is very tardy, but the head does not attain so large a size in hypertrophy of the brain as in chronic hydrocephalus, neither are the fontanelles and sutures so widely open. The skull, likewise, presents some peculiarities in form, which are so remarkable as to have attracted the attention of several observ-

[1] See Mauthner's elaborate tables of the weight of the brain in various circumstances, lib. cit., sect. v.

[2] Lib. cit., 3d ed., Vienna, 1856, vol. ii, p. 430.

[3] See Jenner's valuable Lectures on Rickets, Lect. III, in Med. Times, April 28, 1860, p. 415.

ers. The head not merely shows no tendency to assume the rounded form characteristic of chronic hydrocephalus, but its enlargement is first apparent at the occiput, and the bulging of the hind head continues throughout especially striking. The forehead may, in the course of time, become prominent and overhanging, but the eye remains deep sunk in its socket, for no change takes place in the direction of the orbitar plates such as is produced by the pressure of fluid within the brain, and which gives to the eye that unnatural prominence, and that peculiar downward direction, so striking in cases of chronic hydrocephalus. In hydrocephalus the anterior fontanelle is tense and prominent, owing to the pressure of the fluid within, but when the brain is hypertrophied there is no prominence, but an actual depression in this situation. I have more than once observed this condition in a very remarkable degree, the depression not being limited to the anterior fontanelle, but being observable at all the sutures; and you may notice something of the kind in this cast.

When hypertrophy of the brain occurs in the adult, the symptoms that arise are in great measure due to the compression which the organ undergoes from its bony case being too small to contain it. These symptoms are of course obscure, while, even if the nature of the affection could be recognized, its cure must be hopeless. In the infant, however, and the child whose head is incompletely ossified, the immediate consequences of the evil are far less serious, while some benefit may be expected from the judicious employment of *treatment*, since over-development of the brain in childhood is almost always associated with general disorder of the processes of growth and nutrition. We are not, indeed, acquainted with any means by which we can directly check the morbid increase of the brain, but all our efforts should be turned towards improving the general health, while we interfere directly with the cerebral symptoms only in so far as their urgency may render it absolutely necessary. The child, therefore, must not be dosed with calomel merely because its head is affected, though the deficient secretion of bile may often render the employment of small doses of mercurials necessary. Similar restrictions would apply to depletion, for we have seen that the hypertrophied brain is characterized by a want of blood rather than by its superabundance; but, nevertheless, occasional attacks of cerebral congestion may render local depletion necessary, and the exacerbations of headache, with vertigo and fever, will, if severe, be often benefited by its employment. At one time I tried counter-irritation by means of the tartar-emetic ointment rubbed into the back of the neck, with apparent relief to the head symptoms, in the case of children who were suffering from the indications of hypertrophy of the brain, but the ointment is by no means manageable, and the sores which it produces are often very distressing. I have therefore for some years entirely discontinued its use, and content myself in all cases with the application of blisters; or with the employment of the blistering fluid, which from the rapidity of its action is far preferable when one's patients are children. In young infants, one of our first efforts must be to relieve the brain from the constant irritation to which it is exposed when the child is in the recumbent posture, and the head rests on the yielding and imperfectly ossified occiput. For this purpose we cannot do better than follow the suggestion of a German physician, Dr. Elsässer,[1] and have a small horsehair cushion prepared for the child's head to rest on, a piece being cut out of it large enough to receive the occiput. In cases both of hypertrophy of the brain and of chronic hydrocephalus, I have seen the adoption of this simple contrivance followed by almost immediate cessation of the rotatory movement of the head, and by quiet sleep in its cot, to which perhaps for weeks before the child had been a stranger.

It is not desirable that a child who suffers from this affection should sleep entirely without covering to the head. The profuse perspiration of the head is more effectually checked by a thin linen cap, which may be changed once or twice in the night, while at the same time the child is saved from the danger of catching cold.

While these hygienic proceedings, which have especial reference to the head, are attended to, the child should be daily sponged with salt and water, or with sea-water, if it be possible to remove it to some place on the coast, such as Brighton; or it would probably be benefited by immersion in a tan-bath, in which it should remain for several minutes.[2]

The remedies under the continued use of which I have seen the most good results are the extract of bark, from which you may pass to the preparations of iron—such as Vinum Ferri, or the ferrocitrate of quinine.[3] I have not made much trial of the iodide of potassium, since in all the cases that I have seen some more decided tonic appeared necessary. I have, however, given the syrup of the iodide of iron sometimes with advantage; and in cases where the tendency to rickets was well marked, I have observed a most decided improvement follow the use of cod-liver oil, in doses of a drachm twice a day for a child of three years old. I may just mention that, notwithstanding its nauseous taste, this medicine is usually readily taken by children, some of whom even become fond of it.

With reference to diet, it will probably be desirable, if the child is not weaned, to obtain for it a healthy wet-nurse; while, after weaning, a diet of milk, with an egg once or twice daily, will often agree better than any other food. In cases of this kind, and, indeed, in all where the digestive powers are feeble, a preponderance of farinaceous food is not desirable, while the child may with safety be allowed a little veal broth or beef tea daily, or even a little meat if it have cut some of its molar teeth.

Cases of *partial hypertrophy* of the brain are on record, in which one hemisphere alone was affected, or in which some one or more of the central parts of the brain greatly exceeded the natural size, whilst the

---

[1] Der weiche Hinterkopf, 8vo., p. 205. Stuttgart, 1843.

[2] The tan-bath, which I have employed with very marked benefit in the case of weakly and rickety children among the poor, is prepared, as directed by Dr. Elsässer, by boiling three handfuls of bruised oak bark, tied up in a linen bag, in three quarts of water for half an hour, and adding the decoction to the water of the child's bath. These baths should be applied tepid, and their use should be continued every day for several weeks

[3] See Formulæ Nos. 4 and 5, at p. 57.

rest of the organ deviated in no respect from its normal condition. An instance of the kind you see represented in this drawing of Dr. Mauthner's,[1] in which the right optic thalamus was as large as a hen's egg in a girl of three years old. In cases of this sort sometimes no symptoms are present, and the anomaly is only accidentally discovered after death; whilst in others, although there are indications of cerebral disturbance, yet they are not such as to enable us to determine the nature of the evil of which they are the expression.

There is a condition of the brain the direct opposite of that which we have been examining, in which the organ falls below the natural size, or in which *atrophy of the brain* exists. I do not refer here to those cases where the brain is imperfectly formed, the head exceedingly small, and the child idiotic from birth; but this state of microcephalus appears sometimes to come on afterwards, owing probably, as has been suggested, to premature closure of the fontanelles and sutures. Such a case I saw several years ago, when a woman brought to me her boy, who was three years old, the elder of two children of perfectly healthy parents, none of whose relatives had ever shown any sign of consumption, idiocy, or mental derangement. When born, this boy was perfectly well formed, neither did he present any peculiarity till he was six months old, when his mother began to observe that he did not look any one in the face, and that he seemed to take but little notice of anything. When eight months old, he began to have fits, which had since returned about once a week, being preceded by extreme restlessness for a day or two. The fits lasted for a quarter of an hour; they were attended by convulsive movements of both sides, and followed by drowsiness, which continued for some days. The child ate and drank, though not heartily, and he never seemed anxious for food. He did not distinguish between what was nice and what was nasty, swallowing all things with the same readiness, though deglutition appeared to be difficultly performed. He had cut all his teeth, he seemed tolerably well nourished, and his body and limbs were well formed. He was, however, quite unable to stand; he passed his urine and fæces under him without appearing to take the slightest notice of it, and he seemed destitute of every glimmering of understanding. His mother said that his head was smaller than that of her infant, which was only six months old. It measured 17 inches in circumference around the parietal protuberances, and 11 inches across the head from the centre of the meatus of one ear to the same point on the opposite side. The forehead was extremely narrow, and the head shelved upwards quite in a sugar-loaf shape. All the sutures and fontanelles were firmly ossified, but I have unfortunately omitted to record at what age they became so. I never saw this boy again, but several similar cases have since come under my notice. In all such cases the intellectual faculties are more or less impaired; the condition being sometimes one of the lowest idiocy, but I do not think that there is any invariable relation between the degree of intellectual deficiency, and the degree of smallness of the skull. The poor children who some twenty years ago were exhibited in Lon-

[1] Lib. cit., plate i, and p. 189.

don as Aztecs, furnished a remarkable illustration of the effects of training in bringing out in the case of idiots who were at the same time remarkable *microcephali* some of the lower forms of intelligence and that imitative faculty with which idiots are often singularly endowed. I have nothing more to say about such cases, for their cure is manifestly quite hopeless, and, therefore, though they may interest us as pathologists, they scarcely concern us as practical physicians.

Of much higher practical importance are those instances in which the *brain* of children *wastes during long-continued illness*. The scalp in such cases will usually be found bloodless, the fontanelles collapsed, and the process of ossification will be seen to have been unusually tardy. Fluid will be found within the sac of the arachnoid, and effused into the subjacent pia mater. The brain will be far from filling up the cavity of the skull, so that a knife may be passed in many places between it and the cranial walls. The sulci between the convolutions appear unusually deep, and fluid will be found both at the base of the brain and in the ventricles, as well as in the pia mater. The cerebral substance is pale, and its texture firmer than usual.

The important point about such cases is, that cerebral symptoms and frequently recurring convulsions may be observed in a child whose brain is nevertheless not diseased, but too feeble and too wasted to perform its functions. If, then, you find indications of cerebral disturbance come on in infants who have been exhausted and emaciated by previous illness, you must not interpose too hastily with remedies directed against a supposed disease of the brain, but bethink you whether these symptoms may not be merely the signs of the brain having become unequal to its duties from its having been imperfectly nourished; and do not, without consideration, abandon the tonic plan of treatment which you had been previously pursuing.

It is only in infants that accidents of this grave nature are likely to ensue from the imperfect nutrition of the brain consequent on protracted illness: but symptoms arise in older children, in similar circumstances, well calculated to excite the apprehension of parents. In children who have but lately learned to talk, I have sometimes known loss of speech follow a long illness, the child being too weak to talk, just for the same reason as it is too weak to walk. Occasionally, however, the child apparently regains its previous health, and yet makes no efforts to articulate, even for two or three months. In cases of this kind I have seen parents thrown into great anxiety from the fear lest the child's continued silence should be the result of the intellect having become impaired during its illness. I imagine that in many of these cases the child has forgotten during its illness much of its newly acquired knowledge, and that it is some time before it again feels equal to the mental effort of shaping its ideas into words. But usually, when it begins to make the effort, it recovers its speech rapidly; and you may therefore console the parents with this prospect.

Even a manifest retrocession of the intellectual endowments should not be regarded with too much anxiety, when it has followed some long-continued disease, for it may be the result of mere weakness; the vacant look, the unmeaning laugh, and the silly manner, gradually disappearing as the child gains strength. The brain seems to regain its lower powers, and to perform its humbler functions, before it resumes its nobler office as the organ of the mind.

Partial Atrophy, like partial hypertrophy of the brain, may occur, we know not why, and may be discovered after death, where the existence of cerebral disease had never been suspected; or we may find the explanation of a number of anomalous symptoms, which had existed during life, in a wasted condition of some portion of the organ. This state may be the result of original conformation, or it may come on as the result of disease, in which latter case the substance of the wasted portion of the brain is usually found to be much firmer than natural. We are greatly in the dark as to the nature of the process by which this change is effected; but it is thought in some cases to be the remote consequence of hemorrhage into the cerebral substance, and in others, to be induced by a slow kind of inflammation. One case of this kind has come under my own notice, which, for its rarity, I will relate to you.

The patient was a little girl, aged three years and ten months, the child of phthisical parents, but whose health, though delicate, had never been interrupted by any serious illness until she had an attack of remittent fever in the early part of the spring of 1845: she recovered from it without any bad symptom, and seemed doing pretty well for about a month, when she became sleepy and heavy, and feverish, for which symptoms she was brought to me on May 19th. After being under a mild antiphlogistic treatment for a week, she got better, and was beginning to walk about again, when she awoke one morning with her face drawn to one side—a condition, however, which did not continue. When she attempted to walk, it was noticed that she halted very much on her left leg, and that it sometimes gave way under her, so that she fell down on that side, and then turned round upon her back. She had, besides, but little power with her left hand and arm, so that she could not grasp anything firmly, nor hold it steadily. The child's bowels were at that time constipated: I purged her freely, and sent her into the country, whence she returned in the beginning of August much improved in every respect, though still limping a little with the left leg, and using her right arm in preference to the left. At the end of September I saw her again, she having then a bad impetiginous eruption on the scalp, which was treated with warm poultices and water-dressing; when, on October 6th, she began to limp with her right leg, just as she had previously done with her left; though in other respects she continued pretty well. On October 17th, the affection of the right leg was a good deal less marked; but the child now became unwilling to walk, often turning giddy, and always catching hold of something by which to steady herself. When attempting to walk she often fell down into a sitting posture; and then would sit on the floor, laughing loudly. Fits of uncontrollable laughter often came on without any cause, and the face began to assume an idiotic expression. There was occasionally slight inward strabismus of both eyes, but the pulse was undisturbed; the bowels were regular and the evacuations natural, and the child rested well at night, though her head was often rather hot. A week afterwards there was no new symptom, except that the child kept her neck quite stiff, as though she feared to move it. Her head grew hotter, and she began to have a frequent teasing cough, while her power of walking varied almost every day; she now, too, grew more restless at night. On the morning of the 27th, frequent convulsive twitches of the muscles of the face and extremities came on, and the left eye became permanently turned inwards. She had no sleep in the night; general convulsions came on at 8 A.M. on the 28th and she died convulsed two hours afterwards.

I found some deposit of tubercle in the bronchial glands, but none in the brain, where I had expected to discover it. The left hemisphere of the cerebellum, however, was fully a third smaller than the right; thus presenting an additional instance in confirmation of Schröder van der Kolk's statement[1] as to the greater frequency of unilateral atrophy on the left side of the brain; it was of extremely firm consistence, quite leathery, and on making a section of it, its surface presented a rose tint. The halves of the pons and medulla oblongata were of equal size, as were the two hemispheres of the cerebrum. It was evident, too, that this condition was not congenital, since the two halves of the skull were of equal size, and the elevations and depressions in the interior of its base was precisely similar on both sides. There was a little fluid at the base of the brain, but none in the ventricles; a state of general congestion of the brain and its membranes being the only other remarkable appearances.

The spinal cord could not be examined.

There was no trace of any old effusion of blood in the substance of the cerebellum, though the symptoms that occurred in May, and the subsequent gradual improvement of the patient, are not easily explicable on any other supposition than that hemorrhage had at that time taken place into the substance of the brain. The history of the case presents another difficulty, in the circumstance that the disease was seated on the same side as that to which the symptoms had been chiefly referred. Another problem which I cannot pretend to solve is, why the paralysis should in the first instance have affected the left side, while, on the occurrence of the relapse in October, the right leg was palsied. I must therefore content myself with the bare relation of this history.

[1] In his essay on "Atrophy of the Brain," published in vol. xi of the new Sydenham Society's publications, he states that in 17 out of 29 cases, the affection was situated on the left side of the brain. In his case, however, while the left hemisphere of the cerebrum was wasted, the right half of the cerebellum and the right half of the cord were atrophied. In his case the right side of the body was atrophied; in my case, no wasting of any part of the trunk or extremities was observed, the child's inability to regulate her movements being apparently the chief result of the affection of the cerebellum. S. van der Kolk, in his elaborate essay, regards the affection not as the result of congenital malformation, but as the probable consequence of inflammatory action, occurring sometimes before birth, at other times in early infancy; and the change of consistence of the brain-substance observed in my case bears out the same opinion.

LECTURE XI.

HYDROCEPHALOID DISEASE.—Often succeeds to sympathetic disturbance of brain in course of various affections—Supervening on diarrhœa, pneumonia, and cerebral congestion—Diagnosis in each of these circumstances—Prophylaxis, and treatment.

TUBERCLE OF THE BRAIN.—Its frequency in childhood—Its anatomical characters—Symptoms—Occasionally absent—Generally very obscure—Symptoms of premonitory stage, their great diversity—Symptoms of acute stage also various—Diversities in these respects cannot be altogether explained by the morbid appearances—Occasional recovery where symptoms of cerebral tubercle have long existed—Treatment.

HYDATIDS AND CANCER of the brain.

CLOSELY connected with the state of atrophy of the brain, which we examined in the last lecture, is that condition which is induced if the organ be somewhat suddenly deprived of its usual supply of blood. Even in the adult a profuse loss of blood is followed, as you well know, by extremely severe headache, and by various other cerebral symptoms. In the child, whose brain needs for the due performance of its functions a proportionably larger quantity of blood, the symptoms that follow its excessive loss are of a corresponding gravity. Often, indeed, they present a striking similarity to those which betoken inflammation of the brain; a fact implied in the name of *hydrocephaloid disease*, by which Dr. Marshall Hall, who was among the first to call the notice of the profession to this affection, has proposed that it should be designated.

"This affection," says he, in his admirable essay on the subject,[1] "may be divided into two stages: the first, that of irritability: the second, that of torpor. In the former there seems to be a feeble attempt at reaction; in the latter, the powers appear to be more prostrate. These two stages resemble in many of their symptoms the first and second stages of hydrocephalus respectively.

"In the first stage the infant becomes irritable, restless, and feverish; the face flushed, the surface hot, and the pulse frequent; there is an undue sensitiveness of the nerves of feeling, and the little patient starts on being touched, or from any sudden noise; there are sighing and moaning during sleep, and screaming; the bowels are flatulent and loose, and the evacuations are mucous and disordered.

"If, through an erroneous notion as to the nature of this affection, nourishment and cordials be not given, or if the diarrhœa continue, either spontaneously, or from the administration of medicine, the exhaustion which ensues is apt to lead to a very different train of

---

[1] Republished in his work On the Diseases and Derangements of the Nervous System, 8vo., chap. v, sect. iii, London, 1841. It can scarcely be necessary to refer to Dr. Gooch's paper On Symptoms in Children erroneously attributed to Congestion of the Brain, for another most graphic account of this disorder.

symptoms. The countenance becomes pale, and the cheeks cool or cold; the eyelids are half closed; the eyes are unfixed, and unattracted by any object placed before them, the pupils unmoved on the approach of light; the breathing, from being quick, becomes irregular, and affected by sighs: the voice becomes husky; and there is sometimes a husky teasing cough; and eventually, if the strength of the little patient continue to decline, there is a crepitus or rattling in the breathing. The evacuations are usually green; the feet are apt to be cold."

In early infancy *symptoms* of this kind sometimes succeed to premature weaning, especially if that is followed by an unsuitable diet; but afterwards they are generally induced by some definite attack of illness, either exhausting in itself, or for the cure of which active measures had been necessary. It is important too to bear in mind that they are not equally apt to come on in the course of all diseases, but that those in the early stages of which considerable cerebral irritation has existed, are much more likely to assume the characters of this spurious hydrocephalus when the bodily powers are exhausted.

There is no disorder in which the two conditions of considerable sympathetic disturbance of the brain, coupled with rapid exhaustion of the vital powers, are so completely fulfilled, as in infantile diarrhœa, and in no other affection do we meet with such frequent or such well-marked instances of the supervention of the hydrocephaloid disease.

Some time since a previously healthy boy, aged 18 months, was brought to me suffering from vomiting and diarrhœa, which had existed for three days. After treatment had been continued for two days the purging ceased, but the child seemed to have a distaste for all nourishment, and refused both milk and arrowroot, and the mother made but few attempts to overcome this repugnance; so that for twenty-four hours the child took hardly anything except water and barley-water, and those in small quantities. On the afternoon of the sixth day the child became faint, and seemed so feeble during the night that the mother became much alarmed, and came again to me on the morning of the seventh day. The child's face was then sunken and very anxious; it lay as if dozing, with half-closed eyes, breathing hurriedly; suddenly waking up from time to time in a state of alarm and restlessness, and then in a few moments subsiding into its former condition. The skin was dry but cool, the extremities were almost cold, the lips were dry and parched, and some sordes had collected about the teeth; the tongue was dry, red, and glazed, and coated in the centre and towards the root with yellowish fur. The pulse was extremely feeble. There was very great thirst. The bowels had not acted for twelve hours.

I ordered the child a tablespoonful of equal parts of milk and barley-water every half hour, with the addition of fifteen drops of brandy every hour, and directed that some strong veal broth should be prepared and given every two hours. At the same time, a draught containing ten grains of aromatic confection, half a drachm of the compound tincture of bark, and six drops of sal-volatile, was given every three hours, and a grain of Dover's powder was directed to be taken at bedtime.

Within six hours after the commencement of this treatment the child began to improve; it slept tolerably well in the night, and the next day was lying tranquilly in bed, looking about and smiling cheerfully; the extremities were warmer, and the skin had lost its harshness; the tongue was no longer dry, and the pulse had increased in power. The stimulants were gradually withdrawn; no further bad symptoms came on, and the child was soon convalescent.

It is of great importance rightly to interpret the meaning of the symptoms which attend the first stage of this affection, and to discriminate between the cerebral disturbance of approaching exhaustion, and that which implies the existence of real mischief in the brain.

A little girl was seized with diarrhœa on August 8, which at first was severe, but soon yielded to treatment, and she was again convalescent; when, on the 15th, vomiting and purging returned with great violence, and were attended with much febrile disturbance. On the following day she was still worse in all respects, but was not brought to me again until the 17th. She then looked exceedingly ill; her face was sallow, but with a flush on each cheek, and her eyes were deeply sunk. She lay in a half-dozing state, with her eyelids half closed, and the eyeballs turned upwards, so that nothing but the sclerotica was visible; but from this condition she awoke frequently and suddenly in a state of great alarm, and looking as if she were about to have a fit of convulsions. Her skin was hot and very dry; her pulse very frequent, but not strong; and there was some subsultus of the tendons of the wrist. The abdomen was rather tympanitic; the tongue red, coated with white mucus; the thirst was great, the vomiting very frequent, and the bowels acted two or three times in the course of an hour, the evacuations having the appearance of dirty water.

The child was immediately placed in a tepid bath; an enema containing five drops of laudanum was next administered, and the abdomen was covered with a large bran poultice. The extreme irritability was almost immediately relieved by the warm bath, and still further soothed by the enema. The bowels ceased to act so frequently, and the stomach began to bear small quantities of barley-water and other drinks, which were given cold. In a few hours the imminent danger had passed away, and the child recovered in the course of a few days.

If, in a case of this kind, you fall into the error of regarding the cerebral symptoms as the signs of active disease, and withhold the Dover's powder, or the opiate enema that might have checked the diarrhœa and soothed the irritability, while you apply cold lotions to the head and give the child nothing more nutritious than barley-water in small quantities, because the irritability of the stomach which results from weakness seems to you to be the indication of disease in the brain, the restlessness will before long alternate with coma, and the child will die either comatose or in convulsions.

But it is not only in the course of diarrhœa that errors of this sort may be committed. The early stages of pneumonia are often attended with so much sympathetic disturbance of the brain, as to throw the other symptoms into the background. The child vomits, it refers all its suffering to its head, and possibly has an attack of convulsions almost at the outset. You not unnaturally assume the case to be one of cerebral congestion, and treat it accordingly with free local depletion. On the next day the indications of disordered respiration are more apparent; you think your former diagnosis was incorrect, and probably apply more leeches to the chest to combat the pneumonia you had overlooked. The urgency of the symptoms may be relieved by these means, or, if that is not the case, still the reaction will diminish with the diminished power, and the child for a short time seems to suffer less. But soon the restlessness of exhaustion comes on, and then follow the soporose condition and the apparent coma: you condemn yourself for having overlooked the cerebral mischief, of which you fancy you now have most convincing proof: you renew your antiphlogistic measures, to arrest, if it be not too late, this imaginary hydrocephalus, and your patient dies.

Something of the same kind too may happen in cases where the brain has really been congested, and where the depletion, which you practiced somewhat too freely, was in reality indicated, though to a smaller amount. The restlessness and heat of head may have been diminished by your treatment, and the bowels may have been relieved by the purgatives you administered. In a few hours, however, restlessness returns, though not to so great a degree as before, the child moans sadly when awake, and this suffering state alternates with a drowsy condition, while the stomach, irritable before, now rejects everything almost as soon as swallowed, though the child still seems eager for drink. The previous arrest of very similar symptoms, though but for a few hours, by active treatment, seems to you to indicate the propriety of continuing the same plan, but, nevertheless, the drowsiness deepens into coma, and the child dies, of hydrocephalus, as you suppose—in reality of the *nimia diligentia medici*.

"Forewarned, forearmed," says the old proverb. When head-symptoms come on in the infant, do not judge of their import simply from the present condition of the child, but ascertain its previous history. Learn whether any other members of the family have had hydrocephalus or have been consumptive. Inquire whether this infant has thriven at the breast, or whether it has for some time been drooping; if already weaned, ascertain on what it is now fed, whether signs of declining health soon followed on the change of diet, while it throve so long as it was suckled. Ask what signs of disorder of the bowels there have been, and observe at what times the vomiting comes on; whether only after sucking or taking food, or whether efforts to vomit occur when the stomach is quite empty.

In a case where the symptoms of cerebral disturbance, and those of disordered respiration, come on almost at the same time in a previously healthy child, and so alternate with each other as to render your diagnosis difficult, you will do well to remember that pneumonia often sets in with much sympathetic disorder of the nervous system, and that the disease is much more likely to be seated in the lungs than in the brain. In most cases auscultation will enable you to decide the question, and if you once accustom yourselves to listen to a child's chest as invariably as you would look at its tongue or count its pulse, you will but seldom have to reproach yourselves for the uncertain diagnosis and the vacillating treatment into which, in cases of this description, you will otherwise be too often betrayed. The use of the thermometer too ought to keep you from much of the risk of error to which in former times you would have been exposed. It may be laid down as a rule almost without exception that when in any acute febrile affection of infancy or childhood the thermometer rises within the first two days to 104° ; and remains at that height, not for a few hours only but for twenty-four hours or more, you have to do with inflammation of the lungs and not with any form of cerebral inflammation.

In a child suffering from diarrhœa, you will be prepared to meet with sympathetic disturbance of the brain, and will not allow the occurrence of its symptoms to deter you from adopting the treatment which the diarrhœa requires. If doubt cross your mind as to their signification, and you fear lest mishief be really going on in the brain, it will usually suffice to watch the symptoms closely, in order to detect a want of correspondence between them, which would not exist if true cerebral disease were present. Attention to this point will guard you from error during the stage of excitement, as well as in that of exhaustion and stupor, which simulates the last stage of hydrocephalus.

In no circumstances are mistakes more easily committed, and never are their results more mischievous, than when real congestion of the brain has been somewhat overtreated, and the consequent symptoms of exhaustion are supposed to be those of advancing disease. In such a case, however, it will usually be observed that great faintness had been induced by the first depletion, and that the quiet which succeeded it was that of exhaustion as much as of mitigated suffering. If so, the returning restlessness will probably be the index of the feeble power of the brain, no longer adequate to the performance of its wonted functions, rather than the evidence of active disease of the organ. Nor will the history be the only safeguard from error, but the fontanelle sunk below the level of the cranial bones, instead of being tense and pulsating, the cool surface, and the pulse presenting no other characters than those of frequency and feebleness, will all point to the real nature of the case. You do not need to be told that to deplete in such circumstances would be to destroy your patient—that food is needed, not physic. The sunken powers of life are to be rallied, and as their strength returns, the functions of the brain will again go on harmoniously.

Although the diagnosis of this affection is sometimes attended with difficulty, the *rules for its prevention and cure* are happily very simple. Bearing in mind the possible supervention of the hydrocephaloid disease, you would never keep an infant from the breast, nor put a young child on a spare diet for several days without most absolute necessity ; you would pay especial attention to its food, if the disease from which it suffers be, like diarrhœa, such as interferes directly with its nutrition. Again, you would not trust depletion of a young child, especially if suffering from head affection, to a nurse, but would yourselves exercise the supervision of it. And, lastly, in the treatment of every disease, you would at once suspend the antiphlogistic measures that you had previously been adopting, and resort to the use of stimulants and tonics so soon as any of the symptoms that we have been examining make their appearance.

The state of general restlessness and irritability that attends the early stages of exhaustion is often greatly soothed by the tepid bath, continued for not more than five minutes, for fear of still further depressing the infant's powers. While you secure a free access of air too, you must be extremely cautious to maintain the room at a sufficient temperature; for the power of generating heat is diminished in a very remarkable degree in young animals who from any cause are insufficiently nourished. The irritability of the stomach is best overcome by giving nourishment in extremely small quantities—as a dessert-spoonful of asses' milk for an infant, or of veal tea for an older child, given by little and little every half hour. If the symptoms have succeeded to weaning, a healthy wet-nurse should, if possible, be at once obtained; but as the effort to suck seems sometimes to exhaust the child, and probably thereby to favor vomiting, it is sometimes better at first to give the nurse's milk by a teaspoon. If the exhaustion is very great, and a state analogous to coma is impending, a hot mustard bath is sometimes serviceable in rousing the child; while, at the same time, a few drops of sal-volatile, or of brandy, may be given every few hours. It is desirable, however, to suspend the use of the more powerful direct stimulants so soon as it can safely be done, though a nutritious diet will be necessary for some time. Tonic medicines, likewise, are often of much service, few of which are preferable to the extract of bark, which, dissolved in carraway-water, mixed with a few drops of the tincture, and well sweetened, will be taken very readily by most children. The addition of a little milk to the medicine when taken still further covers any unpleasant taste.[1]

Those cases in which the brain becomes the seat of various *morbid growths* still remain for us to consider, before we pass to the study of affections of the spinal cord.

In the child, as in the adult, the brain may become the seat of hydatid cysts, or of cancerous tumors, or of *tubercular deposits;* but I should not detain you long with their study, if it were not that the last of these three morbid conditions, though exceedingly rare in the adult, is by no means unusual in the child. Thus, while M. Louis met with only a single case in which the brain contained tubercle out of 117 examinations of adults who had died of phthisis; MM. Rilliet and Barthez discovered tubercle in the brain of 37 out of 312 children, between the ages of 1 and 15, in some organ or other of whose body this morbid deposit existed. You will remember that I am not now speaking of cases where tubercle is present merely in the membranes of the brain, producing that granular appearance to which I called your attention when treating of tubercular meningitis; but my remarks refer to separate deposits of tubercular matter in the substance of the brain. These deposits are for the most part distincly circumscribed, of a rounded form, and varying in dimensions from the size of a millet-

[1] See Formula No. 4, at p. 57.

seed to that of a split-pea, or of a bean, or even larger. The largest mass that I ever met with in the brain of a child was almost as big as a hen's egg, but they have been seen much larger. Sometimes there is but a single deposit in the brain, but in the majority of cases there are three or four small deposits, of the size of a millet-seed or rather larger, as well as a single mass of greater magnitude. Sometimes, though not often, the deposits of tubercle are limited to one hemisphere of the brain; but it generally happens that there is a marked preponderance of the affection on one side. The situation of these deposits varies greatly, and they have been found in all parts of the brain, both on its surface and in its interior. The smaller deposits are, I think, most frequently observed on the convexity of the brain, and they are then found closely adherent to the pia mater, to which they remain attached if that membrane is stripped off. They seem, however, to have some connection with the cerebral substance besides mere juxtaposition, since a thin investment of it clings to them, and the place where they were situated may be seen after their removal to be quite uneven. Even when situated at the base of the brain, or in the cerebellum, they often retain this relation to the pia mater; and those larger masses, which generally appear more deeply seated, will often be found, if the convolutions are unfolded, to have been in reality not far removed from the surface. Now and then a distinct, firm, fibrous capsule may be found investing the deposit; but this is oftener absent, or at any rate so delicate as not to be clearly perceptible. I have never seen these deposits presenting throughout the characters of the gray semi-transparent tubercle frequently noticed in the lungs, but once I found the exterior of a small deposit in this stage, while its central part had undergone the transformation into the ordinary friable yellow tuberculous matter—a condition which Rokitansky has also occasionally met with. This appearance too points to the process by which tubercular deposits in the brain increase in size. Fresh deposits of miliary tubercle take place in the layer of connective tissue which is usually found surrounding the mass, while at the same time caseous degeneration takes place in its central or first-formed portion. It is in accordance with this that when softening takes place in cerebral tubercles it begins, just as in deposits of the same kind elsewhere, in the centre, and gradually extends towards the periphery—a condition which I have observed in 5 out of 24 cases. The brain around the softened deposits is almost always of a rose tint and more or less softened, though this alteration seldom extends for a distance of more than two or three lines; and once I observed the cerebral substance perfectly unchanged around a small tubercle, in which the process of softening was already considerably advanced. As a general rule, the brain around deposits of crude tubercle still retains its natural characters; but to this I have seen one exception.

If death usually occurs before the process of softening has taken place in the tubercular deposits, still rarer is it for life to be so prolonged as to give opportunity for the occurrence of that cretaceous transformation by which the disease in other organs is sometimes arrested. MM. Rilliet and Barthez have observed it only twice out of 37 cases of cerebral tubercle; and but one instance of it has come under my notice, in a boy 3½ years old, in whom but one deposit existed, of the size of a large pea, situated in the left hemisphere of the cerebellum. The change was in this instance incomplete, when death took place from tubercular meningitis, succeeding to the sudden cessation of otorrhœa. Had the child lived, however, it is probable that the disease would have been altogether cured, for no tubercles were present in any other organ of the body, with the exception of the bronchial glands; and in them the same curative process was going on.

Cerebral tubercle does not invariably affect the rounded form, but it occasionally extends as a patch, half an inch or more in length, by two or three lines in breadth, immediately beneath the pia mater, and not reaching above one or two lines deep into the cerebral substance, which is usually slightly softened beneath it. Now and then, too, the deposit takes place not in distinct and isolated masses, but in the form of infiltration into the tissue of the brain, which, in this situation, is of a rose-red color, and extremely soft. This condition has come twice under my notice, and was associated on both occasions with abundant tubercular deposits in almost all the viscera.

These tubercular deposits in the cerebral substance are very often, but by no means invariably, associated with that granular state of the membranes which I described to you as occurring in many cases of tubercular meningitis. Thickening of the membranes, and effusion of hyaline matter into the pia mater at the base of the brain—the evidences, in short, of meningitis—are often present, as well as abundant effusion of fluid into the ventricles, and softening of the central parts of the brain. Sometimes, however, the signs of inflammation of the membranes exist without any effusion into the ventricles; and in a few instances the ventricles contain an abundance of fluid, but no softening of the central parts of the brain exists, nor any sign of inflammation of the membranes.

I know but one instance in which tubercle was limited to the brain in childhood, and in that case there was strumous disease of the right ankle: when present in the brain it almost always exists in other viscera, and is but one of the results of that general cachexia which may show itself in any of the various forms of scrofulous or phthisical disease. At the same time there is no uniform connection between the presence of tubercle in the brain, and the existence of advanced general tuberculosis. This is a fact all the more to be borne in mind, since, unless we remember that a condition of good general nutrition of the body does not preclude the deposit of cerebral tubercle, we may run some risk of misinterpreting the symptoms which otherwise would excite our apprehension.

I am unacquainted with any special cause that renders the brain more liable to this disease in childhood, than in adult age, or even in youth. It certainly is not owing simply to the intensity of the tuberculous cachexia, and the consequently greater abundance of the morbid deposit, for I have met with many instances of far more extensive tubercular degeneration than existed in those cases where the brain had become its seat.

Cases are not yet recorded in numbers sufficient for us to determine accurately the time of the greatest liability to this affection: or whether difference of sex exerts any real influence in predisposing to it. Of my own 24 cases, 14 were male and 10 female; 5 were under 2 years of age, 3 between 2 and 3; 5 between 3 and 4; 1 between 4 and 5; 4 between 5 and 6; and of the remaining 6, one was 6½; one, 8; one, 9; and three, 10 years of age.[1]

We come now to the examination of a very difficult question,—namely, that of the *symptoms* of this affection. The difficulty arises from many sources; for sometimes the disease gives rise to no symptoms at all, and its existence is not discovered till after death: and even when symptoms are present, neither their character nor their intensity bears any invariable relation to the extent of the local mischief or its seat; while, lastly, the symptoms that usually betoken tubercle of the brain sometimes exist where no such morbid growth occupies the organ.

Cases in which no symptom whatever marks during life the presence of the morbid deposit in the brain, are very unusual, and but one instance of it has ever come under my own observation. In this case a mass of crude tubercle as large as a walnut was imbedded in the back part of the right hemisphere of the cerebellum, and adhered also to the membranes lining the base of the skull. Much less rare, though still constituting exceptions to the general rule, are the instances of complete absence of all *premonitory* indications of cerebral disorder; symptoms of disease of the brain manifesting themselves suddenly and with violence, and carrying off in the course of a few days, or perhaps even in a few hours, the child in whom tubercle has for months been developing itself. No reason can be assigned for the complete latency of the affection in some instances, or for the sudden supervention of cerebral symptoms in others after the deposit has existed for a long time without giving rise to any indications of its presence. It is true that the brain in the immediate neighborhood of the tubercular deposit does not, to the best of my knowledge, present any sign of softening in those cases which have been characterized by absence of all premonitory signs of cerebral disturbance, and that the tubercle itself always appears in the crude state. This fact at once suggests a plausible explanation of these cases, founded on the assumption that the symptoms, when observed, do not depend simply on the presence of tubercle, but rather on the changes in the surrounding brain. Such an hypothesis, however, is contradicted by the fact, that cerebral symptoms sometimes occur in cases where no perceptible disorganization of the brain has taken place either around the tubercle or elsewhere.

---

[1] The cases recorded by Dr. H. Green, in vol. xxv of the Medico-Chirurgical Transactions, by MM. Rilliet and Barthez, in vol iii of their work, and by Professor Hirsch, of Königsberg, in a dissertation De Tuberculosi Cerebri, 8vo., 1847, added to my own, made up a total of 72, which may be thus arranged:

	Male.	Female.
From 6 months to 5 years, ...	23	14
From 5 years to 10 years, ...	10	14
From 10 years to 15 years, ...	6	5
	—	—
	39	33

In most instances some kind of premonitory symptoms manifest themselves before the commencement of the child's fatal illness; but these are very variable in their character, and often very difficult of interpretation. Dr. Hennis Green, in his very valuable paper "On Tubercle of the Brain, in Children," mentions pain in the head as having been present in 17 out of 20 cases; but this symptom attends upon so many other affections, that taken by itself its diagnostic value is but small. In young children who are unable to describe their sensations, we cannot be certain of the existence of headache; but must be content to infer it from causeless fretfulness, drowsiness, or listlessness. One or other of these indications of disorder of the sensorium was present, however, as the most marked premonitory symptom, in 13 out of 18 cases in which forewarnings of mischief preceded the child's fatal illness.[1]

---

[1] In the following note I have endeavored to bring together the more important points in the history of the 21 cases of cerebral tubercle on which my remarks are founded.

There were no premonitory symptoms of head affection in 6 cases.

No.	Sex.	Age.	Previous history.	Fatal illness.	Duration.
1	M.	4 years.	Convalescent 3 weeks from measles.	Tubercular meningitis.	19 days.
2	M.	1 yr. 5 mo.	Cough for 2 months.	Fits, coma, died in fits.	6 "
3	F.	2 " 6 "	Tabes mesenterica, 4 months.	Fits, coma, died comatose.	5 "
4	F.	10 " 0 "	Constipation, debility, 2 months.	Typhoid symptoms, no fits.	9 "
5	M.	1 " 0 "	Phthisis, 5 months.	Drowsiness, fits, coma, frequent fits.	7 "
6	M.	9 " 0 "	Phthisis, tubercular peritonitis, 7 months	No symptom whatever of brain disorder. Died of tuberculosis.	7 "

More or less marked signs of cerebral disturbance existed in the remaining 16 cases, namely:

No.	Sex.	Age. yr.	Age. mo.	Premonitory symptoms.	Duration.	Fatal illness.	Duration.
1	M.	2	0	Fretfulness.	8 days.	Fit, coma.	99 hrs.
2	F.	8	8	Great drowsiness succeeding to cynanche parotidea.	6 weeks	Fits, for some hours, returned in 5 days, then frequent, drowsy in intervals, coma.	24 days.
3	F.	0	6	Dull, drowsy, suppressed eruption on scalp.	1 mo.	Deepening stupor, fit, coma.	6 "
4	M.	8	0	Drowsy, listless, feverish.	14 days.	Stupor, coma, ptosis of right eyelid, dilatation of right pupil, no fit.	1 week.
5	M.	1	9	Otorrhœa 6 weeks, pain in head, crying at night.	14 "	Vomiting followed by coma, fits, death comatose.	88 hrs.
6	F.	8	6	Otorrhœa 9 months; pain in head on its sudden cessation, and excited manner.	7 "	Several fits, furious delirium, coma.	8 days.
7	F.	6	6	Headache, sickness, constipation.	2 mo.	Supervention of acute hydrocephalus, fits.	16 days.

When headache is present it is yet but seldom that any connection can be traced between the seat of the tubercle and the situation of the pain, which is, for the most part, referred to the forehead. It is often very severe, so that during its continuance the child is entirely taken up with its suffering, and shrieks with the severity of the pain; but it

No.	Sex.	Age.		Premonitory symptoms.	Duration.	Fatal illness.	Duration.
		yr.	mo.				
8	M.	3	6	Habitual rotatory motion of head, pain in forehead, feverish.	2 mo.	Symptoms of acute hydrocephalus, fit 5 hours before death.	13 days.
9	F.	3	0	Fit, left side affected, return in 4 days, twitching of left side.	13 days.	Symptoms of acute hydrocephalus, pneumonia supervened, and caused death.	35 "
10	M.	1	11	Epileptic fits from 7th mo., drowsiness from 16th mo.	16 mo.	Slight fit, followed by coma.	24 hrs.
11	M.	2	0	Head hung to left side since measles.	4 mo.	Two fits, stupor, automatic movements of right side, death comatose.	5 days.
12	F.	3	3	Sudden twitching of right hand, arm, and leg, torticollis, paralysis of right portio dura, last two symptoms disappeared, others improved, no headache.	9 "	Head heavy 10 days, deepened into coma, death comatose from effusion of blood at base of brain.	10 "
13	F.	5	4	Fit, followed by paralysis of right side, 5 months before, and impairment of intellect; febrile attack 3 months, almost constant convulsions 6 weeks.	5 "	Increase of convulsions, deepening of coma, death comatose.	6 weeks.
14	F.	5	0	Headache after measles 4 months, ptosis of right eyelid 1 mo.	4 "	Increase of headache, convulsions 5 days before death comatose.	14 days.
15	M.	10	0	Pain at back of head, and occasional vomiting, emaciation.	6 weeks	Increase of symptoms, but death sudden in sleep. Tubercle 2½ inches in diameter in centre of cerebellum	17 "
16	F.	5	0	Fit, followed by paralysis of left side of face. Nothing more.	4 mo.	Fever, frontal headache, paralysis extending to tongue, gradual occurrence of coma.	24 "
17	M.	5	0	Headache 6 weeks, relieved by occurrence of discharge from left ear in 14 days.	6 weeks.	Cessation of discharge from ear, followed by vomiting and symptoms of tubercular meningitis. No convulsions. No paralysis.	12 "
18	M.	10	0	Paralysis of left arm	4 mo.	Fever, frontal headache, convulsions, drowsiness, death insensible after convulsions.	28 "

does not continue with this intensity for more than a few hours, and on the next day the child will be found to be no worse than usual. Vomiting in many instances attends these exacerbations of pain; and, when this is the case, the absence of any gastric disorder sufficient to account for it will lead you to suspect the presence of tubercle in the brain. In some cases, however, the headache, though severe, does not present this remarkable intensity, while there is so much permanent impairment of the general health, that an occasional attack of sickness does not surprise you. On the other hand you will meet with delicate children in whom attacks of violent headache, sometimes accompanied by vomiting, come on from very slight causes, or apparently without any cause at all, and return at irregular intervals for years together, till they gradually subside as the health becomes more robust; and cease altogether at the age of puberty or sooner. In a doubtful case, the existence of irregularity of the pulse would to some extent govern your decision; though its occurrence in cases of cerebral tubercle is not constant: while I have known children in whom every attack of gastric or intestinal disorder was accompanied by this symptom in a very marked degree. In infants, and in children under two years of age, we of course lose the evidence which is afforded by the patient's complaints of headache, and can only infer it to be present from the occasional loss of cheerfulness, and the attacks of fretfulness and crying. Sometimes too the suffering of the brain shows itself in other ways besides headache. The temper becomes wayward and passionate, or a general dulness steals over all the faculties, and the child grows quite indifferent to what is going on around it. One little boy, aged two years, whom I watched for some weeks before his death, never made any complaint of headache. He was fretful, and cried if moved, but was perfectly quiet if allowed to remain in his chair, where he would sit half dozing for hours together.

Affections of the motor system are often among the early indications of this disease, but neither are they so definite as to present anything pathognomonic of cerebral tubercle. A boy who died at three and a half years old, and in the left hemisphere of whose cerebellum there was a tubercle as large as a pea, had been subject from his earliest infancy to an almost constant and involuntary rotatory movement of the head when in the recumbent posture. And in another boy, who was two years old at death, the head had hung for four months towards the left shoulder before any other symptoms of mischief in the brain appeared: convulsions then suddenly came on, and the child died in 72 hours. Sometimes paralysis of a limb comes on gradually; or, though actual paralysis does not exist, yet the power over one side becomes greatly weakened, and the child drags one leg, or is observed invariably to use one arm in preference to the other. Convulsive movements, however, are the most frequent of the affections of the motor system, and paralysis of a limb or impaired power over it, usually succeeds to their occurrence, and but seldom takes place independently of them. Regular epileptic seizures, attended with equal affection of both sides during the fit, and followed by no impairment of power over any part, are decidedly unusual, and have only once come under my notice; but the convulsive movements generally assume one of two characters. Either they are occasional in their occurrence, attended with insensibility, though the movements are confined to one side of the body or to one limb, the same being affected on each occasion; and these attacks are usually of comparatively short duration, varying from a few minutes to a few hours; or the intellect is unimpaired, but movements like those of chorea affect one limb or one set of muscles constantly. Of this I saw a striking instance in a little girl who died from hemorrhage beneath the arachnoid at the base of the brain when 3½ years old, and in whom numerous tubercles were present in the left optic thalamus, and one in the right hemisphere of the cerebellum. Nine months before her death she was seized, when apparently in perfect health, by twitching tremulous movements of the right hand, which in 14 days extended to the arm, and in a month to the leg, so as to prevent her walking. In 2 months the head was drawn to the left shoulder, and in 4 the mouth to the left side. In 3½ months the head was held straight, and in 5 months the mouth was no longer drawn awry. The tremulous movements diminished, the child began to walk about, and continued to improve till 20 days before her death. She then grew dull, and the tremor returned. In 10 days she became comatose, and continued so, with occasional convulsions, in which for the first time both sides were affected, till she died.

This case illustrates another fact perhaps worth notice; namely, that convulsions affecting one side only are sometimes seen, although tubercle is present in both hemispheres; or in other instances both sides are affected by the convulsions, and yet the deposit is found only in one hemisphere of the brain. Lastly, it may be added, that when convulsions, whether general or partial, attended with insensibility, have once occurred, they are seldom absent for many days together, though to this there are occasional exceptions, in which a pause of many months ensues after the first convulsive seizure; the general health, indeed, being impaired, but no sign clearly indicating the special mischief that exists in the brain.

The transition from the premonitory to the acute stage sometimes takes place gradually, the convulsions becoming more and more frequent, the other cerebral symptoms more serious, and the intervals of freedom from suffering shorter; or the change takes place suddenly, and without such previous increase in the severity of the child's sufferings as to make us anticipate its approaching death; and yet we cannot always discover such differences between the morbid appearances in the two cases as suffice to explain the dissimilar course of the disease. Of the 24 fatal cases of which I have preserved a record, there was 1 in which no sign of disorder of the brain appeared at all, while in the remaining 23 the duration of the acute stage varied from 24 hours to 42 days: being under a week in 8 instances; between one and two weeks in 6; between two and three in 4; twice extending to 24 days; once to 28; once to 35 days; and in one instance convulsions were of perpetual recurrence for six weeks, when at last the child died. In five instances the acute stage was attended by the ordinary symptoms of acute hydrocephalus; once death took place from apoplexy dependent on effusion of blood at the base of the brain; one boy died in his sleep so quietly, that the nurse watching in the ward was unaware of it; once the child gradually sank into a typhoid condition, and died without any convulsion; and twice coma stole on gradually, death again being unpreceded by convulsive movements. In the remaining 13 cases, convulsions took place, though obeying no definite rule as to the frequency of their occurrence, or the intensity of the coma by which they were succeeded.

Wide as the differences are between the effects mentioned as produced by cerebral tubercle in one case from those which are observed in another, and impossible as it is completely to account for them, they are yet, perhaps, not so altogether inexplicable as at first sight they may appear. The size or position of the deposit, or the rapidity of its growth, may in one case produce pressure on the brain, occasion the effusion of fluid, and thus cause the patient's death: or the accidental congestion of the brain following the arrest of some discharge, or the healing of some eruption, or attending on some intercurrent febrile disorder, may render it sensible of the presence of the morbid deposit which it had endured quietly for weeks or months, and all the indications of serious cerebral irritation may at once become apparent. In another case softening may take place in the tubercular mass, and extending to the adjacent tissue, inflammation of the brain may be lighted up; or the deposit not being limited to the brain itself, but affecting its envelopes also, tubercular meningitis may supervene, as it often does, and destroy the patient.

These considerations may serve to explain cases where the tubercular deposit has been found external to the substance of the brain, merely pressing on it, but in no way altering its tissue. Such a case I once saw in the person of a little girl, 10 years old, who for five months had suffered from strumous disease of the knee-joint, but had never manifested any head symptom during her six weeks' stay in the Middlesex Hospital. She was taken home at the end of this time, but had not left the hospital many hours when convulsions of the right side came on, which were succeeded by coma: and this deepened, till in the course of forty-eight hours it became absolute. Convulsions occasionally returned, always affecting the right side, which from the first continued paralyzed in the intervals between their occurrence. She lay thus for eight days without any sign of amendment, and then died. There was a large quantity of clear serum in the lateral ventricles, and much escaped from the spinal canal. There was no disease of the brain, nor any important morbid appearance in the spinal cord; but there was disease about the odontoid process and its articulation with the atlas, with a collection of tubercular matter around it, forming a tumor which, situated in the mesial line, encroached somewhat on the occipital foramen, though pressing but very slightly on the cord. In the quiet of the hospital this disease had produced no symptom; the excitement of her return home kindled the spark, and destroyed the patient.

Bearing these things in mind too, we can account for the sudden death of a child, in whom a solitary tubercle in the brain had already passed into the cretaceous state, but where habitual otorrhœa had ceased suddenly; and we can understand the reason for the intermittent character which the symptoms of cerebral tubercle so frequently assume.[1]

I do not wish for one moment to exaggerate the difficulties that attend the *diagnosis* of this affection; but, at the same time, if we assume that we have to do with an incurable disease we are less likely to use efficient means of treatment than if we feel that there is still some room for hope. While, therefore, I would have you bear in mind that the symptoms which we have been passing in review, especially if associated with indications of tubercle in other organs, render the presence of tubercle in the brain in the highest degree probable, yet they do not afford absolutely certain evidence of it; and further, that the occasional observation of cerebral tubercle which has undergone the cretaceous change, shows that recovery from the disease is not absolutely impossible. Headache aggravated at intervals, and associated with occasional convulsive movements of one limb, and even with attacks of an epileptic character, may occur in children who yet after a time recover, and show by the robust health they subsequently attain to, that some cause of a less abiding nature than tubercular deposit must have given rise to the disturbance of the brain; or on the other hand, though serious cerebral disease may exist, and such as gives rise at length to a fatal result, yet it may appear after death that it was such as would have been mitigated if not cured, by appropriate treatment.

I need not remind you of the value of the ophthalmoscope in doubtful cases, a value which additional experience in its use will probably tend to increase. The appearances which it discovers are such indeed as one might beforehand expect to find; namely, a state of congestion of the optic disk, which is swollen, its outline indistinct, its surface often dotted with tiny ecchymoses, the arteries pale and diminished in size, whilst numerous veins which were before invisible may now be seen enlarged, full, tortuous, or even varicose. This appearance is seldom wanting in cerebral tumors of any size, and is almost invariably present in tumors of the cerebellum, which is, as you will recollect, the favorite seat of tubercular deposits. In doubtful cases I always avail myself of the special knowledge of some colleague expert in the use of the instrument. I advise you to learn to use it for yourselves.

There will, however, in spite of all diagnostic helps, remain cases in which suspicion does not amount to actual certainty, and at any rate we may often palliate when we cannot cure, and protract the life that we are not able to save. You must not therefore remain merely passive spectators of these symptoms; and, if you watch cases of this kind with attention, you will generally find that they afford you some clue to the *treatment* that you should follow. Either there is manifest

[1] See, with reference to the various effects of cerebral tubercle, and the different ways in which it may prove fatal, the excellent chapter on tubercle of the brain in Dietl's work, already referred to, pp. 346–356.

gastric and intestinal disorder, or there are indications of a state of general debility, or there are signs of inflammatory disease in the brain. In the first case, the regulation of the bowels and the careful management of the diet, are obviously indicated; in the second, iron may be given with advantage, and the shower-bath may be cautiously tried, and, if it do not alarm the child, it may often be continued with much benefit. In those cases where there seems to be some slow mischief in the brain, I have once or twice seen recovery take place, contrary to all my anticipations, from the employment of small doses of mercury night and morning, persevered with for many weeks. In such cases, too, counter-irritation to the back of the neck is often followed by the happiest effects. A little girl, 14 months old, was some time since under my care for the frequent recurrence of convulsive attacks of a very anomalous character. So long as a discharge was kept up from her neck by the tartar-emetic ointment, the fits did not occur; but if the discharge ceased for two or three days, they were sure to return.

These are the principles by which your conduct must be governed; but you will find that each case will present some special peculiarity, and will need to be studied and treated for itself.

Tumors of other kinds may exist in the brain in childhood, though they appear to be more frequent in the middle-aged or the old.[1] I once saw a case in which *hydatids* had formed in the substance of the brain in a girl of seven years old; once also I saw *cancer* affecting the brain and its membranes in a boy two and a half years old, and recently a girl aged 8 years died in the Children's Hospital in whom a large mass of *glioma* in the cerebellum furnished an explanation of various signs of brain disease which had succeeded to a fall on the back of the head eight months before her death. But, though such occurrences are interesting from their rarity, I do not know any circumstance, except the absence of the signs of tubercular disease in the patient, by which you could determine during life that certain cerebral symptoms arose from hydatids, or cancer of the brain, and not from tubercle in that organ.[2]

---

[1] Of the 84 cases of non-tuberculous tumors in the brain, which form the basis of Friedreich's elaborate Beiträge zur Lehre von den Geschwülsten innerhalb der Schädelhöhle, 8vo., Würzburg, 1853, none occurred in children under 10 years old; and only 4 in young persons between the ages of 10 and 20.

[2] Dr. Charlton Bastian's excellent article on the morbid anatomy of adventitious products in the brain, at p. 499 of vol. ii of Reynolds's System of Medicine, 2d ed., 1872, ought not to pass unnoticed.

LECTURE XII.

Diseases of the Spinal Cord.—Their study rendered more difficult by the tender age of children.

Irritation and Congestion of the cord.

Inflammation of the Membranes of the Cord.—Not common as a sporadic affection—Illustrative cases—**Inflammation of the Substance** of the Cord—Extremely rare in its acute form—In its chronic form gives rise to symptoms similar to those which occur when bones of the spine are diseased—Cases.

Trismus.—Extremely rare in this country.—Symptoms—Post-mortem appearances—Causes of the disease—Influence of vitiated air—Treatment almost hopeless.

At the commencement of these Lectures I called your attention to the predominance of the spinal over the cerebral part of the nervous system, as constituting one of the grand characteristics of early life. Since then, our daily course of inquiry has brought before us numerous confirmations of this truth, and has shown us how slight a disturbance of the functions of the brain may suffice to destroy the harmony of those which belong to the spinal cord.

To-day we pass from the consideration of those cases in which the brain is the original seat of disorder, and the spinal cord suffers only secondarily, to the study of others, where that organ is primarily affected. I need not remind you how much obscurity hangs over the ailments of the spinal cord at all periods of life; but in the young subject this is not a little increased by the difficulty that attends the observation of some of those symptoms which would be obvious enough in the adult. Thus, for instance, while impairment or loss of the locomotive power in the grown person could hardly escape our notice for a moment, it might fail to attract much attention in a young child, who often totters in his gait, or even becomes unable to walk, if from any cause his health should fail. Or, again, the impaired sensation, or the vague pains in the limbs, which the adult would be sure to tell us of, would be but ill described by a child, even though it had long been able to talk, while terror might cause it to cry if any attempt was made to examine its back, and might thus prevent our ascertaining the presence or absence of tenderness of the spine. These are difficulties, however, which patience and tact will overcome; for not only the diseases of the spinal cord, but the symptoms by which they manifest themselves, are much the same at all ages, the chief difference being that in the one case they strike the eye even of the careless, while in the other, careful observation is necessary for their detection.

Irritation of the cord, however produced, gives rise in the child, as well as in the adult, to impairment of the motor power. A little boy, between two and three years old, remarkably strong and healthy, was observed, without any obvious cause, to fail in his general health, and at the same time to totter in his gait, to become indisposed to move, and, at last, almost entirely to cease walking; and this impairment of his power of walking was quite out of all proportion to the signs of ill health by which it was attended. After watching him for a time, it was discovered that the child had become addicted to the practice of masturbation. This was put a stop to, and he soon regained his health; and with it his power of walking.

In this instance the cause of the irritation of the cord, and of the consequent impairment of its functions, was obvious enough, but cases now and then occur in which symptoms of disorder of the spinal cord manifest themselves without our being able to discover on what they depend. Such cases, too, are all the more important from the circumstance that the symptoms which attend them simulate serious disease, and are likely to lead us into the unguarded expression of a very unfavorable prognosis as to their issue.

On the 30th of December, now many years ago, I saw a delicate boy, between 4 and 5 years old, who had been drooping in health, though without any definite symptom, for a week or two; but had complained of stiff neck for the first time on the previous Christmas Day. This ailment, however, had disappeared and recurred more than once between then and the 28th; since which last date it had been constant, though not always the same in degree, being less marked in the morning, more so towards night. The child looked out of health, and seemed very languid; he moved very cautiously, as if afraid of the slightest jar; his shoulders being raised, his head thrown rather back, and kept most carefully motionless; while he complained bitterly of any attempt to bend his neck, and said that pressure on the upper part of the cervical spine occasioned him much pain. The boy's appearance and manner were precisely those of a patient suffering from disease of the cervical vertebræ; and a most experienced surgeon, who saw the case with me, expressed himself as very apprehensive that the case was a bad one, though whether the disease was in the spinal cord or in the vertebræ he considered to be uncertain. I certainly took a most unfavorable view of the affection; and was much surprised to learn subsequently that after the application of four leeches to the back of the neck, the child went to sleep, slept during the night, and awoke the next morning with the most complete power over the muscles of the neck, showing no pain in moving his head, complaining of no tenderness of the spine, nor did any such symptoms manifest themselves at any subsequent period.

I have since met with several cases of a somewhat similar kind, which I believe to be of rheumatic origin. The symptoms come on too rapidly to be due to disease of the cervical vertebræ, while they are not sufficiently severe to be attributed to inflammation of the spinal cord, or of its membranes. Headache is not present, nor any distinct evidence of cerebral disturbance. Rest in bed, attention to the bowels, diaphoretic medicines, warm applications, and stimulating liniments to the back of the neck, of which there is none better than the Linimentum Belladonnæ, have sometimes removed in a couple of days symptoms that seemed most threatening.

In such cases, as in many others, the results of treatment yield a most important help towards the formation of a correct diagnosis.

Whether in the instance above related the affection was a rheumatic one I do not know, or whether there was some unusual congestion of the vessels of the cord, which the local depletion at once removed, and thus cured the patient. That such a condition existed in the following instance is still more likely, for here there was a local injury amply sufficient to produce it.

In May, 1845, a little girl, four years old, was brought to me by her mother, who said that ten days before, the child had had a fall on her back, while left in the charge of a servant; that on the following morning she was unable to stand or move, unless supported; and that she had ever since continued in the same condition. Her appearance was rather anxious, her face was slightly flushed, skin warm and dry, tongue slightly furred, pulse frequent, and with power. If placed on her feet, she clung hold of her mother, sank down into a stooping, half-squatting posture, and immediately began to cry. She could walk if firmly supported, but hurriedly and unsteadily, stepping on her toes, her legs moving in a semicircle with her toes turned inwards, and one foot being put down just in front of the other. On examining the spine, the integuments from the tenth to the twelfth dorsal vertebra presented a little puffiness, and there was very great tenderness of the spine in that situation; and even when not touched, the child complained of pain in her back. There was no appetite but great thirst, the bowels were constipated, the appearance of the urine was natural, and neither fæces nor urine were voided unconsciously.

She was cupped on the loins to ℥iv, and on the following day was much relieved, moving her legs more readily, and suffering much less from pain in the back. On the 17th she was able to stand, and could walk a little without suffering. Attention was paid to keep the bowels open, and in a few days she was quite well.

Besides cases of this kind, however, in which there is some uncertainty as to the cause of the functional disorder of the spinal cord, others are sometimes met with of a more formidable, though of a less obscure kind. Such are the cases, fortunately by no means common, in which the spinal cord or its membranes are the seat of inflammation.[1]

I shall probably convey to you a more truthful impression of their general characters by relating to you a few of those instances that have come under my notice, rather than by attempting to draw a general portraiture of them from too small a number of examples.

A boy, aged 11 years, of a phthisical family, who seven months previously had had severe and long-continued attacks of headache, was

---

[1] I purposely omit all notice of the epidemic form of cerebro-spinal meningitis, partly because it has never come under my own observation, partly because it does not usually attack young children, and still more because most pathologists regard it as a special disease, not a simple inflammation. I may, however, just refer to an interesting account of an epidemic of the disease which prevailed exclusively among children under 7 years of age, in the village of Barsen, near Neustettin, at the same time with the epidemic prevalence of scarlatina; by Dr. Litten, in J. f. Kinderkr. for 1865, vol. xliv, p. 333.

greatly distressed by hearing of the sudden death of a relation. On the following day he had slight nausea, with pain in the head; but in a day or two he suffered more from pain in his limbs, especially in the calves of the legs, and also shooting from the situation of the coccyx to the middle of the back. He complained, moreover, of a constant pain at the epigastrium, which, as well as that about the lower part of the back, was always much aggravated when the bowels acted; they being, however, usually constipated. These symptoms were associated with great weakness of the legs, which he dragged when walking, and he reached the Children's Infirmary, from which his home was about a mile distant, with much difficulty. On the following day I visited him, and ascertained, on examining the spine, that there was considerable tenderness on pressure from about the middle of the dorsal vertebræ to the apex of the sacrum, but greatest about the lumbar region. There was no intolerance of light, but very distressing sense of giddiness, complete loss of appetite, constant sensation of sickness, and a nasty taste in the mouth. The intellect during the whole illness was only once affected, and then but for a few hours; and the child was remarkably acute, and described his different sensations with great exactness.

The pain in the loins was relieved by cupping; but on the next day the headache was increased in severity, and there was some subsultus of the tendons of the forearms, and a good deal of twitching of the hands. This symptom disappeared after the boy had been depleted copiously by leeches to the head, and after his gums had begun to be affected by mercury, which was freely administered to him; but his pulse, which during the whole of his illness never exceeded 75, sank to 60 in the minute, and its beat became irregular. As the mouth became decidedly sore, first the shooting pains in the back and limbs ceased; then the pulse became regular, and rose in frequency; then the epigastric pain disappeared, and was succeeded for a time by a sense of weight there. By degrees the tenderness of the spine diminished, and finally ceased, and the headache grew less; but his legs long continued weak, so that he could not tread firmly, and the slightest noise, or any kind of over-exertion, brought on an immediate increase of his sufferings. A seton was put in the back of his neck, and the influence of mercury on the system was cautiously maintained for four months before the boy appeared sufficiently well to justify the discontinuance of remedies.

But the disease may run a more acute course, and to a less favorable termination.

A little boy, one year old, who had cut four incisor teeth, and whose health had been habitually good, was brought to me by his mother after three weeks' illness. She told me that he had been suddenly seized with great fever and heat of skin, accompanied, after a lapse of four days, by violent screams. At the outset of his illness he had been cupped at the back of his neck, and leeches had been applied to the head without amendment, and for a week before I saw him all treatment had been discontinued. The child then lay in his mother's lap, frequently crying with a low distressed whimper; his face was usually pale, but occasionally flushed; his head was thrown back, so that the occiput and the back of the neck were nearly in contact with each other.

The sterno-mastoid muscles were rather rigid, though there was no trismus. The hands were clenched, the thumbs drawn into the palm, and occasional attacks came on, in which he uttered a scream, and then bent his body back into an arch. The child sucked eagerly, but frequently dropped the nipple as if in pain; the pupils acted naturally; the pulse was frequent, small, and hard. In the course of the succeeding day frequent convulsive twitchings and startings of the limbs took place, affecting the left arm more than any other part. His face grew pale and more sunken, and the spine became habitually, though slightly, curved forwards, notwithstanding which, occasional attacks of opisthotonos still occurred. The pupils still acted well, but a new symptom appeared, in the labored breathing, which sometimes became so difficult that the child seemed almost choking, while phlegm collected in his throat which he appeared unable to get rid of. This dyspnœa would almost imply that the inflammation had been gradually travelling upwards till it began to involve the origins of the cerebral nerves—a supposition still further confirmed by finding two days afterwards that the eyeballs were in a state of constant convulsive rotation. After this, which was the fifth day from that on which I first saw the child, he was not again brought to me; but, though this case is incomplete, yet it helps to fill up the portraiture of the disease. To complete it, however, I must relate one instance more, in which the results of examination after death confirmed the diagnosis.

Some years ago, I saw a little boy, five months old, of whom his mother gave me the following history: A month before, he had been attacked by shivering (an unusual occurrence in a young child) and, in the night following this seizure, had many fits, during which he screamed much and became very stiff. After they had continued for three days, returning at intervals of an hour or half an hour, a little diminution in their severity followed the use of some medicine prescribed for him by a surgeon; but, even when I saw him, ten or twelve often occurred in the twenty-four hours, though a day would now and then pass without any. The fits were described as presenting the characters of opisthotonos, though in a less marked degree than when they first came on. The retraction of the head by which they were attended at first subsided as they passed off; but in the course of two or three days the tendency to keep the head thrown back became constant, and for a fortnight the head had never been brought out of that position. The mother thought, too, that the child had been blind for that period.

The child appeared well grown and well nourished, and the face was not expressive of particular suffering, but the head was drawn back so that the occiput rested between the shoulders, while the back was bent forwards in a state of perfect emprosthotonos: the legs were drawn up towards the abdomen, the palms of the hands turned backwards and outwards, the fingers clenched, and the thumbs drawn into the palm. On turning the child round on its face, the body formed a complete arch resting on the chin and knees. The whole spine was very tender, and this tenderness was greatest about its upper part. The pupils were dilated and immovable: suction was difficultly performed, though there was no trismus, but the child vomited everything it took almost immediately. The pulse was at this time too rapid and too feeble to be counted, and the child died in a fit of convulsions twenty-four hours afterwards.

On examining the body, blood was found effused, though not in any considerable quantity, within the spinal canal, but external to the dura mater, from the third cervical to the third dorsal vertebra. A thick layer of white lymph was present both under the arachnoid and in its cavity along the whole posterior surface of the lumbar and dorsal portions of the cord, and likewise existed in the cervical portion, though in a less degree. Anteriorly, blood and lymph occupied the whole cervical portion of the sac of the arachnoid, and were effused beneath the membrane; but in the remainder of the front of the cord there were merely patches of lymph beneath the arachnoid. The substance of the cord was apparently healthy. On lifting up the cerebellum, a considerable quantity of serum, with flakes of lymph, escaped from the base of the skull, and the whole under surface of the cerebellum had a uniform coating of white lymph at least a line and a half in thickness, which extended over the medulla oblongata, and was continuous with the deposit of lymph along the spinal cord. The lateral ventricles of the brain were much distended with fluid, in which large irregular masses of yellow lymph were floating. The corpora striata and the fornix were much softened, but the rest of the brain and the membranes at its convexity were quite healthy.

It can scarcely be necessary that I should comment on these cases, either to point out to you the many respects in which inflammation of the spinal cord differs from that of the brain, or to insist on the absolute necessity of active antiphlogistic treatment being adopted at the very outset of the disease.

But besides those cases in which the affection of the spinal cord and its membranes so greatly preponderated, and in which the rapid course of the disease served further to impress on it a peculiar character, others are occasionally met with where the course of the disease is slower, where the symptoms are less exclusively those of disease of the spinal cord, and concerning which it seems almost doubtful whether the membranes of the spinal cord suffer from extension to them of inflammation beginning in the lining of the lateral ventricles, or whether, as indeed I believe to be the case, mischief beginning about the cord is thence propagated upwards.

Such cases are of importance, because, if seen only when far advanced, and considered without reference to their previous history, they often present few points to distinguish them from the more hopeless tubercular meningitis, while at the same time their course is slower, their nature more purely inflammatory, and therefore their treatment may be undertaken with some prospect of success.

A little girl, 20 months old, rather backward in her physical development, and having cut only seven teeth, the last of which appeared at the age of 18 months, was admitted into the Children's Hospital on April 4. Two months previously, while cutting her seventh tooth, her right arm became somewhat stiff, and the power over it rather impaired, a condition which, though improved, had not altogether disappeared at the time of her admission.

On March 24 she vomited, became hot and restless, ceased to talk, and left off all attempts at standing, though her legs did not become stiff, nor were they paralyzed. Her neck became stiff, though she could move her head, she swallowed without difficulty, but had little appetite, her bowels were disposed to be relaxed, her abdomen was not shrunken, her pupils contracted well under light, her pulse was frequent but regular, and there was no return of vomiting after the first day or two of her illness.

On admission the child was in a state of great apathy but not of coma, the surface was not hot, but the pulse 168, though regular. She kept her head somewhat thrown back, but could move it about in any direction, and even bend it forwards. The belladonna liniment was applied constantly to the neck, small doses of the iodide of potassium were given, and the child was fed with beef tea.

For a week improvement appeared to take place in her general condition, but on April 11 the symptoms became aggravated without apparent cause; the pulse sank to 104 and became very irregular in rhythm; divergent strabismus of the left eye became apparent, and the left pupil was more dilated than the right. The child occasionally stretched out its limbs and trunk for a moment quite stiffly, almost like a passing fit of tetanus; but the features were not affected, there was no trismus, and the head was not fixed, though usually retracted.

The pulse sank on the 12th to 80, and its irregularity became more marked, the strabismus varied in degree, the pupils became gradually dilated, and the left usually more so than the right. The application of a blister to the back of the neck was succeeded by an increase of consciousness, and the addition of half a grain of quinine to each dose of the mixture was followed by a still greater apparent amendment, which lasted till the 20th. It was noticed, however, that the stiffness of the right arm rather increased, that the right leg was moved rather less freely than the left, that there was partial paralysis of the left side of the face, and the rectus externus muscle of the left eye, while the left pupil was more dilated than the right.

On the 25th the symptoms had increased. On May 2 the child had lost both flesh and strength; her pupils acted scarcely at all, though they were not extremely dilated, and the strabismus persisted, though it did not increase.

On May 4 a convulsive seizure occurred which lasted for a quarter of an hour, affecting both sides equally. On the morning of the 7th convulsions returned, chiefly affecting the left side, accompanied with much movement of the eyeballs, though with but little distortion of the face. These convulsions lasted for 4½ hours, and in them the child died.

There was no congestion of the vessels of the convexity of the brain. The sac of the arachnoid was dry, the convolutions of the brain were much flattened, and the enormously dilated lateral ventricles contained six ounces of transparent serum. Their lining membrane was coated with a thin layer of very soft greenish lymph, which was already far advanced in fatty degeneration. This lymph was most abundant on the left choroid plexus, and on the walls of the posterior cornua, while in some places it was so thin that it could be made visible only by scraping a considerable surface. The ventricular lining beneath it was perfectly natural, smooth, not thickened, not softened, not extra vascular. In both descending cornua, however, where there was more lymph than elsewhere, it was rather more adherent to the subjacent membrane, and when removed seemed to leave a rather rough surface, on which it was not easy to raise a membrane.

There was but very slight softening of the central parts of the brain. At the base of the brain, from the optic commissure backwards, there was much thick greenish puriform exudation, passing over both crura cerebri, and incasing both lobes of the cerebellum in a thick layer of puriform material, extending also over the inferior surface of the pons Varolii, and both surfaces of the medulla oblongata. There was, however, no softening of the brain-substance.

From the third cervical to the second dorsal vertebra there was much extravasation of blood external to the theca of the cord.

On opening the dura mater, there was a thick layer of lymph of the same kind as in the brain, which invested the whole cord, from the medulla oblongata to the cauda equina.

In the cervical region the substance of the cord was much softened; but it could not be ascertained whether this softening was greater before, behind, or to one side.

Below this point the softening of the cord was inconsiderable. There was no tubercle in any organ of the body.

Now I have seen other cases, in some of which the extent of lymph deposited on the cord was less considerable, and the affection of the ventricles of the brain and of its base also less. Some of these cases, too, have run a slower course, extending over three, four, or even six months. In these the spinal symptoms have been more marked, and those of cerebral disturbance have come on more slowly; convulsions have often occurred, varying in frequency and severity, though usually not of long duration, unattended by much distortion of the features, not limited to one side, not succeeded by paralysis, nor by abiding coma; while even when the children took the least notice of surrounding objects, their condition was one rather of indifference than of insensibility.

The above case, and these observations, will probably suffice to prevent your misinterpretation of these rare instances of cerebro-spinal meningitis, when they come before you in their less rapid forms.

I have not met with any instance of *acute inflammation* and consequent softening of the substance *of the spinal cord*, although there are many such on record. It has been supposed that paralytic symptoms usually attend this affection, while stiffness and spasm of the muscles characterize spinal meningitis; but though this is probably true in many instances, yet it does not by any means hold good in all. Three cases are related by MM. Rilliet and Barthez, where the disease ran its course with symptoms of tetanus and trismus, which continued up to the time of the patient's death. In one of these cases the child died in

36 hours; in the second, in 96 hours; but in the third, a temporary remission having occurred, the patient survived for thirteen days.

I select from Dr. Mauthner's valuable treatise on the Diseases of the Brain and Spinal Cord in Children, a very characteristic case of acute inflammatory softening of the spinal marrow.[1]

A girl aged 11 years, whose occupation as a seamstress compelled her to remain for many hours daily in a sitting posture, with her head bent forwards, while she was at the same time much exposed to currents of cold air, was seized, after she had followed this employment for three weeks, with dragging and tearing pains in the back of her neck. As these pains grew more severe, voluntary power over the arms became impaired, and the paralysis increasing rapidly in spite of the application of leeches to the back of the neck, she was admitted into the Hospital for Children at Vienna, under Dr. Mauthner's care, on December 26. Both arms were at that time completely palsied, flaccid, cool, and almost insensible, the lower extremities still obeyed the will, but the girl was unable to stand firmly. The mind was perfectly clear, the appetite good, deglutition easy, and pulse natural; and in these respects her condition continued unchanged to the very last, except that the pulse became very frequent on the day of the child's death. On the 28th the legs were palsied, and the urine was passed involuntarily. On the 29th, voluntary power over the hands and feet was likewise completely lost, and sensation in them was imperfect. On the 30th, sensation was perfectly lost in all extremities. The child had desire to pass fæces, the bowels not having acted for three days, but she had not power to do so. On the 31st, the sphincter ani was likewise paralyzed, and opened to the size of a shilling. On January 4 the hardened fæces began to fall out of the gaping anus; the respiration was feeble, articulation difficult. On the 6th the child was in much distress, and for many days had scarcely slept at all; the whole left side of the body was completely paralyzed, and only the right side of the chest moved in respiration. Her exhaustion was so extreme that her voice was scarcely audible, but the muscles of the face still retained the power of motion and sensation perfectly, and the intellect was quite clear, though the child died the same night.

The spinal cord presented the only morbid appearance; the membranes being perfectly healthy. The medulla oblongata was as soft as butter, of a yellow color, not retaining a trace of its natural organization; and the same condition existed in the whole of the spinal cord as low as the cauda equina, where it once more resumed its natural appearance and characters.

The *chronic form of inflammation of the cord* will much oftener come under your notice as one of the consequences of caries of the vertebræ. You will remember, too, that this serious result, and the paralysis to which it gives rise, are not produced simply by the distortion of the spine and the mechanical compression of the cord, but rather by extension to it of inflammatory action. You have, then, in these cases, a double danger to combat; both that which arises from the disease in

---

[1] Lib. cit., p. 421, case 117.

the spinal column itself, and that which depends on the probable extension to the cord of the disease which began in the bones. The symptoms of the two affections present likewise so many points of resemblance in their early stages that you can never feel sure that the cord is uninvolved. Of this we have ample proof in those rare cases in which chronic softening of the cord occurs independent of any affection of the bones of the spine. You will find a case that illustrates this fact very well in M. Louis's valuable paper, "On the Condition of the Spinal Marrow in Cases of Caries of the Vertebræ;"[1] and I will relate to you another still more remarkable instance of it, which came under my notice.

On March 31, 1846, a little girl, aged three years and a quarter, the strumous child of unhealthy parents, in whose family phthisis was hereditary, was brought to me by her mother. Nine months previously, her father having taken her in his arms and tossed her, she suddenly cried out that she was hurt, and for several days afterwards refused to walk, and seemed unable to stand, sinking down on her hams if set on her feet. She made no definite complaint, however; no injury was anywhere observable, and in about three weeks she seemed to have recovered her health, and continued well until the middle of March, when her frequent complaints of pain in the neck attracted her mother's attention. The appearance of the little girl, when first placed under my care, was very remarkable; for though the face wore no expression of suffering, yet the neck was so much bent as to give an unusual prominence to the seventh cervical vertebra, and the head was constantly directed downwards. No part of the spine seemed particularly tender; but any attempt to raise the head was forcibly resisted, and seemed to occasion considerable pain. The child walked, though with a tottering gait, and if left alone for a few minutes sank down upon her knees to play. Her constant complaint was of being tired and drowsy, notwithstanding which she slept ill; her appetite was bad, and her bowels were constipated. I regarded the case as one of incipient disease of the cervical vertebræ, and was anxious to make an issue in the back of the neck, but the parents refused to consent to this proceeding. Medical treatment, therefore, was confined to the administration of cod-liver-oil, and afterwards of the syrup of the iodide of iron; but though no fresh symptoms appeared, the child gradually lost strength. On May 12 she was able to walk a distance of nearly half a mile; but on the 14th, though not worse in other respects, she was unable to raise her hands, and was forced to be fed by another person. In the evening she complained of her eyes aching, but nevertheless slept tolerably well till 1 A. M. She then awoke crying and fretful; but on being taken up passed an evacuation, and on lying down again, after a few efforts to vomit, which soon subsided, spoke a few words to her mother, in whose arms she was lying. After breathing in a sighing manner for a few moments she seemed to fall

[1] Mémoires, ou Recherches Anatomico-Pathologiques, 8vo. Mémoire VIII, Observ. i, p. 411. Paris, 1826.

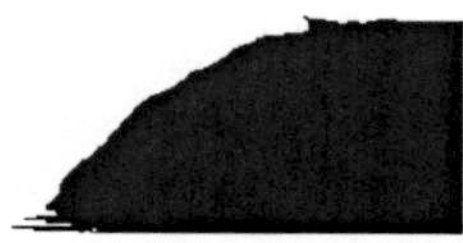

asleep, and in this sleep died so quietly, that her mother was ignorant of it until awakened by her daughter's corpse beginning to grow cold.

On examining the body after death the brain was found to be quite healthy, with the exception of some venous congestion of the arachnoid. The muscles of the back and the bones of the spinal column were perfectly healthy: but on laying open the vertebral canal, the spinal cord, from a level with the third down to the seventh cervical vertebra, bulged considerably, so as completely to occupy the canal, though above and below this its size was natural.

In this situation the two layers of the arachnoid of the cord were firmly connected together by numerous filamentous adhesions, and the membrane itself was opaque and thickened.

The cord in the situation of this bulging had a shining gelatinous appearance, not unlike turbid and badly made jelly, with a yellowish lymph-like matter infiltrated into it. This softening involved the *posterior* columns of the cord much more than the anterior; the bulging, too, seemed due to the posterior columns, though the anterior presented some degree of softening.

Three apoplectic effusions were discovered in the spinal cord. The first was situated just below the calamus scriptorius, and was about the size of a lentil; the nervous matter all around being perfectly healthy. The second, which was larger, was just at the commencement of the swelling of the cord, and partially extended into the sound parts. It just showed through the surface of the cord as big as half a pea, but on longitudinally dividing the cord, was seen to be of the bigness of a kidney bean; and the third effusion just above the termination of the swelling of the cord, was about as large as a big pea. Besides these there were several small ecchymosed spots in the softened parts of the cord, but all the effusions of blood were strictly limited to the posterior columns of the cord.

This case presents many points of interest. The scrofulous diathesis in the family; the probable injury to the spine, followed for a short time by impairment of the motor power, the subsequent occurrence of pain in the bended neck, and the fixed position of the head, all seemed to warrant the opinion that the vertebræ were diseased; but all resulted from inflammatory softening of the spinal cord, while the bones were perfectly healthy. The softening of the posterior columns of the cord, and the extravasation of the blood into their substance, while the anterior columns were in a state of comparative integrity, are occurrences very remarkable when coupled with the impaired motor power.[1] Cases such as this are warnings to us to avoid hasty generalizations on physiological subjects; they show us how hard some of the Sphinx's riddles are to read.

There still remains one affection which we must notice in connection with the diseases of the spinal cord, although it is one whose pathology is by no means thoroughly understood. The *trismus* or *tetanus* of newborn children is a malady which, though frequent in the West Indian

[1] It is almost impossible in so young a subject to ascertain accurately the state of sensation, but there was no obvious indication of its impairment in this case.

Islands, is seldom seen in this country. Four instances of it have come under my own notice, three of which occurred in the Dublin Lying-in Hospital, while for the opportunity of observing the fourth I was indebted to the courtesy of the late Mr. Stone, of Christ's Hospital.

The disease may come on within twelve hours after birth, or, on the other hand, may not occur for several days; but it very rarely makes its appearance after the lapse of a week. I once saw it attack a child fifteen hours after its birth, but in the other case it came on upon the fifth day in one instance, and the sixth in the other two. Though it runs a rapid course, yet its onset is gradual; one of the first things that attracts the mother's notice being in general, that the child does not take the breast when put to it, but utters a whimpering cry, and if the mouth is then examined, it will be found more or less firmly fixed. Sometimes general convulsions come on suddenly, and usher in the other symptoms, but they more frequently follow than precede the trismus. When fully developed, these fits, which come on in paroxysms, are ushered in by a screech, or are attended by some impairment of the respiration, and during their continuance the whole surface becomes livid. The hands are strongly clenched, the feet forcibly flexed on the ankles, and the toes bent, and remain so during the fit, and the trunk is turned back in a condition of opisthotonos: the mouth is generally drawn slightly open, and the lower jaw firmly fixed. When the fit subsides, the muscles do not become generally relaxed, but the child still lies with its hands clenched, and its thumbs drawn into the palm, the legs being generally crossed, and the great toe separated widely from the others, while the head is thrown back, and the opisthotonos continues, though in a diminished degree. The condition of the mouth is peculiar and characteristic. The jaws at first are slightly open, and the corners of the mouth drawn downwards and backwards, but as the disease advances the jaws become quite closed, the corners of the mouth even more drawn down, and the lips firmly compressed against the gums. The power of sucking is early lost, but for some time the child continues able to swallow; at length, however, it accomplishes this with great difficulty, a convulsion sometimes following the attempt, while even that fluid which had apparently been swallowed is for the most part speedily regurgitated. The child dies either during some paroxysm of convulsions, or, seeming much exhausted, it sinks into a comatose condition, and so expires. There are few affections that run so fearfully rapid a course as this; its fatal termination almost always taking place within thirty-six, often within twenty-four hours from the appearance of the first symptoms.

The most frequent *post-mortem appearance* in these cases, and that which I found in the bodies of all the four children whom I observed, consists of effusion of blood, either fluid or coagulated, into the cellular tissue surrounding the theca of the cord. Conjoined with this there is generally a congested state of the vessels of the spinal arachnoid, and sometimes an effusion of blood or serum into its cavity. The signs of congestion about the head are less constant, though much oftener present than absent, and sometimes existing in an extreme degree, while in one instance I found not merely a highly congested state of the [illegible] bral vessels, but also an effusion of blood in considerable quantity between the skull and dura mater, and also a slight effusion into the arachnoid cavity.

In spite, however, of the striking nature of these morbid appearances, I formerly hesitated in referring the symptoms of trismus with certainty to this apoplectic condition of the cord. My hesitation arose from the circumstance that on examining the bodies of infants who died soon after birth in the Dublin Lying-in Hospital, I very frequently found great fulness of the vessels of the cord, and a gelatinous matter, which was frequently deeply tinged with blood, effused around its theca. It therefore became a question whether appearances such as are met with in cases of trismus might not in reality be due to the position in which the bodies had been allowed to remain, resting on the back, and thus be rather the result of simple gravitation than the consequences of the disease. These doubts, however, have been set at rest by the very excellent observations of Dr. Weber, of Kiel,[1] who placed the bodies of infants in various positions before examining them, and thus was able to discriminate between morbid and pseudo-morbid appearances, and who, moreover, although he on every occasion placed children who had died of trismus on their face immediately after death, yet always found intense injection of the minute vessels of the cord and its membranes, extravasation of blood external to the theca, and other appearances similar to those which I have just described to you.

There are few diseases respecting the *cause* of which opinions so various have prevailed as with regard to trismus. Bearing in mind the frequency of external violence as a cause of lock-jaw in the adult, some writers have sought to find in every case the history of a blow or other injury to which it might possibly be attributed; while others have conceived that it depended on awkward management of the navel-string, or on injury of some kind or other inflicted on it. This last opinion has appeared to derive support from some cases in which the umbilical vein has presented the signs of phlebitis: but further observation has shown these appearances to be anything but constant, aud though carefully sought for, they were not found in any of the cases which came under my notice. Moreover, Dr. Mildner, of Prague,[2] who has recorded the results of 46 cases of fatal inflammation of the umbilical vessels in children born in the Lying-in Hospital in that city, states that convulsions occurred in only 5 of the number, and that in no instance had these convulsions the least resemblance to those which characterize trismus. Congestion of the liver, impairment of its functions, and icterus, were among the symptoms which attended it, as well as, in many of the cases, peritonitis, inflammation of the abdominal integuments, purulent infection of the blood and the formation of abscesses in the joints, which occurred 33 times, while in 4 cases hemorrhage took place from the umbilicus. We may, then, fairly conclude that the

---

[1] Beiträge zur pathologischen Anatomie der Neugebornen, 8vo., part i, pp. 7, 68, and 78. Kiel, 1851.

[2] Prager Vierteljahrsschrift, v. 2, 1848; and Schmidt's Jahrb., No. 7, p. 64, 1848.

connection between this disease and trismus is merely an accidental coincidence.

The remarkable frequency of the disease in hot climates, where the heat of the day is succeeded by intense cold at night, favors the opinion that interruption of the function of the skin, by sudden alternations of temperature, is a powerful cause of the disease. In an epidemic of this disease in the Lying-in Hospital at Stockholm, in 1834,[1] there seemed also to be a most marked connection between the periods of its greatest prevalence and the fluctuations of temperature. Nothing, however, can be more satisfactorily proved, than the tendency of a vitiated state of atmosphere to produce it. Where such a condition exists, there trismus abounds, be the peculiarities of climate or temperature what they may. It is very frequent among the children of the negroes in the Southern States of America: it is depopulating the island of St. Kilda, and 64 per cent. of the infants born in Westmannoe, a small islet off the coast of Iceland, die of it between the 5th and 12th day from birth.[2] Dirt, and defective ventilation, are probably almost the only points in common between the dweller in the Southern States of North America and the inhabitants of Northern Europe and the Arctic regions. But, if any further proof were needed that to this cause, and not to some fancied displacement of the cranial bones,[3] this disease is really to be attributed, we are furnished with it in the records of the Dublin Lying-in Hospital, which point out both the evil and its remedy. Sixty years ago, every sixth child born in that institution died within a fortnight after birth, and trismus was the cause of the death of $\frac{19}{20}$ of these children. Dr. Joseph Clarke adopted means to secure the efficient ventilation of the hospital, and the mortality of the children fell at once to 1 in 19¼; and during Dr. Collins's mastership from 1826 to 1833, was only 1 in 58½; and but little more than the ninth part of that mortality depended on trismus.[4]

But though we may hope by wise hygienic measures to avert this disease, yet, when once it has become developed, our prospects of *cure* are so slender that I may almost say the task is hopeless. I have not seen leeches employed, but, bearing in mind the post-mortem appearances, should certainly be disposed to apply them freely at the outset of the disease. I have seen the hot bath used with temporary relief; but though I have witnessed the employment of calomel and of antispasmodics, as assafœtida, and the administration of an enema of gr. iij of tobacco infused for half an hour in ℥viij of water, yet I have never known any of those means followed by even a temporary pause in the symptoms; and the endeavor to excite the action of the skin is the only measure that in the cases which I witnessed seemed to be of the slightest service.

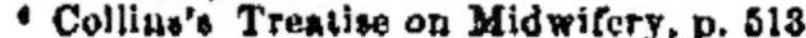

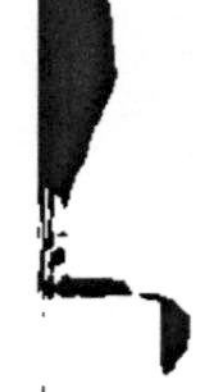

[1] Cederschjold, in Busch's Zeitschrift für Geburtsk., x, 345.

[2] See a very interesting notice, in the British and Foreign Medico-Chirurgical Review for April, 1850, of a work by Dr. Schleisner on the Sanitary Condition of Iceland.

[3] A theory propounded by Dr. Sims, of Alabama, in the American Journal of the Medical Sciences for 1846, and further expanded in the same journal for July and October, 1848.

[4] Collins's Treatise on Midwifery, p. 513.

LECTURE XIII.

CONVULSIONS, independent of organic cerebral disease—Their two forms—The acute form, how distinguishable from those dependent on disease of the brain—Practical importance of the distinction—Rules for their treatment—The chronic form—Relation to them of SPASM OF THE GLOTTIS—Import of this spasm—One of several signs of disorder of nervous system—Relation of these convulsions to processes of development in teething—But exciting causes various—Symptoms—Description of carpo-pedal contractions—Ways in which death is produced—Treatment—Rules for diet and for the regulation of the bowels—Caution with respect to lancing the gums—Occasional necessity for free depletion—Case in illustration—Suggestions as to general management, and prevention of an attack—Use of chloroform—Remarks on some anomalous forms of convulsion, and on the Eclampsia Nutans.

IN the third of these Lectures, when passing in review the different signs of disorder of the nervous system I made some remarks on the subject of convulsions. I tried to show you how their import varies in different circumstances; how at one time they betoken real disease of the nervous centres, at another only betray their irritation from some cause which, if death occur, may yet leave behind no trace such as the skill of the anatomist can discover.

Cases of the former kind have hitherto exclusively engaged our attention, but we must not quit the study of disorders of the nervous system without some consideration of the latter. In the adult, fits sometimes occur independent of obvious cerebral disease; the patient falls to the ground struggling and insensible; but after a time the convulsion ceases, consciousness returns, and the patient recovers. Our anxiety in such cases is much less for the present than for the future: death in a fit is a rare accident, but what we dread is the recurrence of the fits, the weakening of the intellect, the slow impairment of the health which epilepsy brings with it. In the child our apprehension is twofold; for the frailer machinery is more readily brought to a standstill, and the risk of death in the fit is far greater than in the adult; while should the child survive, the convulsions of infancy may issue in the epilepsy of riper years; and, in fact, seem to do so in a very large number of instances.

The convulsions of infancy and early childhood generally assume one of two characters. Either they are sudden in their onset, violent in their characters, frequent in their return, or they come on gradually, and after various forebodings, present less violence, occur at longer intervals, but are not therefore by any means devoid of peril. Cases of the first kind run some risk of being overtreated, from their supposed dependence on active cerebral mischief; cases of the second kind often excite less apprehension than they really warrant, until their symptoms have become manifest in their full intensity.

Some of the most marked examples of the sudden access of violent convulsions which have come under my notice have been in children in whom they succeeded to the sudden drying up of an eruption on the scalp. Even in such cases, however, where we might most readily suspect some direct influence on the brain, the character of the fits is widely different from that which we observe in instances of real cerebral disease. The illness preceding them is neither very marked nor of long duration, while, when the fits come on, instead of only one side of the body, or one set of muscles being affected, sometimes one side is convulsed, sometimes the other, or both are involved equally. Even after the fits have frequently returned, paralysis does not succeed to them, and often neither sleep nor coma, while frequently consciousness returns, even before the convulsive movements have completely ceased, and the pupils, though dilated during the fit, act again almost or quite as well as ever as soon as it has passed off. Vomiting does not precede nor accompany the attack; nor an obstinately constipated state of the bowels; and the abdomen is often much distended with flatus, the endeavor to get rid of which produces troublesome hiccup, while the inspiration is often accompanied by a peculiar crowing sound. There is at no time the burning heat of the head which is observed in active inflammatory disease of the brain; there are not the piercing cry, nor the constant wail, nor the tearless eyes, nor the shrunken abdomen, nor the automatic movements of one side and the contraction of the limbs on the other, which attend upon tubercular meningitis.

These characteristics are such as ought to prevent the by no means unusual error of regarding the attack as symptomatic of active disease of the brain; and under that impression depleting the child freely, dosing it with mercury in large quantities, and at short intervals; a course of proceeding by which all chances of recovery are frustrated, and hopes, small at first, are altogether destroyed.

The state of the child before the occurrence of the fits, and the amount of apparent congestion of the brain, must in cases of this kind determine the question of depletion. Moderate depletion once is often well borne, but the persistence of the fits must not be thought necessarily to indicate the propriety of its repetition. If the attack succeeded to the rapid disappearance of some eruption on the scalp, an attempt may be made to reproduce it by rubbing in every three hours an ointment composed of one drachm of powdered ipecacuanha to an ounce of lard; which generally produces an abundant papular eruption in the course of from 12 to 24 hours. If a purgative is indicated, a single dose of calomel has the advantage of acting surely and speedily, but mercury, given in any other manner or with any other object, is out of place. The flatus by which the intestines are distended is got rid of better by an assafœtida enema than by any other means; while the application to the abdomen of a cloth dipped in a stimulating liniment (such, for instance, as a drachm of oil of turpentine, five drachms of the simple camphor liniment, and six drachms of olive oil), and that covered by a light linseed-meal poultice, both serves as a counter-irritant, prevents the reproduction of the flatus, and relieves that spasm of the abdominal muscles which in many of these cases adds very painfully to the infant's sufferings. These measures having been adopted, you may now, according to the general condition of the patient, prescribe either some carminative medicine with small doses of ether, or of the fœtid spirits of ammonia, or a single dose of Dover's powder, or of chloral if restlessness and excitability have outlasted the other symptoms; or a simple saline, as the citrate of potash, with small doses of the tincture of henbane; or the hydrocyanic acid with a little chloric ether at short intervals—a sedative which, whenever there is a doubt as to the expediency of employing direct narcotics, has always seemed to me of especial value.

Within certain limits, this treatment must of course be modified according to the exact nature of the case, but enough has already been said to mark out the general principles upon which your treatment should be conducted; while even if the attack had seemed at first to present some obscurity as to its cause, a few hours will suffice for its removal, will develop the signs of cerebral inflammation if that were impending, or will bring to light the character of the fever which is making this stormy onset. So long as, notwithstanding the frequency of the return of the fits, recovery is complete after each, so long as the power of deglutition subsists, and the natural hue of the lips and face announces the oxygenation of the blood to be well performed, you may give on the whole a favorable prognosis, though always guarding it by admission of the possibility of the child dying in a fit from that spasm of the glottis, and consequent arrest of breathing, which is the great source of danger in infantile convulsions.

This *Spasm of the Glottis* is, indeed, one of the most remarkable features in many convulsive affections of infancy and childhood; though more especially of that variety to which I have referred as coming on gradually and pursuing a somewhat chronic course.

So prominent a feature, indeed, is it of this latter class of convulsions, that attention has been very generally directed to this one symptom, almost to the exclusion of the other signs of disorder of the nervous system by which it is accompanied, and the various terms, spasmodic croup, child-crowing, spasm of the glottis, and laryngismus stridulus, show how great has been the disposition to regard it as a distinct and independent disease. Hence has resulted the inconvenience, that attention being directed exclusively to the affection of the respiratory function, local causes have been too much sought for to account for the local symptom; defective, if not erroneous explanations of its occurrence have been proposed, and sufficient regard has not been paid in its treatment to the great diversity of conditions under which it may supervene.

The sobbing breathing, or the sense of choking, so characteristic of the hysterical patient, are but instances of spasm of the respiratory muscles similar to those which we observe in the infant, and equally due to the great excitability of the nervous system. In the hysterical girl, fits are frequently superadded to the affection of the respiratory muscles; and in the child, spasm of the muscles of the extremities, giving rise to the drawing of the thumb into the palm, and to the separation of the great toe from the other toes, or to the forcible extension of the foot upon the ankle, is seldom absent; while general convulsions often supervene under slight causes, or even without any apparent reason. In both cases the affections are usually attendant upon important processes of development, since while in the former instance they generally come on about the period of puberty, they oftenest occur in the latter during the time of teething; and this with so great frequency, that in 31 out of 37 cases of which I have preserved a record, the symptoms manifested themselves between the age of 6 months and 2 years, or just at that time when the process of dentition is going on with the greatest activity. The direct irritation of the trifacial nerve in teething has no doubt a great share in the production of the symptom at that time, but I apprehend that we should be in error, if we confined our attention entirely to the local cause, and attributed this, more than any other form of convulsive affection, which occurs at this time, simply to the mechanical irritation of the teeth, pressing on or cutting through the gum. The period of teething, like that of puberty, constitutes one of the great epochs of life; it is a time when great changes are going on in the whole organism—when the animal machine, being in a state of increased activity, its parts are more than usually apt to get out of order. New diseases appear, or such as were before of rare occurrence become frequent; catarrhal affections and disorders of the intestinal mucous membrane are extremely prevalent, and the brain grows more than ever liable to congestion of its vessels. In these circumstances, the various spasmodic affections, of which spasm of the glottis is the most striking and the most important, often occur as the secondary rather than as the primary result of dentition. The child has cut some of its teeth without any symptom of disorder of the nervous system making its appearance, but at length it suffers an attack of diarrhœa, or the bowels are allowed to become constipated, or signs of cerebral congestion show themselves. A crowing sound now becomes audible with the inspiration, and with it some or all of the whole train of convulsive symptoms which I shall presently describe make their appearance. It may be that the gums are not swollen, nor any tooth near the surface just at the moment when the signs of disturbance of the nervous system occurred, but their connection with the process of dentition is not the less undeniable. In many instances, too, though these symptoms may subside as the health improves, yet so great is the nervous excitability of the patient, that they return when he cuts another tooth, and this even without a recurrence of that general disorder which attended them on the former occasion.

The various sources of irritation, however, that give rise to these affections are not limited to the period of teething; and hence they may be met with before the commencement of that process as well as after its termination. By no one has this fact been more clearly stated, or the mode of action of the various exciting causes more successfully explained than by the late Dr. Marshall Hall.

"Spasm of the Glottis," says this distinguished physiologist,[1] "is an excitation of the true spinal or excito-motory system. It originates in

[1] Lib. cit., p. 171.

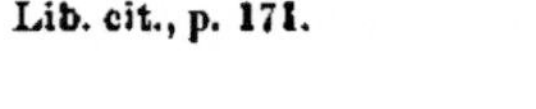

I. 1. The *trifacial*, in teething.
  2. The *pneumogastric*, in over- or improperly-fed infants.
  3. The *spinal nerves*, in constipation, intestinal disorder, or catharsis.

These act through the medium of

II. The spinal marrow, and

III. 1. The *inferior or recurrent laryngeal*, the constrictor of the larynx.
  2. The *intercostals and diaphragmatic*, the motors of respiration."

In illustration of these observations as to the various causes on which these symptoms depend, I may mention that I have seen them in a child ten weeks old as a consequence of improper feeding: in another, aged nineteen months, they followed the sudden suppression of long-continued diarrhœa; while in a third, aged two years, they came on during an attack of purging with severe pain in the abdomen. In another child, aged two years and a half, they seemed to depend on a state of cerebral congestion which succeeded to habitual constipation; in a fifth, aged nine months, they supervened in the course of chronic hydrocephalus; and, not needlessly to swell the list, in a sixth child, who died when two months old, convulsions occurred for a period of six weeks, and eventually occasioned its death, without its having been possible to discover, either from the symptoms or from the appearances found on examination of the body, any cause to which they could be attributed.

But this principle admits of a wider application. Not only are the convulsions which occur during dentition symptomatic of something more than the undue pressure of a tooth against the gum, but in by far the greater number of instances, we have to look deeper than the local cause to which at last the signs of disturbance of the nervous system were due, and find that it is only on the removal of some influence which acted injuriously on the whole constitution that the liability to convulsions ceases. Thus, for instance, in the child brought up by hand, the commencement of teething is ushered in by convulsions, a wet nurse is procured, the convulsions cease; or medical care has failed to relieve the infant resident in London,—it is removed to the country, and the fits previously so frequent disappear.

In spite, however, of the illustration of this fact which the action of remedies affords, it is yet too often lost sight of. The defective nutrition which shows itself in the bowed limbs, and distorted form of the rickety patient, is attended in early life by special proneness to convulsions. So intimate indeed is the relation between rickets on the one hand, and convulsions and spasm of the glottis on the other, that Dr. Gee[1] states as the result of his most careful observations among the out-patients at the Children's Hospital that 48 out of 50 cases of spasm of the glottis presented evidences of rickets; that 19 of them suffered also from convulsions; while further in 56 out of 61 children who were attacked by convulsions before the completion of the first dentition, there were also signs of rickets in a more or less advanced

---

[1] Bartholomew's Hospital Reports, vol. iii, 1867, p. 101.

degree as deduced from enlargement of the growing ends of the bones. It is true that these observations were made among the poor; but it must also be admitted that the minor degrees of rickets are far from unusual even among the children of the richer classes; and I doubt whether even as applied to them these figures would much overstate the truth. It was a partial recognition of the important part played by rickets in predisposing both to convulsions and laryngeal spasm that led a German physician[1] some years ago to think that he had discovered, in the tardy ossification of the skull in such children, an adequate explanation of their liability to disturbance of the functions of the imperfectly protected brain, and putting a part for the whole, wrote by a very pardonable, but not the less mistaken synecdoche, an essay on "The soft Occiput." Again, one of the commonest manifestations of the tuberculous diathesis is glandular enlargement; and the late Dr. Hugh Ley[2] propounded a theory which explained the symptoms of spasm of the glottis by an assumed pressure of the enlarged cervical glands on the recurrent laryngeal nerve. Still more recently, we find a practitioner of considerable experience struck by the connection of spasm of the glottis[3] with enlargement of the liver, and framing a mechanical explanation of the trouble of respiration by the impediment to the descent of the diaphragm which is occasioned by the great size of the organ. Of the frequent coexistence of the enlarged and fatty liver with spasm of the glottis there can be no doubt; but it does not therefore follow that we are to accept the mechanical explanation of the fact which Mr. Hood suggests. Some years ago, my friend and former colleague, Doctor Rolleston, now Linacre Professor at Oxford, wrote a paper which I wish that his modesty had not withheld from publication, in which he shows that this same fatty liver is present in many instances of the hydrocephaloid disease of early infancy; the extreme anæmia, the feeble powers, the rapid sinking under slight ailments, the supervention of signs of disorder of the nervous system (among which spasm of the glottis is by no means necessarily present), being found associated with this grave defect in nature's great alembic, and consequently with imperfect depuration and depraved character of the blood. But modern physiology[4] gives a still graver import to this, as to other morbid conditions of the liver in connection with those disorders of the nervous system in early life which are associated with anæmia or with deranged nutrition. The liver would seem to be not merely a purifier, but an actual generator of the blood; its disease, therefore, interferes immediately with sanguification, and prevents the best devised tonic remedies from exercising that influence which otherwise they would not fail to produce.

---

[1] Der weiche Hinterkopf, &c., von Dr. C. L. Elsässer. 8vo. Stuttgart, 1843.

[2] On Laryngismus Stridulus, 8vo. London, 1836.

[3] On Scarlet Fever and Crowing Inspiration. 8vo. London, 1857.

[4] Funke, Lehrbuch der Physiologie, vol. i, 2d ed. 8vo. Leipzig, 1858, says in § 35, on the metamorphosis of the blood in the liver: "It is the more correct view to regard the liver as an organ the special function of which is the formation of new blood-cells, and to consider the change of the materials which during and probably in consequence of that new formation are excreted from the blood into bile, only as its secondary duty." See p. 147.

It follows then, with reference to all the disorders of the nervous system in early life, that while the mode in which they manifest themselves varies from slight and unimportant causes, and while local accidents may account for their assuming this or the other special form, we must in all instances endeavor to look beyond them to the constitutional ailment, sometimes of one kind, sometimes of another, but always implying some deepseated impairment of nutrition, to which as their ultimate occasion, they are due.

Bearing in mind now what I have just said with reference to the import of *Spasm of the Glottis*,—how it is but one of many signs of the general disorder of the nervous system,—we may proceed to examine the conditions under which it usually manifests itself; the *symptoms* by which it is generally attended. It is a disorder that almost always comes on by degrees; and its early symptoms are seldom such as to excite the alarm of non-professional persons. It does not often occur in perfectly healthy children; but an infant who is attacked by it has usually been observed to be drooping for some time previously, to have lost its appetite, to have become fretful by day and restless at night, and to present many of those ill-defined ailments which are popularly ascribed to teething. At length, after these symptoms have continued for a few days or weeks, a slight crowing sound is occasionally heard with the child's respiration. The sound is something between the hoop of hooping-cough and the stridor of true croup; it must be heard to be known, but when once heard will easily be recognized. Usually it is first noticed on the child awaking out of sleep, but sometimes it is perceived during a fit of crying, or comes on while the infant is sucking. Now and then the first crow is very loud, and, by its resemblance to the sound of croup, at once alarms the family: but this is not generally the case; and its loudness usually increases in proportion as its return becomes more frequent. The spasm may have been excited by some temporary cause, and the sound which is its token may in that case not be heard again; but generally it returns after the lapse of a few hours, or of a day or two. It will soon be found, as its return becomes more frequent, that certain conditions favor its occurrence; that the child wakes suddenly from sleep with an attack of it, that excitement induces it, or deglutition, or the effort of sucking; so that the child will suddenly drop the nipple, make a croupy sound with its breathing, and then return to the breast again. Throughout the whole course of the affection its attacks will be found to be more frequent by night than by day; and to occur mostly either soon after the child has lain down to sleep, or towards midnight, when the first sound sleep is drawing to a close.

At first the child seems, during the intervals of the attack, in as good health as before,—except, perhaps, that it is rather more pettish and wilful; but it is not long before graver symptoms than the occasional occurrence of an unusual sound with inspiration excite attention, and give rise to alarm. Fits of difficult breathing occasionally come on, in which the child throws its head back, while its face and lips become livid, or an ashy paleness surrounds the mouth, slight convulsive movements pass over the muscles of the face; the chest is motionless, and suffocation seems impending. But in a few seconds the spasm yields, expiration is effected, and a long, loud, crowing inspiration succeeds, or the child begins to cry. Breathing now goes on naturally; the crowing is not repeated, or the crying ceases; a look of apprehension dwells for a moment on the infant's features, but then passes away; it turns once more to its playthings, or begins sucking again as if nothing were the matter. A few hours, or even a few days, may pass before this alarming occurrence is again observed; but it does recur, and another symptom of the disturbance of the nervous system is soon superadded, if it has not, as is often the case, existed from the very beginning. This consists in a peculiar contraction of the hands and feet; a state which may likewise not infrequently be noticed during infancy, unattended by any spasmodic affection of the respiratory organs; though it is often overlooked, since unlike the peculiar noise in breathing, it does not force itself on the attention even of the most unobservant. It differs much in degree: sometimes the thumb is drawn into the palm by the action of its adductor muscles, while the fingers are unaffected; at other times the fingers are closed more or less firmly, and the thumb is shut into the palm; or coupled with this, the hand itself is forcibly flexed on the wrist. In the slightest degree of affection of the foot, the great toe is drawn a little away from the other toes; in severer degrees of the affection this abduction of the great toe is very considerable, and the whole foot is forcibly bent upon the ankle and its sole directed a little inwards. Affection of the hands generally precedes the affection of the feet, and may even exist without it; but I have never seen spasmodic contraction of the feet when the hands were unaffected. At first this state is temporary, but it does not come on and cease simultaneously with the attacks of crowing inspiration, though generally much aggravated during its paroxysms. Sometimes a child in whom the crowing inspiration has been heard will awake in the morning with the hands and feet firmly flexed, although he may not have had any attack of difficult breathing during the night. At other times, though but seldom, this state will subside during sleep; while very often it is impossible to assign any reason for its cessation or return. The hands may often be unflexed by bending the fingers, but they will resume their former position on the withdrawal of the force; and such attempts are painful to the child. When the contraction is but slight, children still use their hands; but when considerable, they cannot employ them, and they sometimes cry, as if the contraction of the muscles were attended with pain. Coupled with these carpopedal contractions, the back of the hand and the instep are sometimes swollen, tense, and livid; and occasionally there is slight puffiness about the face. This condition is sometimes more general, and on two successive years the same child was brought to me, in whom these attacks of crowing inspiration were accompanied by a state of tense anasarca of the whole body.[1] The swelling of the hands and feet may be due merely to the

[1] This case presented a remarkable similarity to one described by Dr. M. Hall, at p. 185 of his work on the Diseases and Derangements of the Nervous System, 8vo. London, 1841.

impediment to the circulation presented by the continuous spasm, and will then subside of its own accord as the spasm abates. The general anasarcous condition, of which I have now seen several instances, depends on a different cause. The urine in these cases, if it can be collected, will be found to be albuminous, and under the employment of diuretic and diaphoretic medicines, the removal of the dropsy and the abatement or disappearance of the spasmodic symptoms will take place together.

When the disease has reached a high degree of intensity, a slight crowing sound often attends each inspiration, and the paroxysms of difficult breathing are much more severe; they last longer, and sometimes terminate in general convulsions. The breathing now does not return at once to its natural frequency, but continues hurried for a few minutes after the occurrence of each fit of dyspnœa; and it is sometimes attended with a little wheezing, from the accumulation of mucus in the trachea and larger bronchi during the paroxysm. When this wheezing is permanent, I do not apprehend that it usually constitutes any essential part of the disease, but regard it either as due to an accidental complication with catarrh, which is so frequent during the period of dentition, or as the result of the affection being associated with tubercle in the lungs or bronchial glands, or it may perhaps be owing to a degree of pulmonary congestion, such as takes place in hooping-cough in consequence of the frequent interruption to the regular performance of respiration. The slightest cause is now sufficient to bring on an attack of difficult breathing; it may be produced by a current of air, by a sudden change of temperature, by slight pressure on the larynx, by the act of deglutition, or by momentary excitement. The state of sleep seems particularly favorable to its occurrence, and the short fitful dozes are interrupted by the return of impending suffocation.

The general condition of the child varies much during the existence of these symptoms, but is always widely removed from a state of health. The bowels are almost invariably disordered, constipation being more frequent than diarrhœa. The mouth is sometimes hot, and the gums are swollen—the child is evidently suffering from the process of teething; and this is the state with which spasm of the glottis is perhaps most frequently associated. Sometimes there is evident congestion of the brain, and the face is flushed, the head hot, and the pulse frequent; but these flushes of the face are usually temporary, and the skin is generally pallid. When the affection has continued for some weeks, the countenance often assumes a haggard, miserable aspect; and though it may come on in children apparently in good health, I have never known the health continue good, after the disease, even in a mild form, has lasted for any time.

Death sometimes takes place during one of the paroxysms of dyspnœa, the child being suffocated by the long continuance of the spasm; or at other times the often-repeated difficulty of breathing induces a state of permanent cerebral congestion: general convulsions occur, and the child dies convulsed or comatose, serous effusion having taken place into the ventricles of the brain. Should the child escape both these dangers, and should no tubercular disease of the lungs or bronchial glands exist, recovery is almost sure eventually to take place, though the convalescence is often very protracted, and the attack is apt to return under the influence of the same causes as originally excited it.

The *treatment* of spasm of the glottis must be regulated by the nature of its exciting cause; and this, as you have already seen, varies much in different cases. In infants before the period of dentition, it is usually induced by overfeeding, or by food of an improper kind. Our inquiries, therefore, must at once be directed to ascertain how the infant is fed; and supposing it to be still suckled, it will be wise to interdict any other food than the mother's milk—or, at most, to allow only a little barley-water. Spasm of the glottis, however, occurs much oftener in infants who are brought up by hand, or in those who have been weaned, than in children still at the breast. In such cases, much pains are sometimes necessary in order to ascertain precisely the kind of food that best suits the infant. Two parts of milk, and one of barley-water, sweetened with a little loaf-sugar; or equal parts of milk and of a solution of isinglass, made of the thickness of barley-water, generally agree very well; but much caution must be used in the introduction of farinaceous articles into the child's diet. Asses' milk, which forms the nearest approach to its natural food, must sometimes be given till the child has decidedly improved; while, if it is puny, and does not appear to thrive, and the crowing inspiration continues undiminished, it may become absolutely necessary to restore it to the breast.

The state of the bowels requires no less attention than the regulation of the diet. The tendency to constipation must be combated, not by drastic purgatives, but by mild aperients. Castor oil often answers the purpose very well, but sometimes each dose of it nauseates a child for several hours, and then it is not desirable to employ it if a daily aperient should be needed. Both senna and manna are apt to gripe; and if they should be found on trial to produce this effect, their use must not be persevered in. Few medicines act more mildly or more certainly in children than aloes; and the bitter of the compound decoction may be much concealed by extract of licorice. The bulk of a medicine, however, often opposes a great difficulty to its employment in infancy; and if that is the case, the powder may be substituted for the decoction. If slightly moistened, mixed with a little coarse sugar, and placed on the tongue, it will often be swallowed very readily. The habitual use of mercurials to overcome the constipation is not desirable: their employment is better limited to those cases in which not only the bowels are sluggish, but the evacuations are unnatural in character.

The action of the bowels may be encouraged by rubbing the abdomen twice a day with a liniment composed of equal parts of soap liniment and tincture of aloes; or the bowels may sometimes be induced to act regularly in young infants by the daily employment of a small soap suppository. Enemata, consisting either of warm water or of gruel, may also be given for the same purpose.

Sedulous attention to the diet and the state of the bowels will sometimes effect a cure; but in many instances tonics may be employed with advantage, and none with such decided benefit as the preparations of iron and cod-liver oil. Indeed, if we bear in mind the observations which I have already referred to as to the connection between laryngeal spasm, convulsions, and the rickety constitution, we shall at once have recourse to cod-liver oil as the great remedy for the past, and prophylactic for the future. Removal to pure air, however, or to the sea-coast, is often a tonic of greater power in these cases than all the contents of the laboratory, and one which you will find in some instances to be absolutely indispensable to the child's cure.

All these cares are not less needed in children in whom the process of dentition has already commenced. In them, however, the irritation of teething is often the exciting cause of the affection, and lancing the gums is frequently needed in addition to the other treatment. The relief thus afforded is sometimes very striking; and the frequent repetition of the operation may be necessary to diminish the swelling and tension, and to ease the pain of the congested gum. It is not, however, a proceeding to be adopted, irrespective of all other considerations, simply because the child had begun to cut his teeth when the attack of spasm of the glottis came on. Dentition does not go on continuously from the time when the first tooth is cut until the completion of the whole set, but there are regular pauses in the process, during which its advance is suspended for several weeks together. Thus, for instance, after the appearance of the incisors, there is a pause for several weeks or months before the first molar teeth appear, and then there is another cessation in the process before the child begins to cut its canine teeth. The spasm of the glottis, therefore, may come on during one of these pauses, and be excited by some cause quite unconnected with dentition. Lancing the gums, too, is not well borne in every case, even when it may have appeared to be indicated; and I have more than once been compelled to discontinue it, on account of the pain and alarm which it excited bringing on a violent spasmodic seizure whenever I attempted to practice it.

In some instances the spasm of the glottis is associated with manifest uneasiness in the head. It has been suggested that, in some of these cases, the brain is kept in a state of constant irritation, owing to the deficiently ossified skull being too thin to defend it from injury, while at the same time it affords no adequate counter-pressure to check the overdistension of the cerebral vessels. There is no doubt but that rickety children are peculiarly liable to this affection; and though the constitutional condition of such children has certainly much to do with its production, yet the imperfect bone formation of the cranium probably has a share in such cases in aggravating it. I have seen many instances in which the recommendation that a horsehair cushion should be made for the head to rest on, having a hole in its centre, so as to relieve the occiput from all pressure, has been acted on with manifest advantage. The supervention of attacks of spasm of the glottis, in a case of well-marked chronic hydrocephalus, would call for little change in the treatment, though it must evidently add much to the danger of the patient.

Symptoms of cerebral congestion are sometimes associated with this condition. They are seldom such as to call for active interference;

but the tepid bath and neutral salines, with small doses of hyoscyamus,[1] are often of much service in quieting the general excitement of the circulation, while the occasional application of a leech to the head may be beneficial, especially if general convulsions are beginning to supervene on the attacks of dyspnœa.

It is possible that you may meet with a case in which active depletion is indicated, and you must not allow the consciousness that, as a general rule, it is inappropriate, to prevent you from having recourse to it in such exceptional instances as the following. In this case, indeed, it was found necessary to carry depletion beyond that point which is in general expedient in so young a child.

Some years since I saw a little boy, 2½ years old, who had already suffered from several attacks of spasm of the glottis. A return of the affection had taken place about seven weeks before, though not attended by any very alarming symptoms until after the lapse of a month, when a general convulsive seizure occurred. From this he recovered, and he had for some days appeared to be convalescent from the spasmodic attacks, when his bowels became disordered and a good deal purged, and after they had been so for two or three days his mother noticed one afternoon that his thumbs were forcibly drawn into the palms of his hands. With the exception of this contraction of his thumbs, however, he seemed as well as usual and had a tolerably good night; but immediately on awaking at six o'clock on the following morning he had a paroxysm of stridulous breathing, in which he crowed so loudly as to be heard over the whole house. His face at the same time became greatly flushed, and his hands and feet contracted, as they were when I visited him three hours afterwards. His face was then much flushed, his head hot, his pupils rather dilated, his pulse full and bounding; his thumbs were drawn across the palm; the fingers were not closed, but the hands were forcibly flexed on the wrist; the great toe was drawn apart from the other toes, which were flexed, and the whole foot was stiffly bent on the ankle. The child was then breathing quietly and seemed drowsy, but he screamed out the moment he was touched, as if the least disturbance of his limbs gave him pain.

Eight leeches were applied to his temples, and drew much blood, but without producing any amelioration of his condition. A croupy sound continued to attend his respiration, and he had a fit of urgent dyspnœa, with loud stridulous breathing, between my first visit at 9 in the morning and my second at 5 in the evening. I now bled him from the arm to ℥vj, which subdued the fulness of the pulse, blanched his lips, and diminished the flush of his face, though it did not cause actual fainting. I ordered cold to be applied to the head, and saw him again at 7½ P.M., when I found that he had been lying quiet ever since I left him, and had had some tranquil sleep, without any crowing sound attending the breathing. His pulse was less full, the flush of his face was diminished, the heat of the head was gone, and the contractions of the hands and feet were both less, and less firm.

---

[1] See Formula No. 3, p. 63.

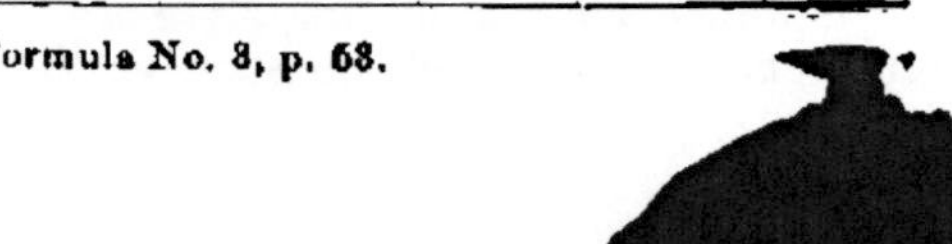

A powder with gr. j of calomel and gr. viij of rhubarb, which had been given in the morning, and had produced one evacuation, was now repeated.

The child had some sleep in the night, and no access of dyspnœa returned, nor did the croupy sound again accompany the inspiration. In the course of the day the spasmodic contractions of the hands and feet greatly diminished, and the child became cheerful. In five days from this formidable attack he was quite well, and continued so for a year, when a slight return of spasm of the glottis took place, in the course of a severe impetiginous eruption on the scalp.

Before concluding this lecture, I will suggest a few cautions, applicable alike to all cases of spasm of the glottis. Sudden excitement, and especially a fit of crying, are likely to bring on the attack, and since there is a possibility of any one of these attacks proving fatal, the greatest care must be taken in the management of the child to avoid all unnecessary occasions of annoyance or distress.

Although the benefit that accrues from fresh air, or from a change of air, is often very great, yet it is very important that the child should not be exposed to the cold or wind, for I have seen such exposure followed by a severe attack of dyspnœa, or by the occurrence of general convulsions. The hazard of such an occurrence is greater in proportion to the severity and long continuance of the affection, and, in such cases, the excitability of the spinal cord, and the irritability of the surface, seem sometimes to become as great as they may be observed to be in frogs when narcotized, whom you may then throw into convulsions by merely shaking the table on which they are placed. It is possible that this condition in the infant may be due to a cause not unlike that which produces it in the lower animal. In the latter, it is manifestly due to the influence on the nervous system of blood impregnated with opium; in the former, a similar influence may be exerted by blood the proper depuration of which has been prevented by the frequent recurrence of spasm of the glottis.

There is also another reason for caution in exposing the child to cold or wind, namely, that the occurrence of catarrh is almost sure to be followed by an aggravation of the spasmodic affection. On more than one occasion I have seen the supervention of catarrh convert a very mild into a very serious attack; and once the exacerbation of the symptoms thus produced was the cause of the infant's death.

The parents should in every instance be made fully aware of the uncertainty that attends this affection—of the possibility of death taking place very suddenly and unexpectedly.

In the paroxysm itself but little can be done. Cold water may be dashed on the face, and the fauces may be irritated, or the finger passed down into the pharynx, so as to bring on if possible the effort to vomit, while at the same time the legs and lower part of the body may be placed in a hot bath.

The remarkable observations of MM. Braun and Chiari[1] on the employment of chloroform in puerperal convulsions, and a short paper

[1] Klinik der Geburtshülfe, &c., part ii, p. 249, 8vo. Erlangen, 1853.

by Dr. Simpson, of Edinburgh,[1] on its utility in the convulsions of children, drew my attention to it, and I have tried it extensively, and in many instances with advantage. In cases where depletion is inadmissible, where the convulsions are not obviously due to organic disease of the brain, while they are both severe in their character and are returning with frequency, the inhalation of chloroform sometimes altogether arrests them. It is also of service in attacks of a more chronic kind, in which, though convulsions are less violent, yet the irritability of the nervous system is extreme, and every change of posture, and every attempt at deglutition, are followed either by threatenings of a fit, or by actual convulsions. Its efficient use, however, is not easy to secure, since it requires the constant presence in the house of some one competent to administer it; while if intrusted to the parents or to a nurse, the fears of the former, and the want of intelligence of the latter, generally render its employment merely nominal. Even when most skilfully administered, too, the efficacy of the remedy soon ceases, if from the return of the convulsions, the necessity should arise for its being given at very short intervals. In these circumstances the narcotism soon becomes very partial, and the fits recur altogether unmitigated by it—a result which I have also observed in puerperal convulsions. I have never seen mischief follow from its use; but its power of doing good seems usually to be more evanescent than that of other sedatives.

Of late years we have become acquainted with two remedies, each of which alone, or the two combined, seem sometimes to exert a marvellous power in controlling convulsions, whether accompanied or not by laryngeal spasm. These two remedies are the bromide of potassium, and the hydrate of chloral; and their most remarkable results are produced in cases where there is no ground for suspecting organic disease, and where there are no distinct indications for treatment beyond such as are furnished by the frequent recurrence of the convulsions. Of the two remedies the bromide has appeared to me the more reliable; but in order to obtain decided results from it, it needs to be given in doses larger than those which are commonly employed: as, for instance, from two to three grains every four hours for a child of one year old, and from three to five grains from the age of three to five. If it does not give earnest of good within the first thirty-six hours, there is little use in continuing it, though it may still be persevered with, with the addition of one or two grains of hydrate of choral. The depressing effects of the bromide must not be lost sight of; and either their occurrence, or the failure of the remedy, may compel us to use the choral in similar doses though at an interval of every six or eight, instead of every four hours. I think, however, that on the whole I have obtained the best results from the bromide every four or six hours, accompanied with a single full dose of chloral every night at bedtime.

There are still a few points connected with the derangements of the nervous system in early life, which require a brief notice before I close this lecture. And first, with reference to cases, happily rare, of violent,

---

[1] Obstetric Works, vol. ii, p. 470, from Ed. Monthly Journal, Jan. [illegible]

causeless, and fatal convulsions in early life, independent of disease of the brain. Such attacks are very unusual after the completion of dentition; sometimes they occur without any apparent exciting cause, but more frequently they follow on some slight error in diet, or on slight exposure to the heat of the sun, or on the drying up of some cutaneous eruption, or of some long-existing strumous sore. They are characterized by the violence of the convulsive movements, by the depth of the coma which succeeds to them, and by the very rapid failure of the child's powers. I think, too, it may be said, that convulsions attended by such circumstances warrant more serious apprehension in children of three or four years old, than in infants of a year or eighteen months. For this the reason doubtless is, that at an age when the nervous system is less susceptible than in infancy, an attack of this kind implies a graver disturbance, and one less likely to pass away. Death in these seizures seems to take place, not from sudden asphyxia, as in spasm of the glottis, but from the slower influence of the perpetual disturbance of the respiratory process, or from exhaustion of the nervous power, just as one sees it do in cases of puerperal convulsions; the skin becoming colder, the pulse more feeble after each attack, and complete collapse being induced within twenty-four, sometimes within twelve hours from the first seizure. With reference to the share which is borne by the imperfect aeration of the blood in destroying the patient in some of these cases, M. Trousseau[1] makes some remarks, distinguished by his usual acuteness. He notices that the state is not dissimilar from that of a person on whom tracheotomy has been performed in the extreme period of croup. The obstacle to the entrance of air may have been removed by the operation, but the consequences of the previous long-continued interruption to the aeration of the blood remain, and they gradually destroy life. Just in the same way, the often-repeated convulsions bring with them great disturbance of respiration and circulation, and scarcely is one fit over when a second and a third return, and leave no time for breathing and the heart's action to resume their regular course. "Thus it happens that when at length a state of calm succeeds to the attack, even though respiration may seem to be regular, it is a delusive calm, and the child dies some hours later without any fresh convulsion, without marked oppression, without the appearance of any new symptom of importance. He dies, if I may be allowed to say so, not of actual asphyxia but of the results of asphyxia."

Far less hopeless are cases, with which we also meet occasionally, of the exceedingly frequent recurrence of convulsions; five, ten, or more taking place every day, for days or weeks together. Such attacks are seldom or never met with after the completion of dentition. The danger to life seems to lessen with the frequency of their recurrence, but there is hazard lest they should end by becoming habitual; while, further, there seems to be a very decided relation between the liability to convulsions in early infancy, and the development of epilepsy in subsequent childhood.

One word, in conclusion, with reference to that peculiar form of

---

[1] Clinique Médicale de l'Hôtel Dieu de Paris, 2ieme éd., Paris, 1865, vol. ii, p. 188.

convulsion, to which, from the movements which characterize it, the name of *Eclampsia Nutans*,[1] or the Salaam convulsion, has been given, and in which some observers have thought they recognized the signs of a special disease. Infants and children affected by it bow the head and bend the body slightly forward, a movement which is repeated with great rapidity, sometimes twenty, fifty, or even a hundred times, and then ceases, but returns once or oftener in the twenty-four hours. During the attack the child seems bewildered, but complete consciousness returns as soon as the movements end; and in one case which was under my care, the infant seemed relieved, and quite bright and happy the moment that the movements ceased. In connection with these attacks, there is a general failure of health, and enfeebling of the mental powers, but they do not tend to destroy life, nor are they connected with any special form of cerebral disease, nor have they any invariable issue.

In one instance that came under my observation, the convulsions gradually lost their peculiar character, became like those of the so-called epileptic *petit mal*, and then finally ceased at about the age of three years, after having continued for a year, though not obviously connected either with the process of teething or with its cessation. Their tendency, however, unquestionably is to pass into confirmed epilepsy, and the bowing of the head seldom lasts for more than a few weeks without some other convulsive movement becoming associated with it. Often it is a slight convulsive movement of one or other arm, but attacks of general convulsions occasionally intervene, and at last they take the place almost or altogether of the previous bowings of the head, and the case becomes one of ordinary epilepsy, with in general very considerable impairment of the intellect. Just the same course is observed to be followed by other partial convulsions, though such convulsions seldom attract attention by their singularity to the same extent as the Eclampsia Nutans. Some years ago I saw an infant, seven months old, in whom attacks of an oscillatory movement of the head from side to side came on just in the same manner, and associated with the same impairment of the general health, as usually attends the Salaam convulsion. The rarity of the latter affection, too, consists not in the nature of the movement, but in its frequent repetition, and I have often observed the first sign of incipient epilepsy in the child to be a sudden bowing downwards of the head, instantaneously recovered from, and just attracting notice by the bruising of the forehead, which had struck against a table or a chair. Next this bowing ceases to be confined to the neck, and the child falls forwards on the ground, though still the attack is so momentary, that it rises again immediately, and it sometimes is not until after an attack of general convulsion has awakened the anxiety of relatives, that any meaning begins to be attached to what was long supposed to be merely the effect of a child's

[1] Four cases of this affection were described by Mr. Newnham in the British Record of Obstetric Medicine, March 15, 1849; two are related by Dr. Faber, in J. f. Kinderkr., vol. xiv, p. 260; two by Dr Ebert, Annalen der Charité zu Berlin, 1850; one by Dr. Willshire, at a meeting of the Westminster Medical Society, March, 1851; and probably others may be found in the medical journals.

heedlessness, or of its not having thoroughly learned to walk. Such cases are but a few illustrations of the fact already so often insisted on, that in the study as in the treatment of the diseases of early life, nothing is too trivial to notice—that the slightest occurrences often have the gravest import.

LECTURE XIV.

Epilepsy.—Its causes—Illustrative tables—Its general character and influence on the mind.—Circumstances which must regulate our prognosis—Treatment—Futility of specifics—General management—Employment of belladonna, and of the bromide of potass.

Chorea.—Not exclusively a disease of childhood—Causes which influence its occurrence—Symptoms—Paralytic chorea—Relation to rheumatism, and to heart disease—Theory of embolism as producing it—Treatment—Estimate of various remedies.

We yesterday studied the convulsions of early childhood in their gravest aspect, as immediately threatening life; but a painful interest attaches to them independent of the anxiety which they excite lest they should prove immediately fatal. That is, the dread of their persistence, or of the child being left with his nervous system so shaken that fits may recur at some later period; that convulsions in infancy or childhood may issue in epilepsy in youth or manhood. Nor, indeed, does this seem to be a groundless fear, for of 68 cases which form the basis of M. Herpin's[1] elaborate work on epilepsy, 17 or 25 per cent. date from the first five years of existence; and of 83 cases of which I have a record in young persons under the age of 12 years, 49 dated back to the first four years of life, 28 occurred between the ages of 4 and 10, and 6 between 10 and 12.

TABLE

Showing Age of Patients at Commencement of Attacks of Epilepsy.

Age at Commencement.	Male.	Female.	Total.
Under 6 months, ...	4	4	8
Between 6 and 12 months, . .	6	5	11
" 1 " 2 years, ...	8	7	15
" 2 " 3 "	3	7	10
" 3 " 4 "	4	1	5
" 4 " 5 "	2	4	6
" 5 " 10 "	13	9	22
" 10 " 12 "	3	3	6
	43	40	83

[1] Du Pronostic, &c., de l'Epilepsie, 8vo., Paris, 1852, p. 336.

In the above table the alleged age at the commencement of epilepsy does not represent that at which some isolated convulsion may have occurred, but the age since which there had been a succession of fits coming on at intervals more or less regular, and without the intervention of any fresh exciting cause. It will be seen that in nearly a fifth of the cases the attacks date back to very early infancy, to a time when the ordinary exciting causes of epilepsy have as yet not come into play, when we must seek for the origin of the disorder in some conditions profoundly affecting the general nutrition, not in such as specially act upon the nervous system. But the gravity of those apparently causeless convulsive seizures which sometimes occur in very early infancy is still further seen, if we bear in mind that in many other cases where epilepsy is stated to have come on during dentition, or even at some later period of childhood, it will be found on close inquiry, that many of the patients had suffered from convulsions in early infancy, although a period of months or even of years may have passed without their return; and the very fact may have been forgotten until our inquiries recall it to the parent's recollection.

In 12 of the cases hereditary tendency to epilepsy was admitted to exist;[1] and I have no doubt but that its real frequency is far greater than the friends of our patients admit; and in not a few instances, especially of the earliest occurrence of epilepsy, a strict inquiry will elicit that other children have had fits during teething, or have suffered from chorea; or that mental peculiarities, more or less remarkable, have been observed in different members of the family. A distinct exciting cause for the attack was assigned in 1 only of the 8 cases in which the fits dated back from the first six months of life; and in that instance they were said, with what truth I know not, to have followed inflammation of the brain.

In 41 of the remaining 75 cases, the attacks were said to have been induced

By fright	in 6	instances.
" injury to the head	4	"
" a fall	1	"
" weaning	1	"
" errors in diet	2	"
" gastric disorder	2	"
" vaccination, ...	1	"
" scarlatina, coming on during convalescence,	2	"
" measles, coming on during convalescence,	1	"
" anger, ...	1	"
" first dentition, ...	19	"
" second dentition, ...	1	"

In one of the above cases the epileptic attacks, which came on during the first dentition, ceased with its completion, and did not recur till the commencement of the second dentition, when they returned frequently and severely. This statement of the alleged causes of epilepsy is imperfect, to a great degree no doubt inaccurate, but still the coincidence

[1] Herpin, *op. cit.* p. 328, estimates the frequency of epilepsy at from four to five times greater in the family of epileptics than in the population at large.

of the attacks in 20 of the 41 cases with the active progress of teething deserves to be borne in mind as a fresh illustration of the peculiar excitability of the nervous system at that important period of development.

In the cases on which my remarks are founded I have not included instances of mere epileptic idiots, in whom the occurrence of fits was only a subordinate and often a secondary manifestation of the general disorder of the nervous system. In childhood, however, more surely even and more speedily than in the adult, the return of epileptic attacks impairs, and at length even completely abolishes, the mental powers. In 7 boys and 5 girls the weakness of the mind amounted to idiocy; in the case of 1 girl there were occasional attacks of maniacal excitement; and in 3 other girls epilepsy coexisted with peculiarities of manner and disposition, such as appeared to me to justify their being regarded as instances of moral insanity. In 28 other cases the child was either duller than the average of children of the same age, or, more painful still, the early dawn of intellect was becoming gradually overclouded with the recurrence of the epileptic seizures, and in 6 of these 28 cases the blunting of the mind was associated with perversion of the character, with violence or obstinacy.

I am aware that these results are more unfavorable than those which are commonly obtained in the case of epileptic adults, and am aware also that it has been alleged on high authority that late rather than early epilepsy is favorable to intellectual failure, and that the duration of epilepsy is by itself without influence on the mental condition of the epileptic.[1] It must be borne in mind that my remarks have reference exclusively to epilepsy in childhood, and that I do not profess to have any such experience as would justify me in speaking about it in the adult. There seems to me, however, to be a very obvious and very sufficient reason for the speedier and graver deterioration of the moral and intellectual character in the young than in the adult epileptic, furnished by the undeveloped state of the nervous system in early life. It stands a shock less well, it bears graver marks of injury in proportion as the shock and the injury are earlier inflicted; while, on the other hand, it may well be that late in life the opposite cause may produce a similar effect, just as one often sees that the two extremes of youth and age appear morally and physically to touch each other. My belief indeed is—and it is this which attaches the gravest import to the apparently causeless occurrence and causeless return of fits in infancy and childhood—that in proportion as epilepsy comes on early will the chances of its being associated with serious disorder of the mind be increased. M. Cazauvieilh,[2] in his elaborate essay on the connection between epilepsy and insanity, states as the result of a comparsion between 26 female epileptics in whom the disease preceded menstruation, and 26 in whom its occurrence succeeded it, that in 19 of the former, and in only 10 of the latter, it was associated with insanity. This fact is always to be borne in mind when consulted about

[1] Dr. Reynolds, in his System of Medicine, vol. ii, 2d ed., 1872, p. 312.
[2] Archives Gén. de Médecine, Janvier, 1826, p. 43.

a case of epilepsy in early life, since it obviously must exercise a great influence upon our prognosis.

To the best of my knowledge, the general characters of epilepsy in childhood agree closely with those which it presents in after-life. I have observed the *petit mal*, as it is termed, continue in children for a period of several months, and finally issue in regular epileptic seizures. In the child, I have sometimes noticed the loss of consciousness during the seizure to be imperfect, and this in spite of very marked convulsive movements; fits with complete insensibility occurring occasionally in the same patient, and being of longer duration though not attended with a greater amount of convulsion, than those in which the loss of consciousness was incomplete. In one instance, attacks of apparently causeless alarm, accompanied by much excitement and incoherent talking, passed in the course of a few months into regular epileptic seizures; in another instance, a girl, who came under my care at the age of 10 years and 10 months, had had an attack of general convulsions when 8 years old, for which no cause could be assigned. Since that time she had been liable to occasional attacks of strange excitement of manner; and these had for six months been attended with a sort of cataleptic condition, in which she stood motionless for a minute or two, wildly staring at vacancy, and uttering a few incoherent words, which apparently had reference to some object she saw, though she could never be induced to describe her imaginings. Eleven months after the commencement of these attacks their peculiar character disappeared, and she began to have regular epileptic seizures, while, in the intervals, her actions and manner, though often rational enough, were frequently those of an insane person. In a boy aged 9, in whom for a year epileptic fits had occurred causelessly, and with a rapidly increasing frequency, until at length three or four came on weekly, and sometimes more than one in a day, a sort of maniacal excitement seized him occasionally, in which he struck other children, though they had given him no provocation. These manifestations of mental disorder are precisely analogous to the momentary delirium observed in the epileptic adult, during which the patient commits some act of gross impropriety, or attacks his friends or attendants, or some bystander, with savage fury, and recovers his consciousness a minute or two afterwards, to learn with horror the act which he has committed.[1] They are, as might be expected, most observable in cases in which epilepsy has not come on till about 5 or 6 years of age, or somewhat later: the convulsions which date from early infancy lead to a more complete obscuring of the mind, and the cases in which they have occurred often present themselves to us as instances of idiocy complicated with epilepsy, rather than as cases of epilepsy producing disorder of the mind by their frequent return. I do not know that the age of the patient makes any important difference in the characters of the epileptic seizure. They

[1] With reference to the relation between epilepsy and affection of the mind, there are some important observations by M. Trousseau in his Clinique Médicale, 2d ed., vol. ii, pp. 69–79; and by M. Falret, in Archives de Méd., 1860, vol. ii, p. 661; 1861, vol. i, p. 461, and vol. ii, p. 421.

seem to be the same, in all essentials, in the child as in the adult. The aura epileptica is often described of their own accord by children; though many are of course too young to explain their sensations, and others, with the strange tendency to exaggeration which one often observes in early life, seeing that their story is listened to with attention, will dress it up with such details as to their young imagination seem most wonderful. In some cases the attacks begin invariably with convulsive movements of one limb. Thus, in a little boy who was some time since in the hospital, the attacks always began with painful convulsive movements of the right hand, which he seized with the left and endeavored to keep still. In a few seconds or a minute these movements ceased; the tonic spasm came on, and then the general convulsive movements as in an ordinary epileptic seizure. These peculiarities seldom last for very long: sometimes for a season one limb is habitually the first to be affected, sometimes another; or the fits invariably predominate on one side, and then, with no other change in the patient's condition, the attack will commence in another limb, or predominate on the other side. Stupor more or less continued, or a heavy sleep, usually follows the attack, but now and then a state of excitement precedes the sleep; a noisy delirium which, but for the tender age of the patient, would be identical with the temporary mania that sometimes follows the epileptic seizure in the adult, and renders him for the time one of the most dangerous class of insane patients.

The question is often put to us in practice as to the probability of fits terminating in epilepsy; or, on the other hand, as to the ground for hope in any case that epileptic attacks which have already frequently recurred will eventually cease.[1] With reference to neither of these inquiries, however, are we in possession of data such as to enable us to give an answer with much certainty. I do not think that those fits of which spasm of the glottis is a prominent symptom, often pass into confirmed epilepsy; long-continued struggling is not a characteristic of them, but more often drowsiness or stupor immediately succeeding to the fits, and heaviness and dulness continuing for some hours after them. It is not the violence of a single fit, nor even the frequent return of fits for a limited time, which warrants the gravest apprehension. It is the recurrence of fits when all observable cause of irritation has passed away; it is their return when the patient is otherwise apparently in perfect health; and hence it is that the statement has been made that attacks of the *petit mal* warrant a graver prognosis than the violent convulsion. As to the prospect of epileptic seizures ceasing at puberty, I fear that the hope is a very groundless one. It is scarcely to be expected that a new period of development should be attended by anything else than a fresh excitement, and an increased disturbance of the nervous system; so that there is more reason for anticipating a deterioration in the patient's condition, than for expecting

---

[1] I am averse to referring to my own writings, but want of room for saying more here compels me to refer to my Lumleian Lectures, "On Some Disorders of the Nervous System in Childhood," 8vo., London, 1871, for further remarks with reference to these and kindred subjects.

an improvement from the changes of puberty. It is true, that if epilepsy comes on while dentition is in active progress, we may hope for, though we cannot with certainty calculate on amendment when teething is accomplished; and though I have no statistics bearing on the subject, yet my impression is, that I have oftener known epilepsy cease spontaneously between the fourth and sixth years than at any other period. In the same way, if epilepsy occurs during the changes that usher in puberty, we may look forward with some degree of cheerfulness to the time when all of those changes shall have been completed. In each of these cases, however, it is not the period of excitement, but the season of repose, on which our hopes are founded; while, to leave the case untreated, in the vague expectation of what at a certain critical epoch of life the healing power of nature may be able to effect, would be to trifle alike with our own reputation and with our patient's prospects of recovery. The first point in every case is obvioulsy to make out, if possible, the cause on which the fits depend; or to ascertain by the most minute observation and inquiry, the peculiarities of health with which their occurrence is associated. The diet, the bodily exercise, the mental pursuits, all need the most rigid investigation: the condition of the bowels, the state of the evacuations, require to be most carefully examined; and the fact of the first dentition having been accomplished is no adequate reason for omitting to watch the process of teething most sedulously. I have seen one or two instances in which convulsive attacks of an epileptic character attended the cutting of the permanent molar teeth; and illustrations of this fact (to which Dr. Ashburner[1] was the first to call attention) are to be found in all our medical journals. In proportion as the fits admit of being traced with probability to causes of a remediable character, may our prognosis be favorable. The severity of the fits is a matter of less importance with reference to prognosis than the frequency of their occurrence; and the oftener they recur, even in a mild form, or the more frequent their forebodings, such as dizziness, or momentary stupor, the less is the prospect of their cessation. In forming our prognosis, also, regard must be had to the state of the child's mind in the intervals between the fits; and the less the intellect seems to be dulled, or the moral faculties perverted, the more encouraging may be our opinion. In judging of this last point it is well to bear in mind that a child who has been liable to any such affection is almost sure to be backward in learning; very likely to be wayward in temper, for his friends will have been afraid to overtax him with work; and they will probably, from fear of crossing him, have indulged many of his caprices. We must judge of his intellect, less by the child's amount of actual knowledge, than by his power of answering simple questions concerning things familiar to him; and must draw our conclusion as to the state of his moral faculties from his general childlike character, his fondness for the same pursuits, his showing the same dispositions, manifesting similar attachments, having similar good and bad qualities to those

[1] In his work On Dentition and its Coincident Disorders, 12mo. London, 1834.

which we observe in other children of his own age, or a few years younger.

With reference to the *treatment* of epilepsy, I know of no specific for it; and the much-vaunted oxide of zinc has proved as powerless in my hands as in those of most who have tried it on the strength of the high encomiums bestowed on it by M. Herpin. I fear, indeed, that it will not be in the search for specifics that we shall light upon the appropriate treatment of a disorder which depends upon causes so almost numberless as epilepsy. We meet every now and then with cases in which some profound impression on the nervous system has been followed by temporary cessation of the fits, and with others in which they seem under the influence of such a cause to have been permanently cured; but the difficulty is how to apply such observations in practice. A girl, aged 10 years, was admitted into the Children's Hospital, suffering from epilepsy, fits of which occurred about seven times in a week. These fits were said to have affected her for a considerable time, though the history given of her was very imperfect. After a month's stay in the hospital, during which time 24 fits occurred, she was attacked by typhoid fever of a mild character, accompanied by abundant rash, but which ran its course in 21 days, unattended by any complication. During the whole course of the fever the fits completely ceased; but on the 31st day from the first complaint of frontal headache and first accession of fever the fits returned, assumed their former severity, and returned afterwards with their former frequency. A boy, 10 years old, suffered from occasional attacks of *petit mal* in February. In the following August the attacks became regular epileptic seizures, which increased in frequency, and in the succeeding March returned several times in a day, and were accompanied by marked impairment of his mental powers and by an unsteady and tottering gait. After a two months' trial of various remedies, and the insertion of a seton in the back of his neck, he left the hospital worse than on his admission. On June 13th he fell in a fit, and struck his occiput a violent blow. A large abscess formed there, which burst of its own accord, continued discharging for a few days, and then healed up. I saw the boy again two years after this accident had happened, and there had then been no return of fits; but the boy had regained his power of walking, and had all the intelligence and cheerfulness that befitted his years. These cases are of interest, they forbid us to despair even when there seems least ground for hope; but I fear they give us little help in our search after remedies, for how are we to obtain any therapeutic agent as far reaching as the poison of typhoid fever, which yet exerted but a temporary influence, or how can we safely imitate the profound shock of the accident concerning which, too, we do not know whether its salutary influence was due to the blow or to the suppuration that followed it? There is of course the most ground for hope, and the fairest opportunity for treatment, when the attacks can be referred to any obvious, or even probable exciting cause. Our first attempts must be directed to its removal; and, according to its nature, depletion may or may not be indicated; or the administration of alterative or purgative medicines may be desirable, and now and then some wisely chosen remedy may in these circumstances remove, almost as if by magic, the cause and its effect together. Unfortunately, however, in a large number of instances, no definite cause is discoverable, and we are thrown entirely upon general principles for the regulation of our conduct. As violent and sudden excitement of any kind will often bring on an epileptic seizure, so the influence of the opposite condition in warding off its attacks is very remarkable; and on several occasions I have received patients into the Children's Hospital, who were reported to have epileptic seizures several times in a day, and who nevertheless remained a fortnight or more in the institution without any attack coming on. The disorder, however, was not cured, but only kept in check by the regularity of the gentle rule to which the little ones are subjected. The order goes for much in these cases; the novelty goes for something too, for almost invariably I have found that after a time the apparent improvement became less marked, and though they continued better than when they first came to the hospital, the children were still epileptic: the advance of the disease had been retarded, but its progress had not been arrested. The quiet which suits the epileptic is not the quiet of listless, apathetic idleness, but the judicious alternation of tranquil occupation and amusement. The mind must not be left to slumber, from the apprehension of work bringing on a fit, but the work must as far as possible be such as to interest the child. It is an observation often made, that adult epileptics who follow dangerous trades, as that of a bricklayer, for instance, scarcely ever have attacks when occupied in their pursuit; and children are rarely seized when at play, but oftenest either when in bed at night, or before getting up in the morning, or when sitting quiet in the evening, tired and unoccupied. The good results, too, which I hear have followed the introduction of gymnastic exercises among the epileptic patients at the Bicêtre, in Paris, point in the same direction. In the occupations of epileptics, therefore, pursuits which not merely employ the mental faculties, but also give work to the hands, such as gardening, carpentering, or the tending of animals, are especially to be recommended; and if by these the mind can be kept awake, the grand object of teaching is answered, and backwardness in reading, writing, or those kinds of knowledge which other children at the same age have acquired, is of very little moment. Many epileptics have an indistinct articulation, and almost all have a slouching gait and an awkward manner. The former can often be corrected to a considerable degree by teaching the child simple chants, which are almost always easily acquired, and practiced with pleasure. The latter may be rectified by drilling, not carried into tedious minutiæ, but limited to simple movements, and the irksomeness of drill is almost completely done away with by music; while I believe that the accustoming a child to the strict control and regulation of all its voluntary movements is of very great importance indeed as a curative agent. Many of these measures could be much better carried out in class than by a child alone, and whatever may seem at first to be the objections to the association of epileptics, I have no doubt but that they would be more than compensated for by its advantages. Epileptic children cannot be educated with such as are healthy for the sake of the latter, but at least equally so for their own; since the different regulations to which they must be subjected, the difference in their education, their amusements, and often in their diet, would be to them a source of ceaseless distress. If educated alone, however, not only do they lose all the advantages of association with other children, though both intellectually and morally this is of great moment, but also they become, far too obviously for their own benefit, the centre around which everything in the household turns, while rules become doubly irksome when apparently made for themselves alone, and not part of a general system to which others besides have to submit. These advantages, however, are not at present to be obtained, and we are compelled to put up with the more imperfect carrying out of our directions, either at the patient's home, or, still better, under the superintendence of some competent person who devotes the whole of his time to the care of the child.

The diet should be mild, nutritious, but usually unstimulating, and as a general rule, should include meat comparatively seldom, and in small quantities. I have certainly seen epileptic fits increased both in frequency and severity by an abundant meat diet, and diminished in both respects when a diet chiefly of milk and vegetables was adopted.[1] This diet, however, must not be adopted invariably, nor in disregard of the patient's general symptoms. In feeble children with cool skin, soft pulse, languid manner, and deficient energy, a generous diet with wine, and the mineral acids with quinine, or small doses of zinc or iron, have certainly proved of service, not only in improving the general health, but even in lessening the frequency of the occurrence of the fits. When the approach of a fit has been usually preceded by stupor, or headache, or drowsiness, I think that I have sometimes warded off its occurence by putting a few leeches on the head; but epilepsy is not to be cured by systematic bleeding, nor by systematic purging, nor, I may repeat, by any of the various medicines which at different times have been employed for its cure, and the very number of which is perhaps the best proof that could be adduced of the inefficacy of all.

There are two remedies which must not be passed over without some special notice—belladonna and bromide of potassium, the latter of which seems indeed to have cast the former into the shade, and to have led to its passing for a time at least into scarcely merited forgetfulness. The action of the bromide is decidedly much more speedy and much more remarkable when it is exerted at all than that of belladonna. It seldom indeed fails within the first few days of its administration to arrest the frequency of the attacks, and now and then it has seemed entirely to prevent them; and the crucial test of

[1] My attention was first drawn to the importance of abstinence from a meat diet in epileptics by Dr. Maxwell, formerly resident physician to the Asylum for Idiots. This caution, too, gains still greater weight from the testimony of Dr. Jackson, of Boston, in America, who, in his Letters to a Young Physician, 12mo., Boston, U. S., 1855, p. 67, insists very strongly on its importance. As already stated, I have little faith in the influence of mere drugs; but I have a yearly increasing confidence in the influence of diet, judicious management, and mental and moral as well as physical hygiene in epilepsy occurring in early life, independent of hereditary predisposition, and unconnected with approaching puberty.

arresting fits by bromide of potass, of suspending the remedy and seeing the fits return, and of once more putting a stop to them by the resumption of the medicine, has on some occasions established its value beyond question. This result has been arrived at by me more frequently in cases of persistent, frequently repeated infantile convulsions than in the distinct epilepsy of childhood, though even here I have had some few apparent successes. In the great majority of cases the amendment, though very marked at first, has not entirely maintained itself; the system has after a time become habituated to the remedy, and after several augmentations of the dose, each of which has seemed to renew the old influence, I have been compelled to discontinue it in consequence of the depression of the pulse, the general loss of power, and the appearance of the peculiar pustular eruption which occasionally follows its long-continued use. In other cases, too, the agent which at first worked wonders ceased to have any influence. The constitution tolerated the increased dose, but so did the disease; the patient continued to take the medicine, but the fits, though once controlled, returned after a time just as before.

Still, with all these drawbacks, the bromide remains the only agent which in my hands has made the least approach to the character of a specific. I always employ it when I can find no distinct indication to guide me. I confess that I use it empirically, for I have found no means by which to distinguish beforehand the cases where the bromide will do permanent good from the other apparently similar but much more common instances in which its influence is merely temporary.

The action of belladonna is much slower, and its results, I fear, are also much more uncertain than even those of the bromide, for all that M. Trousseau could allege in its favor was that he had been "less unsuccessful with it than with any other remedy." I have once seen epileptic seizures of the most marked character and of daily recurrence in a boy of 9 years of age cease under the use of belladonna when they had been entirely uninfluenced by bromide of potass, and I have also seen the frequency of the return of fits diminished under its steady and long-continued use, the best results being apparently obtained by its long-continued administration in small doses for months, not by its employment in large or in rapidly increasing doses.[1]

But if the cause of epilepsy is so deeply seated that it yields so rarely to even the most powerful remedies, it may be inquired whether there are no means of mitigating the severity, or of warding off the occurrence of individual attacks. Something, though I fear not very much, may be accomplished. It suffices occasionally, in attacks of the *petit mal*, to call to the patient in order to cut short at once the condition which might otherwise last for half a minute, and even after actual convulsions have begun to characterize the epileptic fit, I have, in children, seen it equally arrested in the same way. A certain attitude in bed will sometimes bring on a fit on the child waking from sleep, and its careful avoidance will postpone the occurrence. The principles

[1] See, with reference to the use and administration of belladonna in epilepsy, the remarks of M. Trousseau in his Clinique Médicale, 2d ed., vol. ii, p. 95.

implied in suddenly arousing the attention, and thus stopping the fit, may be carried further, and the immediate application of a tight ligature, as a twisted handkerchief, for instance, around the arm or leg, will sometimes entirely arrest a commencing fit, though more frequently it will only postpone it for a few minutes. It is on the same principle that cold water thrown in the face will sometimes retard a fit, or even prevent it, and so long as any of these measures check or mitigate the attacks, they may be persevered in. A trial of chloroform naturally suggests itself to us as a means of mitigating the severity of the attacks. Its influence is too slow to prevent the seizure, for, as you know, to the momentary bewilderment succeeds the tonic spasm, and on that follows the convulsion with the imperfect respiratory movements that attend it, during which the lungs are filled but imperfectly, and the inhalation of chloroform must be very incomplete. Usually, therefore, a convulsive attack would pass away of its own accord long before the influence of the anæsthetic had been produced. In long-continued convulsions, however, I know of no objection to its use, and it certainly is something gained if we can control the violent convulsions, and secure thereby the better peformance of respiration—ends which we can usually attain, though I have found that with each repetition of the chloroform its influence becomes harder to produce, and tends to pass away more quickly.

One last caution I still have to offer with reference to cases where either convulsions have occurred with frequency in infancy, or where actual epileptic seizures, having occurred several times, appear to have ceased for months or even for years. A cause so slight as to seem inadequate to lead to so grave a result will waken the dormant evil, and awaken it to slumber no more. A sudden fright, a fall, the disorder produced by neglect or constipation, a little overstrain of the mind in the endeavor to make up for lost time, will suffice to disturb the balance of the nervous system and to reproduce the fits. You walk on hidden fires; I know not how to avoid the danger which in each case arises from a different source. I can but warn you and urge you to warn the patients' friends of its existence.

Almost every lecture has furnished some fresh illustration of that connection between the development of an organ, or of a set of organs, and their liability to disorder, which characterizes the diseases of early life. The growing brain is readily overfilled with blood, readily emptied of it; cerebral congestion, cerebral hemorrhage are frequent, and so is the opposite state of anæmia, producing as we have seen the signs of spurious hydrocephalus. The balance is so easily disturbed between the different parts of the nervous system, that convulsions occur with a frequency proportionate to the tender years of the patient, assuming all sorts of strange forms; now threatening life in one way, now in another, destroying the child suddenly by spasmodic closure of its glottis, or exhausting it by their violence and their ceaseless return; or, lastly, working a change so subtle that the knife of the anatomist cannot detect it, and yet so serious as to induce their perpetual recurrence, and to convert the once bright and hopeful child into the dull and all but hopeless epileptic.

But we have not yet completed our survey of this class of affections, for there are various forms of impairment of the motor power which are still unnoticed, ailments which indeed rarely threaten life or permanently disturb the mental faculties, but which are yet tedious in their progress, often distressing in their character, and difficult of cure. I shall reserve for another lecture those cases in which there is mere loss of power over a limb, or over some of its muscles, and will now notice those in which that power is imperfectly exercised, in which the will no longer exerts its full control, but the muscles of some parts are left in a state of involuntary activity, though still performing imperfectly their proper duties.

The characters just enumerated are those which mark a disorder with which you are doubtless all familiar, the *Chorea Sancti Viti*, or *St. Vitus's Dance*. It is, however, by no means one of the most frequent affections of early childhood; but its occurrence coincides, as the subjoined table[1] shows, rather with that period of development which intervenes between the second dentition and the completion of the changes that attend on puberty.

Age.	Male.	Female.	Total.
At or under 4 years, ...	4	6	10
More than 4, but not exceeding 6 years,	22	11	33
" 6, " " 10 "	64	142	206
" 10, " " 15 "	87	220	307
Total, ...	177	379	556

It must also be added, that the liability to chorea does not cease entirely with the completion of the changes that accompany puberty, but that it has been computed that a fourth of all cases of it occur during adult life. I believe, indeed, though I cannot prove, that this estimate of the frequency of chorea in the adult is exaggerated, while when it does occur in the grown person, it is probably due either to the influence of some grave internal inflammation, such as pericarditis or endocarditis, or to that peculiar state of the constitution which gives rise to rheumatism, or to both these causes combined, or else to some far-reaching cause which acts on and disturbs the whole nervous system, such, for instance, as the state of pregnancy.

The reason of the greater rarity of chorea in early childhood than subsequently is, I apprehend, to be found in the circumstance that with the progress of growth and the increase of strength the nervous system becomes less impressionable, and the causes which in the infant would have produced a fit, or would have given rise to that more chronic form of convulsive disorder of which spasm of the glottis is a common ac-

[1] Deduced from the cases reported by Dr. Hughes, in Guy's Hospital Reports, Second Series, vol. iv, 1846; by M. Rufz, in Archives de Médecine, February, 1834; and from the statistics of M. Wicke, as reported by Romberg, Nervenkrankheiten, vol. ii, part 2, p. 177.

companiment, no longer produce such grave results. They do not endanger life, they do not even abolish consciousness, but they shake the control of the will over the voluntary movements, and produce chorea. As the boy grows older, his liability to all convulsive diseases diminishes; and as the girl grows older, hers lessens too, but not to the same extent. In her, disorders of a milder kind show themselves with a frequency from which the boy's hardier frame altogether defends him; and chorea occurs only as one form of disturbance of the nervous system, having reference to an earlier stage of development than that at which hysteria commonly appears, when, in connection with the first performance and first consciousness of new functions and a new destiny, the mind and the emotions participate in disorders previously limited to the motor powers.

The attack of chorea is sometimes excited by a violent shock to the nervous system, such as a fright, a blow, or some sudden violent emotion; but even in those cases it is comparatively seldom that it occurs in children previously in perfect health, and the attack of chorea, as far as my observation goes, has never come on until after the lapse of

TABLE

Showing the Age and Sex of 1141 *patients brought to the Children's Hospital suffering from Chorea.*

Age.	Male.	Female.	Total.
At or under 4 years,	21	36	57
Between 4 and 5 years,	19	35	54
" 5 " 6 "	26	45	71
" 6 " 7 "	46	63	109
" 7 " 8 "	38	104	142
" 8 " 9 "	56	132	188
" 9 " 10 "	66	155	221
" 10 " 12 "	75	224	299
	347	794	1141

several days from the action of its alleged exciting cause. For the most part, whether one can point to a distinct exciting cause or no, there has been some previous failure of the general health; such as at an earlier age would have ushered in a fit of convulsions, or an attack of spasm of the glottis. In many instances, too, a minute inquiry into the child's previous history, or into that of his family, will show a special liability to exist to convulsive affections, to chorea, or to epilepsy. The preponderating frequency of its occurrence in girls is but another expression of the same fact, namely, of its association with special excitability of the nervous system.

Just as hysteria, too, comparatively seldom occurs in the robust, but is usually connected with some marked disorder of nutrition, such as anæmia or chlorosis, so, as I have stated, in almost all cases of chorea the commencement of its symptoms is preceded by failing health, by constipation, or by some other form of disorder of the digestive system, or even by some disease intimately connected with defects in the blood-formation, as rheumatism, or one of the eruptive fevers, most frequently the former.

The approaches of the disorder are for the most part very gradual. It is first noticed that the child has certain awkward, fidgety movements, which it seems unable to check; or which, at any rate, it repeats almost constantly, though they may cease for a few moments. On closer watching, it is next observed that these movements are almost or altogether confined to one side, and generally to the arm, the leg being at first almost always unaffected; but my own observations do not confirm the statement that there is any preponderating frequency of affection of the right side either at the commencement or in any stage of chorea. In a few days the leg becomes the seat of these movements also, and the child in consequence stumbles or falls occasionally in walking. Now, too, if not previously, the muscles of the face participate in the irregular movements, and the child almost constantly makes the strangest grimaces, and soon, with very rare exceptions, the affection ceases to be limited to one side, but both legs and both arms, and at length all the muscles of the trunk, become involved.

It is almost impossible to describe the condition of a chorea patient exactly, so much does it vary according to the intensity of the disease in different cases, and so much also in the same case at different times. Excitement increases the movements, fixed attention to any object usually quiets them, while even when severe they generally, though not invariably, cease during sleep.

In some instances the ailment never passes beyond a comparatively mild form; inability to hold objects steadily in the hand, or to keep one or both arms from an occasional twitching movement, with slight momentary distortion of the muscles of the face, or spasmodic motion of the head, being all that is apparent. If the disorder is more severe, both sides are almost invariably affected; the patient is unable to grasp any object, or, holding it for a moment or two, drops it from the hand, which with the greatest effort of will he is yet unable to keep closed. At the same time his gait is so unsteady that attempts to walk are dangerous, or sometimes the power over the legs is so imperfect that the child is quite unable to stand. The face is not merely constantly distorted, but, if the child is desired to show his tongue, he puts it out with difficulty, hurriedly, and imperfectly, while, owing to the affection of its muscles, articulation is stammering and almost unintelligible, and deglutition is also performed difficultly and by sudden gulps. The movements still continue even when the child is lying in bed; those of the lower extremities, indeed, are often most marked in the horizontal position. In the worst cases the intellect is generally dulled, and the child's manner almost idiotic, while if the illness, though not very severe, is yet of long continuance, there is often an imbecility of manner over and above what may be due to the child's inability to control its movements or to articulate with distinctness. My own impression is, that in almost all cases, those alone excepted in which the attack is slight and of very short duration, there is a temporary dulling of the intellect, and instances are sometimes met with where the weakness of the mind is quite out of proportion to the severity of the movements.[1] Now and then the patient's condition is most distressing. It was so in a little girl whom I saw some years ago in the Children's Hospital at Paris. All the muscles of her body were affected; her spine was often bent back in an extreme degree of opisthotonos, while her movements were so violent and so incessant, that it was necessary to place a board three feet in height around her bed to keep her from throwing herself over its edge, and by the violent grinding of her jaws together she had forced almost all her teeth from their sockets.

The violence of the movements of necessity greatly exhausts the muscular power, but there are also cases of chorea in which the loss of power is from the first quite out of proportion to the amount of muscular movement. We know such cases at the Children's Hospital as cases of *limp chorea*, a very good name, which one of our house surgeons gave them, and which describes them as well as the more scientific term of *paralytic chorea*.

In January, 1872 a little girl of excitable temperament, who had had slight twitchings of her limbs for 3 months, which had become more marked for six weeks since a sudden fright, was admitted into the Children's Hospital. The movements thus suddenly increased had again greatly lessened, but in spite of that apparent improvement she had become more and more helpless, and at length could neither stand nor feed herself, nor even talk. The child was fairly nourished, but she lay in bed like a log, quite helpless and sweating profusely, unable to sit up, unable to speak, unable to feed herself, and even when food was put into her mouth it often rolled out again. Her grasp was so weak as scarcely to be felt, her tongue could be protruded only for an instant; her pulse was 120, feeble, and very irregular, and there was an occasional prolongation of the heart's first sound. For a fortnight her state continued almost stationary; she could not indeed be said to be aphasic, for she tried to shape her lips to the sound; but nothing came but the faintest whisper, and usually she was voiceless. By very slow degrees and under the use of Nux Vomica, whether in consequence of it I cannot say, she improved; at the end of 10 weeks she went out, walking very slowly and quietly, and in the country she gradually regained her strength.

Nor are cases such as this of extreme rarity; oftener they are less severe, but sometimes more so, and I have even seen a loss of power for a few days almost as complete as in diphtheritic paralysis. But the power is scarcely ever permanently lost, though sometimes it is very long in being regained. Sometimes too the involuntary movements

[1] See with reference to the mental state of patients suffering from chorea, the discussion in the Académie de Médecine on occasion of a paper on the subject by M. Marcé The hallucinations and the maniacal delirium with which that gentleman appears sometimes to have met, are probably in part due to his field of observation having been a peculiar one, in the Bicêtre and the Salpêtrière, in part to the coexistence of hysteria in some of the cases. My own impression, however, coincides very closely with the opinion of M. Trousseau, who regards disturbance of the intellectual powers as occurring in the greater number of cases of chorea. Bulletin de l'Académie, 1861, April 12, July 5 and 19. See also Trousseau's Clinique Médicale de l'Hôtel-Dieu, vol. ii, p. 139.

have been so slight as not to have attracted the notice of the friends, and the affection perhaps being partial, the child who drags one leg or who uses one arm imperfectly and difficultly is supposed to be paralyzed; and his condition causes great and needless anxiety. The same too may be said about the impairment of the intellect, to which I just now referred, and also to the loss of the power of speech which is sometimes a real aphasia; not silence owing to the difficulty of articulation. Both are but temporary states, though there is no rule by which their duration is governed; one child remaining dull and listless and foolish for weeks after movements have ceased, the other brightening as soon as the movements have lessened, and long before power has returned to the limbs. In the same way the power of speech is sometimes lost; and that neither in proportion to the affection of the muscles which subserve it, nor to the degree of general intellectual dulness; but the memory of words for the time is lost, and the child will labor in search of words to convey the ideas with which its little brain is busy; will look wistfully around as if for help; and then despairingly give up the effort; and yet day by day return to it at intervals till the power comes back again, sometimes by degrees as one may have heard a little bird strive to recover the lost notes of a tune it had been taught, sometimes all at once as a forgotten dream flashes back without effort on our memory.

I might, if I had the time, say much more about chorea in its various phases of violent uncontrollable movement, of impaired muscular power, dulled intellect, and sometimes temporary loss of speech. But there are two complications of the disease so important with reference to our prognosis, and with reference also to our theories as to the nature of the affection, that I must stop to consider them. The first of these complications is rheumatism, the second, disease of the heart: and often, though not always, the two conditions are associated.

The late Dr. Hughes was, I believe, one of the first who drew attention to the existence of a distinct relation between rheumatism and chorea, but it was M. Sée[1] who pointed out how intimate this relation is, and who adduced figures in support of his statement. He alleged that of 109 cases of rheumatism admitted into the Hôpital des Enfants 61 were complicated with chorea. Still more decided is the opinion of M. Roger, justified as every opinion is which he ever expresses by an amount of careful observation and minute clinical research which is all but conclusive.[2] He regards chorea and the heart affection with which it is frequently associated as but another manifestation of rheumatism; he believes that rheumatism does more than predispose to, that it actually produces it, that indeed it is the common cause of chorea, which is a rheumatic symptom just as much as the pains in the limbs or the swelling of the joints, or the inflammation of the endocardium; and, as he justly observes, this view renders the prognosis in chorea far graver than it used to be considered, and brings with it

[1] Mémoires de l'Académie de Médecine, vol. xv.
[2] In the Archives de Médecine, 1866 and 1867.

important practical modifications in the treatment of what used once to be regarded as a mere neurosis.

It has been contended, however, that these statements are too absolute, as is shown by the fact that rheumatism is very frequent in places where chorea is very rare;[1] that even in the same conditions the frequency of chorea and rheumatism is governed by a different law,[2] and that the coincidence of chorea with acute rheumatism is of extreme rarity.[3]

My own notes show 35 out of 93 cases of chorea in children under 12 years of age, in whom the chorea was preceded by rheumatism, sometimes immediately, sometimes several weeks or even months before, and in 4 instances the rheumatism followed scarlatina. In 2 more instances, rheumatism, once preceded by scarlatina, came on during the decline of chorea. The chorea did not in these two instances seem to be modified by the acute disease, though it was in both associated with very grave affection of the heart, but the movements ceased gradually in the course of the convalescence. I have not included in this statement cases where there was merely a rheumatic diathesis in the family, since it may in several instances not have been noted; and I further suspect that my numbers understate the frequency of the rheumatic complication, since I find that my later observations yield a much higher average than the earlier.

But in addition to the cases of distinct rheumatism, 27 in number, in 16 of which there was evidence of heart affection, there were 12 others in which affection of the heart existed independent of any past or present evidence of rheumatism. M. Roger indeed would add these to the other cases, and regard them as instances of rheumatism of the heart, which may exist without equally as well as in conjunction with articular rheumatism. In the majority of cases the heart disease preceded the chorea, but I have observed a very slight and occasional murmur become both loud and permanent in the course of chorea, and have watched the advance of heart disease, and the progress of dilatation take place while the child was confined to bed by the violence of the choreic movements. It has indeed occurred to me to ask myself whether in some of these cases the heart affection may not be due to the disturbance of the organ in its attempts at regular contraction rather than to trouble directly produced by the increase of valvular disease, which in many instances even as shown by post-mortem examination is comparatively small in degree.[4] I must further add, that while mere irregularity of the heart's action may be an occasional and temporary attendant on chorea, a distinct bruit is almost always permanent, and is neither a hæmic murmur, nor a sound "plausibly ascrib-

---

[1] Lombard and Rilliet [illegible] Traité des Maladies des Enfants [illegible] vol. ii. p. 565.

[2] Blache, Mémoires de l'Académie de Médecine, vol. xix. p. [illegible]

[3] Radcliffe, in Reynolds's System of Medicine, [illegible] that while chorea may [illegible] and Steiner, in Prager Viertel[illegible] as being so rare as 4 [illegible] cases.

[4] Dr. Tuckwell, in [illegible]

able to disordered action of the muscular apparatus connected with the valve."

These facts concerning the concurrence of rheumatism and of cardiac disease with chorea whether accepted to the full extent, or whether received subject to those exceptions which some, and I confess that I am of that number, would make to their universal application, add greatly to the gravity of our prognosis. But they do more; for they have suggested a theory of the disorder in support of which strong evidence and much ingenious reasoning have been adduced. The late lamented Dr. Kirkes first propounded the hypothesis of embolism, as explaining by the irritation of the nerve centres from detached fine molecules of fibrin, the production of the disorder. Dr. Hughlings Jackson[1] has tried to advance this theory a step further, and to prove that plugging of the minute vessels of the convolutions near the corpus striatum is the cause of the affection, the tissues not being absolutely destroyed, as in the case of hemiplegia, but undernourished owing to a deficient supply of blood.

Now this theory rests partly on the results of microscopic observations, and these I do not venture to criticize; and can but regret the world of curious scientific research into which I am unskilled to follow. But it seems to me that if propounded as of universal application, the following weighty considerations may be urged against it.

1st. The occasional occurrence of chorea from mere imitation, so that we have sometimes been compelled to change the position of patients in the Children's Hospital from observing the involuntary mimicry by one child of the movements of another.

2d. The extreme rarity of a sudden attack of chorea; the great slowness with which it almost invariably comes on.

3d. The very small number of the instances in which chorea continues limited to one side; and the comparatively short time within which hemichorea almost always becomes bilateral.

4th. The almost invariable recovery of complete power over all the limbs in cases of chorea, and this even in instances where the paralytic character of the symptoms has most predominated; so that I have only two or three times in my life met with cases in which permanent loss of power over a limb could be reasonably referred to antecedent chorea.

5th. The fact that as a general rule, and one with very few exceptions, the second attack of chorea is slighter than the first, and the third than the second; a result wholly unintelligible if organic mischief were the ordinary cause of the attack.

But while I demur to the theory of embolism as capable of accounting for the phenomena of chorea in all or even in the majority of cases, I have no other generally satisfactory explanation to suggest. Fatal chorea is rare, and when death does take place it usually seems to be due to exhaustion produced by the violence and ceaselessness of the

[1] The arguments of different pathologists in favor of the theory of the embolic origin of chorea are well summarized by Dr. Radcliffe in his article on chorea in Reynolds's System of Medicine, vol. ii, 2d ed., pp. 198-206.

movements; it is preceded by a sudden failure of the vital powers, by delirium, or failure of intelligence, and at last by a comatose condition, which seldom lasts longer than a few hours. In such circumstances there does not appear to be anything constant in the appearances discovered after death; and, though congestion of the vessels of the spinal cord and the effusion of blood or of a bloody fluid around the theca of the cord are generally discovered, as they were in the only two cases of the morbid appearances in which I have a record, yet the presence of these conditions is by no means constant, and in some instances a post-mortem examination discovers absolutely nothing to explain the patient's death.[1]

I believe, then, as I have for many years, that chorea falls into the same category with the majority of the convulsive affections of early life; that its phenomena depend on irritation, direct or indirect, of the nervous spstem; and that, consequently, the intensity of its symptoms, and the danger that attends them, are greatly influenced by the exciting cause to which they are due. Idiopathic chorea is therefore almost always less serious than the symptomatic, and the disorder which is excited by some momentary shock generally calls for far less anxiety than that which manifests itself in connection with acute rheumatism, or with inflammation of the heart or pericardium.

It is with idiopathic cases only that I here concern myself, and in the majority of them the question fortunately is less one of whether the patient will recover, than within what time recovery may be expected, and I fear also of what sequelæ may be left behind. The disease is essentially slow in its course, and the average of 117 cases, as reported by M. Sée,[2] is 69 days; the extremes either way, however, vary considerably, for while recovery in the less severe cases is sometimes complete in a month, the convulsive movements persist in others for a period of several months, or longer. Cases of very chronic chorea are, however, usually of the partial kind, the affection having either involved only one limited set of muscles from the outset, or remaining in them after other parts had ceased to be its seat. Not only is chorea slow in departing, it is also very apt to return, and the attacks have been known to recur as often as six or seven times in the same patient, though generally with a progressive diminution in their severity.

In estimating the value of different modes of *treatment*, it must not be forgotten that chorea is one of those affections in which there is a tendency to spontaneous recovery. Not only does this show itself in almost all cases where improvement has taken place up to a certain point under the influence of remedies, but very often the improvement once advanced to this point goes on to perfect recovery with the same rapidity, whether those remedies are continued, modified, or abandoned. Now and then, too, we meet with instances in which even the severer forms of chorea, after bidding defiance to all remedies, spontaneously

[1] Leudet, Sur les Chorées sans Complication terminées par la Mort; in Archives de Médecine, 1853, vol. ii, p. 285: and likewise the most acute and valuable remarks of Dr. Radcliffe on the Pathology of Chorea, at pp. 198–206 of vol. ii of Reynolds's System of Medicine, already referred to.

[2] Op. cit., p. 408.

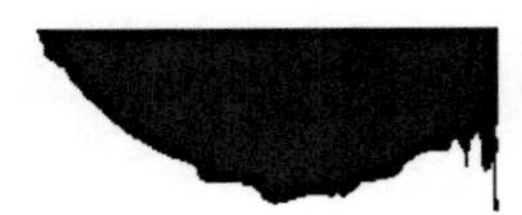

improve when all have been discontinued, and such improvement is as complete and as lasting as that which we ever attain by any mode of medication or by any form of treatment.

Next it is well to remember that there are some forms of choreic movements in which the parts affected vary in the course of a few days, or even within a shorter time, and which consist in winking the eyes, in grimacing, or in twitching the muscles of the face or neck, or in some awkward gait, or awkward gesture, that often occasion much anxiety to parents, but which are best left unnoticed and without any direct treatment. These cases, which are scarcely ever met with among the children of the poor, appear to depend on some temporary irritation of the nervous system, generally, I believe, on mental strain; not of necessity on undue length of the hours of study, or on the difficulty of the tasks imposed, but often on a child's anxiety to make progress, and to keep up with his schoolfellows. In corroboration of this being their cause, I may say that, contrary to the rule which obtains with chorea in general, these movements are much more frequent in boys than in girls. The overmental strain of girls comes later in life, just about the time of puberty, when it produces hysteria, and all sorts of menstrual disorders; but from the age of seven to twelve girls are usually in the nursery or at any rate at home, and are rarely overworked. In cases of this kind, lessening the mental strain is almost always accompanied by a cessation of the twitches, change of air, country amusements, and a generally tonic treatment perfect the cure, and dancing and gymnastics overcome the remains of any awkward habit. But I have never seen any good from calling the child's attention directly to the habit; but, on the contrary, the more his attention is aroused to it, the more in spite of all his endeavors does it become aggravated.

In cases of genuine chorea, usually those of the slighter kind, but yet more definite than those tricks of the facial muscles to which I have just referred, gymnastics are often of great service, and cases in the Children's Hospital sometimes receive no other treatment. They may always be employed with benefit when attention rouses the child to steadier movements of its hands or to a less uncertain gait, and in nothing do two cases of chorea differ more than in this. Notice one child and tell it to take care, and the movements which before it executed tolerably well, become absolutely uncontrollable. Let another see that he is watched, and so long as he attends to what he is about he walks more steadily and grasps more firmly. The great drawback from the success of gymnastics consists in the difficulty of arousing the child's will to activity, for it is not the mere mechanical movement of the limb which suffices, as it does in a stiff joint for which passive exercise is needed; but here it is essential to success that we should be able to evoke the conscious attention of the patient, and that the patient's nervous system should be equal to the effort to attend. Hence it is that gymnastics are of service very much in proportion to the age of the children; hence, too, they are of more use when practiced in a class than by one child alone; and hence, too, music or any simple chant, in time with which the movements are made, helps greatly to fix the attention and expedite the cure.

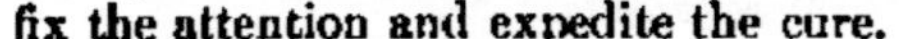

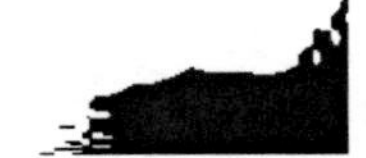

I have never been able to put adequately to the test the employment of gymnastics, or of regulated movements in cases of severe chorea. No one, indeed, who had the honor even of a slight acquaintance with the late M. Blache[1] but must attach the most implicit faith to his statements, but I am not aware that any one has repeated his observations on an equally large scale, and the use of movements seems passing into undeserved forgetfulness. I am quite sure that regulated movements of the limbs, even in cases so severe as to necessitate their being generally kept motionless by bandages at other times, do help in a very important degree the recovery of the patient. I cannot say of my own knowledge what, without other aid, they would effect.

Having spoken about movements in chorea, I must also say a few words about rest. In cases of chorea of even moderate severity I have perpetually seen the ailment aggravated by the child being allowed to be up and about. The sense of intense fatigue which follows an epileptic fit is not all due to the sensorial disturbance: it is owing in no small measure to the violent muscular movements by which it has been accompanied, and in just the same way the unceasing movements of the legs in attempts to walk, or of the muscles of the back in the vain endeavor to sit still, tire the child, and exhaust the muscular power. It is often well worth noticing how much better a child becomes after three or four days' rest in bed in the hospital without any medical treatment having been adopted for its cure; nor less instructive to see how the moment that the child is taken up, the limbs, which before were almost motionless, writhe and twist about in the attempt to stand or to walk. In all cases of considerable severity, therefore, the child should at once be placed in bed, and if the movements are still violent and continuous, their severity is much abated and the child is saved much distress and much subsequent exhaustion by putting splints on the legs and arms and swathing the child completely in soft bandages. As the child gets better they may be removed, but not seldom it is wise to apply them by day, even though they may be removed at night, if, as is sometimes the case, the child should then sleep tranquilly.

It were useless to go over the list of all the medicines which have been vaunted for the cure of chorea. There is of course a large number of cases in which the existence of some distinct indication leaves no room for doubt as to the remedies to be employed. Such are the cases of habitual constipation; such, too, those of marked debility, in which there can be no doubt as to the propriety of administering purgatives in the one case, chalybeates in the other; and there is a period in most instances of chorea during which each of these remedies commonly finds a place. But there still remain a good many cases in which the movements constitute the disease, and in which there is no special indication to guide us. It is in these cases that we meet with the large class of antispasmodic remedies, each of which has been vaunted and abandoned in its turn, and from none of which have I ever seen the slightest benefit. Neither have the sedatives been more

[1] See his paper in the Mémoires de l'Académie de Mèdecine, vol. xix, pp. 598–608.

successful in my hands, except when given in a single dose for the purpose of obtaining sleep; henbane, conium, and belladonna have all been given under my observation, or have been prescribed by myself, and have all proved equally unsuccessful, though I have known them to be tolerated in poisonous doses without any result either for good or evil. I have heard of chloral exerting a marked influence over choreic movements, and it may deserve a larger trial than I have yet given it; though in the cases where I have employed it it seemed to have no power apart from its action in producing sleep; and the bromide of potass, which sometimes acts like a charm in epilepsy, appears to have no power at all in controlling chorea.

The want of accommodation at the Children's Hospital has prevented me from giving a fair trial to the sulphur baths from which French physicians appear to have often obtained very satisfactory results. I am certain, however, that in many instances the violence of the choreic movements is lessened in proportion to the degree to which the action of the skin can be excited; and the extreme dryness of the skin in a large number of choreic patients cannot have escaped general observation. I often employ the hot air bath at night for the purpose of exciting the action of the skin, giving at the same time a diaphoretic dose of antimonial wine, and continue this for three or four consecutive nights, even though the general condition of the patient should be such as to indicate an otherwise tonic plan of treatment.

I have also in a few instances, when the choreic movements were very violent, employed with marked advantage large doses of tartar emetic, as first proposed by Dr. Gillette of Paris, and employed by M. Roger, certainly no reckless practitioners; and approved by M. Trousseau in those exceptional cases for which alone I should reserve it. The plan which they followed consisted in giving three grains of tartar emetic the first day of treatment, six the second, nine the third, then allowing a pause of from three to five days, and recommencing with four grains the first day, eight the second, twelve the third, and so on for three series. When I have employed the remedy, I have begun with an eighth of a grain for a child of ten years old; but by doubling the quantity every four hours, a very large dose is soon arrived at, which is no further augmented so soon as the movements are distinctly controlled; while vomiting, diarrhœa, or failure of the power of the pulse is a reason for its immediate discontinuance. In any case, too, the remedy should be discontinued if marked improvement does not take place within three days, and should not be resumed until after an interval of at least 48 hours. These precautions are all the more needed, since while a sudden failure of power sometimes takes place in chorea quite independent of the treatment adopted, I have met with one instance in which death took place from apparently causeless exhaustion 36 hours after the discontinuance of large doses of antimony, which yet had produced neither vomiting nor purging, and in which the diminished power of the pulse before the child began to die was by no means remarkable.

I should scarcely have thought it necessary to add that I do not recommend this heroic use of antimony except in those cases where the

violence of the movements, uncontrolled by ordinary means, itself threatens life, if it were not that I have been misunderstood and been supposed to advocate this as a common plan of treatment.[1] I ought to add that I have heard of one case in which chloral in frequently repeated doses checked the violent movements in a case of great severity, and should certainly be disposed to give it a trial before employing antimony. I may add that chloroform has in my hands been only temporary in the good it effected, and that its influence to produce even that temporary good was soon exhausted.

The only remedy which has appeared to me to exert any specific power over chorea is the sulphate of zinc, given in increasing doses, as I believe was first done by the late Dr. Barlow of Guy's Hospital. Beginning with one grain or even half a grain three times a day, and increasing the dose by a grain daily, a very remarkable tolerance of the medicine is speedily established, and it is by no means unusual to find 10, 15, or 20 grains taken three or four times a day with perfect impunity. I have never increased the dose beyond the latter amount, thinking that if three weeks' trial, at the end of which so large a dose was arrived at, produced no result, the remedy might be considered to have failed. Neither have I ever increased the dose merely to ascertain how much could be borne with impunity, but have continued the remedy at whatever dose fairly controlled the movements; and if it produced sickness, have continued a smaller dose until the movements were controlled, or till I had become satisfied of its inutility. At one time, in accordance with Dr. Barlow's caution, I was accustomed to leave off the zinc gradually, just as I had increased it; but I have since tried the discontinuance of it abruptly, and have not found any return of symptoms follow from this course.

I have made comparatively few trials of arsenic, probably fewer than I ought to have done, considering the invariable success which some physicians of very high authority have met with in its employment. I have used it in chronic chorea when other remedies had failed, and have found it fail too. I have, however, never given it, as counselled by Dr. Begbie, who used to prescribe it twice a day after meals, increasing the dose daily until the special injurious effects of arsenic became apparent, when he suspended its use for a few days, resuming it again as soon as these symptoms had passed off. Dr. Radcliffe, who has employed it in this way and with success, states that he has often been compelled to discontinue it on account of the gastric disturbance which it produced, and which often became urgent before the remedy had had time to influence the chorea. In these circumstances he suggests a trial of the arsenic hypodermically, from which he has obtained good results on some occasions; and in instances of chorea rebellious to other means, this suggestion, and I may say the same about every suggestion of Dr. Radcliffe's, deserves to be borne in mind.

I have never employed strychnine as a general remedy in chorea,

---

[1] The very kindly critic of my Lumleian Lectures in the Edinburgh Medical Journal for Sept. 1871, seems to me to have fallen into this misapprehension.

in the way in which I employ zinc; for notwithstanding the high recommendation of M. Trousseau, I have felt afraid of it. He himself was accustomed to push the medicine to a dose at which the physiological effects of the remedy became apparent, and speaks of headache, stiffness of the muscles of the neck, pains in the limbs, occasional spasms, and itching of the surface of the body, as indications that the medicine has been carried to the limit of safety. But the twitching of the limbs in chorea prevents our being aware of the occurrence of spasms; while a child's inability to describe its sensations deprives us of another most important guide: and I have seen convulsions occur more than once in young children who were taking strychnine, apparently unpreceded by any of the ordinary physiological effects of the remedy.

On these accounts I have never given it in cases of severe chorea in which the dulling of the intelligence as well as the violence of the movements prevent our learning when the medicine has begun to produce its specified effects. I also very rarely use it in children under the age of seven. I begin with a small dose, increase it slowly, suspend it for two or three days at a time when its administration is long continued; and limit its use almost entirely to cases in which there is loss of power rather than violence of movement. In those conditions in which the limbs cannot be exerted without the irregular movements being at once induced, although these movements are comparatively slight so long as the patient remains quiet in bed, the strychnine has seemed to me sometimes very useful, just as it is in cases of diphtheritic paralysis.

The above are the chief, I do not say that they are by any means the only, remedies for chorea. I have not dwelt on the various indirect means (in the more chronic form of the disorder they are indeed the most important) by which you must endeavor to improve your patient's health. Residence in the country, sea-air, and sea-bathing, a well-regulated but nutritious diet, and generally a careful use of stimulants, when combined with the most sedulous avoidance of overexcitement in any form, often do as much as medicine, or even more, for the restoration of your patient.

In the great majority of cases you may, as I have already mentioned, assure the friends of your patient that the disease will ultimately subside, though it may last for many weeks. Two qualifications, however, you are forced to add to this cheering assurance,—the one that slight causes may occasion its return, and the other that there exists a connection between it and the rheumatic diathesis; and the development of heart disease either with or without rheumatism in the course of chorea is a hazard against which you can furnish no guarantee.

LECTURE XV.

Paralysis.—Sometimes congenital, but this is not true infantile paralysis—Its characteristics—Age at its occurrence—Most frequent during period of dentition—Diagnosis—Identity with spinal paralysis in adults—Prognosis not very favorable—Consequences of its persistence—Treatment—Aids to walking—Modes of exercising the limbs—Galvanism.

Facial Hemiplegia in new-born infants.

Neuralgia in infancy and childhood.

Disturbance of the nervous system shows itself in children as well by loss of the motor power as by the occurrence of involuntary movements; and such an accident as the palsy of a limb naturally occasions parents the greatest anxiety. In the adult, a paralytic seizure is generally the result of very serious disease either in the brain or spinal cord, and the sign of the commencement of a series of morbid processes which issue sooner or later in the destruction of the patient's life. Non-professional persons are aware of this fact, and often suppose that the same rule holds good in the case of the child as in that of the adult; but you may in most instances quiet their fears with the assurance that paralysis in infancy and childhood seldom betokens any peril to life, though the affection is often very slow in disappearing, and sometimes is quite incurable.

Paralysis in childhood occasionally dates from so early a period that there seems every reason for believing it to be the result of some original defect of conformation. In such cases the power over both extremities of one side is greatly impaired, and the limbs on that side are much smaller and less well nourished, and sometimes the defective growth and want of power are evident on the whole of the same side of the face and body. Some years ago, I saw a girl, 18 years old, in whom not only were the left extremities much shorter and smaller than the right, but the left half of the face and body was so likewise. The parents of the girl stated that this inequality in size of the two halves of the body had existed from earliest infancy, and that the defective power over her limbs had not succeeded to a fit, nor to any other indication of acute cerebral disease. The left side was weak, and motion imperfect, but sensation seemed to be unimpaired. The patient in this case was rather deficient in intellectual endowments. In another instance the body was well formed, but the patient, a girl of eight years of age, had had from her earliest infancy but very imperfect use of her right side. She limped with her right leg as she walked, always treading on her toes, with the heel raised considerably above the ground, and turning the foot inwards at every step. She had but very incomplete power over her right arm; the fingers of that hand were constantly flexed and drawn into the palm; and though by a great effort she could extend them, yet the moment her attention was withdrawn they returned to their former flexed position. Sensation was as perfect in the right limbs as in the left, but their wasted condition and smaller size, as compared with the left extremities, showed that their nutrition had been but imperfectly carried on.

It is almost needless to observe, that in cases such as these there is no room for treatment other than the employment of whatever mechanical means may be best calculated to relieve inconvenience or to diminish deformity.

Real congenital paralysis, however, apart from idiocy, is a much less frequent accident than the occurrence of partial or complete loss of power over certain limbs or muscles at a subsequent period. Such sudden loss of power, unattended by any symptoms which endanger life, is so frequent an occurrence in infancy and early childhood as to have received a special designation; and the terms Infantile Paralysis, Spinal Paralysis of Infants, Essential Paralysis, Atrophic Paralysis, Atrophic Fatty Paralysis, all apply to the same affection, either designating one of its special features, or expressing some theory as to its nature. On this one point all are agreed, that there is a form of paralysis frequent in early life, but which differs in its symptoms and its course from any that we commonly meet with in the adult. In many instances its commencement can be traced to some attack, though often a very brief one, of cerebral disturbance, which showed itself, perhaps, by nothing more than a single convulsive seizure, or by an unusual heaviness of the head, that lasted for a day or two, and then subsided of its own accord. In the majority of cases, indeed, the cerebral disturbance that preceded infantile paralysis is neither severe nor long continued; and only two instances have come under my notice in which there seemed to be reason for supposing that it was associated with abiding mischief in the brain. It is therefore of importance to examine an infant carefully, even after a very mild convulsive seizure, in order to make sure that it moves its limbs as freely as before, or that, if its power over them is impaired, appropriate treatment may be at once adopted.

Paralysis sometimes comes on independently of any evident cerebral [illegible] seeming to be induced by the irritation of dentition, or [illegible] the long continuance of a constipated state of the [illegible] in connection with all the indications of general [illegible] to a short feverish seizure, which came on sud[illegible] was in bed at night, and left it with one limb [illegible]. I believe, indeed, that in cases even of the [illegible] of paralysis, there have almost always been some [illegible] disorder of the general health; the few instances [illegible] the immediate action of cold, as from a child [illegible] been followed by paralysis of one or of both [illegible]

[illegible] paralysis in early life calls for, and would well [illegible]ation. Unfortunately, however, the difficul[illegible] into the subject are numerous; and are [illegible] they arise in great measure from the [illegible], which renders it almost impossible adequately to test the value of remedies, or to estimate the changes which time may bring about, either in improving or deteriorating the patient's condition. Of the large number of cases which I have seen, few have continued for more than a few weeks under my observation; so that I am unable to answer, with reference to them, more than a few of the questions which suggest themselves as deserving a reply.

I have spoken of Infantile Paralysis as peculiar in its characters; and I think that it is important before entering on its special study that we separate from it all other forms of palsy which may be observed in childhood, but which with few exceptions are far more frequent in the adult.

First, then, we leave out of consideration all instances in which the loss of power, as in the two cases which I mentioned at the commencement of this lecture, is actually congenital; and next those cases, too, most of which date from birth or from very early infancy, where the paralysis is associated with idiocy; and nervous power is wanting to the limbs just in the same way as it is wanting for the exercise of the faculties of the mind. Neither do cases of simple Facial Paralysis belong here, for they either depend on local injury, as from the pressure of the forceps in labor; or they arise from the same class of causes as produce the affection in the grown person, though I have seen temporary paralysis of the portio dura associated with true infantile paralysis.[1]

The characteristics of infantile paralysis appear to be:

1st. The suddenness of its occurrence.

2d. The absence in many cases of any previous sign of disorder of the cerebro-spinal system, and the fact that when such disorder does occur, there is no constant proportion between its severity and the extent or completeness of the paralysis.

3d. The continuance throughout of undiminished sensation, and the absence in the early stages of the affection of all rigidity or contraction of the paralyzed limbs.

4th. The occasional onset of the affection by severe pains lasting for some hours in the limbs which afterwards become paralyzed, or the existence of greatly exaggerated sensibility of the limbs in the early stages of the affection, and the direct proportion existing between the pain or the hyperæsthesia and the subsequent loss of power.

5th. The tendency of the affection to implicate permanently the lower rather than the upper limbs, and this, even though all should have been paralyzed in the first instance; while in nearly half of the cases the paralysis is throughout limited to the lower limbs.

6th. The direct relation which subsists between the early date of the improvement and its completeness.

7th. The comparative rarity of *absolute* recovery even in the most favorable cases, for not only does a degree of weakness continue, but in many instances one or two muscles of a limb remain almost powerless, even when the others have gained much of their former vigor.

8th. The tendency to retarded growth and impaired nutrition in the

[1] See also Laborde, Paralysie de l'Enfance, 8vo. Paris, 1864, p. 37.

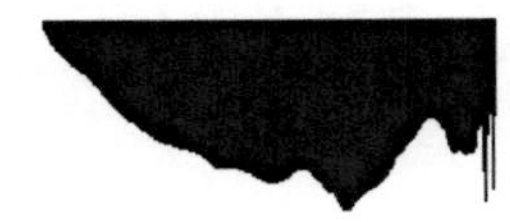

permanently paralyzed limb, to which there is usually superadded a greater or less degree of fatty degeneration of the muscular tissue.

The wasting of the limb, however, does not bear a uniform relation to the degree of paralysis; nor even if the paralysis does not improve is the wasting continuously progressive, but it remains stationary at an uncertain stage, as also does the degeneration of the muscular fibre.

9th. The tendency to the production of deformity in the affected limb; in occasioning which the mere weight of the limb, and the load which it has to support or to move, and which is now disproportionate to its weakened powers, bears, as Volckmann[1] has pointed out, a more important share than mere antagonism between the paralyzed and non-paralyzed muscles. It may be added in further confirmation of this opinion, that when paralysis of either leg takes place in infants or in young children who have scarcely begun to walk, no deformity occurs for months, so long as the child remains upon the couch, but it speedily shows itself when the child begins to make attempts to stand or to walk upon the sound limb, while the weight of the other necessarily remains unsupported.

The following table shows the sex of patients affected with Infantile Paralysis, and also their age at the time of the attack.

	Male.	Female.	
In	1	1	occurred under 6 months.
	0	1	" between 6 " and 1 year.
	12	7	" " 1 year and 2 years.
	3	9	" " 2 years " 3 years.
	3	3	" " 3 " " 4 "
	1	1	" " 4 " " 5 "
	1	0	" " 5 " " 6 "
	1	0	" " 7 " " 8 "
	22	22	

In 32 out of 44 cases, or in nearly two-thirds of the total number, the paralytic symptoms came on between the age of 6 months and 3 years, or in other words, during the time when the process of dentition was going on most actively. In many instances, indeed, it was not preceded by any of the local signs of difficult dentition, but still it is quite apparent that the changes which are going on in the constitution during that important period of development predispose to it, as to so many other affections of the nervous system. But, nevertheless, in two-thirds of the cases, no indications of cerebral disturbance either occurred before the paralysis or came on afterwards, while in only 3 instances were the signs of affection of the brain other than exceedingly transient. With reference to the parts affected—

In 1 case only was the arm paralyzed, the legs not being involved.
18 cases the legs alone were affected, viz., 5 times the right, 5 the left, 8 both.
25 " " and arms were both involved, viz.,
8 " right leg and arm.
6 " left " "
4 " both legs and right arm.
3 " " " left "
4 " " " both arms.

[1] Sammlung klinischer Vorträge, Heft 1. Leipzig, 1870.

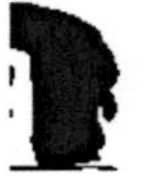

Of these 25 cases there were 13 in which the arm had perfectly recovered while the leg had not; 4 in which the leg had recovered while the arm had not; and 8 in which both had continued paralyzed at the time when the patients came under my care, though these figures do not in the least express what may have been the ultimate issue of the cases.

In almost all instances a certain small amount of voluntary power over the affected side remains after the seizure. Thus, if the arm is paralyzed, the child can move it a little, though with difficulty, and not so as to answer any useful purpose; or if the leg is affected, the child can flex and extend it when lying in bed, or, perhaps, can make some slight attempt at progression if the weight of its body is supported by some one else; and this even though it be wholly unable to stand for a moment without assistance. Owing to this circumstance, the date of the occurrence of paralysis of the lower limbs is very apt to be overlooked in infants who have not begun to walk, so that the affection may not attract notice until it is in reality of several months' duration.

But though the existence of this affection may for a time be altogether overlooked in early infancy, *diagnosis* is not otherwise attended with much difficulty, for the history of the case and the painlessness of the affected limb will at once show that the loss of power over it is not the result of any injury. Often, however, sensation in the affected limb appears to be exalted when the paralysis is recent, the degree of hyperæsthesia in the early stage being in such cases proportionate to the completeness of the loss of power which afterwards is apparent. In some instances, the exaggerated sensibility continues for several weeks, though this is unusual; but when this is the case, the leg being the seat of the affection, and the paralysis incomplete, the existence of hip-joint disease may very likely be suspected. In such a case the child bears all its weight on the healthy limb, turns the foot of the affected side inwards when walking, and stands with the toes of that foot resting on the dorsum of the foot of the healthy side. Still it will usually be found that the exaggerated sensibility of the paralyzed limb varies greatly at different times, while that extreme increase of suffering produced in cases of hip-joint disease, on striking the head of the femur against the acetabulum by a blow upon the heel, and the fixed pain in the knee of the affected side, so characteristic of disease of the hip-joint, are absent; and these points of difference will enable you to distinguish between the two affections. One other important means of diagnosis is furnished by the presence or absence of an increased temperature over the suspected joint. The value of this easy observation in determining the presence or absence of inflammation about any particular spot is dwelt on by Mr. Hilton,[1] in his lectures delivered at the College of Surgeons. I cannot refer to them without recommending them to your most careful perusal, or without expressing my conviction that, more than almost any work which has recently appeared

[1] Lectures on Rest and Pain, 8vo. London, 1863. See p. 64.

on subjects connected with our profession, they bear the stamp of original thought, and of that simplicity which characterizes real genius.

Another important question is, how we may distinguish between forms of paralysis, such as I am here speaking of, and those more serious cases in which the palsy is a sign of organic disease in the brain. In many cases the history of the patient will of itself be sufficient to guard us from error; for if paralysis occurs suddenly, affecting both limbs on one side, and is neither preceded nor attended by any cerebral symptom, it is almost certain that it does not depend on serious organic disease of the brain. Our decision will be more difficult if the loss of power has been gradual, and especially if only one limb is affected; but, if the brain is diseased, we shall rarely find a mere weakening of the motor power; for connected with it there will usually be occasional involuntary tremor or nervous twitching of the limb, or contraction of the fingers or toes, and that independent of the general wasting of the affected limb which takes place in all cases of long-standing essential paralysis, and is then accompanied with contraction, owing to the predominance of the flexor over the extensor muscles. When the paralysis succeeds to convulsions, the case will be still more obscure. In most cases of simple paralysis, however, the palsy comes on after a single fit; while, if it depends on some local mischief in the brain, it is generally preceded by several convulsive seizures, during each of which the limb that afterwards becomes palsied is in a state of peculiar movement, or is sometimes the only part where convulsive movements occur.

And now, having gone with some detail into the various characteristics of infantile paralysis, we come to the question of its nature. Is it, as I have been used to teach, and as my remarks at the commencement of this lecture seemed to imply, an essential paralysis, independent of organic lesion and peculiar to early life, or are its characteristics to be sought in certain changes of the muscular tissue; or is its point of departure to be found in the spinal cord? Is it in fact analogous to or identical with certain forms of paralysis met with in the adult; its one remarkable peculiarity being the frequency of its occurrence; just as all forms of disorder of the nervous system, and especially of the spinal system, predominate in early life; and the other being that disposition to the production of various deformities inseparable from the fact that the paralysis occurs in parts still in a state of growth and development? I believe this last assumption to be correct; that Heine[1] was right when he termed it Spinal Paralysis, and that Laborde and others who have adopted the same view have done good service by leading us to sounder opinions with reference to its nature; though we may still hesitate as to the value to be attached to the alleged microscopic appearances in the substance of the cord. I have been much struck by observing the exact identity of character between the paralysis of infancy, and the paralytic symptoms which have come on in children after a fall on the back, or a blow on the spine, and which were undoubtedly due to spinal congestion.

[1] Spinale Kinderlähmung, 8vo., 1860. Laborde, op. cit.

I do not know that I can better sum up the points of resemblance between the two, or better state my present conviction, than in the words of my friend Dr. Radcliffe.[1]

"It seems to me," says he, "that the peculiarities of infantile paralysis instead of showing that it is unlike paralysis in adults, only show a close analogy to, if not an actual identity with, the paralysis which has been seen to result from spinal congestion. In infantile paralysis the paralysis is partial; in paralysis from spinal congestion it is the same. In infantile paralysis sensation is exaggerated rather than dulled in the paralyzed parts; in paralysis from spinal congestion it is the same. In infantile paralysis the bladder and lower bowel are obedient to the will, so also in paralysis from spinal congestion. In infantile paralysis the limbs are limber, not rigid; so also in paralysis from spinal congestion. In infantile paralysis recovery more or less complete is the rule rather than the exception; so also and very much in the same order in paralysis from spinal congestion. In infantile paralysis 'head symptoms' are exceptional phenomena at any time; so also in the paralysis from spinal congestion. Neither do I know of anything to invalidate the conclusion which those resemblances would seem almost to necessitate, that infantile paralysis is nothing more than paralysis from spinal congestion."

I do not know that one can lay down any decided rules with reference to *prognosis* in these cases as deducible from the sudden or gradual access of the paralysis, though it is my impression that the former, which is the more common mode of onset of paralysis at the time of dentition, warrants a more hopeful view of the case than the latter. The duration of infantile paralysis, indeed, in whatever circumstances it may have come on, is extremely variable. In those instances in which recovery is most complete, amendment generally manifests itself within a few days, and this sometimes wholly independent of treatment, though it oftener occurs under the employment of some simple remedy directed against the symptoms of constitutional disorder with which it was accompanied; so that the same medicine suffices at once to remove the child's indisposition and to cure its paralysis. In other cases, even though all signs of disordered health may pass away with the same rapidity, the child may continue for weeks or months with the power over one side of its body, or over one-half of its face, or one of its limbs greatly impaired; or this condition may persist through the remainder of its life.

The evils resulting from the persistence of the paralysis are also much greater in childhood than in after-life, for the disfigurement which it produces is far more serious. In the course of time the muscles of a paralyzed limb become almost always wasted, and the sinking of its temperature attests its imperfect nutrition; but in childhood the growth of the part also is arrested, or retarded, so that in the course of a year or two the affected limb will be half or three-quarters of an inch shorter than the corresponding member on the opposite side. A little girl had paralysis of her left leg at the age of 1 year and 9 months,

---

[1] In Reynolds's System of Medicine, 2d ed., 1872, vol. ii, p. 708.

after a febrile attack accompanied with pain, and which seemed to have been of a rheumatic character. At the age of 6 years, she having recovered power over her left leg sufficient to walk without a crutch or other support, a line drawn from the anterior superior spine of the ilium to the external malleolus measured 20½ inches on the right side, 19 on the left; the circumference of the right calf was 8½, that of the left 6¾ inches; while, owing to the relaxation of the ligaments about the ankle-joint, a line drawn obliquely from the internal malleolus to the end of the heel measured 2¾ inches on the left side, 2½ on the right. Two years later, a similar disparity between the two limbs still existed; the measurements on the left side yielding 20, 7½, and 3 inches respectively, those on the right side 22, 8½, and 2¾ inches. The arrest of growth, too, had affected the foot as well as the leg, for while the right measured 6½ inches from toe to heel, corresponding measurements of the left foot yielded only 5¾ inches. The relaxation of the ligaments mentioned in this case sometimes exists in even a much greater degree, and tends to increase the deformity and to diminish the usefulness of the limb; and this is generally most marked when the upper extremity is affected. On three occasions I have seen the arm completely dislocated, owing to long-standing paralysis, the ligaments about the shoulder-joint having become so relaxed that the head of the humerus hung quite out of the glenoid cavity; and on measuring the distance from the acromion to the tip of the finger in one of these cases, I found that an apparent elongation of the paralyzed limb to the extent of three-quarters of an inch had thus been produced.

The deformity in these cases, however, depends in the first instance mainly on the weight of the paralyzed limb; next, on the wasting of the paralyzed muscles and the relaxation of the ligaments, and further on the permanent contraction of some muscles when their antagonists are paralyzed. In some cases of long-standing paralysis, the deformities thus produced are very serious indeed, while their removal constitutes one of the greatest triumphs of orthopædic surgery.

It must be borne in mind in estimating the gravity of paralysis in infancy and childhood that the deformities just referred to are not merely the occasional consequences of very serious or very protracted paralysis, but that there is a tendency to their occurrence in every instance; and that the restoration of a very large measure of power to the affected limb furnishes no guarantee against their taking place. From this it follows that in every case of paralysis in infancy or childhood the patient will require the most careful watching during the whole process of recovery—a process not infrequently prolonged over several years; and this the rather, since so long as one set of muscles continues feebler than another, one most influential cause of deformity of the limbs is constantly in operation. But even though treatment be adopted early, and continued long, it must still be owned that the prospects of complete recovery in these cases are far from cheering. I cannot indeed attempt to state the proportions in which recovery takes place, still less to give a numerical estimate of the complete as opposed to the partial recoveries. Whether in hospital or in private practice the majority of cases come under my notice for but a short time, and most of them are instances where either all treatment has been neglected, or where the paralysis has been unusually complete, or the consequent deformity unusually great. I believe therefore that more cases of infantile paralysis get well of their own accord than my individual experience would have led me to suppose, and I believe further that the cases of complete palsy of a limb, or of deformity, irremediable by orthopædic surgery, are less numerous.

One or two observations may be added here with reference to our prognosis in this affection. A certain amount of spontaneous amendment takes place in almost every case; sometimes beginning within a few hours after the occurrence of the paralysis, and going on to the complete restoration of power in the course of a few days, or even of a few hours. Between this, however, which has been termed Kennedy's paralysis, and the true spinal paralysis, I know of no difference in kind, only of a difference in degree; nor do I know of any means by which within the first few hours after its commencement one can tell whether the affection will be temporary or abiding, beyond our knowledge of the fact that the earlier the improvement commences the greater is the probability of its continuance. Usually, even in the worst cases, the amendment begins within a week or two, and is at first very obvious, but soon goes on more slowly, and at last usually comes to a complete standstill, and so continues for months or forever, if no treatment is adopted, except that now the wasting of the muscles and the degeneration of their tissue begin, and continue for an indefinite time, when they too, cease to grow worse, and the child remains for life with a shrunken limb, over which habit and the action of the non-paralyzed muscles at length give it some degree of useful control, greater probably than one might have anticipated, though the deformity still remains unremedied, perhaps irremediable.

Nothing more can be needed than a knowledge of these facts to enforce the necessity for the early adoption of appropriate *treatment.* Its nature must of course vary according to the circumstances in which the affection comes on, and these, as we have already seen, differ very widely; paralysis in one instance occurring during dentition; in another, following one of the eruptive fevers; in a third, succeeding to rheumatic symptoms. There is in the majority of instances an acute stage which, even when short, is generally sufficiently obvious, accompanied with febrile symptoms, sometimes with marked signs of cerebral disturbance; in other cases with severe pains in the limbs, or with marked hyperæsthesia which prevents all attempts at movement. No special rules for treatment can be laid down for this stage, beyond the observance of absolute quiet, the use of antiphlogistic remedies, lancing the gums if the attack appeared to be connected with dentition, the employment of sedatives to relieve suffering, and complete rest of the affected limbs so long as pain is produced by any attempts at movement. A time, however, comes, and generally even in the least favorable cases within a few days, when every sign of acute ailment has passed away, and little remains besides the loss of power to engage our notice. Sometimes no disorder of the general health is present, while in the majority of instances in which any such ailments exist they are limited to a constipated state of the bowels and a condition of general debility. Hence purgatives and tonics are the internal remedies which are most usually indicated, and of these the gentle aperients are more suitable than those of a drastic kind: and preparations of iron and cod-liver oil are usually of greater service than other tonics. There is, however, one tonic which has, and not altogether undeservedly, a special reputation in cases of paralysis, and that is the nux vomica, the employment of which has seemed to me to have been succeeded, in many bad cases, by a rise of the temperature of the limbs, and an increase in power over them. I have not seen it produce those twitchings of the limbs which attend on the administration of strychnine in the adult, but I have seen general and rather severe convulsions come on during its employment, which were followed by no evil consequences, though I cannot say they were unattended with danger. But on this point I have only to repeat the caution which I already gave when speaking of the employment of strychnine in chorea.

Be the purely medical treatment what it may, unceasing efforts must be made so soon as the exalted sensibility has passed away, to bring the palsied limb once more into use, while, when the power is most impaired, we must seek, by the regular employment of passive exercise, and by friction of the limb, to prevent that wasting of the muscles which is sure to follow on long-continued inaction. If the leg is affected, a child who has not very long learned to walk will be taken completely off its feet, while even after power has returned, quite sufficiently to enable it to make some attempts at walking, it will be deterred from the effort by its sense of insecurity, will cry even though carefully supported by its nurse, and will refuse to make the slightest movement. The attempts thus evidently distressing the child are discontinued, and in the hope, too often a vain one, that in the course of months the child will gain more power, much valuable time is thrown away: the muscles waste, and permanent deformity of the limb results. In these cases, two very simple means are often of great service in preventing this untoward occurrence. The baby-jumper, which all infants delight in, exercises the legs most effectually, while as soon as there is even a very moderate return of power in the legs, the go-cart is of great use, since it completely removes all sense of the risk of falling, and the little one, thus convinced of its safety, soon begins to walk again. The go-cart, however, has this disadvantage, that it exaggerates the disposition to lean very much forward in walking, which is observable in all children even for some time after they have learned to walk pretty well: and thus renders the gait very unsteady. So soon, then, as the child can walk tolerably in the go-cart, it is as well to discontinue its use, either entirely or in great measure, and to substitute for it the following contrivance. A little jacket, made of some stout material, lined, and padded under the arm-pits, is put on the child. To it are attached a couple of straps of stout webbing, one end of which is fastened to the front, and the other to the back of the jacket. The straps are of sufficient length to be conveniently held by the child's attendant, and by means of them its weight is supported more or less completely, while in walking the child is not thrown forwards as when stepping in a go-cart. Feeling perfectly safe, the child now perseveres in walking: many of the worst consequences of paralysis are avoided, and a more speedy and more complete recovery is obtained than could at first have been anticipated. If the child is old enough to be taught to walk with crutches (and at five or six years old the lesson is soon learned), it is desirable that as soon as possible it should be furnished with them, for it will certainly make greater and surer progress if entirely dependent on itself, than if its weight is borne, or the possibility of falling prevented, by a nurse or attendant. With all this care, however, it is yet quite possible that some deformity of the leg may take place, calling for the employment of splints or of other contrivances, or even for surgical interference.

When the arm is affected, the principles just laid down are of equal importance, though the mode of carrying them out must, of course, differ. Passive exercise must be strictly carried out: the sound arm must be tied up, either altogether or for a considerable part of the day; coaxing, bribes, and all the inducements which move a little child's heart, must be brought into play as rewards for using the feeble limb. Raising a weight by means of a rope passing over a pulley, is a mode of exercising the arm which can be put in practice even in very young children; while in those who are older, trundling a hoop with the feeble arm is a capital plan for joining work and play. I need not say that much care and much patience are needed in carrying out any of these suggestions, and not a little of that intuitive love for children which teaches those who are its possessors, how to extract fun and merriment from what might in other hands be a most irksome task.

In many cases, however, something more is needed than even the best directed attempts at exercising the paralyzed limb will supply, and this, either from the completeness of the paralysis, or from its long continuance. In these circumstances we generally find the nutrition of the limb greatly impaired, its temperature very low, and its sensibility less acute than natural. In such cases, while rubbing the limbs, and other forms of passive exercise, must be most sedulously persevered in, I think that I have seen benefit from the warm douche to the lower limbs and the sacral region once or twice a day, when steadily continued for weeks together. One objection to the employment of blisters is, that they of necessity preclude perseverance with the douche; and a similar objection, though not to the same extent, applies to the employment of stimulating liniments. In cases of this kind, however, we constantly find that one remedy, though serviceable for a time, ceases at length to be of benefit: so, when improvement under the douche seems to be at a standstill, a stimulating liniment may be tried for a season. I usually employ a croton-oil liniment, or one containing the tincture of cantharides in quantity sufficient to produce a rubefacient effect, but not to blister. Blisters not merely cause much distress by vesicating, but have also seemed to me of more transient benefit than liniments. Galvanism is another remedy from which much good is often derived, but its proper application requires an expenditure of time which it is not always easy to bestow, as well as a tact in its employment scarcely attainable except by long practice. Between the

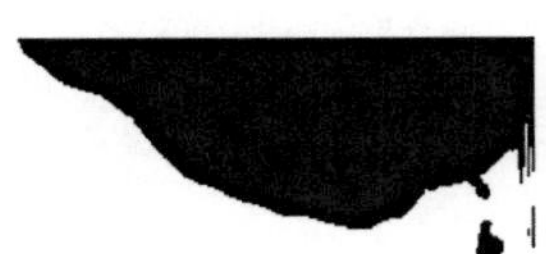

results which follow the ordinary rough mode of employing galvanism and its more scientific application by means of that "localized galvanism," for a knowledge of which we are indebted to Duchenne,[1] the difference is immense, and I look forward to an increased dexterity in the use of the latter as to a means by which we may remedy conditions that hitherto we have been accustomed, and not without reason, to regard as all but absolutely hopeless.

Of late years much has been said about the so-called Swedish Exercises as a means of restoring the usefulness of paralyzed limbs; and though, unfortunately, the direction of them has fallen into the hands of persons not the most likely to maintain the reputation of our profession, we must not on that account undervalue the benefit which they are capable of affording. Two principles seem involved in their employment,—the one, the devising of such movements as shall best bring into play those muscles the power over which is deficient; the other, the calling forth the active exercise of the will in determining them. Of the efficacy of the will, as a subsidiary means of restoring power to the partially paralyzed limb, I have no doubt whatever. Of course in the child, whose will is feeble, and liable to be distracted by very trivial causes, this power is far less energetic than in the grown person; but still it is a power well worth cultivating, and the steady perseverance in it exercised from childhood up to adult age will, I am sure, do more towards the recovery of a paralyzed limb than would ever be imagined from its casual employment on one or two occasions.

It would be useless to go into details as to all contingencies in these cases, or to furnish you with rules for the management of each different degree or stage of this affection. The remarks I have already made will at any rate put you in possession of the principles by which your conduct must generally be regulated.[2]

I may just add one word with reference to cases of *paralysis of the portio dura.* In the child, as in the adult, they usually improve very

[1] For an account of his researches, as well as for most valuable practical information in addition to Duchenne's own treatises, De l'Electrisation localisée, 8vo., Paris, 1861, and Physiologie des Mouvements, 8vo., Paris, 1867, Dr. Reynolds's Lectures on the Clinical Uses of Electricity, 8vo., London, 1871, and Dr. Tibbitt's excellent Handbook of Medical Electricity, 8vo., London, 1873, may be recommended as containing the best and clearest epitome of the present state of our knowledge on the subject.

[2] I have not spoken at all of those rare cases of paralysis which are attended by fatty degeneration of the muscles, and as Cruveilhier has shown, by wasting of the anterior roots of the spinal nerves; since they are by no means confined to early life, nor dependent on causes with which the patient's age has anything to do. The treatise of Dr. Roberts, on Wasting Palsy, 8vo., London, 1858, and his article in vol. ii of Reynolds's System of Medicine, contain a very good abstract of our knowledge concerning this disease, for our first acquaintance with which we are indebted to Cruveilhier. See his essay "Sur la Paralysie musculaire progressive atrophique," in the Archives de Médecine for May, 1853.

Both of this and of the still rarer Pseudohypertrophic Paralysis of Duchenne, cases have been under my observation at the Children's Hospital. The cases were both typical ones, but as they would only confirm facts already noticed by others I abstain from taking up space with their description, for it is so difficult, and yet so important, to avoid swelling the bulk of a book in each successive edition, that I feel it my duty often to omit many things which yet are neither uninteresting nor unimportant.

much; often, indeed, get quite well in the course of time and under treatment directed to the state of the patient's general health, while, in those instances in which the facial paralysis is associated with other forms of infantile palsy, the muscles of the face are almost always those over which power is first regained. You must bear in mind, however, the possibility of the nerve having undergone pressure from some enlarged gland: and if you find reason for believing this to be the case, you may apply a leech in the situation where the nerve passes out of the skull.

Lastly, I may just mention, that infants are sometimes born with facial hemiplegia, as the result of injury to the nerve from application of the midwifery forceps, or, as has in one or two cases been observed, from injury received during the passage of the head through the pelvis without any instruments having been employed. Such occurences are rare, but it is well that you should be aware of the possibility of their being met with independent of any injury to the brain. The paralysis, in these cases, generally disappears in the course of a few days or weeks.[1] In the only instance of the kind which has come under my own observation, the distortion of the face, though very great at birth —one eye being wide open, and the corresponding side of the face powerless, so that the child was unable to suck—had already greatly diminished within forty-eight hours, and disappeared completely in a week.

It would not be right to take leave of this class of subjects without a brief reference to the occasional occurrence of *hyperæsthesia* and *neuralgia* in early life. It is certainly singular, when one considers the extreme liability of infants and children to disorders of the nervous system, that cases of exalted sensibility, frequent as they are in the adult, should in them be so rare. Still I have met with these ailments on several occasions; sometimes preceding the loss of power in limbs which subsequently became paralyzed, and then almost invariably lasting for only one or two days, though I have known exceptions to this, and have observed a state of extreme sensitiveness of the lower part of the spine and of both legs to continue for several weeks, and then gradually to pass away, but leaving the power over the limbs much diminished. Besides these cases, however, I have twice observed in children during teething a state of increased sensibility of the whole surface, but chiefly of the lower extremities, so excessive as to render it almost impossible to move them for the purpose of washing or dressing. For many weeks one of these children could not be moved out of the horizontal position on account of the severe suffering which any change of position occasioned; while the other was thrown into an agony of crying whenever its legs were touched, either to wash them or to put on or take off its stockings. Both of these children, of whom one was ten and the other twenty months old at the time of their coming under my care, were much out of health, suffering from severe

[1] See Kennedy's Observations on Apoplexy, Paralysis, &c., of New-born Infants, in Dublin Journal of Med. Science, 1846; and Landouzy, Sur l'Hémiplégie faciale chez les Enfants nouveau-nés. 8vo., Paris, 1839.

odontitis, with bleeding and spongy gums, and in proportion as their general condition was ameliorated, the excessive sensitiveness lessened, and in the case of the younger infant disappeared in about three months. In the case of that child the symptoms had existed only about a month; in the case of the other, more than three months before it came under my notice. When I last heard of him, he was 2½ years old, greatly improved in health, having cut all his teeth, and his gums having become nearly sound. His limbs had for two months ceased to pain him, and he had begun to sit up for an hour at a time, though he had not made any attempt to walk. In both instances, iron, quinine, and the chlorate of potass were employed, with a moderate use of wine; and it was under this treatment that the improvement, tardy though it was, took place.

Intense neuralgic pain, like that of *tic douloureux* in the grown person, coming and going without apparent cause, is extremely rare in childhood; so uncommon in infancy that I do not remember ever to have met with any instance of pain—severe, obstinate, recurrent—for which sooner or later a distinct local cause was not found. I know, however, of one instance of its occurrence in a little girl aged 10 years, forcing from her shrieks of agony when the paroxysm of pain in her heel came on, but finally ceasing, and leaving behind no impairment of power over the limb, no tenderness on pressure, nor any evidence whatever of local disease. Her health, however, never good, grew worse as she approached to womanhood, and she suffered besides from all those varied ailments of the nervous system which, for want of better knowledge, we commonly class under the head of hysteria. Once, too, I saw a little girl, 7 years old, in whom, after a few days of what seemed like a mild attack of remittent fever, agonizing pain in the head came on, with extreme intolerance of light and sound. The symptoms had been regarded by some medical men who had seen her, as those of tubercular meningitis, and treatment in accordance with that supposition had been adopted without benefit; but it had not escaped the notice of the very intelligent practitioner who had the chief charge of the child, that vomiting had not preceded nor obstinate constipation accompanied these symptoms; that the cries were too vociferous, the suffering too intense, and the occasional intervals of ease too complete to accord with what might be anticipated if organic disease of the brain were present, while, though the treatment had aggravated rather than improved her condition, no additional sign of cerebral mischief had appeared in the course of four or five days, but pain continued as at first to be the only symptom. Regarding the condition as neuralgic, quinine was substituted for the previous antiphlogistic medicines, and the child was at once removed to Tunbridge Wells. Even on the journey the pain lessened in severity, and in a few days had altogether ceased, and the child rapidly regained her health. Two or three cases of a similar kind have also come under my notice in the Children's Hospital, and the symptoms have got better under good diet, perfect quiet, and the employment of quinine. The intensity of the pain, the completeness of its cessation, the persistence of the symptoms, with their non-progressive character, the absence of constipation or of permanent heat of head, as well as of that rapidly advancing emaciation which is rarely absent when active tubercular disease is going on in the brain or its membranes, will generally help us to a correct diagnosis. I have on more than one occasion, when in doubt, experimented for twenty-four hours with quinine, giving a full dose of it every four hours, and have had the satisfaction of finding the experiment succeed, and the symptoms which had seemed to bode such ill, abate and at last disappear under its continued use.

But while cases such as the above are very uncommon, it is by no means unusual for children to have attacks of headache, often of considerable severity, and attended with temporary intolerance of light and sound as the result of slight gastric disorder, or produced by slight overfatigue, or overexcitement. Such attacks closely resemble the sick headache, or the hysterical headache, to which delicate women are liable. They come on suddenly; they do not last above twelve or at the utmost twenty-four hours, they cease spontaneously (though a mild aperient or an alterative dose of mercury accelerates their departure), and, except a little languor, they leave behind them no sign of indisposition. Anxious parents are often solicitous about these attacks, lest they should portend disease of the brain; their very suddenness and their frequent recurrence, however—circumstances which awaken the alarm of non-professional persons—may serve rather to allay your apprehensions when taken in connection with the speedy cessation of each attack, and the absence of any abiding evidence of cerebral ailment in the intervals.[1]

LECTURE XVI.

Night Terrors.—Usually depend on intestinal disorder, not on primary disease of the brain—Their symptoms not to be mistaken for those of incipient hydrocephalus—Sometimes continue to occur for many weeks. Treatment.

Disorders of the Mind in childhood.—Knowledge of them very imperfect—Misuse of the term Cretinism. Mental peculiarities in childhood, how they are obvious in its disorders, which partake of nature of moral insanity, and why they do so. Hypochondriasis, and Malingering in children—Illustrative cases—Suggestions for their management. Moral Insanity—Conditions resembling it sometimes arise from overexertion of mind—Case in illustration, and principles of treatment.—Cases of more aggravated character, and independent of that cause. Mode in which intellect becomes dulled in such cases.

Idiocy.—Difference between idiocy and backwardness, how to be distinguished from each other. Deficiency of our knowledge on the subject of idiocy—Its frequency as a congenital condition overstated—Characteristics of idiocy in early infancy and as the child grows up. Objects of education of idiots—Its difficulties, and principles which should direct it.

It happens sometimes that a child who has gone to bed apparently well, and who has slept soundly for a short time, awakes suddenly in

[1] For further observation on neuralgia in childhood, I must again refer to my Lumleian Lectures.

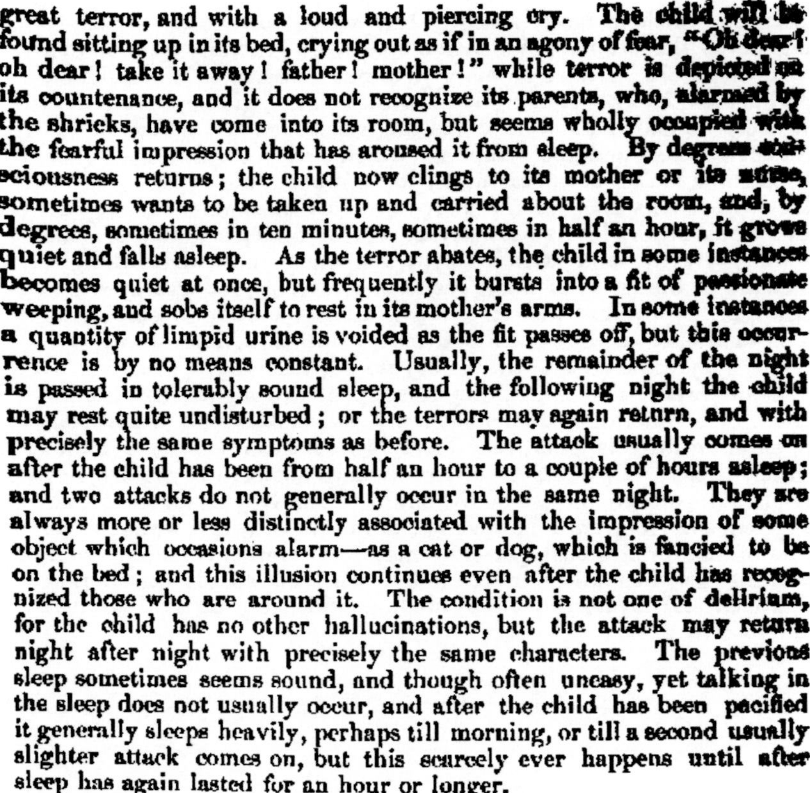

great terror, and with a loud and piercing cry. The child will be found sitting up in its bed, crying out as if in an agony of fear, "Oh dear! oh dear! take it away! father! mother!" while terror is depicted on its countenance, and it does not recognize its parents, who, alarmed by the shrieks, have come into its room, but seems wholly occupied with the fearful impression that has aroused it from sleep. By degrees consciousness returns; the child now clings to its mother or its nurse, sometimes wants to be taken up and carried about the room, and, by degrees, sometimes in ten minutes, sometimes in half an hour, it grows quiet and falls asleep. As the terror abates, the child in some instances becomes quiet at once, but frequently it bursts into a fit of passionate weeping, and sobs itself to rest in its mother's arms. In some instances a quantity of limpid urine is voided as the fit passes off, but this occurrence is by no means constant. Usually, the remainder of the night is passed in tolerably sound sleep, and the following night the child may rest quite undisturbed; or the terrors may again return, and with precisely the same symptoms as before. The attack usually comes on after the child has been from half an hour to a couple of hours asleep; and two attacks do not generally occur in the same night. They are always more or less distinctly associated with the impression of some object which occasions alarm—as a cat or dog, which is fancied to be on the bed; and this illusion continues even after the child has recognized those who are around it. The condition is not one of delirium, for the child has no other hallucinations, but the attack may return night after night with precisely the same characters. The previous sleep sometimes seems sound, and though often uneasy, yet talking in the sleep does not usually occur, and after the child has been pacified it generally sleeps heavily, perhaps till morning, or till a second usually slighter attack comes on, but this scarcely ever happens until after sleep has again lasted for an hour or longer.

Seizures of this kind may come on in a great variety of circumstances, and, according to the cause whence they have arisen, may continue to return for many weeks together, or may occur but a few times. As far as I have had the opportunity of judging, they are never the indications of primary mischief in the brain, but are always associated with some disturbance of the intestinal canal, and more or less obvious gastric disorder.

Some years ago I saw a little boy, aged 11 months, in whom the process of dentition was just beginning, and who for ten days had had slight diarrhœa, with dark and slimy evacuations. He then awoke one night, though before apparently sleeping soundly, with a sudden start, and a scream so violent that all the people in the house heard it. When taken out of bed he continued crying loudly for some minutes, but by degrees grew quiet and fell asleep again, sweating profusely. This sleep was as heavy as it had been before, though the eyes were not always closed during it, but after an uncertain interval of from half an hour to two hours he would again wake with the same loud and terrified scream, and again in a few minutes sink into slumber. The first of these attacks had taken place six days before the child was brought to me: they were increasing in frequency, as many as seven or eight having occurred in the course of a single night, and even during his sleep in the daytime the child was not free from them. He was cheerful, however, at other times; he sucked well, did not vomit, his head was not hot, and the anterior fontanelle was depressed rather than prominent; but the abdomen was rather full, and somewhat tender; the gums were much swollen, and the tongue was rather furred.

The gums were lanced, the child was put in a tepid bath every night: a powder containing one grain of Hydr. c. Cretâ, and one of Dover's powder, was given daily at bedtime, and ʒj of castor oil every morning, and the attack subsided.

Cases of this kind illustrate a point of practice which though important in the adult (you will find it insisted on by Andral in his Clinique Médicale), is still more so in the child. It is, that in many affections of the brain there is a stage quite at the commencement in which depletion may be out of place, but opiates or sedatives will allay the irritation, which, if let alone, would issue in dangerous or fatal congestion, or inflammation.

In the majority of cases of these *night terrors*, the condition of the bowels is one of constipation, not of diarrhœa. Sometimes, after gastric disorder has continued for a few days, in the course of which, perhaps, vomiting may have occurred, an attack of this nocturnal alarm may throw the parents into a state of great apprehension lest disease of the brain should be impending. I have seen a very severe attack of jaundice come on with these symptoms; and in such a case it is important to bear in mind the difference between the sudden, sympathetic disturbance of the brain, and the more gradual approach of tubercular meningitis with the drowsiness the child experiences, and yet the difficulty it has in going to sleep, the restlessness all night long, or the unquiet slumber with the moaning and starting which I pointed out to you when speaking of that disease. If, then, bearing in mind these facts, you find that the child who has had this attack in the night yet does not complain of intolerance of light, or of much or of any headache, and that while the head is cool and the pulse regular, the abdomen is full and hard, and perhaps slightly tender, you will scarcely take the less for the more dangerous affection.

But these symptoms may last for weeks or months together, neither diminishing nor much increasing in severity, so that they seem almost to constitute an independent disease; a view which Dr. Hesse of Altona,[1] who has written a very good pamphlet on it, is disposed to take somewhat too generally.

Such a case was that of a delicate boy, 7 years old, who during the previous twelve months had been cutting his first permanent molar teeth, and for the whole of that time had suffered from attacks of night terrors, which usually came on about half an hour after he had fallen asleep. He then started up with a wild and terrified look, and loud outcries, appearing not to know any one for some time, then

[1] Ueber das nächtliche Aufschrecken der Kinder im Schlafe. 8vo. Altenburg, 1845.

begging to be taken up, and becoming pacified after being carried about for half an hour in his father's arms. As the seizure passed off he used to void a large quantity of limpid urine, and having fallen asleep again, never but once had a second attack of it in the same night, while sometimes none occurred for two or three nights together. In other respects he seemed to be tolerably well, and was a lively and intelligent child, though for about fourteen days before he was brought to me his health had appeared less good, and there were evident indications of gastric disorder. I never saw this child but once again, so I cannot tell you his subsequent history; but his case affords a good illustration of the occasional persistence of these symptoms for a long time without the supervention of any really serious disease.

Although these symptoms may be the result of sympathetic affection of the brain through the medium of the abdominal viscera, still you should watch a child in whom they had frequently occurred with especial care, knowing that long-continued irritation of the nervous centres may, under the influence of comparatively trivial causes, issue in serious disease. Your chief attention, however, must be directed to the removal of the disorder of the intestinal canal; and this should be attempted by gentle means—by the careful regulation of the diet, and the judicious combination of aperients and tonics, rather than by drastic purgatives. Better, too, than either opium or henbane in these cases is a combination of bromide of potass and chloral as a means of allaying the irritability of the nervous system, and obtaining quiet sleep. The attacks usually come on in the early part of the night, so that to secure sleep for the first two or three hours is an almost certain prevention of a seizure. At the same time, too, it is right that the child should not be left in the dark or alone; the affection resembles nightmare, and in childhood dream-images seem to mingle with the waking impressions much more than in adult age. A light burning brightly in the room, and a familiar face meeting the child's eye at once on waking, will do much towards breaking the spell and towards allaying its fears. Harshness in such cases is quite out of place, and few pieces of cruelty can be greater than forcing a timid little child, in whom threatenings of these attacks have occurred, to go to bed in the dark, or to lie there without a candle, while its active imagination conjures up before its eyes, out of the bed-curtains or other objects in the room, the outlines of all sorts of terrific forms.

I have noticed this affection, not merely on account of its own importance as the occasion of much distress to the child, and sometimes also of much anxiety to its parents, but also because from it we may pass by a very fit transition to the brief consideration of some other forms of *disorder of the highest functions of the brain* in early life.

My remarks on these subjects must of necessity be very fragmentary and imperfect; so much so, indeed, that if I knew to what authors to refer you for information concerning them, I should feel that, by sending you to consult their writings, my duty would be best discharged.[1]

[1] For further remarks on the mind in childhood, and on its disorders, see my Lumleian Lectures.

But books will not help you here: and I will try to tell you the little that I know, in the hope that it may at least prevent you from going into practice with the impression that perversion of the intellect may not occur in the child as well as in the adult; or from supposing, if you do meet with a case too striking to be overlooked, that you have done all which can be expected of you in the way of diagnosis when you have pronounced the child an idiot; or all that is possible in the way of treatment, when you have provided for its safe custody.

The first step towards a better knowledge of these affections was taken when that form of idiocy which is endemic in certain localities, and is connected with various disorders of physical development, began to attract general attention. To Dr. Guggenbühl unquestionably belongs the merit of having given the first impulse to this study by his observations on cretinism. Cretinism is, however, but one of many forms of disordered development of the intellect; and there seems to be some risk of our being led into error by the extension of this term to a very large number of cases of idiocy occurring under conditions which have but a very slight resemblance to those which induce the endemic form in Alpine districts. But not only are the causes of idiocy various, and the characters that it presents very different in different cases, but perversion of the intellect or of the moral faculties, as distinguished from mere feebleness of mind, is met with in childhood as well as in adult age, and deserves to be regarded and to be treated as insanity no less in the one case than in the other.

In the first of this course of lectures, I pointed out to you the peculiarities impressed on the diseases of early life by the fact that childhood is a period of development. The peculiarities of the mind in early life are, however, more numerous and more important than even those of the body, and impart their characters to its diseases.

A child's experience is small, his ideas are few, and those are gathered from the world around him, not from his own reflections, while one impression succeeds another with greater rapidity than his feeble memory can hold fast. Hence, in disorders of the mind in early life, we do not meet with the distinct hallucinations, the fixed ideas, which characterize insanity in the adult. But though the intellectual powers are imperfectly developed, the feelings and the impulses are stronger, or at least, less under control, than they become with advancing years; and one great object of education is to bring them into proper subordination. Mental disorders, then, show themseves in the exaggeration of those feelings, the uncontrollable character of those impulses; in the inability or the indisposition to listen to that advice or to be swayed by those motives which govern other children. The affection, in short, is of that kind to which the name of moral insanity is usually given. With this state of mind, however, the child is of course less teachable than others—less able to apply to any form of learning; while fits of passion or of sullenness sometimes for days together put a stop to every attempt at instruction. The disorder of the moral faculties thus reacts upon the intellect; the child learns but little, and consequently grows up ignorant as well as ungovernable till at length either the evidences of insanity become with its advancing years unmistakable, or the mind, growing more obtuse from long want of culture, the case sinks down into one of mischievous idiocy.[1]

Now it is my belief that practitioners in general have not their attention sufficiently alive to some of these forms of mental disorder in early life. They are familiar with the idea of the idiot, as a being incapable of learning anything, unfit to take care of himself, still pleased with the toys of babyhood, but with a heart as stainless and affections as overflowing as the infant's. They are acquainted, too, with the general characters of cretinism, where the mind and body are alike dwarfed and misshapen by the influence of an unhealthy dwelling; but cases such as I have just referred to scarcely attract their notice. They are passed by as anomalies, as painful instances of some extreme badness, or of ungovernable temper, or of strange oddity about the child, from the study of which there is nothing to be learned, and for its remedy nothing to be suggested.

Many of these anomalous cases are, I believe, instances of a kind of mental disorder especially liable to issue in confirmed insanity. I have already assigned reasons for the opinion that affections of the mind in childhood must oftener display themselves in perversion of the moral faculties than in disorder of the intellectual powers; and bearing this in mind, I would always watch with close attention those cases of extremely bad disposition, of unconquerable stubbornness, or unmanageable fury, of which sorrowing parents sometimes tell us, though with but little hope of our suggesting anything that may remove or mitigate their bitter grief.

One of the least serious, though by no means of the least puzzling of these perversions of the moral faculties in childhood, is the disposition occasionally noticed to exaggerate some real ailment, or to complain of some ailment which is altogether imaginary. It is difficult to assign any sufficient reason for this conduct, mere indolence seems sometimes to be the chief motive for it, oftener vanity; the sense of importance in finding everything in the household arranged with exclusive reference to itself appears to have led to it—a feeling which may sometimes be observed to be very powerful even at an exceedingly early age. In many instances a morbid craving for sympathy is mingled with the love of importance, and both these sentiments are not infrequently gratified and exaggerated by the conduct of a foolishly fond mother. Real illness, however, in almost all of these cases exists at the commencement, though the child persists in complaining of its old symptoms long after their cause has disappeared.

I met some years since with a case which illustrates these remarks extremely well. A lad, aged 13, whose family were not very healthy, and who himself had at no period been robust, fell ill nine months before I saw him, with headache and other vague cerebral symptoms;

---

[1] My remarks refer to those slighter forms of mental unsoundness which present themselves to the notice of the ordinary practitioner. The subject of Insanity in early life will be found specially noticed by Dr Conolly in Medical Times, March and April, 1852; and by Brierre de Boismont, Annales d'Hygiène, 2d Series, vol. x, 1858, p. 362.

his illness having apparently been brought on by grief at the death of a favorite sister. This sister, too, had died of some disease of the brain, as had two other members of the family previously, and the anxiety about himself, which a knowledge of these facts naturally excited, was still further increased by his mother's desponding tone, and by the anxiety expressed by her in his hearing lest he should likewise fall a victim to the same disease.

From the very commencement his symptoms had presented a nearly uniform character, and had varied but little in intensity. They consisted of headache, with extreme sensibility to sound, even more than to light, so that if an organ was played in the street he would sometimes rush into another room, and bury his head in a pillow to be out of hearing of the noise. Coupled with this, there was extreme sensitiveness of the scalp and of the hair; for several months he had not allowed his hair to be brushed, combed, or washed, but this sensibility did not extend to the face or the spine.

The boy's appetite was very bad: he not infrequently suffered pain after eating, and for some four months had complained of pain and tenderness in the right hypochondriac and iliac regions; his bowels were constipated, his urine scanty, with considerable deposits of lithates, and occasional pain in voiding it; and erection of the penis sometimes took place during the act of micturition.

The boy was rather small for his age, ill-nourished but not emaciated, his upper lip slightly swollen, his abdomen soft and not at all full, and though he said that he had pain in the right hypochondrium, yet the abdomen was quite as soft there as elsewhere. His pulse was about 113, and very feeble; his tongue moist, slightly coated; respiration was quite good in both lungs.

As he came into the room the lad stopped; he walked feebly and with a slouching gait: but seated himself opposite the light without any apparent discomfort, and answered questions intelligently, though his speech was a little thick and hesitating; and there were slight twitchings of his face as he talked.

The question raised in this case was, whether the symptoms which I have just enumerated did or did not depend upon organic disease of the brain. I believed that no disease existed; for in spite of the long continuance of the symptoms, the boy was confessedly no worse than he had been many months before. Moreover, the absence of any fit, of any paralytic affection, or of impaired power over any limb; the fact that vomiting had never occurred, and that the pulse presented no other character than that of extreme feebleness, negatived, in my opinion, the supposition that disease of the brain existed. Besides, though he complained of so much tenderness of the scalp that the slightest touch of his hair caused extreme distress, yet on several occasions, when the hand had been laid gently on his head without his being aware of it, he made no complaint till he saw the hand. His father also said that he walked better when not noticed than when he was aware of any one's presence; that though he was unable to read, he yet was very fond of playing at cards; and that of an evening, when so occupied, he often seemed quite cheerful and like other children; and moreover, his

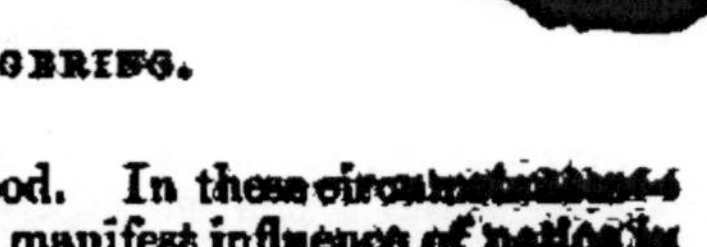

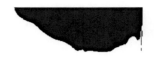

sleep at night was in general tolerably good. In these circumstances the intervals of ease, the quiet sleep, the manifest influence of notice in increasing his ailments, and of amusement in removing them—there seemed to be further and conclusive reasons against the supposition that the symptoms depended on organic cerebral disease.

Treatment of various kinds having been long pursued without any benefit, I recommended the complete discontinuance of all medicines with the exception of the cod-liver oil, to which the boy showed no repugnance, while the very imperfect manner in which he was nourished seemed to furnish a good reason for its employment. His health having previously somewhat improved at the seaside, I advised that he should go thither again, but to a fresh place, and unaccompanied by his mother; that while there all obvious reference to his head, either in general management or medical treatment, should be sedulously avoided, while an endeavor should be made, by fresh occupation, and fresh amusements, to turn his thoughts into a new channel.

This advice was not completely carried out, for an appearance of medical treatment was still kept up, though no active remedies were any longer employed. The boy, however, was sent to the seaside, and without his mother; and three months after, I heard of him as being in no respect worse, and in many better, than when I saw him; and eventually he perfectly recovered.

Another case of a somewhat similar kind may also deserve a brief notice. A little girl, aged 10½ years, whose mother, though a woman of considerable talent, had shown many peculiarities of character, came under my care on account of attacks of headache of the most intense severity. She had suffered from convulsions when 18 months old, and a slight illness at the age of 3 was attended by their return. When 6 years old, she began to suffer from a peculiar spasmodic cough, succeeded in the course of some months by considerable tenderness of the epigastrium. During the course of treatment for these ailments, she began to experience attacks of headache, which, from the age of 8 years until the time of her coming under my care, were reported to have returned frequently and without cause. Apparently nothing could be more arbitrary than the occurrence of these headaches; present at one time with excruciating severity, absent at another for weeks together. A constipated state of the bowels, and a capricious appetite, were the only abiding symptoms of ill-health which existed; but there did seem to be some connection between her occasional residence in a damp situation, and an increase in the frequency and intensity of her headaches.

The first time that I saw her, her countenance was anxious and expressive of intense suffering. She sat with her hand to her head, crying out vociferously, and asserting her inability to move from one room to another; though on being told decidedly that she must walk, she at once rose from the chair where she was crouching, and walked easily and firmly into another apartment. The child's pulse was rather feeble, but otherwise natural; her tongue a little coated, but there were no symptoms of serious illness about her. Sometimes she lay all night grievously complaining of headache; sometimes she slept well, and her sleep was usually more sound if she took some stimulant at bedtime. Accompanying the complaints of headache, there was a loss of interest in all childish pursuits, a waywardness and irritability quite unnatural in a girl of her age; and though now and then roused by some occurrence which interested her, she soon relapsed into her former condition. Sometimes she would rise before six o'clock in the morning, and go for a walk with her maid; while at other times she would lie in bed till a late hour. Her appetite was never large, but there were times when she took food moderately well; while at others she rejected it; and at last absolutely refused to feed herself; so that it became necessary to feed her like an infant. She clung to her mother during the whole of this time with the most exaggerated protestations of affection, but it was obvious that her complaints were always louder and more constant in her mother's presence; and when accidental circumstances took her mother for a few days from home, there was a marked improvement in the child's condition. If I came into the room unexpectedly, the child was often found at cheerful play; but the moment she perceived me, her hand was reapplied to her head, and her moan recommenced. Treatment of the most different kinds had been tried for years; the mother's conviction in the existence of some very serious disease was strengthened by the inutility of medicine, and her sympathy with her child, and lamentations over her sufferings, were often expressed in the child's presence. My opinion that no serious disease existed, that the complaints were exaggerated, that the mind needed discipline more than the body did medicine, that the child's cure would be difficult, if not impossible, so long as she remained with her mother, was unpalatable, and was considered unkind. To turn the attention into new channels; to lay aside ordinary tasks, such as hitherto, when apparently well enough to engage in them, she was set to; to give her the charge of live animals, and to endeavor, by teaching her something of their habits, or something of plants and flowers, which a country residence would have rendered easy—did not seem to be the rules that a doctor was expected to give. Physic was what the mother came to me for, and as I could not undertake the child's cure by drugs, she was soon removed from under my care. She returned home, and in a few days well-marked globus hystericus was added to her other symptoms; she next had general convulsions, though not accompanied by complete loss of consciousness, then hysterical dysphagia, during the continuance of which she was nourished chiefly by enemata of beef tea; and at last these symptoms assumed the character of complete hydrophobia: the appearance of water in a cup caused her to shudder, and the attempt to swallow any fluid produced an attack of general convulsions. This condition lasted for several days; by degrees its worst features subsided, the child regained health, and six months afterwards, when I heard of her, she was galloping about the country on her pony, and cured for the present of all her ills.

Now in cases of this description, and in others of a similar kind which have come under my notice, it is much less the state of the body than that of the mind which excites my apprehension. The constant watching its own sensations, the habit of constantly gratifying every wayward wish and temper under the plea of illness, and the [illegible] indulgence which it meets with in this from a mother's overkindness, exert a most injurious influence on the child's character, and it grows up a juvenile hypochondriac. It is well to be on our guard against the possibility of this occurrence in all the more protracted diseases of childhood; to warn the parents of it, in order that they may join with us in the endeavor to keep the child's mind healthy during the long illness of its body. It is but seldom that this condition comes to be so marked as in the cases which I have related, without very injudicious management on the part of the parents or friends. In such circumstances we often find it necessary to use great caution in conveying to their minds the suspicion which we entertain, and the expression of which they will be disposed to regard as a most unkind and unfounded libel on the child.

Another phase of mental disorder in childhood sometimes presents itself to us as the result of overtasking the intellectual powers. This overwork, too, is by no means in all cases due to the parents unwisely urging the child forward, but is often quite voluntary on its part. Sometimes, too, the friends of the child are so alive to this risk, that they limit the hours of work—a precaution which nevertheless often proves inadequate, from the want of some due provision for turning the thoughts and energies during play hours into some perfectly different channel.

In many of these cases nature happily takes matters into her own management. For a year or two, or more, the mind has grown apparently at the expense of the body; the parents take a fearful joy in their darling's acquirements; and if it should but live, think they, of what remarkable talents will it not be the possessor! By degrees, the extreme quickness of intellect becomes less remarkable; but the body begins to increase in robustness; and a year will sometimes suffice to transmute the little fairy, so quick, so clever, but so fragile, into a very commonplace, merry, rosy, romping child. I may add, that it is well to bear in mind the converse of this; to remember that body and mind rarely grow in equal proportion at one time; that the incorrigible little dunce, though not likely to prove a genius as he grows older, will yet very probably be found at twelve or fourteen to know as much as his playmates. A dull mind and a sickly or ill-developed frame, may make us anxious; but if the physical development is good, the mind will not be likely to remain long below the average standard.

But sometimes the overtasked mind leads to mischief which nature cannot rectify; an attack of cerebral inflammation comes on—often partakes of a tuberculous character, and destroys the patient; or if not, the child sinks under almost any accidental disease. In other instances, however, neither of these results takes place, but the whole nervous system seems profoundly shaken, and the moral character of the child seriously, and even permanently, injured.

A little girl, of whom her mother gave me the following history, came under my notice when seven years old. Never very robust, but quick and clever, her governess took pleasure in urging her forward, though never at the expense of what was supposed to be sufficient rest from study, and amusement suited to her years. However, when 5½ years old, the first signs of overtaxed brain appeared in frequent extreme irritability, and occasional causeless attacks of fury, amounting almost to madness. A few weeks after the commencement of these symptoms, the child began to suffer from chorea, affecting both sides of the body, though not severely; and at the same time she occasionally stumbled, and even fell when walking, though not from the violence of the spasmodic movements; and made complaints of frequent headaches, which were attended with great heat of head.

The chorea disappeared, the child improved altogether, though still having occasional headaches, and retaining much irritability of manner. Her improvement took place during a quiet residence at the seacoast, and a return to London was followed by an attack of influenza and an aggravation of her symptoms, with the exception of the chorea, which did not return. Revisiting the country, she once more improved, but the return to London, and the resumption of her education, even in the most careful manner, were followed by increased headache and more ungovernable temper; and it was in these circumstances that she came under my observation.

She was a fair-haired, delicate-looking child; but with the exception of slight contraction of the left orbicularis palpebrarum muscle, there was nothing remarkable in her appearance. Her pulse was rather feeble; and her mother stated that she was soon tired, and that every day she needed quiet rest upon a sofa for a couple of hours. Occasionally, whether at work or play, she would be attacked with very severe headache, which never lasted for more than a few minutes, but during its continuance incapacitated her, by its intensity, for anything. Equally sudden, and almost equally causeless, were the attacks of fury which she now and then manifested, and which a word, a look, or her favorite companion entering a room before her, or stepping before her up the stairs, would suffice to bring on. At one time she had vented her anger in blows; but though she did not now strike those who offended her, she would burst forth into the most violently abusive language, though seldom uttering above a sentence or two. Sometimes she denied, and her mother believed with truth, that she knew what she had said; at other times she seemed aware of it, and throwing her arms round the person whom she had so addressed, would express her sorrow, and beg to be forgiven. There was still some disposition to fall when walking, though nothing like a fit had ever been observed; and if anything was given to her to hold or to carry, she would not infrequently let it fall. The child's general disposition was amiable; she was very intelligent in her manner, but was morbidly solicitous about her health, and disposed to exaggerate every ailment—a disposition, however, which had been most judiciously controlled by her mother.

In this case, while conceding the possibility that the occasional stumbling in her walk might be the prelude of epilepsy, and that the fits of fury might issue in abiding disorder of the mind, I yet was disposed to entertain a more favorable prognosis—and this, founded in no slight degree on the great good sense with which the child's [illegible] recognised these dangers, and applied herself to guard against [illegible]

As the return to her previous pursuits, even though attempted with the greatest care, was followed on each occasion by a deterioration in the child's condition, I advised that for a time they should be completely laid aside; that she should go into the country; that for [illegible] and music, and history, should be substituted botany, the keeping and managing of pet animals, the studying their habits, and all the [illegible] of quiet occupations which the country offers, especially to those [illegible] friends, as was the case with this little girl, have the intelligence [illegible] derive from them the full measure of advantage which they [illegible] made to yield.

I believe the recognition of the real danger, and the adoption [illegible] proper plan of management, to be of the greatest possible impo[rtance] in these cases; and yet the doing so is often attended with great [diffi]culty. Not merely is the danger at which we hint so fearful, b[ut the] idea of permanent disorder of the mind occurring in childhood [seems] to the parents so strange, even so improbable, that they are dis[posed] too often to think the risk an imaginary one, and to reject the co[unsel] which we offer concerning the best manner of its avoidance. [More]over, the recommendation, which I believe to be a sound one, t[hat in] almost all of these cases the child should be separated from its pa[rents,] while it adds to their distress, diminishes at the same time the p[roba]bilities of their compliance. I am certain, however, that the pa[rents] are very rarely the best persons to carry out the management o[f the] child; often, that they are the very worst to whom it could be in[trust]ed. The very motives which, in the proper relation between p[arent] and child, are the most cogent to induce the latter's obedience, a[re] of a kind to be exposed to the wayward caprices of that child wh[ose] moral faculty is perverted. With the most undeviating kin[dness] there is yet necessary in the management of such a patient a com[plete] impassibility, if I may use the word. "You grieve me," "You [make] me sad by this or that conduct, by this wilfulness, or this fit of [ill temper,"] is in these cases too often but an announcement to the child of a n[ever-] failing mode of annoying those whom he may wish to vex, an[d the] discovery of this power is alone sufficient to weaken their auth[ority] and control. Moreover, the steady undeviating pursuit of a [cer]tain plan for weeks, or months, can scarcely be intrusted with saf[ety to] persons so deeply interested in its issue, so apt prematurely to rejo[ice in] its success, and to diminish their precautions, or equally prematur[ely to] despair of benefit, and therefore to relax in their vigilance, a[s the] parents of the suffering child. Besides all the thousand recolle[ctions] of infancy, which link together parents and children, instea[d of] strengthening, do but fetter their hands if they undertake this offi[ce.]

I should not have thought it necessary to add, that a school i[s not] the place for such children, if I had not sometimes known them sent thither, under the vain expectation that the society of other [chil]dren would amuse, and the necessary regulations of the place would [con]trol and amend them. Ordinary school discipline, however, is in[applic]able to them; occasions of anger constantly abound there, whil[e] frequent outbreaks of fury, characteristic of this condition, can neither be passed over without notice, nor subjected to controlling influence of the proper kind.

The houses of those who receive imbecile and idiot children are, however, not fit places for this class of patients. Their intellect is active enough: they are revolted by the stupidity of those around them, and find a mischievous pleasure in tormenting and annoying them, while no rules can be laid down suited for the management of cases so different as the idiotic and the insane. I believe that children in this condition do best as the only inmates of a quiet family, under the constant control and supervision of some person competent to enter into their pursuits, and to share their pleasures; to whom they may become attached, but whose relation to them will not be so intimate as to place it in their power, even when most wayward, to cause serious vexation or distress. At intervals, as the child improves, it may be allowed to associate with other children; at first in their play, as in dancing, for instance, or in some out of doors amusement—afterwards at other times, and with fewer restrictions; but a course of education, apart from other children, different in its manner and its objects is, I am sure, desirable till the mind has quite recovered its balance, and the power of self-control has been developed and strengthened.

The cases that I have hitherto related were instances of only the slightest degrees of a condition which, if not remedied, may pass into confirmed insanity. I believe the gradations to be almost imperceptible by which the one state passes into the other, and I know of some cases in which the ungovernable temper and occasional fury of the child have changed after puberty to complete mania, which rendered the patient the inmate, and, I fear, the permanent inmate, of a lunatic asylum.

One more history I may add, to show some of the steps by which the change from bad to worse takes place. A girl, 12 years old, an only daughter, pretty, clever, but very vain and very fond of dress, the object of her parents' doating fondness, which she returned with equal affection, was urged by the love of display, and the desire of praise, beyond her powers. She grew wilful, unmanageable, ungovernably passionate; but in spite of this, her expressions of attachment to her mother became stronger and stronger, and on the occasion of her mother's illness it was almost impossible to keep her from the sick-room; and she gave way to fits of fury if ever of necessity denied admittance.

She was now, by medical advice, sent to school, in spite of her most earnest entreaties to the contrary. She remained there two months, during which time she had been extremely unhappy, and returned decidedly worse. The first indication that she showed of positive insanity consisted in lacing her stays as tight as possible over her abdomen, and in tying a handkerchief tight round her body for the same purpose. For this she assigned no reason, but became furious if prevented from accomplishing this purpose. Soon afterwards she had another delusion with reference to the state of her bowels, which she was always trying to relieve, spending sometimes several hours together running up and down stairs to and from the water-closet."

Under a very partial adoption of a plan such as I have mentioned, combined with due attention to the state of her bowels, which were very constipated, considerable improvement took place, and continued for nearly a year. By degrees, however, the ungovernable temper returned, the child's paroxysms of rage became frightful in their violence, and lasted sometimes for hours together, and the desire to be perpetually on the water-closet became as strong as ever. In this condition, about two years from the date of her first showing signs of mental disorder, she died; but of what disease, or in what special circumstances, I am unable to tell.

But it is not only in these circumstances that moral insanity presents itself to us in children. Mental disorder in childhood seems, as I have already stated, almost invariably to assume this character, whatever be the condition in connection with which it comes on.

I once saw a little girl, six years old, who from the age of one year had been subject to fits of an epileptic character, which sometimes were severe, and lasted for several hours, but did not seem to exercise any abiding influence on her general health. They recurred at uncertain intervals of from two to seven months, and though sometimes apparently induced by sudden alarm, often came on independent of any obvious exciting cause. But besides the fits, there were some mental peculiarities about the child which excited her parents' apprehension, and the more so, since the older she grew the more striking did they become.

When I saw her she was a tall, fair-haired, blue-eyed child, and the abiding expression of her countenance was pleasant. She walked awkwardly, however, with her head very much bent down; and when she stood, she kept up an almost unceasing mechanical movement of her hands up and down the front of her dress, or tossed them about not unlike a child with chorea, except that the movements were less violent. Her manner was tolerably intelligent, indeed not without a certain precocious shrewdness, but she laughed once or twice unmeaningly, and on my refusing to give her a toy to keep, which she had amused herself by playing with, she at once struck me.

She was decidedly backward in knowledge as compared with other children; but owing to her condition, had never been taught much. Her parents said that she was quick if she could be induced to apply, but that she would never apply to anything for more than a few minutes. She was said to show a fondness for music; and, though unable to write, it was a favorite amusement with her to scribble over paper in imitation of the writing of her elder sisters.

In disposition she was said to be either an angel or a demon; though fond of her sisters, she would strike them on the slightest provocation, and she had occasional fits of most ungovernable fury.

The advice which I gave with reference to the management of this child was similar to that which I have already given you. It was partially adopted, and with some improvement in her condition, though I do not know what was its ultimate issue. My object in relating the case, was to add another illustration to those already given, of the peculiar character which disorder of the mind assumes in early life, and of the differences between it and mere idiocy or feebleness of intellect. The earlier these symptoms manifest themselves, and the more aggravated their form, the greater will be their influence on the intellectual powers, and the more completely will they interfere with the education of the child, who may in consequence sink in the course of time as low in intelligence as the most hopeless idiot.

Idiocy is unquestionably of much more frequent occurrence in childhood than are those affections of the mind which have hitherto engaged our attention. The term idiocy, however, is a very wide one, including conditions differing remarkably from each other, both in kind and in degree, while not seldom it is misapplied to cases in which there is mere backwardness of the intellectual powers.

Backward children—*enfants arriérés*, as the French call them—constitute a class by no means seldom met with. They generally attain their bodily development slowly, and the development of their mind is equally tardy. They cut their teeth late, walk late, talk late, are slow in learning to dress and to wash themselves, are generally dull in their perceptions, and do not lay aside the habits of infancy till far advanced in childhood. When the time comes for positive instruction, their slowness almost wears out every one's patience; and among the poor indeed, the attempt at teaching such children is at length given up in despair, and, growing up in absolute ignorance, it is no wonder that they should be regarded as idiots. Still, dull as such children may be, and duller still they must needs become if allowed to grow up untaught to manhood, there is a difference between them and idiots, and one which I cannot better describe than in the words of M. Séguin,[1] who has both written and worked so well on this very subject.

"The idiot," says he, "even in the slightest degree of the affection, presents an arrest of development both of body and mind; the backward child does not remain stationary, but his development goes on more slowly than that of other children at his age; he is behind them in the whole course of their progress, and his delay, increasing every day, places at length an enormous distance between them—a distance which, in fact, is insurmountable."

In some of its minor degrees even, this backwardness not infrequently excites the solicitude of parents. I have observed it in children who had been ill-nourished in infancy, or who had been weakened by some serious and protracted illness, even though unattended by any special affection of the brain; but I have also observed it in other instances independent of any such cause. Be the history, however, what it may, the ground on which you rest your opinion that the case is not one of idiocy is this,—that though, at four years old, the child may not seem to be intellectually superior to most children at two, yet in manners, habits, and intelligence it does agree with what might be expected from the child at two; less bright perhaps, less joyous, but still presenting

[1] Traitement Moral, &c., des Idiots, p. 72, 12mo., Paris, 1846.

nothing which, if it were but younger, would awaken your apprehension.

It is well, in all cases of unusual backwardness, to ascertain the condition of the sense of hearing, and of the power of speech; for I have known the existence of deafness long overlooked, and the child's dulness and inability to speak referred erroneously to intellectual deficiency; and have also observed mere difficulty of articulation, partly dependent on malformation of the mouth, lead to a similar misapprehension. In both the instances referred to, the complete inability to keep up intercourse with other children, or the great difficulty in the attempt, had cast a shadow over the mind; and the little ones were dull, suspicious, unchildlike. A similar effect is not infrequently produced by serious illness, even after the time of infancy is passed. The child will for months cease to walk, or forget to talk, if these had been but comparatively recent acquirements; or will continue dull, and unequal to any mental effort, for weeks or months together, and then the mind will begin to develop itself once more, though slowly; possibly so slowly as never altogether to make up for lost ground.

In idiocy,[1] however, there is much more than this; more even than the mere arrest of the intellect at any period. The idiot of eight years old does not correspond in his mental development to the child at six, or four, or two; his mind is not only dwarfed, but deformed; while feebleness of will is often as remarkable as mere deficiency of power of apprehension. Numerous questions suggest themselves to us with reference to this subject; to many of which I can attempt no answer whatever, to none of which can I return anything like a satisfactory reply. The causes of idiocy, the influence which our knowledge of them should exercise on our prognosis, the relations of epilepsy and of paralysis to it, and the extent to which their existence should modify our opinions, are only some among several very important questions to which I can do no more than refer as requiring elucidation.

Down to the present time, the only systematic attempt with which I am acquainted to collect and arrange information on the subject of idiocy, is that which has been made by Dr. Howe, of Boston, by authority of the legislature of Massachusetts.[2] Valuable, however, as such an inquiry is in many points of view, its results can never yield more than mere approximations to truth, and cannot be regarded as positive medical facts. For instance, Dr. Howe states,[3] as the result of his inquiries, that in 420 out of 574 cases the condition of idiocy was congenital; but these numbers, if received as absolutely correct, would, I am sure, lead to a very considerable overestimate of the frequency of congenital idiocy; and it is admitted, indeed, that all cases have been classed as congenital in which the affection dated from in-

[1] It is almost needless to observe, that idiocy is here spoken of independent of that peculiar variety, endemic in certain localities, and which, under the name of cretinism, has attracted so much attention of late years, and has been the subject of several reports, both to the Sardinian, Austrian, and Swiss Governments.

[2] Report made to the Legislature of Massachusetts upon Idiocy, by S. G. Howe, Chairman of the State Commission, 8vo., Boston, 1848.

[3] See pp. 57 and 95 of the Report.

fancy, or early childhood. It is quite certain that a very large number of cases of idiocy date from early infancy; but a sense of hopelessness attaches to congenital disease, which renders it very desirable that this impression should not be adopted hastily; and, though my opinion is necessarily founded on a comparatively small number of cases, I must nevertheless express my decided conviction that instances of really congenital idiocy actually form a minority of the cases of that condition.

The distinct evidence, however, of the really congenital character of idiocy is not by any means sufficient ground for regarding a case as absolutely hopeless, so far as obtaining a very considerable amelioration of the patient's condition is concerned; and no one who saw the children that were exhibited years ago in London, as Aztecs, need despair of being able to teach much even to those whose cerebral conformation is most imperfect. The history most commonly obtained on closely questioning the relations of idiot children, is to the effect that their health having been good up to a certain period, which usually falls within the first year of life, they then had one or more fits, or perhaps a succession of them, recurring at uncertain intervals for one, two, or three years, or even becoming habitual; and that from this date their mental development was retarded in all respects, completely arrested in some; while the signs of idiocy have since then become more marked with each succeeding year. The cessation of these fits, even though once very frequent, does not seem to be by any means generally followed by improvement in the patient's condition; nor, as far as I know, are epileptic idiots, even when the fits date from a very early period, those whose intellectual powers are by any means invariably the lowest. This, however, is but one of the modes in which idiocy comes on; in other instances there is no point in the child's history which can be laid hold of as marking the commencement of this condition; but as the body grew the mind remained stationary, till by degrees the painful conviction that it was an idiot forced itself on the friends; while, again, in other cases some serious cerebral disease which threatened life at two, three, or four years old, or later, has left the mind permanently obscured and weakened.

Even in earliest infancy there is usually a something in the idiot child which marks him as different from babies of his own age. He is unable to support his head, which rolls about from side to side almost without an effort on his part to prevent it; and this often awakens a mother's anxiety long before any other circumstance has excited her apprehension. Next it is perceived that the child does not notice; that his eye does not meet his mother's with the fond look of recognition, accompanied with the dimpling smile, with which the infant, even of three months old, greets its mother. Then it is found to have no notion of grasping anything, though that is usually almost the first accomplishment of babyhood; if tossed in its nurse's arms there seems to be no spring in its limbs; and though a strange, vacant smile sometimes passes over its face, yet the merry ringing laugh of infancy, or the joyous chuckle of irrepressible glee, is not heard. As time passes on, the child shows no pleasure at being put down—"to feel its feet,"

greatly in different cases. Mere verbal memory, too, is by no means a fair index of a child's mental condition; for the idiot may often be taught, parrot-like, to repeat many things of the meaning of which he has not the slightest notion. This sort of acquirement, too, while it exercises but very little influence on the general mental condition, is lost very speedily so soon as the constant teaching is interrupted, and therefore, though not without a certain utility, does not rank by any means among the first objects to which the attention should be turned.

There is not time, however, nor indeed have I the experience to enable me to enter into so wide a subject as that of the education of idiots. I must content myself with having pointed out to you the general characteristics of their condition—the objects towards which your endeavors must be chiefly turned in any attempt at its improvement. I can wish for nothing better than that, before long, the labors of others shall render these observations of mine as superfluous as I know them to be imperfect.

LECTURE XVII.

DISEASES OF THE RESPIRATORY ORGANS, their frequency and fatality.—Peculiarities of the respiratory function in early life—Causes of the rapid pulse and quick breathing in infancy—Feebleness of inspiratory power, and consequent tendency to collapse of the lung.

ASPHYXIA, or still-birth.—Its dependence on interruption of placental circulation—Its degrees, symptoms, and treatment.

IMPERFECT EXPANSION OF THE LUNGS.—Sometimes congenital—Appearance of the lung—Influence of inflation upon it—Its causes and symptoms—Case of its fatal termination—Case of recovery from it—Diagnosis from congenital phthisis—Treatment.

WE now come to the examination of the diseases of those two grand systems of the organism by which the blood is kept in motion, the requisite changes in it are effected, and the animal heat is maintained. Your attention was lately called to the fatality of the diseases of the nervous system in early life as one grand reason for their attentive study; but this argument is still more cogent if applied to the maladies of the organs of respiration and circulation, since they destroy a far greater number of children, and occasion a mortality almost equal to that produced by diseases of the nervous and digestive systems together. It appears, indeed, from our tables of mortality, that very nearly a third of all deaths under five years of age are due to the *diseases of the respiratory organs;* while not above one child in four dies under that age from diseases of the nervous system, and not above one in seven from those of the digestive system.[1]

While the study of these diseases is of paramount importance, we meet with inducements to their investigation which in a great measure failed us in the case of diseases of the nervous system. Peculiar difficulties then attended us, and the truth was veiled in so much obscurity, that we often saw it but indistinctly—sometimes, perhaps, altogether failed to perceive it. The means, however, which have enabled us to bring medical knowledge with reference to the diseases of the chest in the adult, almost to the state of one of the exact sciences, still stand us in stead here; and care and patience will enable us to discover the condition of the lungs with nearly as much certainty in an infant as in a grown person.

Nor is the greater facility of their diagnosis the only circumstance that lightens their study, but a feeling of hopefulness attends their investigation which we often missed in the subjects that have lately engaged our attention. They, indeed, furnished us with interesting pathological studies: we stood around the sick-bed, and watched nature's struggles with disease that was irremediable, and we traced its effects afterwards as we examined the dead body; but the diagnosis of the affection was in many instances but the sentence of the patient's death; and we often felt that, as practical physicians, there was but little for us to do. We shall, it is true, meet with some such affections in our study of diseases of the chest; but, happily, they are few in comparison with those which, in addition to much that would interest the mere pathologist, present still more that will give ample scope for all the skill of the practical physician.

At first sight, it may seem to you that there can be little in the organs of respiration and circulation in early life different from their condition in riper years. And it is true that the part they play is as important at the first hour of existence as in the most advanced old age, and that their structure and functions undergo no such changes as we have noticed taking place in the brain during infancy and childhood; but, nevertheless, they present some *important peculiarities in the young*, with which you must be acquainted before you can hope to treat their diseases with success.

The condition of infancy is one of unceasing development; all the organs of vegetative life have, so to speak, double work to do—not

[1] Table showing the proportion per cent. of deaths from different causes in childhood, in the metropolis, as compared with subsequent life. [Deduced from the 5th and 8th Reports of the Registrar-General, for 1842 and 1845.]

	Under 1 year.	Between 1 and 3.	Between 3 and 5.	Under 5.	5 to 10.	10 to 15.	At all ages above 15.
From Diseases of the Nervous System, ...	30.5	18.5	17.6	24 3	15.1	10.6	10.4
Do., do., Respiratory System	26.9	39 5	33.	32.8	29.5	30.7	38.0
Do., do., Digestive System,	17.5	12.8	5.5	14.1	6.5	8.8	7.7

merely to supply the daily waste, and to remove effete and noxious matter, but to build up that wondrous edifice, the human body. It is probably in great measure on this account that the blood in infancy and childhood runs its course more rapidly, and that the lungs vivify it more frequently than in adult age. We shall probably not be far wrong if we estimate the average frequency of the pulse in the grown person, when making no exertion, at 75, and of the respirations at 18 in the minute.[1] In infants not above a week old, the average frequency of the respirations is 39, and of the pulse 102; but the former may rise to 84, and the latter to 140, as the result of some transient excitement or disturbance, and wholly independent of disease. Until the sixth year the average frequency of the pulse continues at 102; and though that of the respiration diminishes, yet it does not fall below 30. The variations between their maximum and minimum frequency are now, however, circumscribed within limits which grow narrower as the child approaches manhood.[2]

Although the rapid pulse and quick breathing of early life are probably in great measure due to the activity of the vital processes, yet the wide variations in their frequency induced by very slight accidents lead to the suspicion that this is not their only cause, but that both phenomena are to a certain extent indications of the infant's weakness. This suspicion is still further strengthened by our knowledge of the fact, that the quantity of carbonic acid exhaled at each expiration diminishes in proportion as the expirations are more frequent;[3] so that it is plain that the rapidity of the respiratory movements is not of itself a measure of the activity of the respiratory process. But still stronger proof of this fact may be adduced. Animal heat is generated almost entirely by respiration. If, therefore, the activity of the vital processes were in proportion to the rapidity of the breathing, the new-born infant should be warmer than the child, and the child than the youth. But this is not so, for the temperature of health appears to vary but very little after the first week of life; attaining a slightly higher point after that time than it had before, and maintaining it almost unchanged through childhood and adult age; but falling again, though slightly, with far advancing years.[4]

There seems, then, good reason for believing that the rapid breathing of the child is to some extent the result of its more delicate frame, rendering it unable, at a single effort, to inspire as deeply as the more

---

[1] This result is afforded by the numerous and careful observations of Professor Vierordt: see his article Respiration, in Wagner's Handwörterbuch der Physiologie, Part 12, 8vo., Brunswick, 1845, p. 874.

[2] The chief authority for the statements in the text is the valuable essay of M. Roger, De la Température chez les Enfants, 8vo., Paris, 1844, and the more recent confirmatory observations in his Récherches Cliniques, already referred to. The researches of M. Seux, Sur les Maladies des Enfants Nouveau-Nés, 8vo., Paris, 1855, do but confirm, in the main, the results already arrived at with reference to the wide variations in the frequency of the pulse in new-born infants.

[3] See Vierordt's experiments on this subject, loc. cit., p. 887.

[4] The researches of Dr. v. Bärensprung, published in Müller's Archiv., 1851, p. 125, do not confirm the above statement; but they are too few in number to invalidate it, and therefore it is still retained in the text. See § 5 of v. Bärensprung's essay.

robust adult, so that it is compelled, by the frequent repetition of its efforts, to make up for their comparative feebleness. Quite in keeping with this is the small power of resisting cold, or of maintaining an independent temperature, which is a distinguishing peculiarity of early life. If the young of any warm-blooded animal is exposed to a low temperature, its respiration at first increases in frequency; but, if not soon restored to a warmer atmosphere, the nervous energy that should set the respiratory apparatus in motion becomes still more depressed; air enters the lungs imperfectly, the inspirations grow less frequent, and the warmth of the body sinks rapidly down to that of the surrounding medium. Nor is this all; but it often happens if a young infant has been thus exposed to the cold, and especially if this has been done before the respiration had become properly established, that no subsequent removal to a warmer atmosphere will suffice to raise the temperature, or to set in proper activity the respiratory process.

But not merely is the respiratory apparatus more delicate in the child than in the adult—for so are all the organs in early life—but it is feebler, as compared with the work it has to do, with the difficulties it has to overcome; and this constitutes a most important peculiarity in the physiology of respiration in early life, and greatly modifies its pathology.

The interesting researches of Mr. Hutchinson[1] have shown us that in the case of the adult "the resistance to the *ordinary breathing* force, *independently* of the elastic power of the lungs, is equal to lifting more than 100 lbs. at every ordinary inspiration." The elasticity of the walls of the chest which present this resistance is, in proportion to the size of the thorax, nearly as great in the infant as in the adult; but how much smaller is the muscular power by which this resistance is to be overcome! You see proof of it in the ordinary mode of respiration of a young infant, which presents something almost of difficulty. The breathing is quick and short, then after a few seconds there succeeds a pause, and then the hurried respiratory movements begin again, while the slightest disturbance, or the most trivial excitement, will at any time raise the frequency of the inspirations by ten or twelve in the minute. This respiration, too, is almost entirely abdominal; the chest moves but little, its walls are but little expanded, and the ear detects in the respiratory murmur little or nothing of that clear, loud sound which is so characteristic of a subsequent period of childhood, and with which you are all familiar by the name of puerile respiration. This peculiarity of the breathing in early infancy, to which M. Trousseau was, I believe, the first to call attention, is another token of the feebleness of the inspiratory power. As the child grows older, and its strength increases, and its muscular system becomes more developed, the chest expands with each inspiration, and the faint respiratory murmur is succeeded by the loud puerile breathing which is heard as the air enters into the smaller air-cells.

The resistance of the walls of the chest, however, is not the only ob-

---

[1] On the Respiratory Functions, in vol. xxix of the Medico-Chirurgical Transactions.

stacle to be overcome at each inspiratory effort, but the lungs themselves are furnished with an elastic fibrous investment, processes of which dip down into their substance, and form the parietes of the different lobules. If you blow air forcibly into the lungs after their removal from the body, the resiliency of their tissue will expel a large proportion of the air the moment your effort at inflation is suspended. This elasticity of the lungs, then, which has been estimated at offering in the adult male an obstacle to each inspiration equal to 160 lbs., and in the female equal to 120 lbs. avoirdupois, is constantly tending to empty them of air, and constantly resisting the introduction of more.[1] The want of breath, however, puts the respiratory muscles into play; the man takes a deep inspiration, and by this effort he unconsciously overcomes the resistance of the chest and the elasticity of the lungs. The new-born infant feels the same want, and makes the same effort; but its muscular power is small, and its inspirations are often so feeble as to draw the air in some parts only into the larger bronchi, while many of the smaller air-tubes remain undilated, and much of the lung continues in its fœtal state. The blood being thus but imperfectly aerated, all the processes of nutrition go on imperfectly; the vital powers languish, the inspiratory efforts become more and more feeble, the temperature sinks, and the infant dies. But not only may this state persist as the result of imperfect respiration at birth, but cold, or the want of sufficient food, or any other cause that impairs the already feeble muscular power, favors its supervention. As the power of the inspiratory muscles is impaired, the air no longer penetrates into the lungs so far as it once did, while the residual air is gradually driven out of the pulmonary cells by the elasticity of the lung, and portions once permeable to air become in the course of time, altogether useless. Or, an increase of the ordinary resistance to the entrance of the air will have the same effect; and if the pouring out of mucus into the bronchial tubes should much obstruct them, large portions of lung will by degrees become emptied and collapsed, the dyspnœa will grow urgent, and the child will die from symptoms such as in the adult result only from most serious structural disease.

The possibility of a large portion of the respiratory apparatus remaining useless from birth, or becoming so afterwards, without any serious disease of these organs, is a most important element in the pathology of infancy and early childhood. It warns us to be on our guard, during the course of various maladies, against a danger which, in more advanced life, we have not to apprehend; while, at the same time, it teaches us that the dyspnœa, the hurried breathing, and many other symptoms which in the adult would call for most active treatment, may result in infancy from simple weakness, and require stimulating rather than depletory measures.

---

[1] The investigations of Professor Donders, and of Mr. Hutchinson, into the amount of this elasticity of the lungs, though carried on independently, conduct to very similar results: the former estimating it as equal to ℥ix ʒx avoirdupois per square inch as a maximum; the latter estimating it on the average at lbs. per square inch See the researches of Prof. Donders, in the Nederlandsche Lancet, Dec. 1849; and Schmidt's Jahrb., Dec. 1850; and article Thorax, by Mr. Hutchinson, in Cyclopædia of Anatomy and Physiology, vol. iv, p 1058.

Before we proceed to study the diseases of the respiratory organs in infancy and childhood, we must make ourselves thoroughly acquainted with this state of *imperfect expansion of the lungs.* It presents itself to us in two different circumstances.

1st. As a congenital condition: a more or less considerable portion of the lung never having become penetrated by air, but having remained in its fœtal state.

2d. As an acquired condition: portions of the lung which once were freely traversed by air ceasing to admit it; and this not from alteration of structure, but from a simple collapse of the pulmonary tissue.

But, even before this, we must notice that condition in which, on the child's birth, the air fails, for a time at least, to enter at all. The child is born asphyxiated; it does not breathe, does not show the ordinary signs of life, but, to use the common, homely, but expressive phrase, is stillborn.

I said, many days ago,[1] that a stillborn child may present a very great degree of cerebral congestion, or that there may even be actual extravasation of blood within its skull, and that such apoplectic condition may interfere with the success of any effort for its resuscitation, but that, nevertheless, the apoplexy, or the extravasation of blood, is not the immediate cause of its death; but the inability to breathe is.

In some rare cases a child may be stillborn, owing to the existence of some intra-uterine disease affecting it; but it is not with these exceptional cases that we have to do here, nor with those in which a child ill-nourished, or born before its time, dies from mere feebleness. In cases of true *Infantile Asphyxia,* interference with the placental respiration, however produced, is the real cause of all the subsequent phenomena. Hence it is that we see the death of the child follow almost immediately on that of the mother; that the surgeon, waiting for her last breath in order at once to perform the Cæsarian section, scarcely ever succeeds in rescuing her infant. Not otherwise, though more slowly, is the child's death brought about if the mother's system is greatly drained of blood by partial separation of the placenta; for then enough does not remain to produce the necessary oxygenation in the circulating fluid of the child. We see the same result, too, in protracted labors, when the frequent and violent contractions of the womb interfere with the circulation of the maternal blood in the placental sinuses; and though the cause is different, the result that follows is just the same when pressure on the umbilical cord interferes with the afflux or the reflux of the fœtal blood to or from the placenta.

These causes tend to produce an effort at respiration, and this probably in proportion to the suddenness of their operation; and now and then a striking illustration of it is afforded by the *vagitus uterinus*—the unborn babe not breathing only, but even crying, in its mother's womb; while evidence of the unsuccessful effort is oftener furnished by the presence of the liquor amnii in the bronchi of the dead child, or in the large mucous râle which accompanies its first attempts to breathe, if it recovers. The unsuccessful respiratory efforts do but

---

[1] Lecture V, p. 59.

disturb still more the placental breathing; while the longer and the more gravely, in any case, the circulation in the placenta is disturbed, and the oxygenation of the fœtal blood interfered with, the more does the excitability of the medulla oblongata become lessened, and, with it, the prospect of resuscitating the child.

There are, then, different degrees of infantile asphyxia, though, in all, the object to be aimed at is the same; namely, to establish pulmonary respiration as speedily and as completely as possible.

Cases of asphyxia may be divided into two great classes, according as the muscular system has lost its tone, or still retains it. In the latter and more hopeful cases the limbs still yield a degree of resistance, and the muscles of the neck give a partial support to the head; the surface is warm, of a red, often of a livid red color; the conjunctivæ are red, sometimes ecchymosed; the heart and umbilical arteries beat, though slowly, and the vessels of the cord are full of blood. In this condition the mere exposure to air, or some simple irritation of the surface, suffices to excite respiratory efforts, and the child recovers.

This, however, is not always so; and sometimes the child, who was born in what might seem this hopeful condition, and who even had made inspiratory efforts, does not recover. The attempts at breathing become more feeble, and the heart's action grows slower; the muscular system loses its tone, and the limbs their resistance; the surface becomes cool and pale as well as livid; the umbilical vessels cease to pulsate, and the cord grows flaccid; the fœtal mode of existence comes to an end, while pulmonary respiration fails to be established, and the child dies. This different result, the immediate cause of which is the more or less sunken sensibility of the medulla oblongata, is doubtless connected with different degrees and kinds of disturbance of the placental circulation, and with the degree in which fruitless respiratory efforts have been made before birth. I do not know, however, that we are able at present to adopt any definite formula as representing the degree of risk to the fœtus in different cases; for while, on the one hand, we know that in cases of long-protracted labor the child is often stillborn and pale, and with no prospect of resuscitation, even a very short pressure on the cord, in cases of breech presentation or of prolapsus of the funis, suffices to destroy it. In these latter instances, indeed, it is probable that actual extravasation of blood in the cranium may have had a share in producing this result, as well as the mere disorder of placental circulation.

We come now to the practical question of what *treatment* to adopt in cases where the child does not breathe immediately on its birth. First of all, I need scarcely say that, so long as the umbilical vessels are forcibly pulsating, there is nothing to do but to wait patiently and allow the placental circulation to go on undisturbed, until the *besoin de respirer*—I do not know why we should not use plain English, and say till the want of breath—is felt, and efforts at respiration are made by the infant. In many cases the contact of the cold air excites this want; the child attempts to breathe, and, as it does so, the placental circulation diminishes in force, and at length altogether ceases. When this is not the case, but the heart-beat grows slower, and the placental circulation feebler, without any effort at respiration being excited, no more time should be lost, but the cord should be at once divided, and the escape of a drachm or two of blood from its cut surface will often relieve the overloaded heart, and facilitate the establishment of respiration and the flow of blood in its new channels. The first endeavor now, too, should be to arouse the respiratory efforts by stimulation of the surface; as by dashing cold water on the face and chest; by plunging the child for a few seconds in a hot bath at a temperature of 100° or 102°, and then exposing it to the air; by swinging it a few times backwards and forwards in the air, by slapping its nates, by applying ammonia to the nostrils, or by tickling the throat and nares with a feather.

If, however, these measures do not very speedily prove successful, or if the child, when born, is in what may be termed the second degree of stillbirth, with cool, pale surface, and flaccid limbs, and non-pulsating cord, no time must be wasted over these measures, but the endeavor must be made without delay to excite respiration. It might at first seem that this would be best done by direct inflation of the lungs; but experience—at least, the experience of private practice—does not seem to confirm this expectation, and, on the whole, more success appears to follow the attempt to introduce air into the lungs by the artificial imitation of the respiratory movements. To the late Dr. Marshall Hall[1] belongs the credit of having been the first to suggest this proceeding as applicable to the treatment of persons apparently drowned, not by *forcing* the air into the lungs directly, but by *drawing* the air into them by changes of posture which imitate the respiratory movements. The plan of proceeding which he suggested for this purpose has, however, been generally superseded by that recommended by Dr. Silvester, on which a committee of the Medico-Chirurgical Society has reported very favorably.[2] "An inspiratory effect is produced by extending the arms upwards by the side of the head, and restoring them to their original position by the side of the body; or still better, by pressing them on the lower third of the sternum the expanded walls are allowed to resume their previous state, and expiration takes place, the quantity of air expelled being in proportion to that which had been previously inspired."

So long as the surface retains its warmth, and so long as an occasional heart-beat shows that life is not absolutely extinct, these efforts should be persevered with, it may be for several hours; and my own conviction is, that in not a few instances failure is due to want of perseverance rather than to the absolute uselessness of the endeavor.[3]

The stillborn child, however, sometimes recovers only imperfectly; air indeed enters its lungs, but not completely, and we then have to do with congenital *imperfect expansion of the lungs*.

---

[1] Prone and Postural Respiration, &c., 12mo., London, 1857, pp. 24 and 56.

[2] In vol. xlv of the Transactions of the Society.

[3] Schultze, Op. cit., pp. 161–163, suggests another mode of carrying out respiratory movements, which he believes to be still more efficient; but of the merits of which my discontinuance for some years of obstetric practice prevents my being a competent judge.

It is now forty years since Dr. Edward Jörg gave the first clear description of the former of these two conditions, to which he applied the rather cramp name of *atelectasis*, from ἀτελής, imperfect, and ἔκτασις, expansion.[1] We will first study this, since it is the simpler form of the affection, and we shall thereby obtain a clue to the understanding of the second form.

If you examine the body of a new-born infant, or of one that has survived its birth but a few days, you will sometimes find patches of the lung of a dark red color, and depressed below the surrounding tissue, thus giving to the surface of the organ an uneven appearance. These darker portions, which exactly resemble fœtal lung, are solid to the touch, do not crepitate at all under the finger, and sink immediately if thrown into water, while no minute air-bubbles are intermingled with the small quantity of reddish serum which pressure causes to exude from their divided substance. They are not friable nor easily torn, their cut surface is perfectly smooth, closely resembling a piece of muscle, and, if examined under a lens, the pale collapsed air-tubes are seen intersecting their substance, and scarcely distinguishable from the small vessels, which are almost devoid of blood.

If air is blown into a lung some lobules of which have this appearance, it will permeate the collapsed air-tubes; the pulmonary vesicles will by degrees become distended, and the solid lobules will rise to a level with the rest of the lung, will acquire the same color and consistence, and, like other parts of the organ, will float in water. A single inflation, however, is by no means sufficient to render this change permanent, but the moment the tube is withdrawn the air will escape, and the recently distended lobules will again collapse, and sink below the rest of the lung; their color, too, will become dark, though less so than before. Even if, after you have distended the lung to the utmost, you pass a ligature round the bronchi, and allow the lung to dry, a difference will still in general be very perceptible between the size of the air-vesicles which had been inflated by your efforts, and of those which had been distended during life by the natural process of respiration.

The force required thus to distend the collapsed portions of the lung is very variable: sometimes it requires all the force you can possibly exert, and continued for some minutes. If the child had survived for several weeks, the air will penetrate only very imperfectly into the collapsed lobules, while in some parts the resistance will be greater than it can overcome, and the most forcible inflation will be followed by no effect. The situations in which this condition is most frequently met with, are the languette and lower edge of the upper lobes, the middle lobe of the right lung, and the posterior part and lower edge of the lower lobes; and inflation restores these parts to a natural condition much less easily than it does any patches of the same kind in other situations. Whether the impermeability of some collapsed lob-

---

[1] In his dissertation De pulmonum vitio organico, &c., Lips., 1832; and afterwards more fully in his work Die Fötuslunge im gebornen Kinde, 8vo., Grimma,

ules is owing to adhesions having taken place between the opposite surfaces of the minuter bronchi, as has been suggested, I cannot pretend to say, but the supposition is plausible, and microscopical researches, according to which the bronchi of a portion of collapsed lung lose their lining of tessellated epithelium, lend it a still further degree of probability.[1]

It is usual to find, in connection with this state of the parenchyma of the lungs, that the pulmonary vessels contain less blood than usual, that the foramen ovale is unusually open, and the ductus arteriosus but very imperfectly closed. If the child have survived its birth but a short time, the brain is frequently found congested; but otherwise there is often nothing observable more than anæmia of all the organs, together with a general state of atrophy. Sometimes bronchitis attacks a lung thus affected, and besides the presence of mucus in the air-passages, there is then very often a state of congestion of the lungs, which renders the contrast between the collapsed and the healthy lobules less striking.

The *causes* of this condition are not clearly made out. Dr. Jörg has attributed great importance to precipitate labor as a frequent cause of its occurrence, and has suggested a somewhat fanciful theory to explain its mode of production. He conceives that one grand use of the uterine contractions is gradually to enfeeble the circulation through the placenta, and thus to induce in the fœtus that *besoin de respirer* which shall excite the complete establishment of respiration immediately on its birth. If, however, by the very rapid course of labor, the child should be born while the fœtal circulation is still going on with unimpaired vigor, the want of air will not be experienced by the child, and its attempts to breathe will be feeble and imperfect. It is probably better, instead of indulging in speculations of this sort, to content ourselves with the simple statement that when, from any cause whatever, the establishment of respiration at all has been attended with difficulty, there is a very great probability that its establishment will never be complete, but that some lobules only will receive the air, while it will not penetrate into other parts of the lung. The probability of this occurring, too, will be still greater if the children are weakly or ill-nourished when born, or if they are exposed soon after birth to cold or other unfavorable hygienic influences, such as are calculated to interfere with the due performance of respiration.

Cases in which this condition of the lungs exists usually present the history of the child having been apparently stillborn; and, though resuscitated after a time, yet still continuing unable to utter a strong and loud cry like that of other children. Even after breathing has gone on for some time, such children usually appear feeble; and though they may have attained the full term of fœtal life, yet they can scarcely suck, although they often make the effort. An infant thus affected sleeps even more than new-born infants usually do; its voice is very feeble, and rather a whimper than a cry; and the chest is seen to be

---

[1] See a paper on this subject by Prof. Köstlin, in Schmidt's Jarbücher, 1850, No. 1, p. 28.

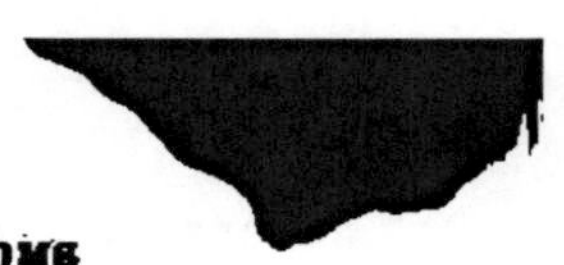

very little, if at all dilated by the respiratory movements. The temperature falls, the skin becomes pale, and the lips grow livid, and often slight twitching is observed in the course of a few hours about the muscles of the face. The difficulty in sucking increases, the voice grows weaker and more whimpering, or even altogether inaudible, while respiration is attended with a slight râle, or an occasional cough; and the convulsive movements return more frequently, and are no longer confined to the face, but affect also the muscles of the extremities. Any sudden movement suffices to bring on these convulsive seizures: but even while perfectly still the child's condition is not uniform, but it will suddenly become convulsed; and during this seizure the respiration will be extremely difficult, and death will seem momentarily impending. In a few minutes, however, all this disturbance ceases, and the extreme weakness of the child, its inability to suck, its feeble voice, and its frequent and imperfect inspirations, are the only abiding indications of the serious disorder from which it suffers. But the other *symptoms* return again and again, till at length, after the lapse of a few days, or a few weeks, the infant dies.

But I will relate a case which may serve to impress these characteristics on your memory. A little boy, three weeks old, was brought to me at the Children's Infirmary, on March 13, 1846. He was puny, emaciated, with a cold surface and bloodless conjunctivæ. His face, which was wizened like that of an old man, was occasionally distorted by slight convulsive twitches; and these fits, as the mother termed them, were, according to her account, sometimes much more severe. The abdomen was tympanitic, and it alone was seen to move during respiration, there being hardly any lateral expansion of the chest. The ear applied to the chest heard but little air entering; and the cry was a stifled whimper, in which none of the inspiratory sound, the *reprise* of French writers, was distinguishable. The child sucked with difficulty, and had wasted ever since its birth, though no diarrhœa existed; but the bowels, on the contrary, showed a tendency to constipation.

The chest was rubbed twice a day with a stimulating liniment, and a mixture was given containing some ammonia and the compound tincture of bark. Under this treatment the child appeared to improve; it began to breathe less rapidly and in a less labored manner, and its cry became louder. The parents, however, were miserably destitute, the mother in an ill state of health, so that her milk afforded but a very imperfect sustenance for the child. From the beginning of April he grew less well, and began to have occasional attacks of general convulsions, in one of which he died on April 26, 1846.

On examining the body, large portions of both lungs presented the appearances which I have described as characteristic of their imperfect expansion; but inflation restored them to a crepitant state. Some patches, however, though they admitted air and assumed the same color as the rest of the lung, yet could not by any effort be dilated so completely as to rise to a level with the surrounding tissue. The foramen ovale was open, the margin of the valve for fully half its circumference not being adherent, although the valve was sufficiently large for its closure. The ductus arteriosus also was quite permeable, although of considerably less calibre than during fœtal life.

This case affords a very good specimen of one way in which the affection leads on to a fatal termination; but sometimes, and probably in those instances in which the affected portion of lung is not so considerable, a less formidable train of symptoms usher in the fatal event. Convulsive twitchings, such as I have before mentioned, do not occur, nor are periodic exacerbations of the symptoms observed; but the child is merely feeble and its breath is short, and it has an occasional cough. It sucks, though with difficulty, but it loses flesh, the bowels become disordered, and medicine is unable to restrain the diarrhœa. The unchecked diarrhœa increases the emaciation and exhaustion of the child, which dies at length worn out and wasted to a skeleton.

Sometimes, too, we meet with cases in which the child eventually recovers, and it is then very interesting to watch the gradual diminution in the frequency and violence of the paroxysms of dyspnœa, while the respiration grows by degrees more equable, and the cry louder, the power of sucking increases, and the child at length attains to perfect health.

A little boy, four months old, was placed under my care by his mother, who informed me that the child had presented in some unnatural position during labor, so that manual interference was required to effect her delivery: and when born the infant appeared dead, and was recovered only after very great difficulty, and after the occurrence of convulsions: the convulsions had since returned almost every day —sometimes, indeed, they occurred several times in the same day— and always came on with greater frequency by day than by night. The attempt to suck often induced them, as did also any rapid movement about the room, or any sudden change of posture. During the fits the child did not struggle much, but he always turned extremely livid about the face and mouth. No fit ever lasted longer than five minutes, and during the intervals between them the child seemed pretty well, except that he often suffered from a suffocating cough.

He appeared tolerably well-grown and well-nourished, and the temperature of the surface was nearly natural. The respiration, however, was very hurried, and was almost entirely abdominal, the chest being hardly at all expanded. The cry, moreover, was feeble, and without *reprise*. There was a considerable want of resonance of both sides of the chest posteriorly, and deficient entrance of air into the back of both lungs. Both the dulness and the scanty admission of air were more obvious in the left than in the right infrascapular region, and some mucous râle was heard in the former situation.

The child was placed in a hot bath, and an emetic was given it every night; the chest, both in front and back, was rubbed twice a day with a stimulating liniment, and the face was ordered to be sprinkled with cold water whenever any threatenings of the fits came on.

At the end of five days the child was better, and the cry louder, though without any distinct *reprise*. Small doses of the ferrocitrate

of quinine were now combined with the other remedies, while the emetics were discontinued, as on some occasions they had appeared to excite the convulsions. First the cry grew louder, then the appearance improved and the manner became more cheerful, then the cough was less troublesome and the breathing less habitually wheezing, and at the same time the chest began to expand more, and the marked dulness of its lower parts gradually diminished. At the end of five weeks, the child was discharged with increased flesh, invigorated strength, and with no ailment more serious than a slight degree of wheezing respiration.

The history of this patient may serve to show us that even very serious symptoms should not lead us to despair of recovery, while it illustrates the importance of forming an accurate *diagnosis* between this affection and congenital phthisis (the only malady with which it is likely to be confounded), lest we either cherish unfounded expectations, or discourage hopes that might reasonably be entertained.

A little care will usually suffice to enable us to distinguish between these two affections, notwithstanding some general points of resemblance between them. The symptoms of the imperfect inflation of the lungs date from the infant's birth: but it scarcely ever happens that tuberculous disorganization of the lung is so extensive in the new-born child as to interfere with the establishment of the respiratory function. But not only do not the symptoms of phthisis appear so early, but they likewise seldom advance so rapidly, as those of atelectasis. Phthisis, too, is not from the beginning attended with the same debility, nor with difficulty in sucking, while it is associated with a febrile action which is quite wanting in atelectasis. The head symptoms, which in so large a number of cases attend the imperfect inflation of the lungs, are absent in phthisis; while, lastly, auscultation would furnish some clue to the real nature of the case: in the one instance there would, in general, be simply a deficiency of air; in the other, respiration accompanied with râles, and often with bronchial breathing.

The *treatment* required by this affection need not detain us long. The importance of maintaining an equable temperature around every child in whom respiration is not duly performed, cannot be too much insisted on; and the power of generating heat being, as you know, much diminished, this temperature ought not to be below 70°, and in bad cases may be even 10° higher. Besides attending to produce this warmth around the child, benefit often accrues from the employment of the hot bath once or twice every day, at a temperature of 100° Fahrenheit, to which mustard may be added to render it more stimulating to the surface. The child should not be allowed to remain longer than five minutes in the bath, and should be enveloped in hot flannels immediately afterwards, to prevent its taking cold. The back and chest should be rubbed twice or oftener every day with a stimulating liniment, as camphor or soap liniment, which may be diluted with a little oil, if it is too irritating to the skin. If the child is very feeble, stimulants may be given, of which there are none better than the compound spirit of ammonia or ether, or the spiritus ammoniæ succinatus, the unpleasant pungency of which remedies is concealed by milk better than by any other menstruum. The daily employment of a gentle emetic of ipecacuanha has, in some instances, appeared to be of service, not merely by relieving the air-tubes of any mucus that may have accumulated there, but by inducing several deep inspirations, and thus aiding the complete establishment of respiration. As the child improves, the more directly stimulating medicines may be withdrawn, and tonics substituted for them, among which few are better than the extract of cinchona.[1] It has the great advantage of not disordering the bowels; a point of no small importance in any case in which diarrhœa is likely to occur. In some cases there is a sluggishness of the bowels, and a deficiency in the secretion of bile; very minute doses of the Hydr. c. Cretâ will often remedy the latter, and the use of a soap suppository will frequently render the internal employment of any purgative needless. The child should be put to the breast unless it is very feeble, but in that case should not be allowed to exhaust its strength in fruitless attempts to suck. It will be better to draw the breast, and give the child its mother's milk by means of a spoon or from a bottle, which latter plan has this advantage, that while it costs the child but little effort to get its food, we avoid the risk of its forgetting how to suck, an inconvenience which attends the use of the spoon if continued for any length of time. Artificial feeding is not at all desirable in such cases, though sometimes, if the child is very weak, it may be necessary at first to give a few drops of brandy in its milk every three or four hours. This plan of treatment must be patiently persevered in, nor must the supervention of symptoms of an apparently acute character induce too wide a deviation from it. The head symptoms in particular must be combated cautiously, lest by too great a solicitude to overcome them we destroy the patient rather than the disease.

LECTURE XVIII.

COLLAPSE OF LUNG THAT HAS ONCE BEEN EXPANDED.—Described as lobular pneumonia by various writers—Its characters—Symptoms and differences from true pneumonia—Observations of Bailly and Legendre—Is not to be regarded as a post-mortem occurrence—Illustrative cases—Instances of its occurrence in the adult—Similar causes tend to produce it at all periods of life—Hence very frequent in old age.

INDURATION OF THE CELLULAR TISSUE.—Its characters—Remarkable reduction of temperature that attends it—Appearances after death—Frequent association with pulmonary collapse, congestion, or sometimes with pulmonary apoplexy—Its cause still obscure—Treatment.

THE condition of the lungs, which we were occupied in examining at the last lecture, is of importance, even if regarded merely as a con-

[1] See Formula No. 4, p. 57.

genital state, the result of nature having failed in the attempt to establish respiration, and to fit the child thoroughly for the new mode of existence to which it is destined after birth. But its claims on our attention are still greater when we bear in mind the possibility of its occurrence in consequence of a variety of causes operating after birth, so that lungs once permeable to air may cease to admit it, and death may at length occur from apnœa without any serious structural change having taken place in the organs of respiration.

Appearances supposed to be the result of pneumonia had long attracted the notice of writers on diseases of children, by the wide differences which they presented from those which inflammation of the lungs gives rise to in the adult.[1] It had been observed that infants and children under five years of age often died after presenting some of the symptoms of inflammation of the lungs, such as cough and difficult breathing, together with more or less extensive dulness of the chest on percussion, and some or other of the auscultatory signs of solidification of the lung. In such cases these peculiar morbid appearances were especially well marked. But while they seemed to prove that these changes in the lung were the consequences of pneumonia, it happened not infrequently that the fever and the pneumonic symptoms underwent a great abatement before any sign of approaching death appeared, or that children, who had seemed to die worn out from various causes, and during whose lifetime no indication of inflammation of the lungs had existed, presented the supposed anatomical evidences of pneumonia in a most remarkable degree. The frequency of occurrences of this kind led to the assumption that pneumonia was an extremely frequent concomitant of almost all the diseases of infancy and early childhood; that this pneumonia was very often latent (that is to say, that it did not manifest its existence by those symptoms which usually attend it); and, lastly, that, owing to causes which were differently stated by different observers, it gave rise to alterations in the lung very dissimilar from those which it occasioned in the adult.

One of the most remarkable peculiarities of this supposed infantile pneumonia led to its receiving the appellation of *lobular pneumonia*, as expressive of the fact that it did not attack a large tract of lung, or the whole of a lobe, at one time, but that it affected isolated lobules, which might be seen of a dark color, solid, often depressed below the surrounding parts, and sinking in water if detached from the healthy tissue in the midst of which they were situated. Sometimes the affection was strictly limited to a single lobule, the boundaries of which could be exactly traced; and though it often happened that a cluster of lobules was thus hard, and dark, and solid, still there was no gradual shading off from the darker to the lighter parts; so that it was evident that, in whatever way the disease extended, at any rate it did not advance by mere continuity of tissue. Sometimes almost the whole of one lobe was thus affected, a few lobules only still retaining a healthy aspect,

---

[1] In the British and Foreign Medico-Chirurgical Review for October, 1864, is a very clear and interesting sketch, by Dr. Willshire, of the progress of knowledge with reference to pneumonia, and conditions of the lung resembling it in early life.

and crepitating under the finger; and it often happened that the bronchi leading to it were full of mucus or pus, while at other times there was marked congestion of the lung; and in the midst of this congested tissue were two or three solid hepatized patches. All these circumstances, as it may be conceived, variously modified the morbid appearances. In the last case the lobular pneumonia was thought to be becoming *generalized;* or, in other words, the inflammation originally limited to certain lobules was supposed to have begun to extend to the adjacent tissues, constituting a kind of transition state between lobular and lobar pneumonia. The lower edge of the different lobes, the whole of the middle lobe of the right lung, and often a very considerable portion, or the whole of one or other lower lobe, were also sometimes found in a state to which, among other names, that of *carnification* was applied, on account of its close resemblance to a piece of muscular tissue. A portion of carnified lung showed the closest possible similarity to a lung that had been compressed by effusion into the pleura. It was dark, tough, solid, contained no air, presented a smooth surface when cut, yielded a small quantity of bloody serum when pressed, and, indeed, seemed almost like a piece of flesh; in all which respects it resembled a portion of lung hepatized by lobular pneumonia, and differed from the lung of the adult when that has been rendered solid by inflammation.

The course of the disease in many of these cases during the lifetime of the patient, and the results of medical treatment, tended to enhance the difficulties which the above-described anatomical peculiarities placed in the way of referring lobular pneumonia to the same category of affections with the pneumonia of the adult. Venesection, leeches, and mercurials, the ordinary antiphlogistic apparatus in the pneumonia of the adult, often appeared to hasten the child's death; blisters rarely effected any good, and the blistered surface often showed a remarkable indisposition to heal. On the other hand, emetics and rubefacients were frequently of service; a stimulant plan of treatment was almost always necessary at an early period, and sometimes seemed to be required nearly from the outset of the affection. The rapidity of the changes that took place in the physical condition of the lung was another peculiarity which rendered the nature of the affection still more obscure; for where air was heard entering freely on one day, none would be perceptible on the morrow, but percussion of that part of the chest would yield a sound of complete dulness. On the other hand, it happened sometimes, though much less often, that dulness was succeeded just as quickly by resonance on percussion, and that breathing became distinctly audible where on the previous day no sound of air was to be heard.

Nothing can show more forcibly the influence of a name, than the fact that this condition of the lungs should have been described by all writers as lobular pneumonia, and that its symptoms should have been attributed to inflammation, while yet it was evident from the concurrent testimony of every one that neither in its progress nor in its results was it similar to inflammation of the lungs in the adult, much less identical with it. Having, however, once been called pneumonia, every person continued to call it so, though often with a full recognition of its peculiarities. Even the close resemblance which the lung presented to fœtal lung, or to those undilated portions which are characteristic of *atelectasis*, was noticed and discussed by myself, and by many far better observers, apparently without a suspicion that both states were identical.

But while the peculiarities of lobular pneumonia were thus generally commented on, it seems strange that no one should have had recourse to the experiment of inflation in order to obtain a solution of some of the difficulties that existed with reference to its nature. This oversight seems the more extraordinary, when we call to mind that this very means had cleared up so many doubts concerning appearances in the lungs of new-born infants, which had once been supposed to be the result of pneumonia in the fœtus, or of some arrest of development. At length the experiment was tried by MM. Bailly and Legendre,[1] and though, as in the old tale of Columbus and the egg, the thing seems so obvious that there is some risk of our underrating the merit of those who were the first to do it, it must not be forgotten that, by that simple means, they have thrown more light on the affections of the lungs in infancy and childhood, than all the writers of the previous ten years together.

MM. Bailly and Legendre state, as the result of their observations, that the appearances to which the name of lobular pneumonia has commonly been given *are in reality produced by an occlusion of the pulmonary vesicles.* This occlusion, say they—and the correctness of their opinion is now universally admitted—is due to the inspiratory power having been inadequate to overcome that elasticity of the lung, which I described to you in my last lecture as constantly tending to empty the pulmonary vesicles of air, and constantly impeding its entrance. Coupled with this, however, there is another cause, the full influence of which had not been recognized till dwelt on by Professor Gairdner, of Glasgow,[2] namely, the presence of the secretions in the bronchi, and the obstacle which they present, sometimes at one point and sometimes at another, to the admission of air. The child inspires, and the secretion, which it could neither expectorate nor expel by coughing, closes the entrance to some small bronchial tube. With the succeeding expiration, a little of the air retained behind this obstacle escapes, and on the next occasion a little more, till at length no single inspiratory effort having been strong enough to surmount the obstruction, while with each expiration the quantity of air behind it is lessened, the vesicle collapses, and its situation is betrayed by the small, dark, depressed spot which may be seen on the surface of the lung, and felt solid or non-crepitant beneath the finger.

In bronchitis, where this secretion is abundant, perhaps excessive, the obstacle to the entrance of air which thence arises becomes, in the case of young children, a very serious source of danger, and the pos-

[1] Nouvelles Recherches sur quelques Maladies du Poumon; in the Arch. Gén. de Méd., Jan., Fév., Mars, 1844.

[2] On the Pathological Anatomy of Bronchitis, &c.: reprinted from the Monthly Journal of 1850 and 1851.

sible occurrence of collapse of the lung must make you very guarded in the expression of your prognosis, even when the symptoms do not appear to be formidable. In such cases, too, the congestion of the pulmonary tissue, and the consequent pressure of the gorged vessels on the air-cells, both favor their collapse and impede their expansion.[1]

But besides these cases, in which the collapse of the lung becomes a grave, perhaps even a fatal complication of disease already existing, there are others in which this condition occurs independently of any affection of the air-passages, and destroys life suddenly and unexpectedly. If from any cause the inspiratory powers are feeble, the obstacle in the air-tubes need be but very slight in order to produce collapse—need, certainly, be nothing more than may be presented by the gradual accumulation in the bronchi of their natural secretions; while in some instances, such as the one which I will now relate to you, the collapse of the lung may be considerable, though the bronchi may contain no appreciable amount of secretion.

A little girl was attacked, when a month old, by very severe diarrhœa, which lasted for three weeks, and then left her greatly exhausted and much emaciated. No return of the purging occurred, and the child lived, though in a state of great weakness, till she was five months old. For the last five weeks of her life she was under my care, and sometimes she seemed, for a day or two, as if she were gaining strength and might recover; but these signs of improvement were never of long duration. Three days before she died, her breath grew suddenly hurried; the dyspnœa was not attended with any cough, but from the time of its coming on, the child's exhaustion increased, and her respiration grew more rapid until her death.

No organ showed any sign of disease, but all presented a most remarkable degree of anæmia. Two-thirds of the upper, and almost the whole of the lower lobe of the right lung, were dark, solid, and non-crepitant; and a few lobules of the left lung presented the same appearance. Inflation restored them to exactly the same state as the rest of the lungs. The bronchi were preternaturally pale, and contained no secretions. It is not possible to say why the child's inspiratory power grew too feeble to fill the lungs at one moment rather than at another, but few would doubt that it had become so just at the time when the dyspnœa occurred. A portion of the lung having become collapsed, the elastic ribs tended to render abortive any faint effort to draw in more breath, and thus the vital flame went out for want of air to feed it.

Sometimes the occurrence of this condition is long preceded by indications of the imperfect performance of the respiratory functions, but yet they go on sufficiently to keep the machinery of life in motion, till some trivial, perhaps some inappreciable cause—a draught of cold air, a little overexertion, the horizontal posture too long continued, the

---

[1] With reference to this point, there are some conclusive experiments of MM. Rilliet and Barthez, recorded in vol. i, p. 427, note, of the second edition of their work on Children's Diseases.

customary food delayed an hour beyond the usual time—sinks them so low that they soon cease forever.

Some time ago I saw a little girl ten months old, who had lost her mother soon after her birth, and had been indebted to a stranger for what should have been a mother's care. She never throve; her chest presented that peculiar malformation commonly called pigeon-breast, and that circular constriction around the base of the thorax, which used to be regarded as due to the direct action of the diaphragm drawing in the receding parts at each contraction; but which Sir W. Jenner's careful observations have shown to be produced by atmospheric pressure acting on the chest-walls just above the upper margin of the liver, spleen, and stomach.[1] But though she was a backward child, and though her respiration was always almost as abdominal as that of a new-born infant, there was no definite evidence of disease till she was nine months old. She then lost flesh rapidly, and began to cough without having had any previous catarrh. Her case seemed to be one of bronchial phthisis.

Four days before she died her breath suddenly became much oppressed, and her cough far more severe than it had been before. The dyspnœa rapidly increased, but her cough soon grew less frequent A few hours before her death her lips were quite livid; she was breathing from 80 to 86 times in the minute, the abdominal muscles acting most violently, but the chest being scarcely at all expanded. Auscultation detected nothing more than some rather large mucous râle in the lung.

After death no tubercle was found in any organ, but large portions of both lungs presented the undilated condition, which disappeared entirely on inflation. The bronchi were pale, and contained very little mucus, but the right side of the heart was greatly distended with coagulated blood, which its thin, pale, and flaccid substance had evidently been unequal to propel with the requisite vigor.

The imperfect respiration had here for some time manifested itself; the vital powers had long been feeble; nutrition had been ill performed, and the heart itself had shared in the general feebleness, till at length the secretion of a comparatively small amount of mucus presented an obstacle to the free entrance of air, which, though slight in itself, was greater than the child could overcome; and the whole machinery of life was thus suddenly brought to a standstill.

In both of these cases the feebleness of the inspiratory power was one chief cause of the collapse of the lung. The result is the same, however, if the obstacle is increased, as if the power is diminished; and hence, as I have already mentioned, the supervention of this state of lung becomes one of the most perilous, while it is one of the most frequent complications of infantile bronchitis. A little girl, previously quite healthy, was seized when ten months old with symptoms of acute bronchitis, suffocative cough returning in paroxysms, and some-

[1] The commonly received explanation of the mechanism by which this deformity of the chest is produced is given by MM. Rilliet and Barthez, op. cit., vol. i, p. 46. The careful observations of Sir W. Jenner are contained in his Lectures on Rickets, in Med. Times, March 17, 1860, p. 262.

times followed by the rejection of a muco-purulent fluid. The symptoms throughout did not seem to allow of depletion; but ammonia, with decoction of senega and tincture of squills, and other expectorants of a stimulating kind, were given with temporary amendment. The child did not, however, appear to have undergone any marked change, either for better or worse, except that she had certainly lost both flesh and strength, when coldness, faintness, and exceedingly labored respiration suddenly came on, and continued till her death, which took place in the course of twenty-four hours.

A few recent adhesions were found on each side of the chest, between the costal and pulmonary pleura. The trachea contained a large quantity of muco-purulent matter, and the same secretion abounded in the bronchial tubes, many of which were filled by it, while nowhere did air-bubbles appear intermixed with it. There was some congestion of both lungs, especially posteriorly; the upper and posterior part of the upper lobe of the right lung, the whole of the middle lobe, and the posterior part and lower edge of the lower lobe, were dark, solid, non-crepitant, and depressed below the adjacent tissue. The same state existed in the whole inferior third of the upper lobe, and the lower edge of the lower lobe of the left lung. On inflating the lung, most of these parts were restored to a perfectly natural condition, but some patches still remained less dilated than the others, and some of the darker, almost violet-colored portions of the lower lobes appeared but little affected by it.

But you may naturally inquire whether any occurrence of a similar kind is ever met with in the adult, since there is certainly no such peculiarity in the structure of the lung in childhood as should render it then exclusively liable to a morbid process from which at all other ages it is exempt. My own experience would not have enabled me to answer this question; but my lamented friend Dr. Baly communicated to me some years ago the particulars of three cases in which he found large portions of the lung in the adult presenting the characters that we have been studying in the child, and, like it, resuming a natural appearance on the insufflation of air into the bronchi. The patients in all of these cases died of fever, attended with dysenteric symptoms; and for some days before their death were in a state of great exhaustion, such as appeared to indicate the free employment of stimulants. In two instances distinct dyspnœa occurred some days previous to death; but though the chest lost its resonance in the situation of the affected parts of the lung, and the breathing there was deficient, yet the minute crepitation of pneumonia was not detected in either case, but merely some mucous râle. In addition to extensive disease in the intestines, this collapsed condition of portions of the lung was found; unconnected with any disease of those organs in one of the cases, combined with the effusion of tenacious mucus in the bronchi leading towards the collapsed portions in a second, and associated with true pneumonia and a state of red or gray hepatization of other parts in a third.[1]

---

[1] The minute accuracy of Dr. Baly's description induces me to subjoin the following particulars of one of the examinations: "No effusion, lungs healthy, ex-

But these are by no means isolated cases; for it would seem that in some diseases which are attended by much depression of the vital power, this collapse of the lungs is by no means unusual. To adduce but one illustration of the fact, it may be mentioned that M. Louis[1] found in nineteen out of forty-six post-mortem examinations of patients who had died of typhoid fever, a condition of the lungs which he calls "carnification," and which it is evident (although he did not try the effect of inflation) was identical with the state so frequent in the child. He describes the parts thus affected as of a deep purple-red, having lost the natural suppleness of the lung, being solid and sinking in water: they were, moreover, tougher than healthy lung; if divided, the section became covered with a reddish fluid, perfectly destitute of air, while the tissue neither resembled that of healthy lung, nor presented the peculiar granular appearance characteristic of lung in the second stage of pneumonia. More recently, too, Professor Gairdner, in his very important essays on the pathological anatomy of bronchitis, already referred to, has mentioned this condition of the lungs as having been of frequent occurrence during the epidemic fever of 1847.

It is true, however, that in these cases the condition of the lung was merely superadded to other lesions in themselves adequate to occasion the patient's death; and hence, though interesting to the mere pathologist, it yet loses much of its value in the eyes of the practical physician. But it will not seem to you that too much stress has been laid on this state, if it should appear that whenever the power of the inspiratory muscles is much diminished there is a tendency to its supervention, so that it alone may be the cause of death; and this, which I have put hypothetically, really does occur in old age.

The term "second childhood" is not a mere figure of speech, expressive solely of the decay of the mental powers, by which the evening of life is obscured and made like the twilight of the mind in early infancy, but it is in many points the statement of a physical truth. Thus, as old age creeps on, and the nutrition is no longer adequate to supply the waste, the respiration loses the character which it presented in the adult, and the extremes of life in this respect present a close resemblance to each other. The muscles of the chest grow too feeble to dilate it fully; the diaphragm becomes, as it was in early infancy, the principal inspiratory muscle, and the vertical diameter of the thorax is that in which its chief enlargement takes place. The ear applied to

---

cept in lower and posterior fourth of right inferior lobe, which is of a dark purple color, is depressed somewhat below the level of other parts, does not crepitate, feels solid, but flexible and tough, almost leathery, and sinks quickly in water: the part having these characters is distinctly defined by boundaries of lobules. The whole lung being inflated, the part just described receives air with greater difficulty than the other parts, but at length becomes distended lobule by lobule, and assumes the same pale red color as the rest of the lungs. The change takes place, as has been stated, lobule by lobule, separate lobules appearing suddenly of the paler color, not merely at the margins of the dark mass, but also in its centre. On cutting through the lungs and tracing the bronchi, it is found that the ramifications of those tubes which go to the dark, contracted, and condensed parts are filled up with tough mucus, from which those going to other parts are free."

[1] Recherches sur la Gastro-entérite., 8vo., Paris, 1829; tome i, pp. 361-364.

the chest no longer detects the puerile breathing of youth, nor the clear vesicular murmur of manhood; but the respiration is coarser, sometimes almost bronchial. There is not occasion, as in infancy, for more rapid breathing to maintain the high activity of the vital processes, but the wornout machinery needs to be put in motion more frequently than in the adult, in order to obtain oxygen enough to support existence; and, accordingly, MM. Hourman and Dechambre[1] found the average frequency of the respiration in 252 old women at the Salpêtrière to be 21.79 in the minute, while in some whose frame seemed most decayed it was far more rapid. Just as in infancy, too, so in old age these respiratory movements are most irregular. Sometimes the parietes of the thorax continue for a long time motionless, and then there succeed a series of rapid movements, while at other times the intervals between the inspirations are irregular, but the inspiratory movements are of the same intensity and duration. Here, then, without pursuing the comparison further, we have ample proof of the many points of resemblance between the physiological condition of the respiratory function in early life and in old age. The respiratory organs, too, in their pathological state, present, as might be expected, the same resemblance; and, accordingly, MM. Hourman and Dechambre[2] notice a state in which the pulmonary parenchyma is of a very deep, sometimes almost of a blue color, or nearly black, non-crepitant, and presenting a smooth surface on a section of it being made. The lung thus altered is often remarkably tough, almost like india-rubber; while under pressure, a viscous fluid, generally of a reddish color, and containing no air-bubbles, exudes from it. The idea of inflating the lung had not occurred to these observers; but they remark, that if portions of lung presenting these characters are dried, the air-cells have a tendency to reappear without having undergone any other change than a well-marked contraction.

I have dwelt long on this pathological condition, though I think not longer than its importance demands; because we shall find that in some form or other it presents itself, modifying the symptoms, determining the prognosis, and influencing the treatment of almost all the affections of the lung in early infancy.

I do not know where more appropriately than here to introduce a brief mention of an affection about whose nature there has been much controversy, and concerning which much obscurity still exists; although there is a marked connection between it and imperfect performance of the respiratory function. Though very rare in this country, *induration of the cellular tissue* is extremely common in the foundling hospitals of the Continent, where so many causes contribute to depress the new-born infant's feeble powers; and I may add, that it happens there with far greater frequency in the winter than in the summer months. The children in whom it occurs are usually weakly, not seldom premature, and its first symptoms generally appear between the first and fifth day

[1] The above facts with respect to respiration in the aged are derived from the interesting papers of MM. Hourman and Dechambre, in the Arch. de Méd. for 1835 and 1836. See especially the number for Nov. 1835.

[2] Op. cit., Mars, 1836, p. 272.

after birth, though occasionally they do not come on till later. In many instances a livid redness of the whole surface is obvious from birth; but the appearance of a circumscribed hard spot on one or other extremity, or on some prominent part of the face, as the end of the chin, or the cheek-bone, is the first sign of the commencement of this affection. Other spots of a similar kind are soon discovered on different parts of the surface; and the body generally, and the hardened spots in particular, are found to present a temperature much below the natural warmth of the body. It appears, indeed, from M. Roger's researches,[1] that a general reduction of the temperature precedes the induration, or, at least, exists in a very marked degree, while the induration is still extremely slight. Sometimes, too, the premonitory loss of temperature[2] may be perceived in weakly children without being succeeded by the appearance of spots of induration. This, however, is exceptional, and in the majority of instances the sinking of the temperature and the extension of the induration advance together, and the warmth of the surface may eventually fall from 100° to 90°, 80°, or even lower. If the induration becomes very extensive, it affects the integuments of the chest and the abdomen, as well as the extremities, and the body feels cold and stiff as though it were frozen.

This condition is, as might be expected, attended with great impairment of the general health, and with a very remarkable degree of emaciation.[3] Children suffering from it are extremely weak, often too weak to suck: their pulse is very small, their respiration abdominal, and their cry is faint and whimpering, wholly unlike that of a healthy infant. In some of the worst cases, too, a bloody fluid is discharged in considerable quantity from the nose and mouth. If the indurated parts are punctured, a small quantity of reddish serum escapes from them, though generally without much diminution of their previous hardness.

If the induration is at all general, death almost invariably takes place; and so great is the fatality of the affection, that, including even slight cases, five-sixths of those children who are attacked by it in the hospitals of Paris, die. In very slight cases, however, if the infant is at once placed in favorable circumstances, recovery need not be despaired of.

The hardness of the surface still persists after death, and the absence of any peculiarity in the effused serum, or of any sign of active disease, left writers generally in much perplexity as to its cause. The venous system is usually found gorged with fluid blood, and this congestion is often apparent in the cerebral vessels, as well as in those of the abdom-

---

[1] Op. cit., pp. 124–151. See also his more recent and more extended observations in his Recherches Cliniques, &c., pp. 405–428.

[2] Hervieux, Sur l'Algidité progressive des Nouveaux-Nés, in Arch. Gén. de Méd., Nov. 1855. Also an essay by Dr. Löschner of Prague on the same subject, in the Jahrbücher für Kinderheilkunde, vol. i, p. 91.

[3] In a paper by M. Elsässer, of Stuttgard, reprinted in the Archives de Médecine for May, 1858, from the Archiv. f. physiolog. Heilkunde, are some very interesting facts with reference to the loss of weight in the course of this affection. The average loss of weight in 53 fatal cases, was ¾ of a pound: the extremes each way being six ounces and two pounds.

inal viscera, particularly the liver. Both the thorax and abdomen also frequently contain a quantity of serum, often tinged with blood—effusions which are evidently of a passive nature, since they are unattended by any trace of inflammation either of the pleura or peritoneum. None of the viscera present any morbid appearances of half so much importance as those which are met with in the lungs, a very great part of which displays those changes to which your attention has already been directed as characteristic of their deficient expansion.[1] This condition of the lungs had been noticed and most carefully described many years ago, as one of the most striking attendants on induration of the cellular tissue. It was thought by some of those who described it to be the result of pneumonia; while other observers, justly insisting on the absence of the other effects of inflammation of the pulmonary tissue, yet drew the attention of pathologists too much away from the chest, where the clue to the solution of the question as to the cause of the affection was to be found, had they but known how to use it. We, however, are aware that many of those appearances once thought to be the result of pneumonia are in reality due to the unexpanded condition of the lung; and we can understand how it may happen, if children are exposed to cold immediately after birth, and then transferred to the ill-ventilated wards of a foundling hospital, and there fed with food far other than that which nature destined for them, that respiration may be but very imperfectly established; that their temperature may consequently fall, and the blood flowing in part through the unclosed fœtal passages may stagnate in its course, may give rise to passive effusions into the great cavities of the body, and to an anasarcous swelling of the surface. I was once disposed to look upon this state of the lungs as furnishing the clue to all the phenomena of induration of the cellular tissue. But the theory must, for several reasons, be given up as untenable, at least in the sense of its affording a constant and sufficient explanation of the causes of the affection. In the first place, changes in the pulmonary tissue are not constant, but are found only in about half of the cases; secondly, in many instances they seem to be consequences rather than causes; in the third place, while the changes are distinctly not pneumonic, they are far from being constantly those of mere collapse, but are at least as often those of intense congestion, sometimes even of pul-

---

[1] The observations of J. A. Troccon, in his dissertation "Sur la maladie connue sous le nom d'endurcissement du tissu cellulaire," 4to., Paris, 1814, are especially remarkable, since he not only described with accuracy the physical condition of the lungs, but even tried the experiment of inflating them, in order to prove that they were not, as had been erroneously supposed, in a state of gangrene. He says: "J'ai insufflé ensuite de l'air dans les poumons par la trachée: aussitôt la couleur noire qui était à leur base s'est changée en une couleur rouge claire, laquelle s'est étendue de proche en proche à mesure que je continuais ces insufflations." After removing a ligature which he had applied around the veins, and allowing the escape of the blood with which the heart and lungs were gorged, he resumed the inflation of the lungs and "les organes de la respiration ont été presque de suite dans un état absolument naturel, et aussi beaux que ceux que l'on voit pendus devant nos boucheries" (pp. 37–8).

It seems strange that neither M. Troccon nor subsequent observers perceived the full bearing of these experiments till similar ones were instituted by MM. Baily and Legendre.

monary apoplexy.[1] Further, one must not forget that while pulmonary collapse takes place in various circumstances, induration of the cellular tissue is limited, or almost limited, to large public institutions; and further, that the extraordinary depression of temperature by which it is accompanied is observed in no other condition whatever, not even in Asiatic cholera.

I need not add, for you will have made the reflection for yourselves, that truth and knowledge are much better served by a recognition of a problem as unsolved, than by straining a plausible explanation beyond the limits that it will bear.

The *treatment* of this affection implies the removal of every cause likely to induce it. Hence warmth stands foremost both as a curative and as a preventive measure. The warm bath may be resorted to as a means of raising the child's surface to a proper temperature, provided its extreme weakness do not contraindicate that measure. Gentle friction with warm oil is a means which has been tried for this purpose with advantage. The child should be nourished with breast-milk, even if it is too feeble to suck, and stimulants, of which white-wine whey is a very good one, will in many instances be needed. Defective respiration being the ultimate source of all the symptoms, the main principles of all your treatment must be the same as have already been laid down for your guidance in cases of atelectasis of the lung; and these it can hardly be necessary to recapitulate.

I should have said more about this affection, its nature and treatment, if it were one with which you were likely to meet often; but, in consideration of its extreme rarity in this country, I may perhaps be excused for passing it over with this cursory notice.

---

[1] Roger, Recherches, &c., p. 411; and a paper on Pulmonary Apoplexy in the New-born Infant, read by M. Hervieux before the Paris Association of Hospital Physicians, in July, 1863, and published in the J. f. Kinderkr. for 1864, vol. xlii, p. 247. One must also not overlook the fact that the lungs in M. Troccon's experiments were gorged with blood, in other words intensely congested, and that it was only after the removal of a ligature, to allow the escape of the blood, that they assumed a perfectly natural appearance.

LECTURE XIX.

INFLAMMATORY AFFECTIONS OF THE RESPIRATORY MUCOUS MEMBRANE.—Comparative rarity of catarrh during the first weeks of life—Coryza—Simple and pseudo-membranous or malignant—Identity of latter with nasal diphtheria—Catarrh, causes adding to its importance in early life—Its treatment—Danger of bronchitis or pneumonia.

Post-mortem appearances of bronchitis—Redness of the membrane—Nature of the contents of the bronchi—Dilatation of their cavity—Extension of the inflammation to the lining of the pulmonary vesicles, producing vesicular bronchitis.

State of the lungs in bronchitis—Frequency of congestion—Carnification of some lobules—Possible extension of inflammation to the pulmonary tissue, producing lobular pneumonia—Suppuration of these patches, producing vomicæ.

ALTHOUGH two lectures have already been devoted to the pathology of the respiratory organs, yet, until to-day, we have not been able to commence the study of their special diseases.

They may be divided into the three grand classes—of the inflammatory, the nervous, and those which result from morbid deposits.

We will examine these in the order in which I have enumerated them.

At every age *inflammatory affections of the respiratory mucous membrane* exceed all others in frequency; and even when the pulmonary substance becomes eventually involved, it is often by the extension to it of mischief which began in the mucous membrane. But in infancy and childhood this is pre-eminently the case, for the delicate and highly vascular lining of the respiratory organs resists but feebly the influence of noxious impressions from without, while it sympathizes most acutely with many morbid processes within.

This extreme susceptibility of the mucous membrane of the respiratory organs in childhood renders its disorders of very frequent occurrence, while we are compelled to study closely the signification of symptoms that may betoken disturbance from such various causes. Something of this sympathy with the affections of other parts exists even in the adult, as we may see exemplified in the cough that attends upon affections of the liver; but in the child the sympathetic disorder of the respiratory mucous membrane is vastly more frequent; and nurses, taught by experience, will speak to you about a tooth-cough, a stomach-cough, a worm-cough; while you will soon find for yourselves that the intestinal mucous membrane is seldom affected without that of the respiratory apparatus suffering too.

It is a curious fact, however, to which Professor Jörg of Leipsic[1] was the first person to call attention, that this extreme susceptibility of the lining of the respiratory apparatus does not exist to the same degree during the first month or two of life as it does afterwards. The ex-

---

[1] Handbuch der Kinderkrankheiten, 8vo., Leipsig, 1836, p. 531.

posure of an infant two or three weeks old to a low temperature or to a vitiated air, will be followed by disturbance of the function of the liver, and the occurrence of jaundice; or, perhaps, by such depression of the muscular power as to render the child incapable of taking a full inspiration, so that its lungs collapse, and it dies from disorder of the respiratory organs, but without the cough or bronchitic symptoms, which would not fail, if it were a little older, to announce the irritation of the mucous membrane of the air-tubes. Why this is so I do not know, but I suppose it to be the result of the generally feeble vitality which renders the lining of the bronchi less susceptible; just as that of the intestine also seems to be at the same period; since, while constipation is frequent, diarrhœa is comparatively rare during the first two months of life.

The mucous membrane of the nares, however, has not by any means this insensibility, and *coryza* is an affection most frequent, and most important, during the first two months of life, when the other forms of catarrh are comparatively rare.

This affection, in its most frequent form, is a source of discomfort rather than of danger. Its most prominent symptom has given rise to its vulgar name of "the snuffles;" for, the mucous membrane of the nares being swollen, the child is no longer able to breathe through its nose as it was wont to do, but is compelled to breathe likewise through its mouth, and its difficult inspirations are attended by a peculiar snuffling noise, which, during sleep, sometimes amounts to a complete snore. As in common catarrh, the secretion from the membrane is at first suppressed, afterwards it flows in an increased quantity, and then at length it is altered in character, and becomes thicker and puriform; when it sometimes dries and forms crusts about the nostrils, which interfere greatly with free respiration, and cause the child much annoyance. At the outset there is often a degree of heat of skin and febrile disturbance, but these symptoms soon subside, and, with the exception of the snuffling respiration the child seems quite well. If the attack is more severe, however, it may occasion a good deal of suffering; for if respiration through the nose is very much impeded or altogether prevented, the child is rendered unable to suck, and so soon as it has seized the nipple and begun to draw the milk, it is compelled to leave it in a state of threatening suffocation. Its distress, too, is further increased by the circumstance that its mouth, being constantly kept open in order to breathe, the tongue and throat become extremely dry, and deglutition, even when the child is fed with a spoon, is often attended with difficulty. Any such severity of the disease, however, is very unusual, though such cases do sometimes occur, and even prove fatal; the difficulty of breathing and sucking together wearing out the patient. In the great majority of instances indeed when this event occurs, something more exists than a simple inflammation of the Schneiderian membrane, since it either secretes a very tenacious mucus in extreme abundance, or becomes coated with false membrane, which sometimes extends even to the tonsils and palate. Cases of this kind are usually associated with extreme depression of the vital powers, and have received on this account the name of *coryza maligna*. I have no doubt of their identity with diphtheria, of which they constitute the form known as nasal diphtheria; though some thirty years ago, when diphtheria was a comparatively unknown disease, their real nature did not strike me as it does now. I shall therefore leave them out of consideration at present, and confine my remarks to that simple coryza which, as I have stated, is usually a source of discomfort rather than a cause of danger.

This simple coryza calls for but little *treatment*, and indeed, treatment appears to exert but little influence over it. It is desirable, however, if there is much difficulty in breathing, that the child be taken from the breast, though it may still be fed with its mother's milk by means of a spoon, since the fruitless efforts to suck aggravate its distress, and should therefore be prevented.

If heat of skin and other indications of fever attend its onset, some mild diaphoretic medicine, with a few drops of ipecacuanha wine, may be given:[1] attention must be paid to the state of the bowels, and in the course of ten days or a fortnight the infant will be found again breathing quietly, and the disease will have subsided. As the secretion becomes thicker, care must be taken to prevent its accumulating and drying at the opening of the nostrils, by which it would cause serious discomfort to the child.

Cases are sometimes met with, in which coryza, though not of a severe kind, is troublesome by its continuance for weeks together. This chronic coryza is, I believe, almost always connected with a syphilitic taint. I have on several occasions met with it when there were not above one or two spots of copper-colored eruption to mark its character; and a few instances of it have come under my notice in which no positive evidence of venereal taint, either past or present, could be obtained, but which nevertheless got well under the use of small doses of the Hydrarg. c. Cretâ.

With the increasing age of the infant there is a growing liability to *catarrh*, and during the period of dentition the susceptibility of the mucous membrane of the respiratory organs appears to have attained its maximum. Slight variations of temperature now induce catarrhal seizures; or even, independently of any such exciting cause, the mere approach of a tooth towards the surface of the gum often gives rise to its symptoms, which subside when the source of irritation ceases. Such attacks often alternate with attacks of diarrhœa, or the two coexist; the symptoms of disturbance of the intestinal mucous membrane, predominating at one time, those of disturbance of the respiratory membrane at another. The preponderance of one or the other affection seems much to depend on atmospheric causes; and children who, during the months of June, July, August, and September, would suffer from diarrhœa, will in precisely similar circumstances in the

---

[1] (No. 8.)
℞. Liq. Am. Acet., ʒj.
Vin. Ipecac., ♏xvj.
Pot. Nitratis, gr. viij.
Syr. Tolutan., ʒij.
Mist. Amygdalæ, ad ℥j. M.
A teaspoonful every four hours. For a child six months old.

earlier months of spring, or the later months of autumn, [illegible] catarrh. From the extreme susceptibility of these two great mucous surfaces arise a large proportion of the ailments, and many even of the serious diseases of infancy. Morbid as well as reparative processes go on most rapidly in early life: the flux of to-day may to-morrow be attended by dysenteric symptoms; the catarrh of to-day may to-morrow have put on the grave features of acute bronchitis.

Now these two circumstances taken together—the extreme susceptibility of the respiratory mucous membrane, and the rapidity with which its trivial disorder sometimes becomes a grave disease—give to the catarrhal affections of infancy an importance such as in more advanced life they do not possess. This importance, too, is still further increased by the tendency of the lung to become collapsed when the entrance of air into its minuter cells is impeded even by a comparatively trivial cause; while in other cases, or even in connection with the collapsed condition of the lung, the inflammatory process may invade the pulmonary cells and the general tissue of the lung, and that which had seemed a slight cold may grow to a dangerous bronchitis, or a still more dangerous pneumonia.

Of catarrh itself and its general characters, little need be said. Allowing for the difference between the ages of the patients, its symptoms are the same as in the adult. Sneezing and running at the eyes and nose, and cough, a hot skin and quickened pulse, attend it. In some children the febrile disturbance with which even a common attack of cold sets in is very severe for the first twenty-four hours or more, and then the more threatening symptoms subside, and the true nature of the affection becomes apparent. At other times, when catarrh is extremely prevalent—epidemic in short—this severe onset is usual; and the affection closely resembles, or is probably identical with, influenza. Often, too, you will find the commencement of an epidemic of hooping-cough preluded by an unusual prevalence of catarrh, the cough by degrees assuming in more and more numerous cases the paroxysmal character and peculiar sound of pertussis. It is unnecessary to allude to the catarrhal symptoms which precede measles; but bearing in mind that that which seems to be a mere cold may turn out to be the first stage of a very serious malady, you are furnished with an additional reason for not slighting it. Lastly, you must not forget that the frequent return of attacks of catarrh is sometimes an indication of that irritable state of the bronchial membrane which the abundant deposit of tubercle in the lungs occasions; and this, again, yields another argument for not neglecting an apparently trivial ailment.

While it is your duty, however, on so many grounds, to watch closely every child, although its indisposition may not seem to be more than a simple catarrh, yet in the way of actual medical *treatment* very little is required. The child must be kept in one temperature; and, if the nursery is an airy room, it is desirable that it be confined to that apartment. If already weaned, it may be well to withdraw some of the more solid articles of diet; if not, care must be taken that the child does not, in consequence of its thirst, suck too much; and a little barley-water should therefore be given it from time to time. A warm

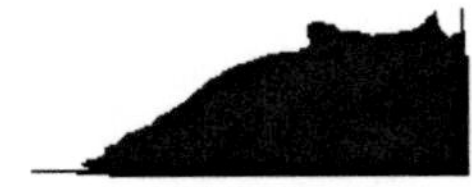

bath at night will do much to allay the heat of skin; and, if the febrile disturbance is considerable, a couple of grains of James's powder, with half a grain of calomel, may be given to a child a year old, at bed-time. During the day a mixture, containing a few drops of ipecacuanha and antimonial wine, with a little of the compound tincture of camphor, if the cough irritates by its frequent return, may be given with advantage; and, as the fever subsides, the spirit of nitrous ether may be substituted for the antimonial wine.[1]

The danger, however, in these cases, is of a more grave disorder of the air-passages coming on; and this brings us to a subject which we cannot pass over hurriedly, namely, the *bronchitis* and *pneumonia* of infancy and childhood.

The study of these affections in childhood is beset by some difficulties which we do not meet with in the adult. The points of difference between bronchitis and pneumonia are sufficiently well marked in the adult for all purposes of practical utility, although many inquiries may be started with reference to the intimate nature of the morbid processes, which we may be unable to answer satisfactorily. Besides, whether the capillaries, or the pulmonary cells, or their parietes, be the structures first attacked, it is clear that they are all involved in pneumonia from a very early stage of the disease; and hence we find it attended from the outset with peculiar symptoms, such as do not occur in bronchitis.

Pneumonia similar to that of the adult is sometimes observed even in early childhood; but it often happens that, though the pulmonary substance becomes eventually a partaker in the disease, yet it is not so at first; but the inflammation, beginning in the larger air-tubes, has passed along them to the smaller bronchi, and then at length involving the tissue of the lung, the case comes to be one neither of pure bronchitis nor of pure pneumonia, but a mixture of the two, which has not inaptly been termed *bronchio-pneumonia.* Another source of difficulty in the study of these affections, as well as an occasion of the great peril that attends them, is the tendency which we have already observed in the lung during early life to become collapsed, and no longer to admit that air without which the changes in the blood cannot take place, and the absence of which naturally aggravates the mischief that the inflammatory disease itself tends so immediately to produce.

I must beg you, therefore, to pardon me if I enter rather more minutely than is my custom into the description of the *morbid appearances produced by inflammation of the lungs and air-tubes* in infancy and childhood.

An increased degree of *redness of the mucous membrane of the bronchi*

---

[1] (No. 9.)

℞. Vin. Ipecacuanhæ, ♏x.
Vin. Ant. Pot.-Tart., ♏xxx.
Tinct. Camph. co., ♏xx.
Mist. Amygdalæ, ℥vij. M.
Two teaspoonfuls every four hours.

(No. 10.)

℞. Vin. Ipecac., ♏x.
Oxym. Scillæ, ♏xl.
Spir. Æth. Nitr., ♏xx.
Tinct. Camph. co., ♏xx.
Aquæ Anisi, ℥viss. M.
Two teaspoonfuls every four hours.

For children of one year old.

is almost constantly observed in the case of children who have died of inflammation of the lungs or air-tubes. There are three sources of error, however, which it is essential to guard against when examining the bronchi with reference to this point. The first is the occasional disappearance of redness after death, even where the presence of an abundant muco-purulent secretion in the tubes bears evidence to the activity of the inflammatory process; the second is the apparent redness of the smaller tubes in cases where the lungs are congested or inflamed, and which may be due, not to the increased vascularity of the bronchi themselves, but to their transparency allowing that of the subjacent tissue to be seen through them. The third is the occasional staining of the mucous membrane, owing to the transudation of the blood through the coats of the vessels after death. With care, however, none of these conditions will lead you astray.

The redness of the bronchi varies much both in degree and extent, and in some cases which have approached to the character of pneumonia rather than of bronchitis, is sometimes limited to the inflamed lobes. In cases, however, in which much bronchitis has existed, very marked redness generally begins about an inch above the bifurcation of the trachea, and pervades all the bronchi, being deeper in the secondary than in the primary tubes, and retaining nearly as great an intensity even in the tertiary branches. It may stop here, or it may extend even into the ultimate ramuscules, or into the pulmonary cells themselves.

In the majority of cases no other change besides this intense redness is perceptible in the *mucous membrane*, but *sometimes it appears both thickened and softened;* and on one occasion, in which a fatal attack of acute bronchitis supervened on a long continuance of the chronic stage of the disease, the bronchial mucous membrane was intensely red, and so thickened as to have an almost villous appearance, and closely to resemble red velvet.

Ulceration of the mucous membrane of the trachea and larger bronchi, which is occasionally met with in the bronchitis of adults, I never observed but once. In that case, a little boy, twenty months old, who had suffered from a not very severe attack of bronchitis, in the course of which, however, he had had occasional difficulty in deglutition, with return of fluids by the nose, died rather suddenly. The only remarkable appearance besides a general redness of the bronchial tubes, consisted in the presence of several small excavated ulcerations or erosions in the upper part of the larynx, just above the chordæ vocales.

Associated with the changes in the mucous membrane of the bronchi there is an *alteration* in the character *of their secretion*. At first, no doubt, this secretion is suppressed, just as we see that furnished by the Schneiderian membrane to be in a common cold; but afterwards it is poured out abundantly, and next ceases to present its natural characters of a glairy mucus; becoming opaque, thick, puriform, or actually purulent, while in a few less common instances the secretion assumes the form and consistence of false membrane, constituting a true croup of the bronchi. Traces of blood are but very seldom observed in the secretion, and the quantity of air-bubbles intermingled with usually in inverse proportion to the thickness of the secretion and its abundance.

But not only are the contents of the air-tubes altered in character, and, for the most part, increased in quantity, but the *tubes* themselves often undergo a marked alteration in their calibre, and *become* greatly *dilated*. This dilatation is usually observable from the secondary bronchi to the minutest air-tubes; the branches often being as large as the parent trunk, or even larger; but that fusiform dilatation which is met with in the adult has never come under my notice. On one occasion, however, in addition to a general cylindrical enlargement of the tubes, many of them presented a marked dilatation about half an inch from their termination; the tube expanding into a cavity big enough to hold half a nut. The interior of these cavities was not perfectly smooth and regular, but its thickened lining was in many parts thrown into folds or wrinkles. The case in which this appearance was observed was the one already mentioned, where the mucous membrane of the bronchi presented so extraordinary a degree of thickening.

Dilatation of the bronchi was once supposed to be the purely mechanical effect of the accumulation of the secretions within them. There is, however, no constant relation between the quantity of the liquids within the bronchi and the degree of their dilatation, and we must look to two other circumstances as being the primary causes of the occurrence. The first of these is the weakening of the muscular fibres of the bronchi by the inflammatory action; the other, the loss of the ciliary epithelium which lines the air-tubes when in a state of health, and contributes by the incessant vibration of its cilia to keep them free for the access of air.

Whenever bronchitis has reached such an intensity as to give rise to the abundant pouring out of thick fluid into the air-tubes, so that the air can no longer permeate them with facility—while this difficulty is still further increased by the loss of the ciliary epithelium, and by the weakening of the contractile power of the bronchi, which would have helped to keep them free—it often happens that the feeble inspiratory power of the child becomes wholly inadequate to fill the lungs, and bronchitis thus becomes the indirect cause of pulmonary collapse.

In some cases, the inflammation of the respiratory mucous membrane extends further than usual along the smaller bronchi, until it involves their extremities and the pulmonary vesicles themselves, when it produces an appearance almost peculiar to childhood, and which has been described under the names of *catarrhal* or *vesicular pneumonia*, or *vesicular bronchitis*. A lung, or a portion of a lung, thus affected, no longer contains any air—it is dark in color, and feels tough, though solid; its surface is beset by a number of small, circular, yellow, slightly prominent spots, of the size of a millet-seed, or smaller, which, on a hasty glance, present a very great resemblance to crude tubercles. A little attention, however, suffices to distinguish between them; for not only do these yellow spots differ from tubercle in their favorite seat being along the lower margins of the different lobes, but on puncturing any of them with the point of a scalpel a drop of pus will exude, and the yellow spot will disappear. Sometimes, too, a minute bronchus may be traced running to its termination in one of these little sacs. It has been suggested that this appearance may be due to the secretions formed in the air-tubes being forced by the column of air which enters in inspiration into the smaller bronchi and pulmonary vesicles, the cavities of which thus become mechanically distended. The opinion that the secretions which occupy these parts are produced at the spot where they are discovered, by inflammation of the ultimate ramuscules of the bronchi, is however, generally entertained, and is supported by very conclusive evidence. Bronchitis often exists unattended with this peculiar appearance; and on the other hand, vesicular bronchitis is met with independent of general inflammation of the air-tubes, while, though usually partial, and often limited to the lower border of one or other lobe, it is sometimes very extensive, and occupies nearly the whole of the lower lobe on either side, constituting the most important of the morbid appearances discovered on examining the chest.

It may, and unquestionably often does happen, that children die of bronchitis alone, and without any notable affection of the pulmonary tissue. But it is much more frequent for the pulmonary substance to bear a part in the morbid process; and this share may either be limited to mere congestion, or may rise in degree until it produces all those consequences which we find attendant on inflammation of the tissue of the lung of the adult.

Some degree of *congestion of the lung* is almost constant if bronchitis is at all severe, for the circulation through the organ is disturbed, the blood flows less freely than natural, and its changes take place more slowly. It stagnates first in those depending parts whence position renders its return most difficult, and the portions of the lung thus affected become by degrees more and more extensive. Dark, solid, non-crepitant patches may be often seen in the midst of a lung thus congested; and until the results of inflation showed that a wrong interpretation had been given to the appearance, these patches were regarded as the centres whence the inflammation was extending to the surrounding tissue. You do not need to be reminded that these are lobules which have collapsed, and become impervious to air; and portions of lung in which this occurrence has taken place seem to have but little disposition to become the seat of active inflammation, and to pass into a state of red or gray hepatization. At the same time it must be borne in mind that this indisposition to active inflammation does not by any means amount to actual immunity from it, and that collapsed lung may sometimes become softened, or even infiltrated with pus.

It does, however, happen now and then that the lung is found in a condition which may justly be called *lobular pneumonia*, as the result of the extension to the surrounding tissue of inflammation beginning in the air-tubes. Patches of lung will then be interspersed through the surrounding pulmonary substance, of a vivid red color, of various sizes, from that of a pea to that of an almond, irregular in shape and not circumscribed exactly by the margins of lobules, as is the case with portions of collapsed lung. This process going on in a number of different situations, the affected parts may at length coalesce, and a pneumonia at first lobular, may thus eventually become generalized. Or, though this should not occur, the inflammation may yet go on in the isolated portions of lung to the infiltration of pus into its substance, or the actual destruction of its tissue, when a portion of the lung will appear riddled with small distinct abscesses, seldom larger than a pea, irregular in form, and communicating more or less evidently with a minute air-tube. They may be distinguished from the vomicæ produced by softened tubercle, partly by the absence of tubercular deposits in other parts of the body, and by their being almost always limited to a single lobe of one lung. Their own characters, however, are sufficiently well marked, for they are altogether destitute of those solid walls which the tubercular deposit forms around a phthisical cavity; though the yellow lymph which often lines them may be mistaken by the inattentive observer for tubercle. MM. Rilliet and Barthez mention having found the pulmonary substance healthy, except in the immediate periphery of these abscesses; but no instance of this kind has come under my own observation, the pneumonia having in each instance become generalized.

The appearances we have been hitherto considering are due almost exclusively to inflammation of the air-tubes; and many of them are peculiar to infancy and childhood. We might next proceed to study the symptoms that betoken their existence; but on the one hand, they seldom exist quite alone, and on the other hand their symptoms present so many points of resemblance to those of pneumonia strictly so called, that it may be better to complete our survey of the morbid appearances that result from inflammation affecting either the air-tubes or the parenchyma of the lung, before we pass to the study of the symptoms that attend the one or the other during life.

The completion of this subject, however, must be postponed to the next lecture.

LECTURE XX.

INFLAMMATORY AFFECTIONS OF THE TISSUE OF THE LUNG.—Lobar Pneumonia—More common in early life than has been supposed—Its general characters the same as in the adult—Some morbid appearances deserving especial notice; viz., subpleural ecchymoses, pneumonic abscess, and emphysema of the uninflamed portions of the lung.

Frequency and causes of inflammation of the respiratory organs—Influence of age—of previous attacks—of various diseases.

BRONCHITIS—ITS SYMPTOMS AND TREATMENT.—A more serious disease than in the adult, and why—Symptoms of capillary bronchitis—Illustrative case—Results of auscultation.

Treatment of bronchitis—Change in the epidemic constitution of diseases and inexpediency of very active measures—General rules for treatment—Treatment of bronchitis in its chronic stage.

INFLUENZA.—Its peculiarities and treatment in early life—Remarks on SPASMODIC COUGH and ASTHMA in children.

WE were occupied during the last lecture with the examination of some of the results of inflammation of the respiratory organs in early life, and considered more especially those changes which inflammation produces in the air-tubes. You were told on that occasion that the disease does not always remain limited to the bronchi or pulmonary vesicles, but that it sometimes involves the substance of the lung, and thus gives rise to the appearance of a number of small circumscribed patches interspersed throughout its tissue, either red, hard, and solid, or gray from the infiltration of pus; while, if the mischief advance one step farther, it may lead to the destruction of the parenchyma of the organ at these points, and thus produce numerous minute abscesses—a condition which has come in a few instances under my own observation. Cases of this kind, constituting true lobular pneumonia, though somewhat less rare than in the adult, are yet of very infrequent occurrence. It is almost needless to remind you that the contrary opinion resulted from persons not having learned till very lately to distinguish between that solidity of the lung which is produced by inflammation, and that which results from the mere collapse of its air-cells.

The exaggerated estimate of the frequency of lobular pneumonia, and the peculiar character of the field presented at the Hospital for Children at Paris, in which the most diligent and most successful students of children's diseases labored, led to an underrating of the frequency and importance of lobar pneumonia such as is met with in the adult; and hence you will find but little said concerning it in many most valuable works of our Continental neighbors. *Lobar pneumonia*, however, is often met with in early life both as an idiopathic and a secondary affection, giving rise to the same morbid appearances as in the adult, and requiring a very similar treatment.

Not only are the physical characters of the lung in lobar pneumonia the same in childhood as in adult age, but the three stages of engorgement, of red and of gray hepatization, are observed with much the same frequency at the one period of life as at the other. I find that after rejecting all cases in which pneumonia occurred as a complication of phthisis, or of acute pleurisy, and in which the results might be modified by the disease to which the inflammation of the lung succeeded, I have a record of 94 cases in which the condition of the inflamed lung was carefully noticed.[1]

In	15	of these cases the 1st and 2d stages of pneumonia coexisted.
"	4	" " 1st and 3d " " "
"	25	" " 2d and 3d " " "
"	14	" " all 3 stages " " "
"	13	" " lung was in the 1st stage only.
"	13	" " lung was in the 2d "
"	10	" " lung was in the 3d "
	94	

This result does not differ very widely from that obtained by M. Grisolle,[2] on an examination of 40 cases of pneumonia in the adult.

In	4	cases the 1st and 2d stages of pneumonia coexisted.
"	3	" 1st and 3d " " "
"	16	" 2d and 3d " " "
"	2	" all 3 stages " " "
"	7	" lung was in the 2d stage only.
"	8	" lung was in the 3d "
	40	

It will be seen, on a comparison of these tables, that the third stage of pneumonia occurs not very much less often in children than in adults, having been met with in the former in the proportion of 56.3, in the latter in the proportion of 72.5 per cent.; and the main difference between the two consists in the greater frequency with which all three stages of pneumonia coexist in the young subject. This peculiarity of pneumonia in childhood is probably due to the tendency which the disease then displays to involve a large extent of pulmonary tissue; and to the same cause we must attribute the frequency of double pneumonia in early life, which, in the cases that came under my notice, preponderated greatly over those wherein only one lung suffered. The well-known law, according to which pneumonia of the right lung is more common than pneumonia of the left, holds good in childhood; nor is the frequency of concomitant pleurisy much, if at all, less in the child than in the adult. The contrary opinion arose from the error to which reference has so often been made, of regarding cases of collapsed

[1] Here, and in many other instances, I purposely abstain from swelling the numbers from which my conclusions are drawn by adding my more recent observations. I do so, because as one grows older, especially in consulting practice, the field in which one labors becomes more and more an exceptional one, and one but little suited for the application of the numerical method. I believe, however, that the conclusions to which the figures above given point are correct.

[2] Traité de la Pneumonie, 8vo., 2d ed., Paris, 1864, p. 17.

lung, either with or without bronchitis, as instances of red hepatization of the pulmonary substance.

Instead of inflammation of the lungs being less active in the child than in the adult, there are some facts which would seem to lead to a directly opposite conclusion. Such are the frequency with which, in fatal pneumonia in children, ecchymoses are found beneath the pleura covering the inflamed lung, the more common occurrence of pulmonary abscess in early than in adult life, and the very extensive emphysema which is often observed in those parts of the lung to which the inflammation has not extended.

The *subpleural ecchymoses* appear to result from the rupture of some of the minute capillaries of the lungs in consequence of the great disturbance of the circulation through them. They are usually small, like petechiæ, but occasionally they attain a large size, and now and then they even extend a little way into the tissue of the lung, constituting little spots of pulmonary apoplexy, about the size of a millet-seed, or even a little larger. They are most numerous on the posterior surface of the lungs, and especially in parts where the lung has become hepatized, though by no means confined to those situations.

The termination of pneumonia in *abscess of the lung* is so rare an occurrence in the adult, that Laennec did not meet with it above five or six times in the course of several hundred examinations of persons who had died of inflammation of the lungs. In the child, however, the case is otherwise, for abscess of the lung has come under my observation in four out of the ninety-four examinations of cases of pneumonia, on which my present remarks are founded. In one of these cases, that of a boy, aged 20 months, who died on the fourteenth day after the commencement of his illness, the following appearances were observed: The upper and middle lobes of the right lung were connected with each other, and with the walls of the chest, by adhesions which were chiefly recent. Nearly the whole of the upper lobe was solid, and sank in water. It was of a mottled reddish-gray color, in which gray predominated; it broke with a granular fracture, and was readily reduced to a dirty putrilage. Near the apex was a portion the size of a walnut which was already soft and in a state of quagmire. The upper two-thirds of the middle lobe were in the same condition as the upper lobe; the lower third was emphysematous. In the centre of the middle lobe was a cavity the size of a bean, irregular in form, intersected by the remains of some vessels, lined by a thin layer of yellow lymph, and surrounded by lung in the third stage of pneumonia; but neither in that lobe nor in any part of the pulmonary tissue was there the least trace of tubercle. The lower lobe of the right lung was in the first stage of pneumonia; the left upper lobe was quite healthy; the left lower lobe was in a state of mingled red and gray hepatization. Two cases occurred in children who had suffered for some weeks from hooping-cough, and in both the lungs contained numerous semi-transparent, gray, tubercular granulations. One of the children was a boy five years old; the other a little girl aged two years. In the case of the former, the abscess, as large as a walnut, was situated at the lower border of the upper lobe, extending a little into the lower lobe. In the latter it was of the size of an unshelled almond, and occupied a similar position with reference to the right upper and middle lobes. The characters of the abscess were the same in both instances, being situated almost immediately beneath the pleura: from which a wall of lung not above two lines in thickness separated it. Its cavity was partly filled with a yellowish, puriform, very tenacious fluid, like very tenacious pus, and which did not bear any resemblance to softened tubercle. It was not lined by any membrane; there was no appearance of tubercular deposit in the hepatized lung in its immediate vicinity, which was generally in the second stage of pneumonia, nor was it situated near to, nor in communication with, any large bronchial tube. In the fourth case, that of a boy aged eleven years, who died of pyæmia, consequent on exposure to cold and wet, the purulent deposits were not limited to the lung-substance, although they were associated there with general pneumonia, and with several patches of pulmonary apoplexy.

The *emphysematous condition* of the uninflamed portions of the lung, in cases of fatal pneumonia in early life, seems to be connected with the rapidity of the advance of the disease. It is usually most obvious at the anterior part of the upper lobes of the lungs and at the margin of the other lobes, and always bears a marked relation to the shortness of the patient's illness, and the extent of lung which has been rendered unavailable for purposes of respiration. The cases, however, which terminate most rapidly are not those in which the *direct* results of inflammation are the most extensive, but rather those in which collapse of a considerable portion of lung has taken place; and the emphysema, which is met with also in many cases of vesicular bronchitis, is consequent less on the inflammation than on the collapse by which it is accompanied. Its occurrence in those circumstances affords therefore an illustration of that modification of the *inspiratory* theory of emphysema so clearly propounded and so ably supported by Professor Gairdner of Glasgow;[1] and which regards the overdistension of the air-vesicles of one part of the lung as a necessary compensation for their collapse, and the consequent diminished bulk of another part, while the enlargement and the capacity of the thorax during inspiration remain the same, or at any rate are but slightly modified.[2]

The *causes* which give rise to inflammation of the lungs and air-tubes are, to a great extent, the same at all periods of life; so that we need not devote much attention to the special study of those which

[1] On the Pathological Anatomy of Bronchitis, &c., 8vo., Edinburgh, 1850; and Edinburgh Monthly Journal, vol. xiv.

[2] In the second and third editions of these lectures I stated that the amount of emphysema bore a "marked relation to the shortness of the patient's illness, and the extent of lung which had been invaded by the inflammation." A careful re-examination of the accounts of my post-mortems of cases of pneumonia and bronchitis, convinces me that the statement as now modified is more correct in point of fact, while at the same time it harmonizes perfectly with Dr. Gairdner's theory of emphysema. That theory, however, is, I am convinced, applicable only to one class of cases, while of another equally numerous, Sir W. Jenner's *expiratory* theory (see his paper in vol. xl of the Medico-Chirurgical Transactions) offers the true solution. To this reference will be made when the subject of hooping-cough comes for consideration.

tend to produce it in childhood. It should be borne in mind, however, that the fluctuations in temperature, or the biting wind, or the cold weather, which may be encountered with impunity by the robust adult, may prove most deadly when they act on the feeble frame and delicate organs of the child. Hence it is, in great measure, that inflammation of the respiratory organs is so much more frequent, and so much more fatal, in childhood than in adult age, and in infancy than in childhood. The fact is well shown by the Reports of the Registrar-General for the years 1842 and 1845, from which it appears that 67.1 per cent. of the total mortality from inflammation of the lungs and bronchi, in the metropolis, took place in persons under fifteen years of age; 63.2 per cent. under five; 57.1 under three; and 28.7 per cent. under one year. But the tendency to these affections, as is shown in the following table, is not greatest in the first month of life, diminishing in proportion as the child advances in age and increases in strength; but the time when they are most prevalent coincides exactly with the time when the susceptibility of all the mucous membranes is at its highest point, namely, the period of dentition.

TABLE,

Showing out of 299 cases of children dying from various diseases, in whom I carefully examined the thoracic viscera, the number of instances in which the lungs, bronchi, and pleura presented no sign of recent inflammation, and also those in which signs of it were discovered. [The first line represents the former, the second the latter class of cases.]

Under 1 mth.	From 1–6.	From 6–12.	From 12–18.	From 18–2 yrs.	From 2–3.	From 3–4.	From 4–5.	From 5–6.	From 6–7.	From 7–8.	From 8–9.	From 9–10.	From 10–11.	From 11–12.	Total.
5	18	17	15	6	22	17	8	12	5	11	5	4	8	2	145
	8	10	15	18	23	16	15	13	8	10	11	3	4	5	154

This table illustrates the fact mentioned in the last lecture, that when the child is first born, the mucous membrane of the respiratory organs is endowed with but little of that susceptibility which it afterwards acquires, and that accordingly those diseases whose point of departure is from that membrane are far less frequent during the first six months of life than they become during the succeeding eighteen months; while from the completion of the second year up to the time of puberty, they go on diminishing in frequency and fatality. And there are important practical inferences which may be deduced from the facts we have just mentioned. They teach us not only that a catarrh is a much more serious thing in infancy than in adult age, but also that it is more serious at one period of infancy than at another, and they warn us to guard a child, during the time that the process of teething is going on, with double care against all causes that are likely to excite inflammation of its respiratory organs.

There are some diseases which, after having occurred once, confer on persons an immunity from subsequent attacks. This, however, is far from being the case with bronchitis or pneumonia in early life, but the susceptibility of the respiratory organs appears to increase in exact proportion to the frequency with which they have already suffered,[1] and a child who has once been attacked by inflammation of the lungs or air-tubes is more likely to have a second attack brought on by a slight change of temperature than another who had never suffered from it would be to experience a seizure from a much graver cause. With advancing age this susceptibility seems to wear out—the child outgrows it; but we should act most unwisely if we were to sanction exposure to the cold with the view of hardening a child against its influence.

The importance of inflammatory diseases of the respiratory organs depends not merely on the frequency of their occurrence as idiopathic affections, but also on their tendency to supervene in the course of other maladies. This tendency, though very evident at all ages, is especially remarkable in early life, as is apparent from the fact that in only 25 per cent. of the cases enumerated in the table was the inflammation an idiopathic affection. When we come to the subject of measles, hooping-cough, croup, diarrhœa, and typhoid fever, it will be necessary to study these secondary attacks of bronchitis and pneumonia with attention, since they constitute frequent and serious complications of those diseases against which it behooves us to be most anxiously on the watch.

We will now pass to the study of the *symptoms of bronchitis*, and will commence with the examination of the most simple form of inflammation of the air-tubes—namely, that which develops itself out of ordinary catarrh. In such a case the child has for some days seemed to suffer from nothing more serious than a common cold; but by degrees instead of the cold and cough subsiding, the heat of skin becomes more considerable, the cough tighter, more frequent, and more painful, the child sometimes crying after each cough: the pulse becomes more rapid, the respiration wheezing, hurried, and often somewhat irregular. These graver symptoms in many instances steal on very gradually, and among the poor it by no means seldom happens that the disease has already attained an advanced stage, and the condition has become one of very considerable peril, before the parents, never very observant of those ailments that are not attended with acute suffering, take the alarm. The flush of the face and the heat of the skin become increased, the respiration grows more labored, and the cough more troublesome towards evening; and the first hours of the night are usually very restless, but the child then falls asleep, and often dozes tranquilly for some hours; it then generally awakes with its respiration very oppressed, for the secretions have been accumulating in the smaller bron-

[1] In a tract on Pneumonia in Children, published thirty years ago in the British and Foreign Medical Review, I mentioned that of 78 children who came under my care for inflammation of the lungs, 31 were stated to have had previous attacks of the disease; 21 once; 4 twice; 2 four times; and 4 were said to have had it several times, though the exact number of seizures was not mentioned. Of these 31, 10 were under two years of age, 10 between two and three, and the remaining 11 between three and six The same fact is noticed by the most recent writer on pneumonia in childhood, Ziemsen (Pleuritis und Pneumonie im Kindesalter, 8vo., Berlin, 1862, p. 153), though his numbers do not represent it as of quite such frequent occurrence.

chi, and have now begun to impede the entrance of the air. An attack of cough probably comes on, which very likely ends in vomiting and the rejection of some mucus, and then by degrees the breathing becomes more easy, and the child may for a short time seem comparatively cheerful. The temperature of the surface, though increased, is variable; and if the disease continues for several days, perspiration will be observed occasionally to break out on the body, while the pulse, though quickened, is not very much accelerated, and the tongue continues moist throughout. The ear detects nothing in the chest besides a mixture of rhonchus, sibilus, and largish crepitation; the dry sounds preponderating at the upper, the moist at the lower part of the chest, and being vastly more abundant behind than in front. Now in the adult a condition such as this would excite but little apprehension, but in the child it must be borne in mind that nothing more is needed than a copious secretion of mucus in the bronchi, or a feeble condition of the vital powers, to prevent the air from freely entering the pulmonary vesicles, and thus to induce the collapse of a large portion of the lung. Thus it is, at least as I apprehend, that we must explain many of the instances in which urgent dyspnœa, and all the symptoms of serious pulmonary disease, have developed themselves in the course of a few hours out of what had seemed to be nothing more than a rather severe cold, or a bronchitis of moderate intensity. This too accounts for the occasional sudden supervention of dulness on percussion, and of bronchial respiration in the child; so that you may discover them in the morning in a situation where overnight the percussion was good, and no sound was heard of graver import than large crepitation; changes which, unlike those dependent on solidification of the lung from inflammation, you may find, as has been remarked by Dr. Gairdner, unaccompanied by any exacerbation of the febrile symptoms. This rapid change in the auscultatory phenomena has been noticed by Sir W. Stokes as occasionally happening in the pneumonia of the adult.[1] That distinguished physician offered no explanation of the occurrence; but we can now understand what is its true import, and what the reasons are for its being met with so much oftener in the child than in the adult.

But, notwithstanding this danger, which is great in proportion to the youth of a child, most cases of idiopathic bronchitis that come on gradually, developing themselves out of previous catarrhal symptoms, have a favorable termination; and, as a general rule, it may be stated that an attack which is long in arriving at its acme is seldom very dangerous in its character. Pure idiopathic bronchitis occurring in an otherwise healthy child, usually subsides in the course of a few days, leaving the patient with an increased susceptibility to the influence of those causes which brought on the first attack, and perhaps with a degree of debility, the recovery from which may be protracted for many weeks.

There is, however, a form of acute bronchitis which is often, though not always, idiopathic, that runs its course with much rapidity, and generally tends to a fatal termination. In this, the *suffocative catarrh*

[1] On the Diseases of the Chest, 8vo., Dublin, 1837, pp. 311 and 327.

of some writers—the *capillary bronchitis* of others—the smaller air-tubes throughout the whole or a considerable portion of the lungs are attacked either in connection with the larger bronchi, or independently of them; and the inflammation, which is very intense, usually terminates in the abundant secretion of pus, or in the formation of false membrane that nearly obliterates their cavity, or, involving the pulmonary vesicles themselves, it gives rise through a considerable extent of the lungs to those appearances which have been described under the names of vesicular pneumonia and vesicular bronchitis.

Its attack is sometimes sudden, though in the great majority of cases it is preceded for a few days by the ordinary symptoms of catarrh, or it supervenes on that condition of bronchial irritation which accompanies or follows one or other of the eruptive fevers. In these latter circumstances there is either a progressive though rapid increase in the severity of the bronchitic symptoms, or there is a sudden outbreak of fever and dyspnœa, and the cough becomes all at once frequent, short, and hacking. The disease soon attains a very considerable intensity; the face becomes anxious and oppressed, the eyes heavy, the manner depressed; the respiration very hurried, generally irregular, and interrupted by the cough, which frequently seems to occasion pain. The restlessness is often extreme, and the position which the child assumes very variable; but, in whatever attitude it may have placed itself, it does not like to be disturbed, and endeavors at once to return to its former posture. If spoken to, the child's answers are hurried, and its manner impatient, as though it were too much taken up with its suffering, or with the business of respiration, to be able to reply to questions. Sometimes it will say that it feels stuffed, or will complain of distress about the sternum, or of pain at the epigastrium; while pressure on the abdomen, by interfering with the free descent of the diaphragm, always produces much discomfort. There is no appetite; and, though at first the thirst is very considerable, yet the child soon ceases to take much drink, for it wants breath to swallow fluids in any quantity, and therefore does little more than moisten its lips. At the same time the tongue is moist, and either differs but little from its condition in health, or it has a thin coating of yellowish fur; the bowels are usually constipated, and not only is nausea or vomiting seldom present, but emetic remedies often fail of their ordinary effect when given in the course of this affection. As the disease advances the cough becomes less hacking, though it continues very frequent: it sometimes puts on a paroxysmal character, and returns in fits somewhat like those of hooping-cough, except that each fit of coughing is shorter, does not terminate with a whoop, and is seldom attended with expectoration. Even if the cough is accompanied by expectoration, it is seldom that anything is spit up more than a little mucus tinged with blood, or now and then a little pure blood, while in a few instances small shreds of false membrane are intermingled with the mucus. For a time the respiration grows more and more hurried and paroxysms of dyspnœa continue to occur at irregular intervals almost to the last. In these paroxysms the child's distress and restlessness are extreme, and it sometimes throws itself wildly about the bed. The breathing does not, however, go on increasing in rapidity until the patient's death; but, after the disease has reached its acme, the respiration often grows less frequent, though more irregular and more variable. The face loses its flush, and, instead, acquires a livid hue; the cough becomes smothered, and occurs less often; the pulse gains in frequency and fails in power; and though there is often a diminution of the restlessness, yet, if able to talk, the child will generally say that it is no better. As death approaches, though the respiration grows more labored and more abdominal, yet the child's suffering generally diminishes, or a state of somnolence gradually steals over it, in which it lies till roused by an attack of cough or by a paroxysm of dyspnœa, and then, after a struggle for breath, it subsides into its former drowsiness. The struggles for breath grow feebler with each returning paroxysm, the drowsiness becomes more profound, and the patient dies.

Though the indications afforded by auscultation and percussion are often sufficiently characteristic of this disease, yet there are some circumstances which may occasionally render their information doubtful. The child is sometimes so extremely alarmed, and the sensibility of its surface so much increased, that we have much difficulty in percussing the chest: but we shall usually be able to distinguish this from the painfulness of the walls of the thorax which attends pleurisy by finding that it is not limited to one half of the chest, but that it is felt equally on either side, and as much in front as behind. If we can succeed in percussing the chest, however, it will be found to yield a natural, sometimes even an increased degree of resonance, while little, if any, difference can be discovered between the sound afforded by the upper, and that given out by the lower part of the chest; or, should such be perceived, it is generally due to pneumonia having supervened. The ear detects a scanty transmission of air, attended at first with rhonchus and sibilus, but soon with a universal subcrepitant râle, heard most distinctly on the child making a deep inspiration. By the term subcrepitant râle, it can hardly be necessary for me to say that a sound is meant smaller in character than large mucous râle, but larger than the true small crepitation of pneumonia. As the disease advances, the only change that takes place consists in this subcrepitant râle being replaced by a large mucous râle, the result, not of any improvement in the child's condition, but of the air scarcely penetrating beyond the larger bronchi; for you will still hear the smaller sound during the deep inspiration that follows the attack of cough.

This form of bronchitis is one not only very dangerous, but likewise very rapid in its course to a fatal issue. One little girl in whom it came on while convalescent from an attack of measles fourteen days before, died within forty-eight hours; and a boy of 7½ years old, in whom the disease was idiopathic, died in less than four days from the appearance of any serious symptom. These, however, are instances of a rather unusual rapidity in its course; and from five to eight days, which is the estimate of its duration formed by M. Fauvel, who has written a very valuable essay on the disease,[1] is probably not far from the true average.

[1] Recherches sur la Bronchite Capillaire, &c., 4to., Paris, 1840; republished in a more extended form in vol. ii of the Mémoires de la Société Médicale d'Observation, 8vo., Paris, 1844.

But we may now pass to the treatment of *bronchitis*, and in reconsidering the rules which I shall lay down for your guidance, I am struck by the different conclusions to which more than thirty years of the practice of my profession have led me from those which I adopted at the outset of my career. It is, I believe, but rarely, at the present day, that depletion is indicated in bronchitis or pneumonia; and tartar emetic needs to be given more sparingly than in former years, and acts with less certainty in cutting short at its very outset the inflammatory action. And yet, when looking back on the records of cases where I abstracted blood freely, and gave antimony in large doses, I cannot admit that my practice then was a mistaken one, that the recoveries which then took place were the result of accident, or that, in counselling now a different course, I am merely following the fashion or the prejudice of the age.

"If any one," says M. Trousseau, with reference to this very subject, "reads with attention the remarks of Sydenham and of Stoll on the change of the treatment of disease which the differences in the epidemic constitution of successive years rendered necessary, he will be sure to arrive at two conclusions: first, that any physician must have but a very narrow view of his art, who, in spite of the change of constitution, continues still to treat all diseases in the same way; and next, that the change of epidemic constitution exerts an immense influence on the action of the same remedies in a disease whose local manifestations continue unchanged."

You will now understand, gentlemen, why it was, when I told you at the beginning of this lecture, that the necessity, nay even the utility, of depletion in pneumonia did not seem to me well established, that I made a point of adding *just at present*. I did so, because it so happens that now for the past several years we are in the midst of an epidemic constitution in which diseases do not require this remedy, though formerly they did require it, and though in the course of time they will no doubt stand in need of it again.[1]

But besides, I believe that with advancing years all practitioners become disposed to attach more importance to the hygiene of the sick-room; to the temperature of the air which the child breathes, to the perfection of the ventilation, to the posture of the patient in bed, to the regulation of the diet, the avoidance of all causes of irritation and distress; and the favorable issue of the case not seldom justifies the apparent overcaution in these respects to which experience seems to lead.

The confidence sometimes expressed in nature's healing power is, however, altogether misplaced, unless accompanied with every care to place the patient in the most favorable conditions for that power to be exercised. These conditions once secured, the severity of the attack of

---

[1] Clinique Médicale, 2d ed., vol. i, p. 744. See also on the subject of depletion generally the remarks of Sir T. Watson at vol. i, p. 241–258 of the 5th edition of his Lectures. If, however, I might criticize one whom I so much respect, I should express surprise that he, on whom more than on any other English physician of this day Sydenham's mantle has fallen, should take so little heed of Sydenham's doctrine of the varying epidemic constitution in different years, or terms of years.

bronchitis must govern the further treatment. In a healthy child, at the outset of a bronchitic seizure of moderate intensity, small doses of calomel, antimony, and ipecacuanha, given every four hours for the first twenty-four or thirty-six hours, are often extremely useful. This combination usually acts on the bowels slightly as well as on the skin, and often notably abates the febrile disturbance. The mercurial should then be discontinued, but small doses of antimony or of ipecacuanha should still be continued in a saline mixture. In addition to these means, the breathing is often much relieved by the application of a large warm linseed poultice to the chest, or of a large piece of spongio-piline wrung out of hot water; either of which may be made more stimulating by the addition of a third or fourth part of mustard to the poultice, or by sprinkling some stimulating liniment over the spongio-piline.[1] These applications should be frequently renewed, and should be continued for twenty-four or thirty-six hours together, while any marked increase of difficult breathing must be controlled by the application of a mustard poultice between the shoulders, or to the front of the chest; a proceeding which has this great advantage over the use of a blister, that it will admit of frequent repetition. After the first day or two the abundance of the secretion poured out into the bronchi not only increases the discomfort of the child, but is a positive source of danger, inasmuch as it tends to favor the occurrence of pulmonary collapse. An emetic once or twice a day is the great means of relieving this discomfort, and warding off this danger. The emetic selected should be one of ipecacuanha in preference to antimony; or even the sulphate of zinc if the ipecacuanha, as happens sometimes, while it fails to vomit, should act upon the bowels.

Your attention has more than once been called to the remarkable tendency of the nervous system in early life to sympathize with the affections of other parts. This tendency is often very evident in inflammation of the respiratory organs; and accordingly you must not always take the degree of dyspnœa in a case of infantile bronchitis as a measure of the severity of the disease, since it may be only an evidence of the sympathy of the nervous system. In the majority of instances, it is towards evening that this acceleration of breathing comes on, accompanied with a state of general restlessness, and usually with an increase, though not to an extreme degree, of the heat of skin; but yet if you listen carefully to the chest you will find no deterioration in the results of auscultation. In the infant, too, you will probably perceive in the half-closed eyes, and in the thumbs drawn into the palm, indications of the disturbance of the nervous system.

The evening warm bath often relieves this symptom very much, and if the amount of the secretion in the bronchi is not so considerable

---

[1] (No. 11.)

℞. Lin. Camph. co., ℥j.
Tinct. Lyttæ, ʒij
Tinct. Opii., ʒij. M. Ft. linimentum.

The pungency of liniments often compel us to employ them to the posterior part of the chest only, or to rub the front of the chest with a much weaker liniment than that which is used for the back.

as to contraindicate its use, a dose of Dover's powder given afterwards will soothe the child and obtain for it a few hours of quiet sleep. The emetic and the mustard poultice will in other cases be followed by the same result, while it must be borne in mind that a constipated state of the bowels on the one hand, or the irritation of teething on the other, may give occasion to a hurry of respiration, which will at once cease on the administration of a dose of castor oil, or on lancing the gums.

The combination of a direct sedative with each dose of the medicine which the child takes must be had recourse to cautiously, and must have reference rather to the relief of the irritating cough than to the control of any very marked symptom of nervous dyspnœa, since, whenever in these cases the blood is imperfectly aerated, risk attends the frequent employment of narcotics. On this account the chloric ether is often so useful an adjunct to the cough mixture; while of the more direct sedatives the compound tincture of camphor is preferable to any other preparation of opium, and the tincture of henbane is perhaps still safer; the Dover's powder in a fuller dose being reserved for the evening exacerbation of dyspnœa.

After the first few days, sometimes even very early in the attack, comes the necessity for supporting the child's strength, and for watching carefully against that collapse of the lungs which in infancy is the grand source of danger. Ammonia must now be added to the expectorant mixture which the child was previously taking, or it may be given in combination with the decotion of senega[1] and tincture of squills, if secretion in the bronchi is very abundant, while once or twice in the twenty-four hours the attempt must be made to unload the air-tubes by the administration of an emetic.

The maintenance of the child's strength by food, and often by stimulants, becomes now, too, a matter of the greatest moment. Veal broth or beef tea, given alternately with white whine whey, or brandy added in a small quantity to all the food which the child takes, becomes necessary so soon as a feebler pulse, or diminution of temperature of the extremities, or a more labored respiration with an increase of mucus in the air-tubes, accompanied by a diminution or suppression of the cough, gives token of failing power. One troublesome symptom, very apt to supervene in this condition, and which sometimes frustrates all our endeavors, is an obstinate diarrhœa, that exhausts as well as distresses the child. The chalk mixture with tincture of catechu sometimes suffices to check it, but, should this fail, an opiate enema will very generally succeed in arresting it, provided it has not been allowed to continue unrestrained for more than a few hours.

During the patient's convalescence, great care is needed to avoid a relapse, which is the more apt to recur and the more likely to be serious

---

[1] (No. 12.)

℞. Decoct. Senegæ, ℥ij ʒv.
Ammon. Sesquicarb., gr. xij.
Tinct. Scillæ, ♏xvj.
Syr. Tolutan., ℥iij. M

A dessertspoonful every four hours. For a child from two to three years old.

in proportion to the tender age of the child. In the case of teething children, it is by no means unusual for a fresh attack of bronchitis to occur just as each tooth approaches the surface; a circumstance which renders it specially important to watch over the period of convalescence with the greatest care. If the season of the year admits of it, a change of air has more decided influence in removing the remains of any bronchitic attack than medicine, though for the most part the cough will gradually cease, and the child regain its health, under the influence of preparations either of bark or of iron. Sometimes, however, bronchitic symptoms continue for a long period, the expectoration being copious and puriform, while the child loses flesh, and the relatives become not unnaturally apprehensive lest it should be phthisical. Their fears may be well founded, but at the same time that you would recommend change of climate to some warmer country in the winter, or to the sea-coast during the summer, you would, as I shall hereafter point out to you when speaking of phthisis, be warranted in taking a much more favorable view of such cases in a child than in the adult.

Before concluding this lecture, it may be as well to say a few words on the subject of *influenza*, or epidemic catarrh, as we observe it among infants and children. Catarrhal epidemics, indeed, not infrequently occur among the young at a time when there is no general prevalence of the same class of ailments in the adult population, and they do so especially just before the commencement of an epidemic of measles or hooping-cough, and for a short period after its outbreak. Such catarrhs, however, are not in general very severe, and are important chiefly as forewarnings of the more serious disorder by which they are often succeeded.

This affection assumes, on the other hand, a more serious character when influenza is generally prevalent; and children are attacked, not especially, but in common with persons of all ages. It is then often very severe, and in many instances presents notable peculiarities, with a description of which I prefer occupying your time to repeating over again the description of how ordinary catarrh assumes by degrees the graver features of bronchitis, and the bronchitis, in its turn, becomes associated with pneumonia. Of course, in every epidemic of influenza, there are many instances of this occurrence, and, in every case, we need watch most carefully for its indications. But the anomalous forms of influenza are of no less moment. Of these, one of the most remarkable is characterized by the intensity of the febrile disturbance as contrasted with the comparative unimportance of the chest symptoms, so that the ailment sometimes runs its course more like a severe attack of ephemera than like an affection in which the organs of respiration are implicated. In such circumstances I have even known convulsions occur in very susceptible children, and be followed by a state of intense overpowering drowsiness, which, though unaccompanied by other signs of cerebral disturbance, continued for twenty-four hours, and then gradually subsided, being succeeded either by a slight feverish condition or by the ordinary catarrhal symptoms, and those not always of great severity. The convulsive seizures are, indeed, exceptional, and of decidedly rare occurrence; but the burning skin, the extremely frequent pulse, the irresistible drowsiness, are by no means unusual; a child going to bed a little ailing, sleeping heavily during the night, seeming unable to get up in the morning, and continuing apparently overpowered by the disorder for the ensuing twenty-four hours, but then recovering with great rapidity.

It is not, however, by any means constant for the disorder of the nervous system to be thus limited to the sensorium; for, in very many instances, the respiration is greatly disturbed; and with the burning skin and heavy head there are associated acceleration of breathing, and imperfect aeration of the blood, such as we may often observe in hooping-cough. This disorder of breathing too will often be found to be utterly out of proportion to the gravity of the auscultatory signs, which generally consist in a large diffused rhonchus, equally audible over the whole of the chest.

The danger, indeed, frequently consists less in the occurrence of pneumonia or in the advance of bronchitis than in the supervention of a state of collapse, such as in epidemics of influenza not infrequently carries off the aged. In the influenza of 1856 many instances of this kind came under my notice, by no means exclusively among infants, but at least as often among children between two and three years of age, in whom the attack set in with considerable nervous dyspnœa and heat of skin (symptoms which on some occasions had undoubtedly been treated with overactivity before the patient came under my notice), but in the course of two or three days the fever suddenly disappeared, and was succeeded by a state of extreme depression, with a cool, moist skin, a very feeble pulse, and labored respiration. In this condition the children, though quite conscious when roused, lay generally dozing, while, though the somewhat livid hue of the lips and surface seemed to imply the existence of some serious mischief in the lungs, there was often nothing to be heard but a large moist râle. When this state was well marked, the symptoms of exhaustion usually went on increasing, in spite of the free employment of stimulants, and terminated fatally on several occasions in the course of forty-eight hours, and within a week from the commencement of the illness.

One more point deserves notice, and that is the frequent tediousness of the convalescence from influenza; an irregularly remittent febrile condition, with complete loss of appetite, and much impairment of strength, often remaining behind. These symptoms, however, disappear, and sometimes rapidly, under the beneficial influence of change of air and preparations of quinine.

The cautions to be borne in mind in the *treatment* of influenza are sufficiently apparent from the remarks which have just been made. The danger in these cases is oftenest that of doing too much; of misinterpreting the nervous element, which plays so important a part in the production of the symptoms; and of regarding the dyspnœa, the hurried breathing, and the rapid pulse, as the necessary evidence of active inflammation of the lungs or air-tubes, calling for vigorous treatment to subdue it. Both depletory measures and the employment of large doses of antimonials are out of place, and the indications are best answered by maintaining a uniformly warm temperature in the room, by giving gentle diaphoretics, with small doses of ipecacuanha, and of some opiate, such as the compound tincture of camphor, or Dover's powder, if the cough is very troublesome or the nervous dyspnœa considerable. Counter-irritation by large mustard poultices to the chest will often relieve any great access of difficult breathing; and the evidence of auscultation should be very decided to justify a recourse to stronger measures, while it must be borne in mind that the necessity for ammonia, ether, and wine is by no means unlikely to occur, and that the first appearance of those signs of exhaustion which I have just described must be taken as an indication for their immediate employment.

There are two or three other conditions which may perhaps be best briefly mentioned here, before I close this lecture. One of them is the *spasmodic cough* often heard in children as the result of gastric or intestinal disorder. Its common character cannot be better described than by its well-known name of *tussis ovilla*, loud, hoarse barking. This character, however, is not invariable, for sometimes it is a short, dry, frequent cough, of which the child seems almost unconscious, ceasing for the most part during sleep, and also generally stopped by taking food. Auscultation discovers nothing, but in a good many instances there is slight redness of the fauces and soft palate, and the long and relaxed uvula appears to have a share in keeping up the irritation. It is enough to be aware of this condition in order to provide for its appropriate treatment, and to dissipate the anxiety of the patient's friends.

Aperients, alteratives, the mineral acids as tonics, and preparations of bark or quinine, with, in many instances, change of air, do more for the ailment than the whole range of sedatives. Sometimes, too, the cough is arrested when the uvula is long, or the soft palate relaxed by the application of the glycerin of tannin, or by the occasional use of a solution of ten grains of nitrate of silver in an ounce of distilled water.

There is also a peculiar form of paroxysmal cough which one sometimes meets with, though I do not know any one who has specially described it, except Professor Vogel of Dorpat, who, in his very excellent Manual on Children's Diseases,[1] speaks of it as the *Night Cough of Children*. It is a cough which comes on exclusively at night, not when the child first lies down, but after a few hours of sleep, from which, indeed, it does not wake up at first, but only after coughing for a time. It is a short, teasing, irritable cough—dry, not paroxysmal, not accompanied by expectoration, nor occasioning dyspnœa. After lasting for an hour or two it ceases, and does not recur until the next night, when it comes back with just the same characters as before, and thus continues, with occasional intervals of quiet for a night or two, even for weeks together, not apparently seriously affecting the child; though the disturbed rest at night tells somewhat on it, and it loses the look of health which it had before.

The limitation of the cough to the night-time, the absence of any

[1] Lehrbuch der Kinderkrankheiten, 4te. Auflage, 8vo., Erlangen, 1869, p. 267.

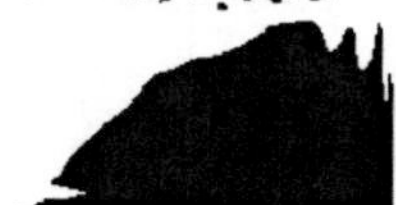

sign of chest affection in spite of the continuance of the ailment, and the patient's condition, one of ailment rather than of illness, characterize it. It is a nervous cough, and, like affections of that class, is cured by change of air, by bark and quinine, by good diet with moderate stimulation; while a cure is often hastened if the habit is broken through by a rather full dose of the bromide of potass and chloral at bedtime for a few consecutive nights.

Dr. Salter, in his classical work on *Asthma*,[1] states that in 71 out of 225 cases the disorder dated back to the first ten years of life, and in 11 of the number it came on under the age of one year. My own observations confirm his statements as to the frequency of the affection in early life; and recently Dr. Löschner of Prague[2] and Dr. Politzer[3] of Vienna have called attention to its occurrence in infancy. The characters which it presents are much the same at all periods of childhood, and do not differ from those of spasmodic asthma in the adult. It is not an ordinary sequela of hooping-cough, even though that affection should have left the child with emphysematous lungs; but it is not infrequently developed out of frequent attacks of bronchitis dating back even from very early infancy. In the majority of cases, however, its spasmodic character does not become so marked as to attract notice until the age of five or six, or even somewhat later, while many of the children in whom asthmatic symptoms then come on will be found to have previously been extremely liable to attacks of a half-spasmodic cough—the *laryngite striduleuse* of French writers, the laryngeal spasm by degrees diminishing as the disposition to spasm of the air-tubes comes on. In other instances the asthma has succeeded to extensive eczema, and so marked is the connection between the two conditions, that I have never known eczema to be very extensive and very long continued without a marked liability to asthma being associated with it. It cannot, however, be said that the two conditions always alternate, the asthma being worse when the cutaneous affection is better; but the radical cure of the eczema is usually followed, though often not till after the lapse of three or four years, by the cessation of the liability to asthma.

Catching cold, which in other children would produce ordinary catarrh, seldom fails in children with a predisposition to it to be followed by an asthmatic seizure, though it often comes on independent of previous catarrh, constipation and indigestion being two of its most frequent exciting causes. When the asthmatic habit is once established, the attacks are apt to recur at uncertain periods, without any exciting cause, and at all seasons of the year, though undoubtedly spring and autumn are the times of its greatest frequency, especially the former. If the attacks are not exceptionally severe and frequent, their tendency undoubtedly is to cease about or rather before puberty—or from the age of twelve to fifteen years. The probability of this being the case de-

---

[1] On Asthma. 2d ed., 8vo, London, 1868, p. 112.

[2] Aus dem Franz Josef-Kinder-Spitale. 2ter Theil, 8vo., Prag, 1868, No. vii, pp. 144–158.

[3] Jahrb. f. Kinderheilk., 1870. 3ter Jahrg., 4 Heft, p. 377.

pends very much on the success of the endeavors to stave off the attacks; but yet our prognosis may, on the whole, be a favorable one.

I do not dwell either on the symptoms of the asthmatic seizure or on the treatment, for, to the best of my knowledge, neither the one nor the other differs from what we observe and practice in the case of the adult. We use all remedies, however, with greater hope; while a sojourn for three or four years in a climate which suits the child (and three times out of four that climate will be found in a moderately sheltered seaside place, with a sandy soil, such as Bournemouth) is not infrequently successful in entirely overcoming every disposition to asthma throughout the whole remainder of the patient's life.

LECTURE XXI.

PNEUMONIA, ITS SYMPTOMS AND TREATMENT.—Symptoms of pneumonia frequently present a mixed character when it supervenes on bronchitis—Idiopathic pneumonia—Approach of first stage generally gradual—Characteristic peculiarities in mode of sucking and of respiration—Attack sometimes sudden. Symptoms of second stage—Results of auscultation—Reasons for rarity of true pneumonic crepitus. Symptoms of third stage—Convulsions often precede death—Their import—Occasional imperfect recovery—Auscultatory phenomena of this stage.

Nature of modifications in symptoms produced by association with bronchitis. Diagnosis from bronchitis—Pleurisy—Hydrocephalus—Remittent fever—Intestinal disorder during dentition.

Treatment—Expectant treatment—Depletion—Tartar emetic—Limitations as to its use. Mercury—Its importance—Danger of salivation very slight. Diet—Antiphlogistic in the early stages—Caution as to sucking—Stimulants often needed in advanced stage. Blisters not desirable.

It was stated in the last lecture, that the supervention of inflammation of the substance of the lungs constitutes one of the chief dangers of infantile bronchitis. Pneumonia, however, is not to be regarded as being invariably a secondary affection; for, in some cases, while the disease of the air-tubes is but trivial, the pulmonary substance is the seat of serious inflammation; and in other instances the air-tubes are altogether unaffected, or at least are involved only in common with the other constituents of the lung. In either case, there are peculiarities enough, both in the symptoms observed and in the treatment required, to render the separate study of pneumonia indispensable.

When pneumonia supervenes, as it by no means seldom does, on previous catarrhal symptoms, the disease often comes on insidiously, and develops itself so gradually out of the preceding trivial ailments that it is not possible to determine the exact date of its attack. At other times, indeed, there is a sudden and well-marked increase of the fever and dyspnœa, and an aggravation of all the symptoms, sufficient clearly to point out the date of the supervention of the pneumonia. But, even though this should be the case, yet, if there were much bronchitis previously, the affection of the air-tubes will often mask that of the lung to some degree; and the case not presenting the symptoms either of pure bronchitis or of unmixed pneumonia, will assume some of the characters of each, and merit, both by the phenomena attending it during life, as well as by the appearances found after death, the name of *bronchio-pneumonia*. Cases of this mixed character occur most frequently during the period of teething, when the mucous membranes are especially susceptible. We will return to notice some of these peculiarities hereafter, but we will first examine the *symptoms* that attend a case of *idiopathic pneumonia*, where the pulmonary substance has been affected from the outset, and has not merely become involved by the extension to it of mischief commencing in the bronchi.

In almost all of these unmixed cases, a condition of general feverishness, exacerbated towards evening, with fretfulness and pain in the head, precede the more marked symptoms. The child is either restless at night, or, if it sleeps, its repose is unsound; it talks in its sleep, or wakes in a state of alarm. Sometimes from the very commencement, at other times, soon after the appearance of these febrile symptoms, cough comes on; at first, short and hacking, frequently not causing the child any uneasiness, and so slight as scarcely to excite the notice of the parents, and not at all to awaken their anxiety. Loss of appetite and increase of thirst are early observable: the bowels are usually constipated, and vomiting is not infrequent, especially in infants at the breast. The tongue and lips are at the same time of a florid red; the tongue is less moist than usual, and is generally coated in the middle with a thickish white fur. In these symptoms, indeed, there is but little to mark the real nature of the case, or to point to the organ whose disease has kindled the fever in the system; for the slight cough, if not overlooked, may yet be attributed to irritation of the bronchi, sympathetic with derangement of the stomach or intestines. The respiration too is not always much hurried at this early period; while, in the young child, both its frequency, and that of the pulse, are much modified by position; and the results of auscultation are not uniform, and may sometimes afford no information at all. Even now, however, there are some signs which to the attentive observer will convey much information, and information all the more valuable from our being furnished with it chiefly in those young infants in whom the diagnosis of the disease is attended with most difficulty. The seat of the mischief is shown to be in the respiratory organs by the child no longer breathing through the nares, while the tongue is applied to the roof of the mouth as in health; but by its breathing through the open mouth also, whence the tongue early acquires an unusual degree of dryness. This same inability to respire comfortably through the nares causes the child to suck by starts: it seizes the breast eagerly, sucks for a few moments with greediness, then suddenly drops the nipple, and in many instances begins to cry. As the disease advances, these peculiarities in the mode of sucking and of respiration often become more striking; but it is at its onset that they are most valuable, since then we have fewer indications to lead us right.

It is not, however, thus gradually that pneumonia always comes on; for sometimes a child who has gone to bed well, or merely a little poorly, wakes in the night in a state of alarm, refusing to be pacified, with a flushed face and burning skin, and hurried breathing and short cough. This sudden supervention of pneumonia is not so often met with among infants at the breast as among children from two to four years old. Often, though not always, this severe onset of the disease has appeared to depend on the pneumonia being associated with extensive inflammation of the pleura; but sometimes the symptoms which at first seem so threatening soon subside, and the affection, in its subsequent stages, presents no peculiarity, and is not by any means remarkable for its severity.

This *first stage* of pneumonia passes, for the most part, by degrees into the *second*, in which the nature of the affection is generally obvious to all. The momentary cheerfulness which before existed has now passed away; infants now no longer wish to be removed from the cradle, or from the recumbent posture in their nurse's arms, and older children have quite lost all interest in their play; they become drowsy, ask to be put to bed, and cry if taken up. The hurry of the respiration is now abundantly evident; the *alæ nasi* are dilated with each inspiration, the abdominal muscles are brought into play to assist in its performance, and any change of posture renders the breathing more labored and more hurried. The cough has become much more frequent; it is still hard, sometimes is evidently painful, so that the child cries with each cough; at other times it is an almost constant short hack. The bright flush of the face, and the florid tint of the lips, are gone, but the heat of skin continues; for the persistence of an almost unvarying high temperature throughout its course is, as M. Roger has shown, one of the characteristics of the pneumonia of the child as well as that of the adult.[1] It is a pungent heat, which becomes more sensible the longer the hand is kept in contact with the surface; and so great is the elevation of temperature, that M. Roger found it average almost 104° Fahr. in ninety-seven experiments, while in some cases it greatly exceeded this degree. Though so intense, however, this heat is unequal at different parts—the extremeties being cool, or even cold, while the body is hot; but there is no moisture on any part of the skin. The face now assumes a puffed, heavy, but anxious appearance, and when the child is very young, or the pneumonia very extensive, the lips put on a livid hue, which is also very evident around the mouth, while the face generally is pale. The thirst usually continues very urgent, but children at the breast still vomit the milk. This is apparently owing to their thirst being so urgent as to lead them to suck too greedily, and thus overload their stomach, since, while they generally vomit almost immediately after leaving the breast, they do not reject small quantities of fluid given them from a cup or a spoon. The disease of the lungs now betrays itself most strikingly in children at the

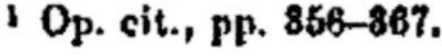
[1] Op. cit., pp. 356–367.

breast, for as often as they attempt to suck, the respiration becomes at once greatly hurried; they drop the nipple, panting, from their mouth, or, having seized it, have not breath sufficient to make the vacuum necessary to bring the flow of milk.

The results of auscultation, though variable, are now sufficiently obvious. Crepitation is now heard, often in both lungs, and generally in their lower and posterior parts—seldom, however, the minute crepitus such as we hear in the pneumonia of the adult, but that sound known as the subcrepitant râle. The comparative rarity of true pneumonic crepitus in inflammation of the lungs in infancy is a point not to be lost sight of: often, however, if you keep your ear to an infant's chest, and wait till it takes an unusually deep inspiration, you will hear the true crepitus of pneumonia just for a moment when the air enters the pulmonary vesicles; and then again you will lose it when the child breathes as it was doing before, and you will hear only the subcrepitant râle. If the inflammation has attacked only one lung, you will perhaps be struck by the loud puerile breathing in the healthy organ, which is thus compelled to perform a double function. If both are involved, you may almost overlook the disease, since you have not the aid afforded by contrast; unless, as sometimes happens, the mischief on the one side is so far advanced as to cause bronchial breathing, while on the other side crepitation alone is audible. This bronchial breathing is sometimes heard associated with the subcrepitant râle, or with large crepitation, while at other times the ear detects nothing but the whiff of air through the larger air-tubes; and often this alone is audible on an ordinary inspiration, while on a deep breath being taken the subcrepitant râle will be at once perceptible. In the child we lose all the information which, in the adult, is afforded by the different modifications of the voice sound; for the shrill or querulous tone of a suffering child, and the words often uttered in very different keys, afford, even when the child is old enough to talk well, results far too uncertain to be trustworthy.

Percussion sometimes yields a very manifest dulness on the affected side; and this dulness is usually most evident in the infrascapular region. At other times, however, no such marked results are afforded, but the lower parts of the chest give a somewhat duller sound than the upper, and the impression communicated to the finger is that of greater solidity below than above the scapula. This last sign is often very valuable, since it may be perceived at a time when the ear cannot clearly detect actual dulness on percussion.

Death may take place in this, the second stage of pneumonia, if a very extensive portion of lung has been involved in the disease, or if it is associated with much inflammation of the pleura, or if the pneumonia has been grafted on severe bronchitis. The pneumonia which supervenes on measles, or which comes on in a child debilitated by previous illness, sometimes terminates unexpectedly in this stage, and on an examination of the body after death the lung is found scarcely to have passed beyond the first stage of pneumonia, except in a few portions of but limited extent; though still larger tracts will probably be found in the state of collapse, and to the sudden supervention of this condition the fatal event is probably in great measure due. It is important, therefore, to bear in mind that in weakly children, a pneumonia of even very small extent will often prove fatal: hence the great importance of watching most sedulously against all those intercurrent affections of the lungs which come on in the course of diarrhœa, measles, or typhoid fever.

But the pneumonia may be free from any of the above-named complications, and then, if unchecked by treatment, it will pass into the *third stage*. The respiration now becomes more labored, and, though its frequency is sometimes diminished, it will be found to have become irregular; several short and hurried inspirations being followed by one or two deeper, and at longer intervals, and these again by hurried breathing. The cough sometimes ceases altogether, or if not, it is less frequent, and looser, since it is now produced by the child's efforts to clear the larger air-tubes from the accumulating secretions. The voice is often lost, the patient speaking only in a hoarse whisper; while children who were just learning to talk will frequently maintain complete silence, as if conscious that they have no breath to waste in words. The face looks sunken, the extremities are cold, and though the trunk retains its high temperature almost to the last, yet the skin often loses somewhat of its previous dryness, and clammy sweats break out, especially about the head. The pulse is extremely frequent and small, and the beats so run into each other that it is almost impossible to count them. The child is sometimes very restless at intervals, tossing about from side to side as much as its reduced powers will permit; but it usually lies in a state of half-consciousness, though sensible when spoken to, and fretful if disturbed. If raised hastily from the recumbent posture, or if put to the breast, the great increase of dyspnœa which is immediately produced shows how seriously the respiratory organs are affected. In many cases, too, the livid hue of the face and of the nails is a further proof of the great impediment which exists to the decarbonization of the blood; and once I saw purpurous spots appear on the arms and hands thirty-six hours before the death of a previously healthy child of a year old, in whom an attack of idiopathic pneumonia terminated fatally on the seventeenth day. This condition seldom lasts above two or three days; for either life becomes gradually extinct, without the supervention of any new symptom, or convulsions occur, which are followed by fatal coma, or the child recovers for a few hours only to suffer a second attack of convulsions, and a return of coma, in which it dies. It can scarcely be necessary to remind you of what was said some time since with reference to the import of convulsions, and to their being in many cases merely a token of disturbance of the functions of the brain, such as delirium is in the adult. The former symptoms in the child, and the latter in the adult, betoken in a case of pneumonia that the brain is suffering from the circulation through it of imperfectly aerated blood.

The third stage, however, does not always advance thus uninterruptedly to a fatal issue, but a kind of imperfect recovery sometimes takes place. A diminution is obvious in the more alarming symptoms; the patient begins to express some desire for food as well as for drink, and even has occasional gleams of cheerfulness. The cough, which in many instances had almost or altogether ceased, returns, but is short and hacking, although there is sometimes a good deal of mucus in the larger air-tubes. The dyspnœa is no longer urgent, though the breath is habitually short. The skin is hot, dry, and harsh, and evening exacerbations of fever often occur; the tongue is red, dry, and sometimes chapped, or presents small aphthous ulcers at its edges; diarrhœa is not infrequent; the child wastes daily, and dies in the course of a week or two, worn out and exceedingly emaciated.

The auscultatory signs of this third stage of pneumonia are in the main those of the second stage, except that the bronchial breathing usually becomes both more distinct and more extensive, occupying situations where either the subcrepitant râle, or even large crepitation, had previously been heard. As it extends, too, it becomes audible in front as well as behind, and both it, and dulness, on percussion, may be perceived in the infra-mammary as well as in the infra-scapular region, to which at first they are almost always limited. The bronchial breathing is generally much more extensive on one side than on the other, and sometimes it is heard throughout the whole posterior part of one side of the chest; but it is exceedingly unusual to find bronchial breathing confined to the upper part of one lung, except in cases where there existed previous tubercular disease of the organ, and then the pulmonary tissue may become solidified under the influence of an amount of disease which otherwise would be inadequate to produce this result.

The symptoms that attend the third stage of the disease usually are the result of the lung having passed into the state of suppuration. I say usually, for sometimes recovery eventually takes place even from a condition apparently desperate, and in such cases the degree to which disorganization of the lung had actually advanced must always remain uncertain.

The results of auscultation do not help us, any more than in the adult, to determine with certainty the amount of injury that the lung has sustained, while we are deprived almost entirely of that information which in the grown person is afforded us by the changes in the appearance of the sputa. In some cases of rapidly fatal pneumonia I have seen a frothy secretion collect about the mouth; but this was evidently not furnished by the air-tubes, but was merely the saliva which the child was unable either to spit out or to swallow. The cough of pneumonia being generally short and not paroxysmal, we have not so much chance of seeing the sputa as in the case of acute bronchitis, and children even of five or six years old seldom spit out the matters that they expectorate, but almost always swallow them.

When resolution of hepatized lung takes place, the changes in the physical signs of the disease are much the same as are perceived in the adult. I have not, however, in any instance detected a return of true pneumonic crepitation, but subcrepitant râle in most cases became audible, and in a few instances large crepitation. In either case mucous râle was eventually heard, and it often continued for many days after the lung had in other respects recovered its natural condition; apparently much as, in the pneumonia of the adult, prolonged expiration often persists for a long time after all the other signs of disease have disappeared.

At the commencement of this lecture reference was made to cases in which the symptoms of pneumonia are modified by those of the bronchitis with which it is associated. In such cases there is from the very outset a marked degree of dyspnœa and distress, and the face presents from the first a livid hue. The cough is less short than in simple pneumonia, but it comes on in paroxysms which greatly distress the patient: the respiration is more hurried and more irregular, and this irregularity comes on at an earlier stage of the disease. Large crepitation and subcrepitant râle are generally heard very extensively in both lungs, but true pneumonic crepitation is unusual. A preponderating affection of the lower lobes is seldom perceptible; and, since these cases usually tend to a rapid termination, death sometimes takes place before either dulness on percussion, or bronchial breathing, has become distinctly audible.

Such are the characters generally presented by pneumonia in early life, and these are usually so well marked as to render it impossible either to overlook the disease or to mistake its symptoms for those of some other malady. This, however, is not invariably the case even when the inflammation of the lungs occurs as an idiopathic affection, while in those instances in which it comes on in the course of other diseases, it very often remains latent, and much acuteness of perception, as well as much patient observation, is necessary for its detection. We will pass over for the present the consideration of secondary pneumonia, since to understand all the varieties that it presents would require a previous acquaintance with those diseases in the course of which the inflammation of the lungs supervenes. When we come to the study of hooping-cough, croup, measles, remittent fever, &c., I will endeavor to point out the period at which, in each of these maladies, pneumonia is most to be apprehended, and the symptoms that indicate its attack; but for the present we will confine our notice to those cases in which the inflammation of the respiratory organs occurs as an idiopathic affection.

The points of *difference between pneumonia and bronchitis* have already been dwelt on so fully as to render it unnecessary to recapitulate them. In many cases they are too obvious to admit of your falling into error, but in others they are so shaded off that it is difficult to determine whether the characters of one or the other predominate; and we are forced to conclude that the two exist together, the one obscuring the otherwise well-marked features of the other.

In the child, as in the adult, some degree of pleurisy exists in a large proportion of cases of pneumonia, though sometimes so slight as to be scarcely noticed; whilst in other cases, though a little friction-sound may be heard for a short time, yet it is evident that the danger [illegible] is occasioned by the mischief in the lung, and not by the [illegible] the pleura. Sometimes, however, inflammation of the [illegible] chief, if not the sole cause of the patient's danger, and [illegible] sirable to know even at the outset, whether the lung or its investing membrane is the part chiefly affected.

An attack of *pleurisy* is much oftener marked by complaint of severe pain in the chest, than is an attack of pneumonia; or if the child should be unable to express its feelings, the seizure is not infrequently announced by violent and continued screaming. Sympathetic disturbance of the brain is more frequent and more severe at the onset of an attack of pleurisy than of pneumonia, and the attendant restlessness is greater. Auscultation, too, fails to discover the crepitant or subcrepitant râle which characterizes pneumonia, but air enters the lung on the affected side much less freely than on the other, and a friction-sound may perhaps be distinguished; though this is by no means invariable, and even when present it may easily be mistaken for rhonchus. It may be laid down as a rule, subject to but few exceptions, that whenever a child is suddenly seized with symptoms which, while they indicate some affection of the lungs, are yet unattended with the auscultatory signs of pneumonia, the disease from which it is suffering is pleurisy; and this probability is rendered almost a certainty if, while the child bears percussion on one side of the chest, it cries and struggles on the slightest attempt at percussion on the opposite side.

The error of taking a case of pneumonia for one of pleurisy, however, or the opposite, is of comparatively little moment; but there are other diseases for which pneumonia may be taken, in which the error of diagnosis will lead to serious, and perhaps fatal mistakes in treatment.

These mistakes, too, may be made at almost any stage of the disease. The symptoms of *disorder of the brain* may throw those of the lung affection into the shade; and the disease may not only begin, but may even run a large portion of its course with so great an amount of cerebral disturbance as to mislead the unwary practitioner. It is especially in pneumonia of the upper lobes that this predominance of disorder of the nervous system is most remarkable, the attack even setting in, as that of acute pleurisy does sometimes, with convulsions, while great stupor with delirium in children old enough to present this symptom, marks its subsequent progress. The cough may be short, or altogether suppressed, and the hurried breathing is not unnaturally referred to the supposed affection of the brain; while a hasty auscultation fails, even if resorted to, to discover the real nature of the case, to which MM. Rilliet and Barthez gave the appropriate name of "cerebral pneumonia."[1] If, however, we are on our guard against being misled, there are two symptoms, which, even independently of that careful auscultation which should never be omitted, will usually preserve us from error. One is, the extremely high temperature from

[1] Op. cit, 2d ed., vol. i, p. 526. More recently, too, some very valuable remarks on this subject have been made by Professor Steiner in Jahrb. f. Kinderheilk., 1869, p. 357. I cannot but doubt, however, whether the internal otitis to which he attaches such importance as the occasion of the head symptoms in many of these cases was other than a purely accidental complication of the pneumonia, or the pneumonia a complication of it. In many instances, undoubtedly, most marked symptoms of cerebral disorder are present where yet the lungs are the exclusive seat of disease.

even the outset, and its steady continuance; and the other, the great and constant acceleration of breathing, unlike the hurried, yet irregular and unequally rapid respiration which attends acute affections of the brain or of its membranes. But besides these exceptional cases in which a mistake is half excusable, there are others in which, especially in infancy and early childhood, the inflammation of the lungs is sometimes overlooked, and the symptoms are regarded, until too late, as those of tubercular meningitis. The vomiting, the pain in the head, the restless nights, with talking in the sleep, which attend the onset of almost all the acute affections of childhood, the fever, and the constipated state of the bowels common to both diseases, lead to this error. The cough in some cases of pneumonia is so slight as scarcely to be noticed, while even if present it may be taken for that sympathetic cough which is sometimes present in the early stages of tubercular meningitis; and the child, if questioned, may complain of his head, and of nothing else. But still there are circumstances which would lead the attentive observer, independently of auscultation, to detect the real nature of the case. The vomiting that ushers in an attack of pneumonia, though sometimes violent, seldom continues long, and is unattended with that permanent nausea and irritability of the stomach which are so marked in the first stage of the brain disease. The evacuations in pneumonia are natural; the tongue is of a much more vivid red; the pulse is much more frequent, its beats are not irregular, the heat of the skin is far greater, far more constant, and more remarkable on the trunk than about the head, and the thirst is generally urgent. If these indications, however, are overlooked at the commencement of the attack, and if auscultation, by which the error might still be set right, is neglected, it is probable that each subsequent occurrence will be misinterpreted, and that the real nature of the disease will not be understood until it is revealed by the post-mortem examination. More or less sympathetic affection of the head is seldom wanting in pneumonia to confirm the preconceived erroneous notion; while, as the child grows worse, the difficulties in the way of making a careful auscultation increase. Convulsions sometimes occur even several days before the patient's death, and the head symptoms may appear, especially to a prejudiced observer, to be much more striking than any which indicate affection of the lungs.

It sometimes happens that the sympathetic *disturbance of the stomach and bowels* is so considerable as to obscure the chest symptoms, and the case is taken for one of enteritis; or perhaps, if the heat of skin and sensorial disturbance are considerable, for what is loosely termed remittent fever; and this latter error is especially likely to be committed if the upper lobes of the lung are the seat of the inflammation. The vomiting at the outset of the disease, the pain referred to the abdomen, with the evident increase of discomfort on pressure, the red tongue, with its disposition to dryness, and the diarrhoea that exists in these rather exceptional cases of pneumonia, are the symptoms which tend to lead into error; and this error may be confirmed on the practitioner finding that at least temporary relief follows the application of leeches and poultices to the abdomen. With reference to the complica-

of pain in the belly, which seems often to have a large share in inducing this error, it must be remembered that the statements of children with reference to the seat of pain are very vague, and that they frequently speak of the belly when they mean the chest; while the impediment to the descent of the diaphragm occasioned by pressure on the abdomen, especially if this pressure is either sudden or considerable, will almost always excite expressions of uneasiness when the organs of respiration are in any way affected. It is in careful auscultation that your chief safeguard against these mistakes will consist; but you will find besides, that by accustoming yourselves to look not at one or two prominent symptoms only, but at the relation which each bears to the other, many of the chief difficulties in the way of forming a correct diagnosis will disappear.

It may perhaps seem to you that much of this is very dry and rather needless detail; but unfortunately my own case-books would enable me to illustrate each of these errors of diagnosis against which it is my endeavor to guard you. One more caution I would offer you, and that is, not to overlook the *pneumonia* which sometimes comes on *in children while teething*. Unless you are on the watch for it, its early symptoms will probably fail to excite your apprehension, since they will be regarded as the result of that sympathetic irritation of the air-tubes which so often accompanies dentition, and the time for action will thus be allowed to pass unemployed. The disease comes on most frequently in weakly children, is unattended by much constitutional reaction, and often runs a somewhat chronic course: while its nature is further obscured by the tendency to diarrhœa which exists during dentition, and which is now excited by the thoracic affection. The purging often becomes the most striking symptom, and all means are employed to suppress it, and to check the vomiting which generally attends it. These efforts, however, are unavailing; the child wastes daily, and its skin hangs in wrinkles about its attenuated limbs, while the abdomen becomes tumid from the collection of flatus in the large intestines, and tender on pressure, and the tongue grows red, dry, and chapped, or covered with aphthous ulcers. The cough now perhaps attracts notice; but both it and the bronchial breathing in the lungs are probably looked on as indications of phthisis, and the doctor consoles himself with the belief that he has failed to cure the disease because it was irremediable. At last the child is worn out, and dies, and great is the surprise to find no tubercle in any part of the body, no disease in the intestines, but pneumonia, with purulent infiltration in both lungs—a disease which ought to have been detected, and which probably might have been cured.

When speaking of the treatment of bronchitis in early life, I felt it to be my duty to explain to how large a degree changes in the character of disease had led to a modification of my practice. But in the case of the *treatment of pneumonia* we have to consider even more than this, and to decide whether the adage "Optima est medicina, medicinam non facere," does not include, as some have contended, all that we need know with reference to it. This allegation has been made: it has been asserted that in the young the tendency to recovery from uncomplicated pneumonia is so invariable, that the physician has nothing more to do, after having established his diagnosis, than to watch how nature brings about the cure, and to abstain from disturbing processes which his interference can only mar.[1]

Dr. Barthez[2]—a name which we cannot mention without stopping for a moment to pay the tribute due to the memory of his worthy fellow-laborer, Rilliet, who passed away so suddenly, so prematurely for science, if not for his own fame—addressed a communication to the Academy of Medicine of Paris in April, 1862, the object of which was to vindicate the expectant treatment of pneumonia in early life. In this paper he states, that of 212 cases of lobar pneumonia occurring between the ages of two and fifteen, in the course of seven years, at the Hôpital Ste. Eugénie, two only had a fatal termination, although no approach to active treatment was adopted in more than a sixth of the number. M. Grisolle, so deservedly high an authority on the subject, seems inclined to accept the conclusions of M. Barthez for children above the age of four, and for young persons up to the age of five and twenty, but demurs to its applicability at a more advanced age; or, in other words, where his own largest experience commences, and his own personal responsibility weighs upon him most heavily, he hesitates to stand by a mere spectator of the combat between disease and nature for the mastery. M. Barthez sums up his conclusions very decidedly, though with just moderation, and it is fairest to state them in his own words: "The only positive rule which I am anxious to lay down is this: that it is scarcely ever useful, and still less is it necessary, to employ very active treatment in the idiopathic pneumonia of children, and that it is especially important to abstain as much as possible from the repeated abstraction of blood, since its evident effect is to weaken the children uselessly, and to protract their convalescence considerably."

Now I have no statistical data to oppose to the statements of M. Barthez. I meet with idiopathic pneumonia in an early stage much more rarely now than I did formerly, when I was physician to the Children's Dispensary in Lambeth, or when I had charge of some of the out-patients of the Children's Hospital; and in the case of most of the patients who are admitted with pneumonia, the disease has long since passed the stage in which active treatment would have been admissible. The same, too, applies to the cases that have come under my notice in private consultation; though at the same time it must be allowed that the very rarity with which idiopathic pneumonia has fallen under my observation in private, says much for its tendency to spontaneous subsidence when the patient is placed in favorable hygienic conditions.

But I confess that I cannot forget the good results which I saw years ago from the abstraction of blood at the outset of an attack of pneumonia in previously healthy children, in whom fever, short cough,

[1] For the history of opinion with reference to the expectant treatment of pneumonia, see Grisolle, La Pneumonie, 2d ed., Paris, pp. 564–578.

[2] Reported in the Bulletin de Thérapeutique, 8vo., Paris, 1862, vol. 62, pp. [illegible]–374.

and hurried breathing had come on suddenly, and unpreceded by catarrhal or bronchitic symptoms. It is conceded, by writers even at the present day, that depletion employed at an early period lessens heat of skin, abates hurry of breathing, and relieves distress; and to these admissions I should be disposed to add that, in some instances, it cuts short the disease. I do not, however, think that after the first twenty-four or thirty-six hours this result will be obtained, and should not advise depletion at a time when small crepitation has become generally diffused, still less when dulness or bronchial breathing is perceptible; nor should I advocate a repetition of bleeding in any case when the good which it appeared to have effected had passed away.

But if I cannot admit that the abstraction of blood in the early stage of pneumonia is never indicated, still less can I allow that antimony is in no case to be employed, even though the symptoms do not seem to justify depletion, or though the time for having recourse to it may have passed way. So long as the breathing has not become bronchial, or the heat of skin and hurry of respiration continue, and the vital powers of the child are manifestly unimpaired, even though the diffusion of small crepitation through the lungs proves the inflammation to be very general, I believe that antimony is likely to prove of essential service. I mean here antimony employed for its own specific action, and not merely given as an adjunct to other treatment. Given in a dose of gr. ⅛ every ten minutes till vomiting is produced, in the case of a child of two years old, and continued afterwards every two hours for a period of twenty-four or thirty-six hours, it subdues the fever and abates the dyspnœa in a most remarkable manner; the minute crepitation becomes larger, and, as M. Trousseau says, "there is no stage of convalescence;" the child dangerously ill yesterday is all but well to-day; and nothing but our experience of the real importance of the previous symptoms would satisfy us that we had not misread their meaning, nor overestimated their gravity. But I must add that antimony thus employed usually accomplishes its purpose in twenty-four, or at the most in thirty-six hours; and that with the establishment of its complete tolerance comes the signal for its discontinuance, or at least for a change in the mode of its administration, and the results of auscultation must now in great measure determine our subsequent conduct. Should that inform us that the physical condition of the lung has greatly improved, as well as the general state of the patient, the use of the remedy may be persevered in at longer intervals, as every four or every six hours. If the signs of inflammation are advancing, and have become perceptible in portions of lung previously free from disease, mercury must be employed, which may be combined with small doses of antimony, while large doses of that remedy may still be given to combat any sudden increase of fever or dyspnœa that may chance to supervene. If, notwithstanding a manifest diminution of the fever and reduction of the dyspnœa, bronchial breathing should have become distinctly audible, mercurials must at once be substituted for the antimony; and the existence in any case of extensive or well-marked bronchial respiration should be regarded as of itself contra-indicating the antimonial plan of treatment. It is not my intention to say, that after the supervention of bronchial respiration antimony ought never to be given, but only that it should not be employed except in small doses, and in combination with other remedies.

In cases where the symptoms do not set in with such violence as to indicate the necessity for very large doses of antimony, or in which the disease has passed that stage where antimony so given is likely to be beneficial, *mercurials* may be used with great advantage. In cases of the former kind, from two-thirds of a grain to a grain of calomel, combined with two grains of James's powder, may be given every six hours to a child two years old. If the case is of a graver kind, and bronchial breathing has become perceptible notwithstanding depletion and the administration of tartar emetic, the calomel must be given more frequently—as every four or three hours, combined with small doses of Dover's powder and tartar emetic, if the child is not so depressed as to render the use of the latter medicine inexpedient. Sometimes the combination of antimony with the mercurial is at first well borne, but afterwards it becomes desirable to discontinue it on account of the sickness that it produces, or on account of the debility of the patient. The diarrhœa which the calomel excites may usually be checked by increasing the quantity of the Dover's powder, or by an occasional dose of chalk mixture. There are some troublesome cases, however, in which the stomach and bowels are so irritable that scarcely any medicine can be borne; and in them, as well as in cases of neglected pneumonia, where the proper time for active treatment has been allowed to pass by, and the child has become exhausted while a large extent of lung is impervious to air, much benefit sometimes follows the persevering use of mercurial inunction, or the employment of that convenient substitute for inunction, the mercurial belt, on which the ointment should be renewed every twelve hours. In infants and children under five years of age, the gums hardly ever become affected by mercury, even though most energetically employed; and it has only once occurred to me to meet with an instance of profuse salivation, or of dangerous ulceration of the gums, as the result of the employment of mercury in pneumonia. Such accidents, however, do now and then occur, and have been known to terminate in fatal gangrene of the cheek, or in necrosis of the jaw. On this account, therefore, you must watch the condition of the gums in infants and children to whom you are administering mercury, just as you would do in the case of the adult, and diminish or discontinue the remedy on the first indication of their being affected.

The *diet* of children in the early stages of pneumonia should be sparing; and infants not weaned should have some less nutritious food than the mother's milk, which their thirst will otherwise lead them to take more abundantly even than when they are well. If the pneumonia is severe, it is better to give even the mother's milk with a spoon, rather than to allow the infant to suck, since the very act of sucking is injurious, and taxes to the utmost the respiratory function, the organs of which it is desirable to keep in as unexcited a state as possible.

But though the treatment of inflammation of the lungs requires a strict antiphlogistic regimen in the early stages of the disease, yet in many, perhaps in most cases, there arrives a period in which a [illegible] diet is no longer suitable—in which your main efforts must be directed to support the constitutional powers, rather than to subdue the inflammation. If you forget this, it may happen to you to overcome the mischief in the chest, but to lose your patient from carrying too far, or from continuing too long, the very treatment which, within proper limits, was most salutary. No point in the management of the disease is more difficult than the seizing the exact moment when the employment of stimulants becomes necessary; and no general rule can be laid down for regulating their use. If, however, the patient were beginning to be much purged, if the respiration were growing more labored and irregular, though diminished in frequency, and if the pulse were becoming more frequent, and above all, smaller and smaller, it is high time to resort to their use. Wine is as indispensable in such cases in the pneumonia of the child as in that of the adult; and it may be necessary to give it even to infants at the breast. Ammonia may also be advantageously administered in this stage of the disease, either in a mixture with the decoction of senega,[1] or dissolved in milk, which conceals its disagreeable pungency better than any other vehicle. If diarrhœa does not exist, strong beef tea or veal broth is the best form in which nutriment can be given; but if the bowels are relaxed, arrowroot, or the *décoction blanche*[2] of the French hospitals, should be substituted for it.

In conclusion, it may be well to offer a caution with reference to the employment of *blisters*—a measure to which we often have recourse with advantage during the resolution of pneumonia in the adult, but which is not advisable in young children whose lungs have been solidified by the disease. The sores which blisters form are very apt in weakly children to take on an unhealthy character; and the disposition to this accident appears to be greater after inflammation of the lungs than after almost any other disease; and especially in those cases of secondary pneumonia that supervene on measles. For any such counter-irritation, I am accustomed to substitute the constant application of warm linseed-meal poultices. These afford great relief to the patient, and I imagine answer by their soothing influence, the chief purpose aimed at by the use of cold compresses to the chest, which appear to me objectionable, not only on account of the child's repugnance to their use, but also on account of the necessity for frequently disturbing the patient in order to renew them.

I am bound, however, to add that these objections are not based on personal observation; and that many German physicians[3] of deservedly high reputation advocate this mode of treatment, though rather as a means of abating fever than of importantly modifying the course of the disease. I must further say, that the evidence in favor of the use of cold for this purpose, and also for its soothing influence when steadily applied, is so strong, that I do not consider myself altogether free from blame for never having given it a trial.

---

[1] See Formula No. xii, p. 279. [2] See Note, p. 57.

[3] Especially Ziemmsen, Pleuritis und Pneumonie im Kindesalter, 8vo., Berlin, 1862, pp. 273–281.

LECTURE XXII.

ŒDEMA OF THE LUNGS.—Occasionally comes on in the course of scarlatinal dropsy —Severity of the symptoms, and their sudden accession—Difference between characters of œdematous and hepatized lung—Treatment—Importance of venesection—Occasional exceptions to its use—Chronic œdema, or carnification.

GANGRENE OF THE LUNG.—Case illustrative of the disease—Is not the result of mere intensity of inflammation—Unattended by any pathognomonic symptom.

PLEURISY.—Its symptoms and morbid appearances similar to those observed in the adult—Auscultatory signs of it, and their changes as recovery advances—It occasionally simulates other diseases, as affections of the head and of the abdomen—Evidences of auscultation less conclusive than in the adult, and why.

Latent pleurisy—Occasional sudden death in these cases—Various modes in which pleurisy proves fatal—Other terminations of the disease—Empyema—Deformity of the chest from pleurisy—Spontaneous opening in chest—Its tendency to remain fistulous.

Treatment in the acute stage—Importance of depletion and antiphlogistic measures —Management in subsequent stages—Question of paracentesis considered—Minute rules laid down for its performance and for after treatment—Its dangers—Reasons against leaving cases to nature—Deformity of chest after pleurisy.

BEFORE we proceed to the examination of some other forms of inflammatory disease of the respiratory organs, it may be convenient to notice two conditions of the pulmonary tissue, which, though not the direct results of inflammation, yet are closely connected with it. One of these conditions is *acute œdema of the lung;* the other is *gangrene* of its substance.

It is unnecessary to occupy your time with any detailed account of that anasarcous state of the lungs which is sometimes met with in connection with general dropsy of long standing, or with some old disease of the heart and great vessels. In such cases, the œdema of the lungs is a secondary affection, and has very little share in producing the patient's death. But it occasionally happens that children are attacked by intense dyspnœa, and other symptoms of disorder of the respiratory organs, which terminate rapidly in death; while it is discovered, on an examination of the body, that the thoracic viscera generally are free from disease, but that the tissue of the lungs is loaded with serous fluid. Laennec[1] refers to such an accident as probably accounting for the occasional sudden supervention of extreme dyspnœa in children recovering from measles; but the late much-lamented M. Legendre[2] was, to the best of my knowledge, the first person who clearly proved the connection between the symptoms observed during life, and the state of extreme œdema of the pulmonary tissue after death.

This *œdema of the lungs,* though it sometimes destroys life very speedily, is seldom, if ever, a purely idiopathic affection, but occurs generally as one of the complications of that acute anasarca which not

[1] On the Diseases of the Chest, translated by Dr. Forbes, 4th edition, p. 166. London, 1834.

[2] Recherches sur quelques Maladies de l'Enfance, 8vo., pp. 324–352. Paris, 1846.

infrequently succeeds to scarlatina; and even then it is not of very common occurrence. M. Legendre records only four cases, all of which were observed in children who were suffering from anasarca after scarlatina; but several instances of it have come under my notice since the publication of his observations, in all of which it supervened during scarlatinal dropsy. In some of these cases it came on while the children were laboring under a great degree of anasarca; while in others the dropsy had greatly abated before the thoracic symptoms appeared. Indications of slight mischief in the chest, such as frequent dry cough, some degree of dyspnœa, with rhonchus and sibilus, or scanty crepitation, preceded the more serious symptoms for two or three days. The patient, in short, had seemed to be suffering from a bronchitis of moderate intensity, when suddenly extreme difficulty of respiration supervened, attended with very hurried breathing, orthopnœa, and most tumultuous and violent action of the heart, though with a feeble pulse. The cough continued, being still short, and quite unaccompanied by expectoration. Auscultation in such circumstances does not seem to give account of mischief sufficiently serious to explain the alarming nature of the symptoms. It may be thought that air enters the lungs less freely than it should do; but the crepitation heard is scanty, bronchial respiration is not perceptible, neither is the resonance of the chest on percussion diminished unless fluid has at the same time been effused into the pleura. Nevertheless, if relief is not soon afforded, the child's sufferings in a few hours amount to perfect agony; the difficulty of respiration and the tumultuous action of the heart continue; the lips and face become perfectly livid, but the intellect remains clear, and the child complains of great distress, referred to the heart or epigastrium; till at length death takes place suddenly, which it sometimes does within twenty-four hours from the appearance of these alarming symptoms. At other times the approach of the disease is more gradual, dyspnœa being augmented in paroxysms, but on the whole increasing with the increase of the general anasarca, and proving fatal in the course of five or six days.

On examining after death the bodies of children who have died of this acute œdema of the lungs, some transparent serum is usually found in the chest, and a few deposits of lymph on the surface of the lung sometimes betoken the existence of slight inflammation of the pleura. The lungs themselves are of a deep red color, firm, and destitute of air through a great extent of their substance, not breaking down so easily as lung in a state of true hepatization would do, but giving exit when cut into to a most abundant quantity of reddish serum, mixed with very few air-bubbles. If the lung is punctured, the fluid will by degrees drain out, and the organ will recover much of its natural flaccidity, while, if air is blown into the bronchi, the pulmonary tissue will completely resume its light color, and will crepitate as in a state of health. These experiments show that the fluid is not actually incorporated with the substance of the lung; and M. Legendre explains the sudden occurrence of alarming dyspnœa in some instances by the assumption that it is due to compression of the air-vesicles by the rapid pouring out of fluid into the cellular tissue by which they are surrounded. The supposition, however, that the fluid is in these cases entirely external to the pulmonary vesicles does not appear to be well founded, for watery fluids[1] will pass by endosmosis from one part of the lung to another, and will even transude through the pleura. The general effect, however, is the same, whether the chief accumulation of fluid be within the air-cells or external to them, for in either case the free entrance of air is impeded; while the severity of the symptoms depends upon the rapidity with which the œdema has taken place almost as much as upon its degree. In cases where it comes on towards the close of some chronic affection, there is often no dyspnœa nor any aggravation of the patient's sufferings to mark its occurrence, while, when it takes place suddenly, not only are the symptoms most urgent, but the right auricle and ventricle are found after death enormously distended with coagulated blood—a token of the difficulty with which the heart had discharged the functions to the performance of which it at length became wholly unequal.

In every case of anasarca after scarlatina, the possibility of the supervention of this condition must be borne in mind, and every endeavour must be made, by the employment of diaphoretics and antimonials, and by the use of the hot-air bath, to maintain the action of the skin, and to relieve thereby the congested kidneys. If in spite of care, or, as the oftener happens, from want of it, these symptoms should occur, your course of *treatment* must be governed by the child's general condition. If its employment is not absolutely contraindicated, free venesection will be found to bring the same remarkable and immediate relief which it affords to those most urgent symptoms that follow the escape of air into the pleura; and the relief is probably in both cases brought about in the same manner. After depletion, large doses of tartar emetic should be given, since there is no other remedy that so speedily or so effectually reduces the urgent dyspnœa. In the subsequent management of the case, just such remedies are required as would be best calculated to relieve the general dropsy; and, as that decreases, the œdema of the lungs will likewise diminish and disappear.

Very often, however, especially among the poor, the œdema of the lung comes on after long neglect of the patient's symptoms, or after some course of treatment altogether inefficient has been adopted; and the cold extremities, the livid surface, and the feeble pulse forbid all depletory measures, and render the use of any depressing remedy, such as antimony, altogether inappropriate. In such circumstances, a directly opposite plan must be adopted: a large mustard poultice must be applied to the chest; stimulants must be given abundantly, such as the nitrous or sulphuric ether, wine, or brandy; and sometimes it is necessary to continue these measures for several days, while some mild diuretic, such as the tartrate or citrate of potass, or the benzoic acid, is the only medicine which we can venture to employ. On one or two occasions I have found reaction speedily follow the use of stimulants, and have even been able in six or eight hours not only to discontinue

[1] See the remarks and experiments of M. Barthez, in a note at p. 188 of vol. ii of his and M. Rilliet's work on Diseases of Children.

them, but have even ventured to take blood from the arm; and the relief which followed justified the wisdom of the course. These, however, are exceptional cases, and care is often needed, on the other hand, lest the child should sink from the too early withdrawal of the stimulants.

It would be wrong, perhaps, to leave this subject without some notice of the views of M. Baron[1] with reference to certain alterations in the lungs, and in other parenchymatous viscera, which he believes to be due to chronic œdema of their tissue. He describes a state of *carnification* in which the substance of the organ becomes dark, firm, and compact, as if from compression; but instead of these changes being attended by any diminution of its bulk, its size is actually increased. This alteration, though observable both in the liver and spleen, is naturally most striking when it exists in the lung, and was found by M. Baron, in all instances, either coexisting with dropsical effusions, or present in cases where such effusions had previously existed. He believes it to be due to long-standing œdema, and to depend on changes in the tissue which the infiltration of fluid brings about in the course of time. The tendency of this condition, when the lung is the part affected by it, is to compress the air-cells, and interfere with the entrance of air; but nevertheless in many cases there were no symptoms announcing its existence during life, and air was found in the pulmonary vesicles after death—a fact which goes far to substantiate the correctness of Dr. Gairdner's opinion, that positive obstruction of the bronchial tubes is necessary to prevent the entrance of air into the lung; that the mere elasticity of its tissue, or congestion of its vessels, is not adequate to occasion this result. I will not, however, dwell further on these opinions, which involve questions of morbid anatomy more than of practical medicine, and the rather since I have no observations of my own bearing on the subject.

My experience of *gangrene of the lung* in childhood is extremely limited, for only one case of it has come under my notice. The particulars of it, however, may be worth relating, since they illustrate very well the symptoms which the disease usually presents, and the circumstances in which it generally occurs.

A little girl, three years old, the child of healthy parents, who had previously had good health, with the exception of a severe attack of inflammation of the lungs when two years old, began to droop in health, to cough, and to have shortness of breath, on February 11, 1843. No treatment was adopted until the child was brought to me on the 15th. Her breathing was then more oppressed, her general condition more cast down, and her strength more reduced than is usual in so short a time from the commencement of an attack of pneumonia, which had not set in with very severe symptoms. Four leeches were applied beneath the right scapula, and half-grain doses of calomel and Dover's powder were given every three hours. Slight relief succeeded to the bleeding, but this was of but short duration; and the child did not seem to be either better or seriously worse until the 19th, when she appeared to be losing strength. The mercury was now discon-

[1] In the Gazette Médicale for 1851; and republished in the Journal für Kinderkrankheiten, vol. xviii, March, 1852.

tinued, and ammonia and nourishing diet were freely given. On the 20th, the gums both of the upper and lower jaw began to swell; by the next day they were ulcerated; the breath became very fetid, and a discolored, stinking fluid ran from the mouth. The thoracic symptoms continued much the same, not at all increasing in intensity, and the cough growing looser than before; but the child became paler and more exsanguine, and continued to lose power. The ulceration of the gums extended to the fold of the lower lip, and three of the incisor teeth fell out before the disease was finally checked, on February 26, by the application of pure nitric acid. The child did not appear to suffer pain, but was very restless, and continually harassed by efforts to vomit, during which she rejected nothing but an offensive mucus. She was extremely indisposed to take either wine or any nourishment for four days before her death, which took place, apparently from exhaustion, on March 1, nineteen days after the commencement of her illness.

On an examination of the body after death, the left lung was found perfectly healthy, with the exception of some emphysema of its upper, and considerable congestion of its lower lobe.

The right lung, which consisted of only two lobes, was universally solid and non-crepitant, with the exception of about a fourth of the upper and inner edge of the lower lobe, which was emphysematous. The two lobes were connected together by a layer of yellow lymph. The exterior of the lung generally was of a dark grayish-red color, with irregular patches of yellow deposit beneath the pleura, some of which were nearly half an inch in length and a quarter in breadth; besides which many small purulent deposits were contained within the pulmonary vesicles, as in vesicular bronchitis. The upper part of the upper lobe, and a small portion near the diaphragmatic surface of the lower lobe, felt soft and boggy to the touch. On cutting into the upper lobe, a cavity was opened as large as a hen's egg, very irregular in form, intersected in various directions by the tubes and vessels that crossed it; from which, as well as from the walls of the cavity, portions of lung hung in shreds. The cavity contained a small quantity of dirty, grayish-yellow putrilage, which exhaled a most fetid odor. The substance of the lung in the immediate neighborhood was in a state of far advanced purulent infiltration, and other parts of the lobe were in an earlier state of the same condition; besides which, small collections of puriform fluid, not bigger than a split pea, were found in various parts of its substance. The state of the lower lobe on the whole resembled that of the upper, but the cavity in it was not larger than a marble, and contained a small quantity of yellow pus, of a less fetid character than that in the upper lobe. The bronchial glands were swollen, soft, of a homogeneous aspect, and a gray color; but neither in them, nor in either lung, nor in any organ of the body, was there the least trace of tubercular deposit.

Although there was in this instance a larger amount of inflammatory disorganization of the lung than is usually met with in connection with gangrene of its substance, yet the symptoms noticed during the patient's lifetime were precisely such as are generally observed in cases of that

description. The child was attacked with symptoms of pneumonia, which, however, were far from being severe; but, nevertheless, by the fifth day from their commencement, the greater part of the right lung had become impervious to air, and percussion over the right side of the chest, on February 15, yielded an almost entirely dull sound. Even then the child's strength seemed much reduced, and in the course of a few days more she sank into a state of great weakness. Throughout the whole course of the disease, there was the same absence of striking indications of the extent to which the respiratory organs had suffered, and this even after a large portion of the lung was completely disorganized. The most remarkable phenomena were those which betokened the general loss of power in the system, while the appearance of gangrenous ulceration about the gums tended to prove the correctness of the opinion which refers the disease to some peculiar alteration of the circulating fluid rather than to the violence of the inflammatory action. Another circumstance which tends to support this opinion is, that gangrene of the lung much more frequently supervenes on the pneumonia that comes on in the course of the exanthematous fevers, than on idiopathic inflammation of the lungs. The disease, too, occurs far more rarely in children who are well fed, and who live in pure air, than in those who are surrounded by unfavorable hygienic conditions. Hence it results that this, as well as other forms of gangrene, are met with in the Children's Hospital at Paris with far greater frequency than elsewhere, and that they sometimes show a tendency to become epidemic in that institution.

There is no symptom that can be mentioned as of constant occurrence in gangrene of the lung in children, and as pathognomonic of the disease. That peculiar fetor of the breath on which so much reliance is placed in cases of gangrene of the lung in the adult, sometimes loses its value in the child, as it did in the case just related, by the coexistence with it of gangrene of the mouth. It happens, too, not infrequently, that the characteristic odor of the breath is altogether absent in cases of gangrene of the lung—a circumstance for which it is not easy to account; though of the fact there can be no doubt, since it rests on the authority of MM. Rilliet and Barthez.

Should you meet with any case in which you apprehend that this condition of the lung is present, you would adopt a tonic and stimulant plan of treatment, as affording the only chance, and that a very slender one, of saving the patient's life. Sir W. Stokes's suggestion, too,[1] for the administration of chlorine, in the form of the chloride of lime or soda, should not be forgotten, since if the remedy did nothing else, it might diminish that fetor of the breath, which is a source of very great suffering to the patient.[2]

Pleurisy, or inflammation of the investing membrane of the lungs, is a disease which received until comparatively lately much less attention

---

[1] Op. cit., p. 359.

[2] For the fullest account of pulmonary gangrene in children, the reader is referred to vol. ii of 2d edit. of Rilliet and Barthez, pp. 404–421; and to the most elaborate work of Dr. Steffen, Klinik der Kinderkrankheiten, 8vo. Berlin, 1869, vol. ii, pp. 47–94.

than its importance deserves. Some writers on the diseases of children, indeed, have left it altogether unnoticed on account of its supposed extreme rarity in early life; though this opinion is certainly erroneous so far as regards that secondary pleurisy which comes on in the course of pneumonia, and which is almost, if not quite, as frequent in childhood as in adult age. It is true that acute idiopathic pleurisy, unconnected with pneumonia, or in which the inflammation of the lung bears but a very small proportion to that of the pleura, is an uncommon affection during the first years of childhood; and that as a cause of death its rarity is extreme. According to the Reports of the Registrar-General, of 202 fatal cases of pleurisy that occurred in London in the years 1842 and 1845, only 14, or, 6.3 per cent., took place in children under five years old; while you will not have forgotten that 63.2 per cent. of all fatal cases of pneumonia are alleged on the same authority to have befallen children aged less than five years. It may be doubted whether this statement, which rests only to a comparatively small extent on the results of post-mortem examination, does not underestimate the frequency of idiopathic pleurisy in early life. But, be this as it may, the rarity of the disease unquestionably diminishes after the first years of infancy are passed; while its importance as an occasional complication or sequela of other affections, and more particularly of scarlet fever, and the frequent obscurity of its symptoms, are reasons for devoting to it more than a passing notice.

In fatal cases of pleurisy in childhood, the *appearances found after death* are precisely the same as are met with in the adult. Adhesions between the costal and pulmonary pleura, and between the different lobes of one or other lung, associated sometimes with very intense redness of parts of the membrane, are hardly ever wanting, and in connection with them a small quantity of transparent serum, often of a reddish tint, is sometimes effused into the cavity of the chest. In other cases the effused matters are entirely solid, and both the surface of the lung and the interior of the thorax are coated with a distinct investment of lymph; or, in addition to the deposit of lymph on the lung, fluid is poured out into the chest—no longer transparent serum, but either a sero-purulent fluid in which flakes of lymph are floating, or more rarely healthy pus. The most frequent complication of pleurisy is with inflammation of the lungs; besides which, it occasionally happens, when the left pleura has been the seat of inflammation, that the disease extends from it to the pericardium, which on four such occasions I have found lined with lymph, partially adhering to the heart, and containing a sero-purulent fluid.[1]

[1] In 118 cases in which the above-mentioned consequences of recent inflammation of the pleura were observed after death in non-phthisical subjects, they existed in the following combinations:

Recent adhesions and deposit of lymph,	30
Serous effusion existed alone,	22
" " " with adhesions, or deposits of lymph,	18
Sero-purulent effusion, or effusion of pus,	48
	118

In 89 of the above 118 cases, the affection of the pleura, though sometimes [illegible]

The main *symptoms* that attend the disease, as well as the *physical signs* of its existence, are the same at all ages. There are, however, some circumstances peculiar to early life, which, unless you are on your guard, may serve to obscure the real nature of the affection. The history of a case of acute pleurisy in childhood is generally something to this effect: A child previously in perfect health is suddenly attacked by pain referred to the chest or to the upper part of the abdomen, so severe as to occasion it to cry aloud; perhaps attended at first by vomiting, accompanied with fever, a rapid pulse, and hurried respiration interrupted by frequent short cough, which evidently occasions pain, and which the child labors, though in vain, to suppress. After a few hours the severity of the pain subsides; but the fever, hurried respiration, and cough continue, and the child, though usually it looks heavy and seems drowsy, yet becomes extremely restless at intervals—cries and struggles, as if in pain, and violently resists any attempt to alter its position, since every movement brings on an exacerbation of its sufferings. The posture which it selects varies much: sometimes its breath seems disturbed in any other than an upright position; at other times it lies on its back, or on one side; but whatever be the posture, any alteration of it appears to cause much distress, and is sure to be resisted by the patient.

The probabilities are that, if you auscultate the chest of a child in whom these symptoms exist, you will hear good breathing through the whole of one lung. On the other side, the motion of which in breathing will be seen to be less extensive, and performed in a slightly jerking manner, the air will be found to enter less freely, though unaccompanied by any moist sound, perhaps unattended by any morbid sound at all; or, possibly, a rough sound like a rhonchus may be audible on this side, and for this you may very likely at first take it, though with more attention it will be discovered to be a friction-sound. A day or two later you will detect a sound like that of bronchial breathing,[1] as

siderable, appeared to be secondary, and subsidiary to that of the lung itself. In the remaining 79, the pleura was the chief seat of the mischief, the lung being either simply compressed by the quantity of the effused fluid, or its inflammation being secondary in extent and importance to that of which the pleura bore evidence.

The following were the circumstances in which the affection of the pleura came on in the latter 79 instances:

Idiopathic,	in 21
After Scarlatina,	32
" Measles,	1
" Typhus,	1
" Typhoid,	1
" Diphtheria,	3
" Pyæmia,	1
" Pericarditis and endocarditis,	10
" Peritonitis,	3
" Ascites with diseased liver,	2
" General dropsy, diseased kidneys,	3
" Disease of cervical vertebra,	1
	79

[1] Rilliet and Barthez were the first to insist on the constant occurrence of bronchial breathing as one of the earliest auscultatory signs of the existence of pleurisy in childhood. See vol. i, p. 554, of the 2d edition of their work.

you pass your ear from above downwards along the posterior part of the chest, while the friction-sound, if it had previously been audible, will have disappeared; and still lower there will be an utter absence of all sound. In most instances, however, no friction-sound is to be heard at the commencement of the attack, though it becomes perceptible on its decline, but a bronchial character of the respiration will be perceived as one of the earliest auscultatory signs of the disease. The walls of this side of the chest, if their tenderness do not prevent your trying percussion, will yield a much less resonant sound than usual; while, at the same time, a distinct sense of solidity will be communicated to the finger, and the vocal fremitus will either be indistinct or altogether absent.

The first auscultatory evidence of improvement is often furnished by the reappearance of friction-sound, or by its beginning to be heard for the first time. It is usually perceived first about the upper and back part of the affected side, and descends by degrees in proportion as the air enters with more freedom, and as the thin layer of fluid which has been poured out becomes absorbed. This process of absorption obeys no rule as to the time which it occupies; so that a friction-sound may be heard in some cases only for a few days, in others for several weeks. The very long persistence of a friction-sound, however, always raises the suspicion that tubercular deposit has taken place on the surface of the pleura. It is very rare for a friction-sound not to be heard over at least some small extent of surface, but in some instances, when very little fluid has been poured out, the costal and pulmonary pleura speedily become adherent, and in such cases little or no friction-sound may be heard. With the gradual return of the pleura to a healthy state the rubbing-sound passes away; but for some time after all other traces of the attack have disappeared, a somewhat harsher character of the breathing, and a marked dulness on percussion, continue. The dulness on percussion, too, far exceeds that which the disparity between the amount of air admitted into the two lungs would seem to account for, and has, to the best of my knowledge, never yet received a thoroughly satisfactory explanation.

The symptoms by which an attack of acute pleurisy is ushered in, point sometimes rather to the head than to the chest. The child is seized with vomiting, attended by fever and intense headache: it either cries aloud, or is delirious at night, or screams much in its sleep, and, when morning comes, complains much of its head, but denies having any pain whatever in its chest, while the short cough and the hurried breathing may be thought to be merely the result of the cerebral disturbance. Sometimes, too, the cough is altogether absent, and the acceleration of the breathing so slight as not to suggest the idea that serious mischief is going on in the chest. Under the impression that the child is suffering from cerebral disease, auscultation is omitted, or at least practiced hastily and superficially, and consequently serves but to confirm the erroneous diagnosis. It often happens, indeed, that in these cases no friction-sound is perceptible, and that you have no other indication to guide you aright besides the feebleness of the respiratory murmur on the affected side. The child, too, fearful of taking a deep inspiration, fills neither lung completely, so that the information usually gained by comparison of the breathing in one lung with that in the other is in great measure lost. Still, the presence of feeble respiratory murmur at the lower part of one lung, when coupled with the sudden accession of acute febrile symptoms in a previously healthy child, points almost invariably to the existence of acute pleurisy; while a careful consideration of the patient's history and general condition will, even irrespective of the results of auscultation, go far towards preventing you from falling into error. The onset of the illness has been far too acute, attended with far too much febrile disturbance, for a case of tubercular meningitis, while many of the signs of cerebral mischief which might be expected in a case of simple encephalitis have not presented themselves. The heat of head is not greater than that of the rest of the surface: the cries with which the disease set in have not ended in coma. It happens but seldom that convulsions mark the commencement of the disease; but if they had occurred at the onset, they have not since returned; neither twitching of the muscles, nor strabismus, nor retraction of the head, is present; and though the child may cry (as children when ill and fretful often do) at the curtain being undrawn and the candle brought near it, yet there is no real intolerance of light, while in spite of its fretfulness, the intelligence is not otherwise perverted. Error indeed is easy, but to avoid it requires in this, as in most instances, not so much great acuteness as great care and great patience.

The pain with which pleurisy sets in is sometimes referred not to the chest, but to the abdomen; and its commencement may be attended with vomiting and purging. This mode of onset of the disease is especially likely to be observed in cases of diaphragmatic pleurisy, and more particularly if the inflammation is seated on the right side; and in this latter case, bilious vomiting is often one of the most marked of the early symptoms. Pressure on the abdomen, too, not only in these, but frequently also in other cases, occasions a considerable increase of suffering; and you may thus be led to overlook the existence of the pleurisy, and to allow your attention to be entirely directed to the abdominal symptoms. Some years since a boy seven years of age was admitted into the Children's Hospital in the sixth week of a pleurisy of the right side, which had terminated in empyema, for which paracentesis was afterwards successfully performed. He was reported to have had inflammation of the bowels, and the marks of recent leech-bites in his right iliac region bore witness to the diagnostic error which auscultation would have avoided. In any such doubtful case, it is well to bear in mind that children, long after they can talk, describe the nature and seat of their sufferings very inaccurately; and if, as often happens in these cases, they refer the pain to the right hypochondrium, you should not forget that pain in that situation is at all ages much oftener connected with inflammation of the pleura than of the peritoneum; and lastly, that the increase of discomfort produced by pressure on the abdomen may be due to the additional impediment thereby offered to the already laboring respiration. The careful auscultation, which I need not say should never be neglected, will generally save you from error, but in a case of diaphragmatic pleurisy you are rather left to infer the nature of the disease, from the non-correspondence of its symptoms with those of any other ailment, than enabled to decide upon its character from any positive sign of mischief in the chest with which your ear makes you acquainted. The heat of skin, the frequency of the pulse, and the hurry of the breathing, are such as to exclude the suspicion of almost all affections of the abdomen, while not only do not the general characters of the attack tally with those of acute peritonitis, but there is no such tenderness upon even slight pressure, no such tension of the abdominal walls, no such dread of the slightest movement, as characterize that disease. Your great safeguard will be found, in such a case, in the right interpretation of the general symptoms, and in the recognition of the fact that, when attended with acute febrile symptoms, the mere imperfect entrance of air into the lung is itself a valuable indication of inflammation of the pleura. The danger, in cases of pleurisy in early life, is, however, not simply that of overlooking the existence of mischief in the chest, but also of referring that mischief to a wrong cause. The fever, and cough, and dyspnoea, may be so marked as to render the former mistake impossible; but auscultation, unless you rightly interpret the information it affords, may not guarantee you against the latter. It is not by any means a matter of indifference whether you take a case of pleurisy for one of pneumonia, or whether, in a case of bronchitis, which may for some time have been under your care, you recognize the inflammation of the pleura which may have supervened, or see in the increased urgency of the chest symptoms merely an exacerbation of the previous ailment. The error, indeed, is one not so likely to be committed in a case of idiopathic pleurisy that you may have watched from the commencement, but it is one into which you may very probably fall in those instances where pleurisy succeeds to the exanthemata, especially to scarlet fever, and less often to measles. Cough and hurried breathing, and rhonchus, with some crepitant râle, may have already existed for some time, and in these circumstances a friction-sound, even if it should become audible, is very likely to be unnoticed. But, besides this, the unequal breathing so characteristic of early life, as the result of which air may seem one hour to enter one lung imperfectly, while a few hours subsequently the deficient respiration may appear to be on the opposite side, naturally leads you to undervalue the importance of mere deficient respiration. But, if the bronchial character of the breathing forces itself on your attention, the probability is that, without any further consideration, you may put that down as an unequivocal proof of the advance of pneumonia, and altogether overlook the pleurisy of which, in this instance, it is an indication.

It is the more important to bear in mind the possibility of error, since some of the means of distinguishing between pleurisy and pneumonia on which we rely much in the adult are less available in the child. It is so difficult to induce children to speak several words consecutively in the same tone, and their voice is often so feeble, as to deprive us in great measure of the information which the different resonance of the two sides of the chest would otherwise afford. For the same reason, too, the difference of vocal vibration, as perceived on applying the hands to either side of the chest, is often by no means so manifest in children as in grown persons. The experiment, however, is one which should never be omitted, since the information which it yields, provided it do not fail altogether, is as valuable in the one case as in the other. Two more hints may perhaps be of service in helping to keep you from error; first, that the limitation of the physical signs of affection of the chest to one side, of itself raises a presumption that that affection is inflammation of the pleura, not of the lung; and second, that the bronchial breathing which is perceived at an early period of an attack of acute pleurisy is attended by diminished resonance on percussion rather than by that absolute dulness which is perceived when the substance of the lung itself has passed into a state of hepatization.

But there are also cases of *latent pleurisy* in the child as well as in the adult; cases in which there are vague symptoms of feverishness, with perhaps a little cough, and nothing more; nothing to call special attention to the chest, nor even to suggest the existence of grave ailment anywhere. In young children the symptoms are attributed to teething, in those who are older to worms, or to gastric fever; terms which cover a large amount of carelessness, ignorance, and indolence. I know of no means infallibly to preserve from error, besides those simple rules which have grown almost wearisome by frequent repetition. Bear in mind, with reference to teething, that there are pauses in the evolution of the teeth; that it does not follow because a child has not yet cut all its teeth, that dentition must therefore at any particular moment be in active progress. Next, that how much soever the presence of worms may interfere with a state of perfect health, febrile symptoms are not indicative of their presence; and in the third place, that, with the exception of the exanthemata and of ague, and very rarely of typhus, typhoid fever is the only essential fever to which children are liable. In other words, fever is symptomatic of disturbance somewhere; it behooves you by careful examination to make out where; and in order that you may not fail to discover the seat of the disturbance, you must never omit auscultation.

A little girl, two years and two months old, had slight cold and a cough, which seemed so trivial that medical care was not sought for; and when at the end of a fortnight a purulent discharge took place from the right ear, that was looked on but as another evidence of the dependence of the ailment on dentition. At the end of three weeks, as she did not recover her customary health, a doctor was called in, who found her breathing quietly, with no cough, but looking worn and ill. She slept well during the night, and the following day seemed much the same, except that she was rather more fretful, so that she would not allow of any attempt at auscultation, and her pulse had suddenly fallen from 120 to 72 beats in the minute. She slept pretty well during the night, but the next morning, when taken up, as was her wont, she laid her head on one side against the nurse's bosom, and died without a struggle or convulsion.

I was present at the post-mortem examination, which disclosed no morbid appearances whatever in the brain. There were, however, nearly six ounces of reddish serum in the cavity of each pleura, though without any deposit of false membrane on their surfaces. Some portions of the lung were in a state of collapse; there were some white clots on the right side of the heart, while the left side was empty and contracted.

Few symptoms had here called attention to the condition of the child, who at length died suddenly in consequence of the effusion into its chest, and probably from the sudden change of posture on assuming the sitting position.

This case has a twofold interest, partly from the latency of its symptoms, partly from the suddenness of its termination; and the possible sudden termination of a case of pleuritic effusion is perhaps less borne in mind than it should be.

A little boy, not quite three years old, whose health had never been very robust, was brought as an out-patient to the Children's Dispensary in Lambeth on June 11, 1847, on account of a chronic impetiginous eruption on his scalp. On the night of June 12 he suddenly became hot, and his chest was much oppressed, but on the following day he was well enough to be out at play in the garden, and on the 15th was drawn a mile and a half in a perambulator to and from the dispensary when I saw him for the first time. He looked pale and ill, was feverish, and breathed with a wheezing noise, but there was nothing about him indicative of serious mischief; and in the hurry of prescribing for a large number of patients, I regarded him as probably a phthisical child, who had caught cold recently. I ordered some simple medicine for him, and at one P.M. he returned home. At three o'clock the same afternoon he suddenly became much worse, was very faint, breathed with extreme difficulty, and died at eight o'clock the next morning. Some serous fluid was present in the abdomen, and about six ounces in either pleura, by which the lower lobes of both lungs were so compressed as to be almost destitute of air.

But again, death may, as in the first case, be almost immediate; and this sudden death, be it observed, takes place chiefly in instances where the inflammatory action has not been intense, and where the effusion is simple serum. A little boy, aged eight years, was attacked by moderately severe scarlatina. Slight anasarca appeared on the 19th day, which had somewhat increased, but was accompanied by no urgent symptom on the 22d day, when he walked a distance of two miles without suffering serious fatigue. After a rather restless night he rose to relieve his bowels, and there was so little suggestive of danger in his condition that his mother left him for a few minutes alone. On her return, his bowels had acted scantily, and he seemed faint. He was replaced in bed, when he immediately began to struggle feebly, and in a few minutes was dead.

The lungs were compressed by abundant serous effusion in each pleura, and the pericardium also contained four ounces of fluid, but there were no other morbid appearances except some congestion of the kidneys.

This very sudden death is unquestionably a rare result of pleurisy, but nevertheless, the disease in early life is by no means unattended with danger; and my own impression is that a fatal termination of acute idiopathic pleurisy is by no means of such rare occurrence in early as in adult life. In most of those cases, however, which I have seen terminate fatally, the disease though it began in the pleura, did not continue limited to it, but extended either to the pulmonary substance or to the pericardium. I have, indeed, in these circumstances known a case of pleurisy prove fatal within four days from the first appearance of its symptoms.

Besides these cases, others require notice in which the pleurisy neither proves immediately fatal, nor terminates on the other hand by speedy recovery. Here the effusion which takes place produces an even greater degree of deformity of the chest in the child than in the adult, since its more yielding walls give place more readily. The immediate consequence of the effusion is of course to produce an enlargement of that side of the chest into which the fluid is poured out, while at the same time the respiratory movements on that side are almost entirely abolished, and the intercostal spaces are bulged outwards, or at least are raised to a level with the surface of the ribs; though in the child the amount of fat beneath the integuments renders this less obvious than in the adult. The heart's apex, too, will be displaced from its natural position, and will be felt beating either outside the left nipple, or far to the right of the mesial line, according as the one or the other pleura is the seat of the effusion; while, if fluid is poured out abundantly in the right pleura, the liver may often be felt forced down far below its ordinary situation; or if into the left, a similar change may be discovered in the relations of the spleen. As the one side, however, is expanded by the effusion of fluid, the other also increases very appreciably in the course of ten days or a fortnight, as the result of the extra work thrown on the healthy lung, which has to perform its functions not for itself only but also for the other, whose action is impaired, or it may be almost completely arrested. With the commencement of the absorption of the fluid the affected side begins to shrink; and in the course of time from being half an inch to an inch larger than the healthy side it becomes at least as much smaller; it grows flatter in the infra-clavicular region; the spine itself yields, its upper convexity being directed towards the healthy, its lower convexity towards the contracted side. The hypertrophy of the healthy lung produces a bulging of the corresponding side, the shoulder of which is thrown up, while the other is proportionately depressed, and a very remarkable degree of deformity is thus produced. Gradually with the lapse of time, a sort of restorative process seems to be set on foot, the steps of which have not been sufficiently studied; but by it the spinal curvature and the flattening of the upper and front part of the chest are lessened, in proportion as air permeates the lung more freely; and in many instances, a comparatively slight degree of deformity remains the only evidence of what had seemed to be almost irremediable mischief.

This, however, is a result which it does not seem possible to calculate on with any certainty, for there can be no doubt but that in the large majority of cases of acute pleurisy in early life in which effusion takes place, either pus is poured out at once, or the fluid very speedily becomes purulent, and consequently inapt for absorption, though by no means incapable, as was once imagined, of being absorbed.[1] In these circumstances, we usually find the chain of occurrences to be somewhat as follows. After the first acute attack which has terminated in the effusion of fluid, the more active symptoms abate, the fever subsides, and the child enters on a state of semi-convalescence. This, however, does not last above a week or ten days, when, without any fresh accession of acute symptoms, the child begins to suffer from notable dyspnœa, grows unable to lie at all except on the affected side, while the superficial veins on that side become greatly enlarged, the integuments somewhat œdematous, and the whole surface so tender that even the gentlest percussion cannot be tolerated. These symptoms indicate that the matter is about making its way outwardly, which it does usually by perforating the chest-wall, though the empyema now and then empties itself into a bronchus, of which I have seen four instances; and has been known to burst through the diaphragm into the abdominal cavity, and thus to produce fatal peritonitis. In by far the majority of cases the matter is discharged externally through the chest-wall, almost invariably through the anterior wall of the chest, and mostly in the fourth or fifth interspace and a little outside the nipple. Increase of the tenderness of the chest-wall, and then bulging of the integuments in one or other intercostal space, precede the distinct pointing of the abscess, which, whether opened or allowed to burst of itself, will almost invariably continue fistulous for a great length of time; the profuse discharge exhausting the patient, and the rapid contraction of the side producing great and often remediless deformity. This external opening, too, is not infrequently an indirect one, the matter having burrowed between the pleura and the chest-wall for some distance before it escaped externally.

Thus, in the case of a boy, aged eight years, who died eighteen months after the first symptoms of pleurisy on the left side, and fourteen months after the formation of a pleural fistula between the first and second bones of the sternum, which remained open till his death, and another between the sixth and seventh rib, which ceased to discharge nine months before that event, a post-mortem examination disclosed the following state of things:

The old sinus between the sixth and seventh rib did not extend for more than a quarter of an inch, and terminated without entering the chest. That between the bones of the sternum opened at once into a number of sinuses which led for at least an inch upwards and downwards in several directions, and then pierced the chest-wall to run along in a similar manner in the substance of the costal pleura, which was like cartilage in appearance, and at least three-fourths of an inch in thickness; and all these sinuses were filled with pus.

[1] In Mr. Hilton's work, already referred to, will be found many instances of the absorption of the contents of abscesses. Perhaps the most interesting is that related at p. 375, in which the small amount of solid residuum found on the patient's death after the lapse of some months, was ascertained by chemical examination to be absolutely identical with the constituents of pus.

To sum up then. Speedy recovery when little fluid has been poured out; tardy recovery when it has been more abundant; and followed in most instances by deformity, which time tends gradually and imperfectly to remove; occasional sudden death when serous fluid has been poured out rapidly and in large quantity; escape of the fluid in most instances when purulent through the chest-walls, in obedience to the laws which govern the course of an abscess, wherever situated: such are the different issues of pleurisy in early life. How these facts bear upon our treatment of the disease is the question that we have next to consider. Before doing so, however, I must just add one word of caution with reference to the diagnosis of pleurisy and empyema in childhood. This caution, too, concerns not the difficulty of discovering the condition, but the culpable carelessness with which it is often overlooked by practitioners, who satisfy themselves with determining that their patient has inflammation of the chest as they term it, and never take the trouble to inquire further into its nature; and at last are taken by surprise, either by their patient's unexpected death, or by the unlooked-for escape of the matter with which one side of the chest was filled, through some external opening. There are no cases in which it happens to me to have to screen the mistakes of others so often as in cases of pleurisy and empyema; and I venture to use one of the privileges of age, in order to entreat the younger members of my profession never to allow themselves to fall into habits of inaccuracy. The limits of our knowledge are narrow enough; we need not circumscribe them still further by our own indolence.

The causes which have already been referred to as modifying in very important respects the *treatment* of bronchitis and pneumonia, have also exercised their influence over the treatment of pleurisy. But, nevertheless, I am fully convinced that considerable activity in the early stage of the disease best averts danger, and most economizes the patient's strength. In almost every instance, indeed, that has come under my observation, where the issue of acute pleurisy has been unfortunate, either all treatment had been neglected until the children were past hope, or the nature of the complaint had been mistaken, or the treatment followed had not been sufficiently active. The same statement, too, may be made with reference to those cases in which paracentesis of the chest became necessary. By active treatment, I imply depletion in all cases in which the child's previous health has been good, in which pleurisy is idiopathic, the symptoms are at all urgent, and the patient is seen before the occurrence of effusion. In children of five or six years old, general depletion is to be preferred, and the relief to the breathing may be taken as the indication for stopping the flow of blood. If after the lapse of four or six hours the pain and dyspnœa return, leeches should be applied to the affected side, and four or six leeches will seldom fail to give permanent relief. In the case of younger children local depletion alone will suffice, but that should not be practiced too timorously, since the most relief is procured when the abstraction of blood answers to some degree the purpose of a general bleeding. After depletion our chief reliance is to be placed on calomel, which should be freely given in combination with opium or Dover's powder, while a warm poultice is constantly applied to the affected side; and an attack of pleurisy thus treated will often be cut short in thirty-six or forty-eight hours.

In many instances, however, the child's previous health does not warrant, or the severity of the symptoms is not such as to indicate, these very active proceedings. In these circumstances a mustard poultice to the chest will often give immediate ease; and on its removal a linseed poultice may be applied, and renewed every four hours, so as to maintain the effect of a gentle counter-irritant. At the same time the iodide of potassium may be given in combination with a saline and diuretic,[1] and continued steadily for several days; while its action may be seconded by a small dose of mercury, given once or twice a day, as one grain of calomel, or three of gray powder, for a child of six years old. The mercurial may be discontinued at the end of a week, but the iodide of potass may be persevered with for two or three weeks; the abatement of all febrile action, and the diminution of the effusion, indicating the time when it may be given with less frequency. Often, however, after the symptoms have subsided, the affected side remains dull, and the respiration scanty for several weeks together; and now is the time when the use of blisters, or still better the painting the side with tincture of iodine, seems to be of much service in promoting the absorption of the fluid; while cod-liver oil given twice a day, is a useful means of maintaining the nutrition of the child, and of counteracting that tendency to the development of tubercular disease which is so apt to manifest itself in cases where pleurisy has passed into a chronic stage.

Sometimes, indeed, in spite of remedies perseveringly employed, one side of the chest continues full of fluid; and the question then comes before us whether it will not be expedient to let out that fluid by mechanical means. I believe that so long as the child's health is improving, or at least not deteriorating, as the temperature, which falls after the first onset of acute pleurisy, has not begun to rise again, as the respiration is not growing more hurried, nor the cough more troublesome, as the chest-walls have not become tender, nor the superficial veins notably enlarged, and there is no sign of pointing anywhere, while careful measurement of the chest proves the effused fluid not to be on the increase, we may persevere in the employment of the means already indicated. I believe, however, also, that we shall best consult the interests of our patient by evacuating the contents of the pleura, so soon as any of the above-mentioned favorable conditions cease, and that we shall err if we delay until the supervention of intense dyspnœa leaves

---

[1] (No. 18.)

℞. Potassii Iodidi, gr. xij.
Potassæ Nitratis, gr. xxx.
Spt. Æth. Nitr., ʒj.
Liq. Taraxaci, ʒiij.
Tinct. Scillæ, ♏xxx.
Tinct. Digitalis, ♏xxiv.
Aquæ, ad ℥iv. Syr. Aurantii, ℥iv. M. ft. Mist.

A tablespoonful every four hours. For a child six years old.

us no choice, or until the pointing of the empyema externally allows us to do no more than anticipate, by a very few days, the completion of the process which nature herself has undertaken.

In 48 out of 88 post-mortem examinations, in which fluid was found in the pleural sac, that fluid was purulent; and if the cases were excluded in which either the fluid was very inconsiderable in quantity, or in which its effusion was secondary to scarlatinal dropsy, we should find that in almost every instance the pleura contained pus. In 34 out of 38 of my cases in which paracentesis of the chest was performed the fluid was purulent. In one of the four exceptional cases the effusion followed scarlatinal dropsy, in a second it succeeded to measles, in the other two the pleurisy was idiopathic, but paracentesis was in one instance had recourse to on the 8th, in the other on the 14th day from the commencement of the child's illness. In the latter of these two cases, it became necessary to repeat the puncture 18 days later, and the fluid was then becoming turbid. It is indeed my belief that in almost every instance of idiopathic pleurisy in which fluid is poured out in considerable quantity, that fluid either is originally purulent or becomes so very speedily. The possibility of the absorption of pus is indeed no longer disputed, but at the same time pus is inapt to be absorbed, and its absorption is sure to be tedious; while the longer the lung continues compressed by it, the more likely is it to become bound down permanently by lymph, to become altered in texture, and incapable of being again permeated by air. If to this we add the constitutional symptoms which never fail to be excited by the presence of a large abscess; the risk of pyæmia inseparable from it; and the great probability, nay the almost certainty, that in the course of time nature herself will decide the point, and make an opening in an undesirable situation which will empty the pleura but imperfectly, while it will remain fistulous for months or years, difficult to close, aggravating the deformity of the chest, wearing the strength by the constant drain of matter; we have, I think, a number of reasons more than sufficient to justify the comparatively early performance of paracentesis.

While these reasons tell very strongly in favor of paracentesis, I know of no valid arguments against it; and I believe there are now very few dissentients from its performance.[1] It is true that we cannot regard each case of successful tapping, as one in which a life has been saved that would otherwise have been lost; since the frequency with which we meet with pleural fistula, shows the extent of nature's resources; while at the same time it points out the proceeding which art can anticipate with so much advantage. Still more rarely—in the child, I believe, very rarely—and usually only after much and prolonged suffering, the matter finds its way into an air-tube, the empyema is spit up, and the patient recovers. But if each successful paracentesis

[1] It seems strange, however, to find a man of the large experience which Professor Vogel, of Dorpat, undoubtedly possesses, saying in his Lehrbuch der Kinderkrankheiten, 4th ed., 8vo, Erlangen, 1869, p 263, "I have not met with any instance where paracentesis was urgently required, and have therefore never had recourse to it."

does not represent a life saved, still less does each failure represent a life destroyed; and the common, and I believe, on the whole, correct estimate of one death in every four cases of tapping of the chest[1] in childhood, tells usually of too tardy an interference, or of some inevitable complication, and very rarely indeed of any added risk which the operation brought with it. This fact receives one of its best illustrations in the difference between the results of tapping in private and in hospital practice. Of six cases in which the chest was tapped under my direction in private, all recovered; and the only one who did not regain health was a little boy, from whose right pleura I removed six ounces of pus when he was only seven months old, and who died of general tuberculosis three months later. In hospital practice, on the other hand, fifteen out of thirty-four cases died, or very nearly half. But one of these patients died of intercurrent scarlatina; in two the pleurisy was consequent on scarlatina; in two others on measles; three died from caries of the ribs or sternum, consequent on undue delay in the performance of the tapping; and four died of tuberculosis. If I were to state, indeed, in as few words as possible, my experience of paracentesis of the chest in pleurisy, I should say that I have in no single instance ever regretted its performance, but have often been sorry that I did not have recourse to it sooner.

What, then, may we lay down as the indications for tapping the chest? First, it ought to be had recourse to in every case of urgent dyspnœa, accompanied with effusion into the chest, where there is reason for believing that great, even though only temporary, relief would be obtained by the evacuation of the fluid. It is not often, however, that we meet in children with any considerable amount of passive effusion in the cavity of the chest, except in cases of dropsy succeeding to scarlatina. In those cases, too, the pleuritic effusion is usually associated with so considerable an amount of previous œdema of the pulmonary tissue, that we are very likely to be disappointed in obtaining the relief that we anticipated. Even here, however, I do not believe that the mere fact of tapping the chest makes any appreciable addition to the gravity of the patient's condition.

In the next place: in any case of acute pleurisy, in which, however early it may be in the disease, there is fluid in quantity sufficient to modify the form of the chest, or to produce displacement of the viscera, the child at the same time suffering from cough, distress, or dyspnœa, the fluid should be at once let out. The chest ought also to be tapped even independent of those symptoms of constitutional disturbance, if the effused fluid should remain stationary for three or four days in spite of treatment; and I believe that, even though nature might eventually have accomplished the absorption of the fluid without this intervention, recovery will take place more speedily as well as more surely in consequence of the tapping.

---

[1] The latest statistics, those of Steffen, in vol. ii of his Clinic der Kinderkrankheiten, p. 598, yield this result. They are founded, indeed, on only 59 cases; but I doubt whether a comparison of larger numbers would lead to any very different conclusion.

In these cases, or in any others in which there is a possible question as to the presence of fluid, or as to its exact situation, it is well to puncture the chest, in the first instance with a hypodermic syringe, by which, even if the lung should be pricked, no harm can be done; and to be guided in our subsequent proceedings by the information thus obtained. The presence of fluid having been ascertained, the trocar may be introduced in the fourth or fifth interspace, and about two inches outside the nipple, unless there should be some special reason for choosing some other position. On the whole, I prefer a Thompson's syringe, with a tube of vulcanized india-rubber attached to it, by which the fluid may be evacuated under water, to any more elaborate contrivance, such as the aspirator, or Bowditch's syringe. I do so for several reasons; of which one of the chief is the great importance of simplicity in the instruments, and in the performance of an operation which is even more likely to be required at the hands of a country practitioner than at those of a hospital surgeon. In the next place, a certain degree of practice is needed in the use of the aspirator, while there is always risk when Bowditch's syringe is employed, lest the process of exhaustion be carried too far, and blood be drawn after the pleura has been emptied of its contents; an accident which I have witnessed more than once.

I do not think that the complete emptying of the pleura is by any means essential to the success of the operation; neither has my experience led me to believe that in cases where the fluid is serous, the accidental entrance of air leads to its becoming purulent, or that it produces any of those formidable consequences which have been attributed to it. Inasmuch, however, as our object is to place the patient in the best possible condition for obtaining the complete absorption of any fluid that may still be left behind, for avoiding its re-collection and for facilitating the expansion of the compressed lung, I avoid, as far as possible, the entrance of air into the chest, and close the wound. Supposing the fluid let out to be serum—which, however, it rarely is in idiopathic pleurisy in childhood—a single tapping may suffice, and recovery may be both uninterrupted and speedy. Even though the fluid should be purulent, it yet does not follow of necessity that a second tapping will be required, for sometimes the operation is followed by steady, though more gradual improvement. In many cases, however, where the fluid was originally serous, and in most where it was purulent, a second, and even a third tapping is necessary; while the smaller the quantity of fluid evacuated, and the longer the interval between each successive tapping, the better the prospect of the patient's recovery. The indications for each tapping are in the main the same as those which guided us in its first performance, though, as a rule, in spite of the presence of even a larger quantity of fluid, the dyspnœa is less urgent, the cough less troublesome, and the symptoms altogether less grave than they were on the first occasion. The heart often fails to regain its natural position immediately on the evacuation of the fluid, so that the evidence afforded by displacement of the viscera ceases to guide us; while, if the lung did not rise immediately on the first performance of paracentesis, the affected side speedily falls in. In consequence of this, instead of the affected side

free exit of the pus; and in such circumstances a canula must be substituted for the wire. I have not found it desirable to attempt any plan of drainage by means of a distant counter-opening kept patulous by a tube or other contrivance introduced into it. I tried it, indeed, on two occasions, but the proceeding appeared to be a severe one, and the opening at the back of the chest became unhealthy, and it was necessary to close it. Even without any such counter-opening, in all cases where the operation has not been too long delayed, the fluid lessens by degrees, and finally ceases to be secreted as the lung gradually expands on the one side, and the yielding chest-wall falls in to meet it on the other. The only instances in which it has seemed to me to be desirable to make a second opening have been cases of neglected empyema, in which there is a circuitous sinus leading to a fistulous aperture into the chest. In these circumstances it is sometimes useful to make and to maintain a second direct opening into the chest at a distance of two or three inches from the first; and the free escape of the matter being thus provided for, the fistula will close in time, and no great difficulty will in general be experienced in the closing of the second aperture. I do not, as a general rule, wash out the chest; for if the opening is free, the pleural cavity in general remains tolerably empty; while I have not found that those iodine injections which greatly modify the secretion from a simple serous cyst have any influence on that poured out by a pyogenic membrane. But whenever the discharge is specially offensive, I always wash out the pleural cavity first with warm water, and afterwards with a weak solution of iodine, or of carbolic acid, either of which greatly lessens any bad odor.

There still remain two questions with reference to these cases: the one of which concerns the causes of death in chronic empyema, and the other the reason why it is inexpedient to leave the evacuation of the fluid to nature.

The causes of death are generally one or other of the following:

1. The supervention of inflammation either on the side originally affected, or still more frequently on the opposite side; an accident which may occur at any time, though rare when the disease has passed completely into a chronic state.

2. The occurrence of ulceration of the pleura and the extension of the mischief to the ribs or sternum, producing necrosis; an accident far from being very uncommon.

3. The failure of constitutional power, in consequence of the continued drain on the system, though this occurs far less often than might have been expected.

4. The development of general tuberculosis, which I believe to be the most frequent of all causes of death from chronic pleurisy.

The reasons why it is inexpedient to leave the evacuation of an empyema to nature have already been indicated in what I have said, but they may perhaps be summed up under the following heads:

1. The needlessly protracted suffering, as well as the additional risk, to which the patient is exposed.

2. The extreme probability that the opening which nature makes

will be in a situation unfavorable for its eventual closure, and the further likelihood that it will be circuitous, and not direct.

3. The risk that the ulceration of the pleura, which precedes the formation of the opening, will not be limited to one spot, but will occur at several; that it will extend to the periosteum, denuding the ribs or sternum at different parts, and thus leading to their caries.

4. The certainty that the false membrane lining the chest and covering the lung will be more extensive and thicker than if the fluid had been let out; that the discharge is therefore more likely to persist; that the lung, long compressed and firmly bound down, will be less capable of expansion; and that the resulting deformity will be far more considerable.

In all cases of effusion into the chest, whether it has been tapped or not, some deformity is sure to take place; due in part to the falling in of the wall of the affected side, partly to the expansion of the opposite side, owing to the increased development of the sound lung, which has a double duty to perform. I was accustomed once in all cases to resort to mechanical contrivances almost from the first, in order to control this deformity, and to prevent as far as possible the occurrence of great spinal curvature. I am now, however, convinced that in the great majority of cases this precaution is needless; for even when the contraction has at first been most marked, a disposition to its spontaneous removal almost invariably becomes apparent in a few months, and at the end of a year or two all traces of it have almost always disappeared. To this rule, indeed, one must make an exception in most cases where the opening remains fistulous, though even here we meet with instances where the lung gradually rises, and a small circumscribed collection of matter remains shut off from the general chest cavity; an inconvenience rather than a grave trouble. Still these are happy exceptions; and an opening which communicates with the general cavity of the chest leads almost always to deformities which tax all the skill of the orthopædic mechanician, and too often vainly, to rectify.

LECTURE XXIII.

CROUP.—Reasons for not studying it earlier in the course—Discrepancy of opinion with reference to it—Two distinct though allied diseases included under the name.

LARYNGEAL CROUP; OR CYNANCHE LARYNGEA.—Causes of the disease—Its frequency in childhood, in the male subject, in northern climates, in rural districts.

Post-mortem appearances—Variations in the extent of false membrane in the air-passages—Changes associated with it—Affection of the fauces and soft palate.

Symptoms—Occasional sudden onset—Catarrhal stage—General course of a fatal case—Occasional delusive appearances of amendment—Evidences of suffocation—Changes in tracheal sound.

Duration—Prognosis.

Treatment—Importance of abstraction of blood—Directions for its performance, and for the administration of tartar emetic—When and how mercurials are to be employed—Modifications in treatment produced by alterations in epidemic constitution—Importance of not exaggerating them, and of not confounding in their treatment croup and diphtheria.

In strict propriety the very important disease which we are now about to investigate, ought to have engaged our attention immediately after we had completed our study of infantile bronchitis. Two reasons, however, independent of mere convenience, have led me to postpone till now the consideration of the subject of *croup*. One of these reasons is, that its gravity is often greatly increased by the association with it of inflammation of the lungs—a complication the importance of which it was essential that you should thoroughly understand; the other is, that croup, though an inflammatory disease, is not without a very evident spasmodic element in every case: so that it may very appropriately form a sort of transition between the inflammatory and the spasmodic diseases of the respiratory organs.

It can scarcely be necessary to tell any of you that croup is the English name for the disease designated by scientific writers *cynanche trachealis*, or *cynanche laryngea*. It consists in inflammation, generally of a highly acute character, of the larynx or trachea, or of both, which terminates in the majority of cases in the exudation of false membrane more or less abundantly upon the affected surface.

The formidable nature of the symptoms by which it is attended, and the rapidity with which it tends to a fatal issue, have led many of the ablest physicians to devote much time and attention to the study of croup. It might, therefore, be anticipated that our knowledge of a disease which betrays itself by very manifest and highly characteristic symptoms, and which gives rise, when fatal, to changes easily appreciable after death, should, by this time, be very definite and settled. With reference to many of the more important points in the history of the malady, writers are now, indeed, pretty well agreed; but croup, like many other diseases that depend to a great extent on atmospheric and telluric causes, is modified in many of its symptoms by peculiarities of air, water, and situation. The affection assumes one character among the poor of a crowded city, and another among the children of the laborer in some rural district; or varies in both in accordance with what Sydenham calls the epidemic constitution of the year.[1]

[1] I have preserved a record of 23 cases of croup that came under my notice at the Royal Infirmary for Children between May, 1839 and April, 1849. Of these 23 cases 11 were idiopathic, 12 secondary; five of the former and two of the latter recovered. In two of the idiopathic cases that recovered, a scanty formation of false membrane was observed upon the velum and tonsils, but no such appearance existed in the other idiopathic cases. Three of the six fatal idiopathic cases were examined after death: in two the false membrane was confined to the larynx; and there was but little injection of the trachea or bronchi: in the third case there was great redness both of the trachea and bronchi, and a large quantity of purulent secretion in both, and ulceration of the mucous membrane of the larynx, but no false membrane. Of the twelve secondary cases, one supervened in the course of pneumonia; in the other eleven, croup appeared as the sequela or concomitant of measles, and ten of the twelve terminated fatally. In the cases which recovered, and in three of those which terminated fatally, there was no false membrane on the velum or fauces, but

If, therefore, you find that my account of the disease varies in any respect from the description given by some other writers, or from the results of your own observation hereafter, do not too hastily assume either that your teacher has been mistaken, or that your own observation has been incorrect. The difference may be nothing more than a fresh exemplification of the old story of the shield, silver on the one side and golden on the other, about which the knights in the fable quarrelled.

There are, indeed, two diseases which have often been included under

---

in the other seven, false membrane was present in those situations as well as in the larynx, and twice this false membrane extended into the œsophagus. Six of the fatal cases were examined after death: in one there was no false membrane anywhere, but intense redness of the larynx, trachea, and bronchi, with an uneven granular appearance of the larynx, and ulceration about the epiglottis. In the other five cases the larynx contained more or less false membrane, and its surface was ulcerated; and in four of the cases the palate and tonsils were inflamed and coated with false membrane In all these five cases, pneumonia existed in both lungs, and four times it was found to have reached in some parts the stage of purulent infiltration.

These results, which differ in so many respects from the conclusions of many most excellent observers in this country, approach much more nearly to those obtained in the Hôpital des Enfans Malades at Paris. The district in which my observations were made is low, with defective sewerage, open drains running close to many of the houses; and most of the patients were the children of poor parents, who occupied only one room, and who consequently were placed in most unfavorable hygienic conditions.

I may further add, that with the change of my field for observation since the opening of the Children's Hospital in 1852, a more sthenic form of the disease came under my notice; and in some of the fatal cases which occurred in that institution under my care, a complete false membrane not only lined the trachea, but extended even into the tertiary bronchi. This state of things continued for some five years, and then once more the disease assumed an asthenic character as it increased in frequency; and became associated with diphtheria, in which latter disease it for a time almost completely merged. The following abstract from the tables of the Children's Hospital is not without interest as illustrative of these changes in the epidemic constitution of the time since it was opened. I need not say that it is not to be taken as illustrative of any other fact:

Date.	Total Admissions of In-Patients.	Cases of Croup.	Cases of Diphtheria.
In the year 1852,	143	0	0
1853,	187	4	0
1854,	251	2	0
1855,	263	8	0
1856,	309	15	0
1857,	325	11	5
1858,	380	4	6
1859,	411	4	5
1860,	384	0	8
1861,	577	10	15
1862,	543	7	17
1863,	571	2	23
1864,	581	7	11
1865,	658	6	7
1866,	786	8	10
1867,	618	5	7
1868,	719	7	12
1869,	709	5	8
1870,	691	4	1
1871,	678	2	8
Total,	9804	106	128

the common name of croup, though the points of difference between them are at least as numerous and as important as are those in which they resemble each other. Of these two diseases, the one is almost always idiopathic, the other is often secondary; the one attacks persons in perfect health, is sthenic in its character, acute in its course, and usually proves amenable to antiphlogistic treatment; the other attacks by preference those who are out of health or who are surrounded by unfavorable hygienic conditions, and is remarkable for the asthenic character of the symptoms which attend it. The one selects its victims almost exclusively from among children, is incapable of being diffused by contagion, is governed in its prevalence by the influence of season, temperature, and climate, but rarely becomes, in the usual acceptation of the term, an epidemic; while the other attacks adults as well as children, is propagated by contagion, and though it occasionally occurs in a sporadic form, is susceptible of widespread epidemic prevalence. The one is developed out of catarrh, and the amount of disease of the respiratory organs is the exact measure of the danger which attends it; while the other affects the organs of respiration secondarily, its peril is often altogether out of proportion to the degree in which they are involved, and death itself may take place although they are altogether unaffected. In this latter ailment, too, a long train of sequelæ not infrequently remains after the local symptoms have been dissipated: the evidence of its affinity to the class of blood diseases rather than to that of simple inflammations. Cynanche Trachealis, Cynanche Laryngea, are the appellations of the former; Home[1] and Cheyne[2] and Albers,[3] its historians; Angina Maligna, the Garotillo, Morbus Strangulatorius, Diphthérite or Diphtheria, the synonyms of the latter; Severinus,[4] Ghisi,[5] Bard,[6] Starr,[7] Rumsey,[8] Bretonneau,[9] Trousseau,[10] and Jenner,[11] some of the writers who have most carefully described it.

Different, however, as the two diseases are, there are yet between them points of similarity no less striking—

Facies non una, nec diversa tamen,

and the diagnostic difficulties which are thus almost inevitable, are still further enhanced by the not infrequent simultaneous prevalence of both affections.

---

[1] An Inquiry into the Nature, Cause, and Cure of the Croup. 8vo., Edinburgh, 1765.

[2] On the Pathology of the Larynx and Bronchia. 8vo., Edinburgh, 1809.

[3] De Tracheitide Infantum. 4to., Lipsiæ, 1816.

[4] De pædanchone maligna, &c., in De recondità abscessuum naturà, p. 518. 4to., Lugd. Bat., 1724.

[5] Lettere mediche; la seconda contiene l'istoria delle anghine epidemiche degli anni 1747 e 1748. Cremina, 1749, 4to.

[6] An Inquiry into the Nature, &c., of the Angina Suffocativa, in Transactions of American Philosophical Society. 4to., vol. i, 2d ed., Philadelphia, 1789, p. 388.

[7] An account of the Morbus Strangulatorius, in Philosophical Transactions, vol. xliv. 4to., London, 1752, p. 435.

[8] Transactions of a Society for the Improvement of Medical and Surgical Knowledge, vol. ii.

[9] De la Diphthérite. 8vo., Paris, 1826.

[10] Clinique Médicale, &c., vol. i, pp 312–450.

[11] Diphtheria, its Symptoms and Treatment. 12mo., London, 1861.

It will be my endeavor to describe, first, that disease which used at least to be the more frequent in this country, and then to give the best account in my power of that other malady, which is a yet more formidable visitant, and one less within the power of medicine to control.

Croup, or Cynanche Laryngea, in the form which it usually assumes in this country is essentially *a disease of early life;* for it appears from the Fifth Report of the Registrar-General, that while 1022 out of 98,391 deaths in the metropolis and twenty-four town districts, took place from croup, 1013, or 99.9 per cent., of those deaths occurred before the age of fifteen; and 879, or 87.9 per cent., before the age of five years. Of 100 cases of croup occurring among the in-patients of the Children's Hospital, 84 took place in children under five years of age, and only 16 in children between the ages of five and ten. 58 of the patients were males, 42 females. It has been attempted to explain this great frequency of croup in early life by the imperfect development of the organ of the voice before puberty. This, however, can scarcely be admitted as a valid explanation, since it does not at all account for the extreme rarity of the disease after five years of age. The preponderance of male over female children among those who are attacked by croup, is another fact which, though confirmed by the experience of all observers, has never received any adequate explanation.[1]

Croup appears to be *influenced by peculiarities of climate and locality* much more than most diseases of the respiratory organs. Though not entirely confined to northern climates, it prevails but seldom in the southern parts of Europe, and is even less frequent in the southern than in the northern counties of England. In Kent, Surrey, and Sussex, the deaths from croup are to the deaths from all causes in the proportion of .9 per cent.; while in the four northern counties, Durham, Northumberland, Cumberland, and Westmoreland, which contain an equal population, the deaths from this cause are in the proportion of 1.6 per cent. It is endemic in particular localities; and residence near the sea, proximity to the mouths of large rivers, a moist soil and a damp atmosphere, have been enumerated as greatly predisposing to the disease. The influence of these local peculiarities has probably, in some

---

[1] From the Fifth Report of the Registrar-General, it appears that, while the deaths of males under 15 from all causes, are to the deaths of females from all causes as 11 to 10, the deaths from croup are as 15 to 10. Of 249 cases that came under Gölis's observation at Vienna, 144 occurred in males, 105 in females; at Geneva, under Jurine's observation, 54 males and 37 females died of croup, between the years 1791 and 1808; and the relation of the sexes at Berlin among the deaths from croup between 1838 and 1849, was, as nearly as possible, as 6 to 4; the actual numbers being 545 male to 459 female children. See Hönerkopff über die Anwendung des schwefelsauren Kupferoxyd's gegen Croup. 8vo., Leipzig, 1852.

It may be noticed as a point of difference between croup and diphtheria that no such special liability of the male subject to its attacks is observed in the case of the latter disease. The proportion, indeed, would seem from the 24th Report of the Registrar-General to be almost reversed, since while 2821 male deaths, and only 2076 deaths of females, took place from croup in 1861 throughout England; 2450 female deaths, and only 2064 male deaths, occurred from diphtheria. M. Roger, in his valuable essay on diphtheritic paralysis, notices the same fact, of the equal liability of both sexes to diphtheria, or that if any difference exists between the liability of the two sexes to diphtheria, it is the female sex which suffers the most; in the proportion of about 5 to 4. See p. 462 of vol. i of the Archives de Médecine for 1862.

instances, been overrated; but still it cannot be denied, for a most striking illustration of it is afforded by the comparative rarity of croup in towns, and its frequency in rural districts. In the county of Surrey, exclusive of the metropolitan districts, the mortality, from all causes, under five years of age, is little more than a third of the mortality in Liverpool, and little more than half the mortality in London. But the total mortality, under five years of age, from croup in the county of Surrey is to that in Liverpool nearly as 3 to 2, and to that in London as 2 to 1; so that out of 100 children dying under five years of age from all causes, more than four times as many will have died from croup in Surrey as in Liverpool, and exactly four times as many as in London.

Variations in the condition of the atmosphere, and peculiarities of situation, not only influence the frequency of the occurrence of croup, but they likewise greatly modify its character, and determine to a considerable extent the nature of the lesions which it produces. The chief *morbid appearances*, however, are always discovered in the larynx, trachea, and air-tubes. They consist of redness of the mucous membrane, which is often thickened, sometimes abraded or ulcerated, and very generally covered with a more or less abundant exudation of false membrane. This exudation, however, though so generally met with as to have suggested to medical writers the terms angina polyposa, angina membranacea, as appropriate designations of croup, is neither invariable in its occurrence, nor of a uniform extent in all cases. It is found in the larynx oftener than in the trachea, and in both more frequently than in the bronchi. Nevertheless, in many instances, the secretion of false membrane is so extensive as not only to line the larynx and trachea, but even to reach into the minuter air-tubes, forming a complete cast of many of their ramifications. There appears to be some connection between the circumstances in which children become attacked by croup, and the extent of false membrane in the air-passages, which a post-mortem examination reveals. In rural districts, where the disease wears throughout a sthenic character, false membrane is deposited in greater abundance and over a greater extent of surface than is usually observed in the case of the poor in this metropolis: while, on the other hand, we find in London a condition of unhealthy ulceration about the larynx; ulceration, and the deposit of false membrane about the tonsils and palate in many instances, appearances which are seldom met with in children placed in circumstances more favorable to health.[1]

In cases of croup that have come under my own observation, the formation of false membrane in the larynx has seemed almost invariably to precede its deposit in the trachea; and not infrequently it has been found constituting a tough, continuous membrane in the former situation, but growing less tenacious in the upper part of the trachea, and passing gradually into a thick, puriform mucus, interspersed with

[1] It is open to question how far one is justified in classing such cases with true croup; whether they do not approach more nearly to *diphtheria*, or whether at least they do not form a sort of connecting link between the two diseases.

shreds of lymph. I have usually observed the false membrane lining the whole of the larynx, and reaching down to the lower edge of the thyroid cartilage, while the trachea contained nothing else than a puriform matter, or glairy mucus, sometimes of a reddish color. In some instances the false membrane has been confined to the upper part of the larynx, lining the lower surface of the epiglottis, blocking up the opening of the sacculus laryngis, and covering the chordæ vocales, but not extending any further. When first secreted, the false membrane is firmly adherent to the mucous lining of the air-passages, but after a time a secretion of a puriform character is generally poured out, which detaches the membrane from its connections; and it is after this occurrence has taken place that tubular pieces of false membrane have sometimes been expectorated. This detachment of the false membrane from the subjacent surface takes place more frequently and more completely from the interior of the trachea than from that of the larynx. On removing the false membrane from the trachea, the lining of the tube is seldom found to present any change other than an increase of its vascularity, which, though sometimes very considerable, does not bear any certain relation to the amount of false membrane present. The greater difficulty in removing the false membrane from the larynx depends upon the more extensive alterations which the lining of that part of the air-tubes is usually found to have undergone. It is generally red and swollen, especially about the edges of the rima glottidis and the arytenoid cartilages, and the opening of the sacculus laryngis. Small aphthous ulcerations are also frequent in the two former situations; and occasionally, the ulceration being more extensive, the whole of the larynx, on detaching the false membrane that lined it, presents a worm-eaten appearance.

It seldom happens that the bronchi are perfectly free from disease; but even if the trachea should contain no false membrane, and should present but few signs of inflammation, they are almost always much congested, and contain a muco-purulent or purulent secretion: though false membrane is seldom found in them, except when it is continuous with a similar adventitious structure in the trachea.

Pneumonia, in all its stages, is far from being unusual, and is a complication especially to be feared in those cases where croup occurs as a secondary affection in the course of measles.

The cavity of the mouth and the fauces do not present any invariable alteration in cases of croup. Congestion about the fauces and soft palate is of frequent occurrence, sometimes coupled with a scanty deposit of false membrane in those situations, or the tonsils are found in a state of ulceration. In that form of croup which succeeds to measles, there is moreover in many instances a condition of unhealthy inflammation, and aphthous ulceration of the mouth and gums; a slight speck of ash-colored false membrane covering each little ulcer. In many of these cases I apprehend that the laryngeal affection does not come on in consequence of extension to the air-passages of disease beginning in the mouth, but that the disease is the same in both situations; though the accident of the locality renders that a serious disorder when seated in the larynx, which is but a trivial ailment when affecting the mouth.

Cases of this last kind have been called cases of ulcerative laryngitis: they have always come under my notice associated with the exudation of false membrane, and I suspect their affinities are with diphtheria rather than with true croup.

Whatever be the circumstances in which croup comes on, the *symptoms* resulting from disease obstructing the channel of the larynx and trachea by false membrane, or inducing a spasmodic closure of their aperture, must always be to a great extent the same. Its mode of onset, however, is very variable. Sometimes, especially in those forms of croup that prevail among healthy children living in the country, the disease is announced by few, if any, premonitory symptoms; but the affection of the larynx is apparent from the very outset, and attains, in the course of a few hours, to a high degree of intensity. Some years since I saw a little boy, about seven years old, living at some distance from London. He had overheated himself at play during the afternoon of a hot day in August, but went to bed apparently well at eight o'clock, and soon fell asleep. At ten, he began to breathe with the peculiar noise characteristic of croup, and presented all the symptoms of the disease before midnight.

In his treatise on croup, Professor Gölis, of Vienna,[1] relates the case of a little boy, four years old, previously in perfect health, who having gone out of an overheated room into the open air, during an extremely cold winter's day, was seized while walking with all the symptoms of most violent croup, which proved fatal in fourteen hours.

This sudden onset and rapid course of the disease, however, are of rare occurrence, and croup generally comes on gradually, attended in *its first stage* by but few symptoms that could distinguish it from ordinary catarrh. Slight fever, drowsiness, suffusion of the eyes, and defluxion from the nares, attend it. The respiration is not perceptibly disturbed, and the cough, though frequent, presents no peculiar character. There is, besides, occasional complaint of slight sore throat, or of uneasy sensation about the larynx, but so slight as scarcely to attract attention, and not sufficient to cause any alarm.

The duration of this stage is very variable: nor is there any regularity in the mode of its transition into *the second stage*. In the majority of cases, indeed, the transition takes place gradually; but thirty-six hours seldom pass without the supervention of some symptom which, to the well-schooled observer, would betray the nature of the coming danger. Most symptoms may continue unchanged, perhaps scarcely aggravated, but a slight modification takes place in the character of the cough, which now becomes attended with a peculiar ringing sound, difficult to describe, but when once heard not easily forgotten. This peculiarity in the cough very often precedes any change in the respiration, and may sometimes be so slight as scarcely to attract the parent's notice at the time, and to be remembered only when the full development of the disease leads to inquiries as to how the attack came on. Soon after this modification of the cough has become per-

[1] De rite cognoscendâ et sanandâ Anginâ Membranaceâ, 8vo. Viennæ. Observ. iv, p. 141.

ceptible, or even simultaneously with it, the respiration undergoes a change no less remarkable. The act of inspiration becomes prolonged, and attended with a stridor as difficult to describe, but as characteristic of the disease, as the tone of the cough. It often happens that these two pathognomonic symptoms first come on, or at least first excite attention, in the night, and that a child who at bedtime was supposed to ail nothing, or at most to have a slight cold, awakes suddenly with ringing cough and stridulous breathing, frequently in a state of alarm, and with marked dyspnœa. Through the whole course of the disease, indeed, an obvious tendency exists to nocturnal exacerbations, and to remissions as the morning approaches. In whatever manner these symptoms may have come on, they will not continue for many hours without being attended by increase of fever, by acceleration, and soon by difficulty of respiration. The skin becomes hot and dry, the face flushed, the breathing hurried, the cough frequent, the pulse full and quick, the child dull, fretful, and passionate. For a few minutes, indeed, it may appear cheerful, may turn to its playthings, and breathe more naturally, though the peculiar respiratory sound never ceases altogether. Soon, however, the dyspnœa returns with increased intensity; the whole chest heaves with the inspiratory effort, which is more prolonged, and attended with great stridor. During it perspiration breaks out at every pore, and the veins of the neck and face become greatly distended. Short and forcible expiration follows, and after this state of dyspnœa has lasted for some minutes, an interval of comparative ease succeeds. The child now often falls asleep exhausted; but during sleep, the sound attending respiration is heard in an exaggerated degree. Though the drowsiness is great, sleep is uneasy, and frequently interrupted by violent startings, in spite of which the child may still sleep on. After some minutes he awakes in a state of terror, to pass through another paroxysm similar to the preceding one, though more severe. The cough does not increase in severity in proportion as the disease advances; it is unattended by expectoration, or at most a little mucus is spit up, but without any relief. Although the paroxysms of dyspnœa are not dependent on the cough, they are sometimes provoked by it, and the two or three inspirations next following an effort of coughing are often attended with increased stridor. From the first appearance of the more marked symptoms, the voice is hoarse, cracked, and whispering, or in young children is either totally suppressed, or, if their voice is not actually extinct, at least their disinclination to speak is so great that they will reply to questions only by signs, and cannot be induced by any persuasion to utter a word.

There is almost always much eagerness for drink, and deglutition is generally well performed. The fauces are often red, though their redness bears no direct proportion to the intensity of the croupal symptoms; and there is frequently considerable tenderness of the larynx. The tongue is red at the tip and edges, but coated in the centre and at the back with thick white fur; the bowels are rather constipated, and the appetite for food is entirely lost.

As the disease advances, the paroxysms become less marked, or rather, the intermissions grow less distinct, and the child is constantly [illegible] with the effort to respire. The cough now sometimes ceases altogether, and the breathing frequently becomes sibilant rather than stridulous. The child throws its head back as far as possible, in order to increase the capacity of the trachea; the chest is heaved violently at each effort to inspire, during which its lateral region becomes flattened, and all the soft parts of its parietes recede, indicating the inadequacy of the attempt to fill them; and the larynx is depressed forcibly towards the sternum, while the abdominal muscles co-operate energetically in expiration. The face is heavy and anxious, the eyes are dull, the lips livid, the skin dry, and the extremities cold; or clammy sweats bedew the surface. The respiration is hurried, unequal, and irregular, and the pulse is very frequent and very feeble. Though no remissions now occur, there are frequent exacerbations, in which the child throws itself about, and puts its hand to its throat, as though to tear away some obstacle to the admission of air, while helpless, hopeless agony is depicted on its countenance. In the midst of these sufferings the patient dies, or coma or convulsions come on, and close the scene.

It is not always, however, that *the last stage* of croup is attended by such distressing symptoms. The treatment employed may seem to have mitigated the severity of the disease; the restlessness may give place to ease, the burning skin may grow moist, the respiration may become tranquil, the cough loose with but little clangor; expectoration may be easy, and a wheezing, attended with a very slight croupy sound, may be the only indication of the dangerous disease under which the patient is suffering. This apparent amendment may continue for a few hours, and then be succeeded, without any assignable cause, by the return of all the former symptoms, and soon be followed by death; or, the mitigation of the disease may be accompanied with great drowsiness, which, however, does not excite alarm, since it is very naturally attributed to the exhaustion produced partly by the disease, partly by the remedies. During sleep, the respiration is deep and tranquil, like that of a person in a sound slumber; it is, indeed, attended by a kind of wheeze, but presents little of the croupy stridor; and when awake the child is quite sensible, and even cheerful. After a time, however, it becomes difficult thoroughly to rouse him; his pulse grows more rapid, the moisture on his skin changes almost imperceptibly to a cold clammy sweat, and convulsive twitchings of the angles of the mouth occasionally disturb the repose of his features. Silently, but surely, the exudation has been making progress, and when the alarm is taken, it is too late; the stupor deepens, and the child dies comatose, or rouses only to spend its last hours in the vain struggle for breath, and embittered by all the painful circumstances which ordinarily attend the suffocative stage of croup.

Auscultation yields us information in cases of croup with reference to two important points; namely, the amount of obstruction to the entrance of air into the lungs, and the extent of disease of the air-tubes or substance of the lungs which accompanies it. At first, air is heard entering the chest freely, and unattended by any morbid sound other than that stridor which is produced in the larynx. If the lungs should continue unaffected, no other morbid sound will be heard; but as the disease advances, the same negative results will be obtained from auscultation as are yielded by it in cases of emphysema—a feeble respiratory murmur belying the loud resonance on percussion. Often, however, respiration is attended from the commencement with the sonorous rhonchus of the first stage of bronchitis, though masked to some extent by the croupy noise in the trachea. Even in cases where the disease was originally confined to the larynx or trachea, inflammation almost always extends to the bronchi; often, also, to the substance of the lungs, so that mucous or subcrepitant râle generally becomes perceptible during its course, often attended by impaired resonance on percussion over the lower part of the chest. Air, however, may enter so imperfectly as not to fill the smaller bronchi; and these sounds may be quite unperceived, unless the auscultator listens at the moment when the child makes an unusually deep inspiration, such as often follows a fit of coughing. The pneumonia, too, in all cases that I have observed, was double, and the resonance consequently nearly equally diminished on both sides of the chest. Hence the importance of comparing the sound elicited by percussion of the upper with that given out by the lower part of the chest—a point to which you will remember that your attention has already been called on several occasions.

The changes in the tracheal sound which attend the progress of the disease may be traced with great distinctness by applying a stethoscope to the larynx. Some writers have thought that they recognized in its variations the indications of the formation of false membrane, and that these changes also afford a means whereby to judge of its extent. I believe that usually, when false membrane has been extensively formed in the larynx, the tracheal sound becomes less stridulous and more sibilant; but I noticed on one occasion those alterations in the tracheal sound which are supposed to indicate the presence of a very extensive deposit of false membrane, although no false membrane was either expectorated during the patient's lifetime, or discovered in the inflamed larynx and trachea after her death. We must conclude, therefore, that the changes in the tracheal sound do not afford absolutely certain evidence of the existence of false membrane, and that still less can they be regarded as safe criterions of its extent.

It is difficult to state with precision the *duration* of a disease such as croup, since its premonitory symptoms vary greatly, and its fatal termination is often in great measure due to the concomitant or consecutive bronchitis or pneumonia. When the laryngeal affection goes on to destroy life, it is seldom that more than forty-eight, or at the most seventy-two hours elapse from the full development of the croupal symptoms to the fatal event; and, allowing the ordinary duration of the premonitory stage to be about thirty-six hours, the disease will be found to run its course in from four to six days. Twice I knew death take place within thirty-six hours from the occurrence of the first croupal symptoms; and on a third occasion within thirty-seven hours; but these are instances of unusually rapid termination of the disease. Treatment sometimes partially subdues it; but it returns, and the relapse, in the course of a few hours, proves fatal. Now and then the acute symptoms subside, and the disease assumes a chronic character; but

this has very rarely come under my notice in idiopathic croup, though it is more common in that form of the disease which we shall have hereafter to notice as constituting a serious complication of measles.

The *prognosis* of croup must always be guarded, and is generally unfavorable, since the disease is unquestionably one of the most dangerous to which childhood is liable. Much depends upon the patient being seen at an early stage of the disease; and the prospect of recovery is generally very small if no treatment should have been adopted until after the full development of the symptoms. The presence ot bronchitis, and, still more of pneumonia, adds greatly to the dangers of the affection, and would induce us to form a very unfavorable opinion of the chances of recovery. A second attack of croup is generally less serious than the first; and cases in which catarrhal symptoms have preceded the seizure for several days are more amenable to treatment than those in which the premonitory stage has been short, or altogether absent. Diminution of the dyspnœa in the intervals of the cough—a louder and looser cough, attended with expectoration or vomiting of muco-purulent matter, intermingled with shreds of false membrane—a less suppressed voice, less anxiety, and less restlessness—all indicate that the disease is abating. Much caution, however, must be exercised in drawing a favorable conclusion from a diminution of the severity of the symptoms, until such improvement has continued for twenty-four hours at least. In all but the most acute cases of croup the remittent character of the disease is very apparent; and it is well to bear in mind that the fatal termination usually takes place with extreme rapidity, when an exacerbation of the symptoms follows soon after a manifest remission of their intensity.[1] It can scarcely be necessary to remind you that extinction of the voice, suppression of the cough, the change from stridulous to sibilant breathing, and increased difficulty of respiration, all show death to be surely and speedily approaching.

The danger of being lulled into security by the apparent improvement of a child who has been attacked by croup, is so serious, that before proceeding to consider the treatment of the disease I will relate to you a case by way of caution. On the 25th of June, a little girl, four years old, became hoarse and lost her appetite, though she did not appear otherwise ill. On the 27th she seemed less well, and in the night was very restless, and had difficulty of breathing. On the 28th respiration was more difficult, and though she had but little cough, she seemed sometimes in danger of choking. In the night a croupy sound accompanied her breathing, and violent attacks of dyspnœa were of frequent occurrence.

On the 29th she was taken to a surgeon, who gave her some medicine, after each dose of which she was sick, and this sickness was followed by much relief, and by an almost complete cessation of the croupy sound. This improvement was thought to have continued during the 30th; the child slept quietly during the night, and was

[1] "Mox post symptomatum remissionem recidivantes, brevi ac certâ morte demuntur." Gölis, lib. cit., p. 164.

considered so much better by her parents that she was brought by them to the Children's Hospital at 9 A.M. on July 1st. As she lay in the lap in a sitting posture, her countenance was pale and livid, her respiration was sibilant, her surface cool, her pulse very frequent and feeble, but there did not appear to be any of the distress usual in the advanced stages of croup. At 9 A.M. she was admitted; at 6 P.M. she died; though no great distress nor violent struggle for breath preceded her death. The extensive deposit of false membrane in the trachea and bronchi showed that, in spite of her apparent amendment for a season, disease must all the time have been advancing, unsuspected by her friends, overlooked even by her medical attendant.

In no disease is the prompt employment of appropriate treatment more important than in croup, since in none does the use of remedies sooner become unavailing. Even in cases where the attack is merely apprehended, but where catarrh exists, attended with a slight ringing cough, such as often indicates the commencement of croup, the patient should be watched most sedulously, and visited not merely by daytime, but also late in the evening; and attention should be particularly directed to the character of the respiration during sleep as well as in the waking state. The child should at once be placed in a warm bath, be confined to bed, be placed on a spare diet, and should take an emetic of ipecacuanha and antimony, to be followed by some mild saline medicine, containing slightly nauseating doses of antimonial wine.[1] At the same time the air which the child breathes should be both warm and moist, the temperature of the room being steadily kept up at 65°, while the moisture of the air is easily maintained, by a kettle boiling on the fire, with a long roll of paper, or, still better, a tin tube attached to its spout, which serves to direct the steam into the apartment. These simple precautions, useful in diminishing the irritability of the air-tubes when croup is merely threatened, are, I need scarcely say, of still greater moment when the disease is fully developed.[2] By these measures, which should be observed with especial care if the premonitory symptoms of croup appear in a child who has previously suffered from the disease, or in whose family a liability to it exists, you may often succeed in warding off the attack.

A far more energetic plan must be resorted to if the disease sets in with violence, or if, the indications of its approach having been either

---

[1] (No. 14.)

℞. Potassæ Bicarbonatis, gr. xl.
Acidi. Citrici, gr. xx.
Vin. Ant. Pot.-Tart., ℥iss.
Vin Ipecac., ♏xx.
Syr. Limonum, ℥iiss.
Aquæ, ℥iiss. M. ft. Mist.

A dessertspoonful every 3 or 4 hours. For a child two years old.

[2] At the Children's Hospital, so much importance is attached to the maintenance of a warm and moist atmosphere around the croup patient, that we are accustomed to inclose the bed with curtains, and to introduce within them the steam from boiling water, so as to maintain uniformity of moisture and temperature if necessary for days together. Many contrivances have been employed for this purpose. My colleague, Dr. Gee, has devised a very ingenious one, which we always use at the Children's Hospital.

overlooked or unchecked, the symptoms should have attained their full development before the patient came under your notice. The abstraction of blood, and the administration of tartar emetic, are the two measures on which your main reliance must be placed; remembering that if relief do not come soon it will not come at all—that there is not danger only, but death, in delay. I have never met with an exception to the rule which prescribes the free abstraction of blood in every case of severe idiopathic croup, when seen at an early period, and before the purple lips and livid countenance, and failing pulse, announce the long-continuance of a serious obstacle to the free admission of air into the lungs. Even in very young children local depletion forms in these cases but a poor substitute for general bleeding, for it is not merely the abstraction of a certain quantity of blood that is needed, but its removal in such a manner as most speedily to produce an effect on the system. Bleeding from the jugular vein is preferable in these circumstances to venesection in the arm, since the latter often fails in children under three years old; and the blood never flows so freely as when taken from the jugular vein. It is not easy to state in figures the exact quantity to be abstracted, since the child's previous health, the intensity of the symptoms, and the effect produced by the flow of the blood, must all be taken into account in determining when to stop. Dr. Cheyne says, "The removal of three ounces of blood from a child between one and two years of age, or of six ounces from a child from eight till ten, generally appears to make a sufficient impression on the disease; and this is a sufficiently near approach to a correct estimate of what is usually needed. The effect of free venesection is often very striking, and as the blood flows, the respiration may be seen to become notably easier. But though the relief thus afforded is very great, it proves but temporary; and unless followed by other remedies, the symptoms will often regain their former intensity in the course of four or six hours. I have not seen any instance in which the repetition of general bleeding appeared indicated, but I have occasionally employed local depletion with advantage a few hours after the general bleeding; though, if you follow up the first loss of blood by the free employment of tartar emetic, you will generally be spared the necessity for further depletion. It has been recommended that leeches should be applied to the top of the sternum rather than to the windpipe, since difficulty may be experienced in arresting the bleeding if applied in the latter situation, as children are very intolerant of pressure in that neighborhood. The caution is worth bearing in mind; but if you superintend the application of the leeches yourselves, which in such a case you certainly ought to do, the advantage of drawing the blood as nearly as possible from the affected part will more than make up for the risk of some slight difficulty in stopping its flow.

To accomplish any real good by means of the tartar emetic it must be given in doses of an eighth, a quarter, or half a grain every ten minutes until vomiting is produced; and the same doses should afterwards be continued every half-hour, until decided and permanent relief has been afforded. The dose that at first caused vomiting may, after it has been repeated a few times, cease to excite it, in which case we must increase it, and not rest satisfied with tolerance of the medicine having been established, since its utility appears to be closely connected with its emetic power. Nauseating doses of antimony have not seemed to me to check the disease so surely, while they cause a greater depression of the system, and thus mask the approach of the fatal event. A striking illustration of the superiority of emetic over nauseating doses of medicine is given by M. Valleix,[1] who states that, in thirty-one out of fifty-three cases of true croup, ipecacuanha and antimony were employed in full doses as emetics, and of these thirty-one cases fifteen recovered; while of the twenty-two cases in which their use was but sparingly resorted to, only one survived.

If, after antimony has been thus administered for four or six hours, no satisfactory measure of improvement should have appeared, local depletion may be resorted to. If the croupal symptoms, on the other hand, should have begun to abate, the antimony may be given at longer intervals; but you cannot be too much on your guard against being misled by temporary improvement, and abandoning the medicine too soon. Its use likewise is not to be relinquished by gradually diminishing the dose and substituting a quantity sufficient only to induce nausea for that which caused vomiting, but a full dose should be given every hour or two hours, instead of every half-hour, and if amendment continues, the interval may be prolonged to three, four, or six hours. It is now, after the severity of the disease has been subdued by antimony, that the time has come for the administration of calomel. From the very commencement of the attack, mercurial inunction may be had recourse to every two or three hours; or a flannel bandage, on which two drachms of mercurial ointment have been spread, may be swathed around the abdomen of the patient; but the action of mercurials is far too slow to overtake at its outset a disease which tends so rapidly to a fatal issue. At this period, however, calomel seems to have a twofold utility; it counteracts the tendency to the formation of false membrane in the air-passages, and prevents or subdues that inflammation of the lungs which is so frequent and so fatal a complication of the disease. I usually employ it in doses of half a grain or a grain in children from two to five years old every hour or two hours, in combination with minute doses of ipecacuanha, but interrupting its use at intervals in order to give an antimonial emetic. The appearance of any exacerbation of the croupal symptoms, however, would lead me at once to discontinue the calomel, and to return to the emetic employment of antimony.

It is not unintentionally, nor from any oversight, that I have allowed my observations on the treatment of true croup to remain unaltered; expressing the opinions which I formed, and the practice which I adopted, thirty years ago. Both indeed have been modified, just as the treatment of bronchitis and pneumonia has been modified, by the changes in the epidemic constitution of disease which recent years have brought with them, and which have been especially marked since the second epidemic prevalence of cholera in this country in 1848 and

---

[1] Bulletin Général de Thérapeutique, Oct. 1848, p. 246.

1849. But with every allowance made for these changes, I still believe that a decided antiphlogistic treatment (by which I mean the employment of antimony in emetic doses, the subsequent administration of calomel, and if the case be seen at the very outset, the recourse to actual depletion) is indicated in almost all cases of acute idiopathic croup.

I have full notes of 114 cases of croup or diphtheria, though very many more have come under my observation in consultation, when I have seen them one, two, or three times. The earliest date borne by these notes is July, 1840, and for the first ten subsequent years all cases, with the exception of those secondary to measles, were treated by me with uniform activity, in accordance with the principles laid down by Dr. Cheyne, and to which reference has already been made.[1]

About this time, however, I find from my notes evidence of a gradual falling off in the activity of my treatment, and this in spite of my field of observation having shifted to a district in which disease generally, and croup among the rest, presented a more sthenic character than it wore in the low-lying district to the south of the Thames. I notice less frequent employment of depletion, and at the same time recourse to cauterization of the throat, a proceeding to which I was led in a measure by Dr. Horace Green's remarks on cauterization of the larynx in croup, and which therefore had by no means constant reference to the presence of false membrane about the fauces.

For some years past I have given up the charge of out-patients at the Children's Hospital, and almost all the cases of croup which I see in private I see in consultation, and consequently when some symptom of special gravity has already arisen. It may perhaps be due in part to these circumstances that I have met with no occasion for depletion during the past ten years. I have, however, met with not a few instances of idiopathic laryngeal croup, which, in the hands of younger practitioners who thought of nothing but diphtheria, were being plied with stimulants and perchloride of iron, and were saved by antimony, by emetics, and the use of mercurials.

In Germany, in spite of the prevalence of diphtheria there as well as here, the old form of inflammatory croup still prevails; and some of the older practitioners[2] have raised their voice against the tendency to ignore its existence, to assume that diphtheria is the one only form of croup, that the observers of five-and-twenty or fifty years ago committed a mistake in supposing that antiphlogistic treatment was ever called for, or that stimulants could possibly be out of place.

My object is to warn against the same errors, to insist on the difference in character between cynanche trachealis and diphtheria, and, as a consequence, on the necessary difference between their treatment.

There is, however, one point which it is important to remember in

---

[1] The peculiarities of this form of secondary croup, and its relation to the then so-called diphtheritis, were noticed by me, and illustrated by cases, in the Medical Gazette, Aug 25, 1843.

[2] Among them is especially deserving of notice a short paper by Dr. Clemens, of Frankfort, in J. f. Kinderkrankh., vol. xxxvi, June, 1861, p. 359.

the management of the severe cases of croup, lest you fall into the error of overtreating your patient; an error not less hazardous than the opposite one of too great inertness. The disease, as you know, has a marked tendency to exacerbations and remissions, even independently of any physical change in the condition of the respiratory organs. You must not, therefore, allow the return of more difficult breathing, after a period of comparative tranquillity, to lead you at once to the inference that the child is worse, and that necessity exists for renewed and increased activity of treatment. It is very possible that the increased dyspnœa may be merely spasmodic; that immersing the child in a hot bath will give immediate and most signal relief; and that if you auscultate the chest afterwards you will find the air entering the lungs in as large a quantity as before, and unattended by an increase of morbid sounds.

The administration of calomel is not necessary in every case of croup, for when seen early, and treated with due activity, its symptoms are sometimes completely removed in the course of a few hours. But though we may sometimes be warranted in suspending all active treatment for a season, yet we must watch our patient with most untiring care for some days after the decline of the acute croupal symptoms, and at each visit our attention must be directed to the condition of the lungs, in order that we may at once put a stop at its very commencement to that inflammation of the smaller bronchi and of the pulmonary substance which so often disappoints the fairest prospects of recovery. Its treatment does not differ from that of ordinary bronchitis or pneumonia, except that depletion is not generally indicated, and that it not infrequently becomes necessary to support the patient's strength even from a very early period.

Your own good sense will suggest to you the care and watching which are required during convalescence from croup; the necessity of withdrawing your remedies cautiously, and of awaiting the complete disappearance of all hoarseness, and the cessation of all cough, before you allow the child to breathe the external air. In cases where the peculiar croupal sound continues with slight cough, long after every other sign of mischief about the larynx has subsided, you will often find it of service to paint the neighborhood of the larynx every day with the tincture of iodine; a mild, but in the circumstances a very efficacious form of counter-irritation.

It still remains for us to inquire into the treatment of cases in which we have not the good fortune to encounter the disease at its outset, but in which we have to combat it when it has already reached the second stage.

This subject, however, must be reserved for our next lecture.

LECTURE XXIV.

CROUP continued.—Treatment of the more advanced stages of the disease—Tracheotomy—The difference between the results obtained by it in England and in France, and its probable cause—Objections to its performance—Reasons for not regarding them as conclusive—Inquiry into the object of the operation—Indications for its performance—Its dangers—And how they are to be obviated.

IN the last lecture we were occupied with the consideration of the management of those cases of croup in which the patient is seen early, and in which his condition warrants the employment of powerful antiphlogistic measures. He may, however, be seen too late for such means to be allowable or they may have been tried in vain. If antimony ceases to vomit, or if it is rejected immediately and without effort, the fluid thrown up being unmixed with phlegm or false membrane, while the temperature sinks, the lips grow more livid, the pulse becomes more frequent and feeble, and the paroxysms of dyspnœa are undiminished in severity; or if the respiration, though less laborious, is attended with a sibilant instead of a stridulous sound, it is evident that by continuing the medicine we may destroy the patient, but shall fail to cure the disease. A totally different plan of *treatment* must at once be adopted, though with but slender hope of success.

An attempt should be made to arouse the child from the state of collapse into which it is sinking, by placing it for a few minutes in a hot mustard bath, and emetics of the sulphate of copper should at once be administered. The sulphate of copper has been considered by some writers to be possessed of a specific influence over croup. I cannot, however, take this view of its action. It has seemed to me to be nothing more than an emetic of great power, and therefore especially applicable in cases where considerable depression exists, where the stomach has consequently lost much of its irritability, and where tartar emetic would probably not act at all, or if it did, would be injurious from its depressing action. Alum has been recommended in similar circumstances, and I dare say would answer equally well, though perhaps there is some advantage in the smaller bulk of the sulphate of copper.[1] I am accustomed to give it dissolved in water in quarter or half-grain doses every quarter of an hour till free vomiting has been produced, but have never trusted to it alone, in the same way as in an earlier stage of the disease I am used to rely on tartar emetic. I employ it with a twofold purpose: first, to obtain the stimulant action of an emetic; second, to prevent, if possible, the accumulation of false

[1] Alum has been used and strenuously recommended in these circumstances by Dr. Meigs, of Philadelphia; and the experience of his son, Dr. J. Meigs, as recorded in his work on Diseases of Children, seems fully to bear out his father's recommendation. He gives a teaspoonful in honey or syrup, every 10 or 15 minutes, till free vomiting is produced. See Meigs and Pepper, op. cit., 4th ed., 1870, p. 99.

to be much alleviated, the respiration to be rendered far more easy, and expectoration for the first time to accompany the cough. In any case, if very manifest relief were not observed within six hours after the abstraction of blood and the administration of antimony, while further depletion did not appear justifiable, I should apply a blister to the throat.[1]

It was to be expected that the probable utility of *bronchotomy* in cases of croup should suggest itself to the earliest observers of the disease. For many years, however, after it was first advocated on theoretical grounds by Dr. Home, the value of the operation was not put to the test; and even for a long time after it had been tried, but one instance was recorded of any other than an unsuccessful result.[2] In the year 1825, M. Bretonneau, of Tours, saved the life of a little girl when in the last stage of croup by performing tracheotomy. Eight years afterwards a second operation was performed and a second success obtained by M. Trousseau, and in the subsequent five-and-twenty years the operation was had recourse to in France nearly 500 times, and about a fourth of the patients on whom it was performed recovered.[3] This proportion, too, may be taken as representing very nearly the present rate of recoveries after the operation of tracheotomy in early life, when had recourse to either for croup or diphtheria.

The results of the operation in this country are, however, far less favorable than those which have been obtained in France, and many attempts, though none to the best of my judgment altogether satisfactory, have been made to account for this difference. I once thought that the difference between the characters of the disease in the two countries might account for the different results of tracheotomy; that the diphtheritic form of croup which prevailed in France might be more amenable to mechanical relief than the sthenic variety, associated with bronchitis or pneumonia almost from the outset, which was more frequent in this country. Recently, however, the character of the disease in the two countries has become more closely assimilated, without influencing the great preponderance of successes on the other side of the Channel. Sir W. Jenner[4] suggests that the greater frequency of rickets

---

[1] This opinion being opposed to that of men such as Sir W. Stokes and Mr. Porter, I feel it necessary to appeal in support of it to the authority of Gölis, lib. cit., p. 118; and Albers, De Tracheitide Infantum, p. 127; and not to rest it solely on the results of my own experience.

[2] In this case the operation was performed in the year 1782 by M. André, of London, on a little girl, five years old. The particulars are related in a dissertation published at Leyden in 1786, by Mr T. White, whence they are extracted by Dr. Farre, and appended as a note to a paper of his on Croup, at p. 338 of vol. iii of the Medico-Chirurgical Transactions.

[3] The most recent statements with which I am acquainted of the results of tracheotomy in France, are those of MM. H. Roger and Sée, which yield 126 recoveries to 446 operations, or 27 per cent. during the last seven years Gaz. Hebdom., Nov. 12, 1858, p. 789. The somewhat more recent estimate given by M. Roger, in his paper on Diphtheria already referred to, does but confirm on the whole the accuracy of his previous conclusions. M. Trousseau, in his Clinique de l'Hôtel Dieu, 2d ed., vol. i, p. 438, which was published in 1865, states that down to that time he had performed tracheotomy more than 200 times, and more than a fourth of the cases had had a successful result.

[4] Op. cit., p. 80.

in this country, and the consequent greater flexibility of the chest-walls; as the result of which mechanical power is wanting to draw air beyond the fluid which from any cause finds its way into the bronchial tubes, has much to do with the different results obtained in the two countries. Something, too, is unquestionably due to the earlier stage of the disease in which the operation is resorted to on the Continent[1] than in England, so that while in this country a successful tracheotomy represents a child snatched from inevitable death, in not a few of the instances of its performance in France other means might have been tried, and would probably have controlled the disease. Still, if these facts detract something from the apparent value of the operation, they at least show that in itself it is not attended by serious dangers; and statistics prove that, in as far at least as the diphtheritic form of croup is concerned,[2] there is no sort of connection between an increase of frequency in the performance of tracheotomy and a higher mortality from the disease. Further, it must be conceded that the somewhat premature performance of tracheotomy is not without some compensating advantage, by the relief it affords to that spasmodic action of the muscles of the glottis which endangers the patient's life, independently of the extent of false membrane in the glottis. My own personal experience of the results of tracheotomy is exceptionally unfavorable, inasmuch as I have to record but seven recoveries out of thirty operations. In most of these cases the disease had already reached an advanced stage when the patients came under my care, and the operation was resorted to as a doubtful remedy, holding out a chance of recovery when otherwise none appeared.[3] I suspect indeed that it will be found that the date of performance of the operation has more than anything else to do with its result. In New York tracheotomy appears to have been performed in general at an early stage of croup, and 213[4] cases yielded 50 recoveries, a proportion as high as that obtained in Paris. My own experience too points in the same direction; the first 16 of my cases yielded but 1 recovery, the second 14 gave 6.

In spite, however, of the unfavorable issue of many of my cases, I am so far from being opposed to tracheotomy, that the euthanasia which it secures, even when all hope of cure is gone, seems to me cheaply purchased by its performance. As a remedial measure, my chief anxiety is to make out the indications that may justify me in having more timely recourse to it in future. The discrepancies of

---

[1] In illustration of this fact two cases may be noticed, recorded in the Journal de la Société Médicale d'Indre et Loire, extracted and commented on in the Bull. Gén. de Thérapeutique, Octobre, 1842.

[2] Roger and Sée, loc. cit.

[3] The thesis of M. Millard, De la Trachéotomie dans le cas de Croup, 4to., Paris, 1858, illustrates extremely well the almost invariable fatality of tracheotomy when performed on young children. Of 124 cases in which the operation was performed at the Hôpital des Enfans between January, 1857 and July, 1858, 29, or 24 per cent., had a favorable issue. But of twenty children under two years old who were operated on none survived; and of 36 between two and three only 5: the remaining 24 recoveries having been obtained in children between the ages of three and nine.

[4] As stated by Dr. Jacobi, of New York, in 1868, in a paper referred to by Meigs and Pepper, op. cit., 4th ed., 1870, p. 106.

opinion which have prevailed with reference to it are, I think, partly due to an overestimate, on the part both of its advocates and opponents, of the ends which it is proposed to attain by it. In itself, tracheotomy in croup is not a *curative* proceeding, nor can its performance warrant the discontinuance of those measures previously resorted to, whose object was to overcome the disease of the larynx and trachea. It professes to remove in some cases the danger of immediate death from suffocation, and thus to give time for nature and art to do their best in overcoming the inflammation of the air-passages, or in obviating its results. That it should prove inefficacious to accomplish this in cases where false membrane has extended to the extreme bronchi, is no argument against its performance in the present state of our knowledge, though it furnishes a cogent reason for the endeavor to perfect our diagnosis, so that our failures may be lessened by our less often attempting the impossible, or at least by our performing the operation with the avowed object of mitigating suffering, not of prolonging life.

The questions that call for determination in any endeavors to estimate the value of tracheotomy are, *first*, whether the danger arises from causes which in certain instances tracheotomy, and that alone, can remove; and *secondly*, whether the dangers attendant or consequent on the operation are themselves of such a kind as to outweigh its advantages. If these inquiries should be answered in favor of the operation, we may then endeavor to determine by what means its danger can be most effectually lessened, and those cases be best discriminated in which the benefits of the proceeding are likely to be most signal.

It has been objected by no less an authority than Dr. Cheyne, that inasmuch as three-eighths of the aperture of the larynx have been found free in fatal cases of croup, there must have existed during life room enough for the entrance of air; or that, in other words, the suffocative symptoms of croup do not depend on a cause which tracheotomy can remove. The operation, however, is not performed merely on the mechanical principle of removing from the windpipe a quantity of matter which prevents the entrance of air into the lung; but it is done rather to obviate the dangers of that spasm of the glottis which the inflammation or the deposit of false membrane occasions, and which will not cease until either the inflammation is subdued, or the spasm relaxes with the approach of death. Even the narrow opening made into the trachea—often much narrower than the aperture of the larynx, though diminished by swelling or encroached on by false membrane—suffices, for a time at least, to admit all the air which the patient needs, and the dyspnœa is relieved. The larynx is now at rest, while the air entering continuously, and without effort, duly oxygenates the blood; and the child is thus placed in a condition in which all remedial agents would seem much more likely to tell upon it, than when it was in a state of impending suffocation.

Tracheotomy, then, in cases of croup, answers a twofold end, and one not by other means attainable.[1] It removes in some instances a

[1] I purposely pass with this slight notice the proposition of M. Bouchut (originally suggested, indeed, by the famous Dessault) for the so-called "*tubage de la*

positive mechanical obstacle to the entrance of air into the lungs, while in all it puts a stop to that spasm of the glottis which interferes with respiration as much as the actual deposit of false membrane, though not so constantly nor with equal peril.

Now, it may be asked, what evils are there attendant on the operation that counterpoise these indisputable benefits? To this inquiry it does not seem to me that the opponents of tracheotomy give any sufficient answer. It is admitted on all hands that in itself the operation is not attended by serious hazard; while the uncertainty as to its issue depends, not on any defect in the proceeding, but on an imperfect knowledge of what cases are within the power of art to succor, and what are beyond the help, not of tracheotomy only, but of all other measures likewise. The shock of the operation is seldom serious except in cases where it has been delayed to the very last moment; serious hemorrhage is a very rare accident, and is generally due to the unskilfulness of the operator, while the dysphagia which occasionally follows is a troublesome rather than a dangerous occurrence; one, too, which is not encountered until the canula has been worn some days, and which is a result of the disease rather than of the operation; or, in other words, is due to the paralysis of the soft palate which follows diphtheria, and has no relation whatever to the laryngeal affection for which tracheotomy was resorted to, any more than to the tracheotomy itself. The gravest charge against it is that it is apt to induce serious bronchitis, or, at any rate, to aggravate any previously existing inflammation of the lungs or air-tubes. I am not altogether certain that there is not some ground for this accusation, but on the other hand it must be borne in mind that these very diseases are the ordinary, almost invariable, complications of croup, however treated; and further, that they are not ordinary sequelæ of tracheotomy when resorted to in other circumstances, as in cases of acute laryngitis, or of œdema of the glottis.

But if we come to the conclusion that in cases of croup which have not yielded to ordinary medical treatment, and in which there seems reason to anticipate a speedy death unless the inability to fill the lungs with air can be soon relieved, the operation of tracheotomy does not superadd some peculiar danger of its own more certain and more des-

glotte," or introduction of a tube within the canal of the larynx, in order to keep a passage permanently free for the entrance of air, and thus to do away with the necessity for the performance of tracheotomy in croup. M. Trousseau's Report on the subject to the Academy of Medicine at Paris, most temperately, but at the same time most conclusively, exposes the fallacies of M. Bouchut, and shows the small practical value of the suggestion, as well as its almost complete inapplicability to the treatment of croup Of seven cases in which this proceeding was resorted to five terminated fatally, and in the only two patients who recovered tracheotomy was performed. The proceeding is very difficult to accomplish, while in some instances the presence of the tube within the glottis could not be tolerated by the patients, and its removal was necessary; and though M Trousseau admits its possible utility in cases of œdema of the glottis, and of simple laryngitis, I should doubt whether even in these instances the presence of a foreign body within the opening of the larynx would not be likely to produce a most mischievous irritation of the diseased organ, and such as would far exceed that which would be excited by a tube in the trachea.

perate than those by which the patient is already surrounded, it then becomes our duty to resort to it; and this not at the last moment, but so soon as ever we feel that our remedies are too tardy to overtake the disease. In such circumstances, to gain time is to gain everything, and it is just this which tracheotomy places within our reach. It is not possible to fix absolutely what rate of mortality may be fairly expected to follow an operation performed in circumstances such as those which call for tracheotomy; for that, unlike most surgical proceedings, does not remove the disease for which it is had recourse to, it does but give the constitution another chance of battling with it; and many of the deaths after tracheotomy are, strictly speaking, far from being instances of failure of the operation. The operation may have done all that it could do, but false membrane may have extended far beyond the opening in the trachea, or the bronchitis may have reached the capillary air-tubes, or the pneumonia may have involved the pulmonary substance too extensively for recovery to be possible. We may hence deduce a limitation to the performance of tracheotomy which I cannot state better than in the words of its great advocate, M. Trousseau,[1] who "forbids the performance of the operation in any cases where the danger to the child appears to depend on disease of the general system rather than on the affection of the larynx or trachea." But in cases where no such contraindication exists, it is yet evident that the issue of the operation must be in a great measure controlled by the age of the patient, by the fact of the disease being idiopathic or secondary, by the extent of the disease of the respiratory organs generally, and that this influence must be of a kind which no surgical dexterity or medical skill can do much to control or to modify.

Some circumstances may, however, be borne in mind as influencing the result of tracheotomy, while at the same time they are not beyond the control of the medical attendant.

The *first* of these concerns the size of the tracheal tube, a point the importance of which was first insisted on by M. Trousseau. He explains the occasional speedy and apparently causeless disappearance of the amendment that at first succeeds the operation of tracheotomy, by the inadequate size of the canula which is frequently employed and which does not provide for the permanent admission of a sufficient quantity of air. The air admitted through even a small canula is enough to afford temporary relief, but not enough for the continued discharge of the functions of the organism; and the return of hurried breathing, and the reappearance of the livid hue of the surface, betoken the imperfect depuration of the blood. "Take," says he in illustration of this fact, "a quill, and, closing your nostrils, endeavor to breathe entirely through it: at first you breathe easily enough, but soon your respiration becomes laborious; and at length you are fain to throw away the quill, and with open mouth once more to fill your lungs completely. Now precisely this is what happens when an opening of inadequate size is made into the trachea; air enters readily, and without the interruption which the spasm of the glottis occasioned;

[1] Archives Gén. de Médecine, Mars, 1855, p. 257.

but it does not enter in sufficient quantity, and hence the return of the symptoms and the patient's death." Acting on this principle, M. Trousseau used to make a larger opening into the trachea, and to introduce a larger canula than had previously been customary; and this practice I believe to be now gaining ground among persons who have omitted to acknowledge their obligation to M. Trousseau for the suggestion. One word, moreover, must be added against the needless exaggeration of M. Trousseau's wise caution. It is, as Mr. Marsh has pointed out in his admirable paper on Tracheotomy in Children,[1] the size of the aperture of the glottis, not that of the trachea, which regulates the quantity of air inspired.

The *second* of these precautions has reference to the necessity of surrounding the child after the operation with a warm, moist atmosphere, such as alone it ought to be allowed to respire; though, unfortunately, this is very much neglected, not in hospitals only, but also in private practice. The importance of attention to this point, and also to keeping the canula free, cannot be overstated; and yet these little things are overlooked or intrusted to unskilful hands, because they seem too trivial for such large issues to be dependent on them.

The *third* caution which I would urge is, that medical treatment must not be suspended, nor necessarily modified, after tracheotomy has been performed. The operation, indeed, seems so heroic a measure, and when it yields relief, the relief is so speedy and so striking as to occasion some risk of its being forgotten that the disease has not been removed by it, that its danger has only been postponed, and that the indications for treatment continue the same after tracheotomy as they were before.

A word or two with reference to the after-management of cases of tracheotomy will comprise all that I have to say on this subject. My own patients have rarely lived long enough after the operation for me to become practically familiar with many of the difficulties which arise some few days after its performance. These, however, apart from such as are the consequences of the supervention or increase of the disease of the respiratory organs, are twofold, and arise from the condition of the wound, and from the occasional supervention of difficulty of swallowing.

One of the reasons for seeking to remove the canula as early as possible is supplied by the irritation of the edges of the wound which its long-continued presence is apt to produce. I saw the death of a child take place from this cause on the 11th day after the otherwise successful performance of tracheotomy by my colleague, Mr. Athol Johnson; and it was ascertained after death that, in addition to the destruction of several rings of the trachea, an abscess had formed in the anterior mediastinum which communicated with the external wound by sinuses that burrowed between the trachea and œsophagus. In fat children the unhealthy state of the edges of the wound is partly produced by the canula remaining deeply sunk in the flesh; an evil which would perhaps be lessened by the use of a long canula with a [illegible]

[1] St. Bartholomew's Hospital Reports, vol. iii, 1867, p. 331.

shield; or else by the employment of one "*à lorgnette*," as it has been termed by its inventor, M. Paul Guersant; that is to say, capable of being lengthened by pulling it out, like a telescope or an opera-glass. Besides this, the covering the wound with lint thickly spread with spermaceti ointment, and placing over that a piece of oiled silk so as to defend it as far as may be from irritation, and from the external air, as well as the touching its edges daily with the nitrate of silver, are the most important means of maintaining its healthy condition.

Another of the dangers of the operation depends on the abrasion of the mucous membrane of the trachea by the end of the canula, and its consequent ulceration. This danger, however, is almost, although perhaps not quite invariably, prevented by M. Lüer's modification of the canula, which was introduced to general notice by M. Roger. This modification consists in the canula being movable on the shield, so that its position shifts with the varying attitudes of the child.

The difficulty of deglutition is an inconvenience which usually comes on about the fifth or sixth day after the operation; that is to say, at the time when the larynx, though now free from the false membrane which before occluded it, has not completely recovered from the effects of the disease, but a state of partial paralysis of its muscles remains, which allows food, and especially liquids, to enter the air-tubes. This accident, which is by no means invariable in its occurrence, has probably little or no relation to the operation. It is a result of that paralysis of the soft palate and muscles of the pharynx which sometimes succeeds to diphtheria, and which, from being a troublesome accident, is converted by the previous tracheotomy into a dangerous complication. If the patient is sufficiently intelligent to admit of M. Archambault's suggestion[1] being adopted, and will place the finger on the opening of the tube, and endeavor to breathe quietly though the larynx when swallowing, it is very likely that the want of harmony between respiration and deglutition will be overcome in many instances, though, according to M. Trousseau's experience, by no means in all. In the majority of cases, however, we are compelled, by the tender age of our patients, to confine ourselves to feeding them as far as possible on solid, or at least on pultaceous food; rejecting all drink as far as possible, and giving it, when absolutely necessary, in small quantities, and either immediately before or a considerable time after food.[2] In some instances, M. Guersant[3] has found the use of the stomach-pump, or of a tube introduced through the nares, necessary to convey food safely into the stomach; though happily such are exceptional cases; while generally the larynx recovers itself in three or four days, and deglutition is then no longer attended with difficulty or danger.

It happens now and then that, after apparent recovery from croup or diphtheria, difficulty is experienced in the withdrawal of the canula, and that we are compelled to allow it to remain for an almost indefinite time. The cause of this difficulty is not always very obvious. At first

---

[1] L'Union Médicale, Juillet, 1854.

[2] Archives Gén. de Médecine, Mars, 1855.

[3] Notices sur la Chirurgie des Enfants, 8vo. Paris, 1864, pp. 34–48.

it seems to be owing to some impaired action of the laryngeal muscles; which having been thrown out of gear as it were by the operation, and in diphtheria partly also by the subsequent paralysis, are long in regaining their power of harmonious action. It is in inspiration that this condition is most marked; and while air passes out readily by the mouth; and inspiration too goes on fairly well for a short time, the ability to inspire continuously through the larynx is wanting. In some cases the child may even be able to breathe tolerably by the mouth during the daytime, and when quite quiet, but can no longer do so if hurried or excited; and no sooner falls asleep than it is seized with urgent dyspnœa; which subsides only on the reintroduction of the tube.

It is therefore a wise precaution, before attempting the final removal of the tube, to try how far the child is able to breathe with the orifice of the canula closed by a plug, and then to withdraw it at first in the daytime only; a competent person being at hand to replace the tube immediately if the respiration begins to be more hurried, and not to await the occurrence of severe dyspnœa.

But besides these cases, where the difficulty is but temporary, and is overcome by a little time and patience, there are some instances in which a distinct mechanical obstacle exists to the entrance of air. M. Guersant speaks of having met with perfect occlusion of the larynx after tracheotomy by the adhesion of false membrane to the vocal cords, and recommends that the larynx should be swept out by a little piece of lint introduced through the canula, and carried from below upwards so as to detach any adherent deposits.

He confesses, however, that the proceeding has not always been successful, and instances are on record in which the larynx has remained permanently obstructed, so that it was altogether impossible to remove the canula. In a patient of my own, operated on for diphtheritic croup, it was not until after the lapse of fourteen months, and after a variety of means had been resorted to by my colleague, Mr. Thomas Smith, to widen the canal, and to keep it pervious, that she was able entirely to lay aside the canula. Now, seven years after, she continues perfectly well, though her voice is gruff and low.

To Mr. T. Smith's most interesting paper[1] I must refer for a further detail of this case; and of all the difficulties he encountered, and how he overcame them; as well as for the particulars of other similar cases which may be found scattered through our medical literature.

---

[1] Medico-Chirurgical Transactions, vol. xlviii, 1865, p. 227.

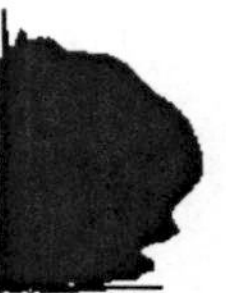

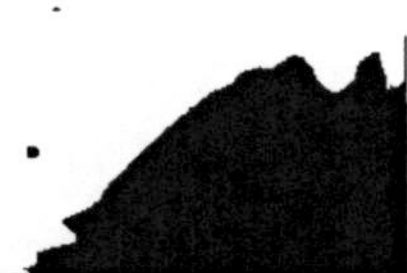

LECTURE XXV.

DIPHTHERIA, OR ANGINA MALIGNA.—Not a new disease—Its anatomical characters—Mode of extension of the disease—Its relation to true croup—Characteristic peculiarities of each disease.

Symptoms of diphtheria.—In its milder form, insidious supervention of croupal symptoms—In its severer forms, frequently associated with albuminuria—Peculiar depression which attends it—Evidence of its affinity to the class of blood diseases—Paralytic symptoms which follow it—Relation between it and scarlatina examined—Evidence on both sides of the question stated—That in favor of their non-identity considered to preponderate.

Treatment.—Local applications—Constitutional measures—Necessity for tonics and stimulants.

Modified form of the disease.—Usually a complication of measles—Its symptoms and treatment.

LARYNGITIS STRIDULA, or croup with predominance of spasmodic symptoms—Not a distinct disease, but results from constitutional peculiarity—Illustrative case.

Instances of spasmodic cough and affection of larynx, from irritation in lungs.—Intestines—Brain—Note on thymic asthma.

REFERENCE was made in the last lecture to a second form of disease, resembling croup in some respects though differing in others, alike but not the same, and calling therefore for a separate notice. This other disease, Angina Maligna, Diphtheritis, or more correctly Diphtheria, is no new malady,[1] but one which, though always prevalent, forces itself occasionally upon general notice by the formidable symptoms that sometimes attend it, by the rapidity with which it then runs its course, and by its selection of several victims from one town, one village, or one family. At such seasons it wears a character which seems so different from that which it assumes in its milder forms as to render it almost impossible to believe that the slight sore throat which caused only a trivial inconvenience, and hardly required any medical treatment, is one with the malignant disease, whose local symptoms are often cast into the shade by the grave constitutional disorder that attends them.

In each case, however, its essential anatomical characteristic is the same, and consists of redness, and swelling involving the tonsils and soft palate, and accompanied within a few hours by the exudation on their surface of a dense white false membrane, appearing in little points or spots, which speedily coalesce, and form a uniform investment to the

---

[1] Starr's unpretending account of the disease at Liskeard, a century ago, details all the most characteristic features of diphtheria. the false membrane on the fauces, its extension to the air-passages, its appearance on blistered surfaces and upon the skin behind the ears, leave scarcely a symptom wanting to prove the identity of the two affections. Those who wish to pursue the question will find all necessary information in Fuchs's Historische Untersuchungen über Angina Maligna, 8vo., Würzburg, 1828.

part where swelling and redness were first apparent. The white color of the original deposit is speedily lost as fresh exudation is produced; and the membrane becomes gray or blackish as the air acts upon it, or as blood from the congested mucous surface beneath stains it. Speedily too it splits up into shreds, which, hanging down at the back of the fauces, produce that appearance of a sloughing tissue which imposed upon the early observers, and obtained for the disease the name of Angina Gangrænosa.

If detached from its connections, a number of minute bloody points on the subjacent tissue attest the firmness with which the false membrane adhered to it; but beyond increase of their vascularity the parts do not in general display any marked alteration. I doubt, however, whether that rigid classification which would refer to a separate category all those instances in which there exists distinct erosion or ulceration of the mucous membrane beneath the exudation is either practically useful or pathologically tenable; for while the surface of the tonsils is not invariably free from ulceration, I believe that in a very large proportion of the instances in which the exudation extends into the air-passages the mucous lining of the larynx is distinctly eroded, and small specks of ulceration are discernible about the edges of the glottis.

Coupled with the condition of the fauces there is usually a swelling of the submaxillary glands, and of the adjacent cellular tissue, as well as to some extent also of the parotids. This swelling, however, though very rapid in its formation, and equally so in its disappearance, is seldom so considerable as that which often attends upon scarlatina; it has but little tendency to terminate in abscess, and still less to assume the brawny hardness, and the extremely indolent character, which often add so much both to the suffering and the danger of that disease.

Although the soft palate and tonsils are the parts on which the deposit is first observable, it often does not remain limited to those situations, but its tendency is to extend by mere continuity of tissue to the mouth, the pharynx and œsophagus; to the larynx and trachea, and also occasionally upwards to the nares. Affection of the mucous membrane of the mouth, and the deposit of exudation on the tongue or on the inside of the cheeks or on the surface of the gums, are exceptional occurrences. I have met with such deposit only on four occasions, and I believe that at all times it is far more frequently absent than present. In two instances, though the mouth was free from false membrane, the œsophagus was lined by it for two-thirds of its length; the subjacent mucous surface showing but very slight increase of vascularity, and the exudation being but very loosely connected with it. In one case, although the œsophagus was perfectly normal, the stomach was lined by a thick false membrane, intimately adherent but terminating abruptly both at the cardiac and pyloric orifice. False membrane was in this case deposited also on the tonsils, velum, upper surface of the epiglottis, pharynx, root of tongue, in the nasal fossæ, and in the larynx as low as the cricoid cartilage. The disposition of the false membrane to affect the nares seems to vary much in different epidemics. It has very rarely come under my notice in this country in its most characteristic form as a distinct false membrane, though a discharge from the nostrils similar

to the scarlatinal coryza is present in almost all cases of severe diphtheria. M. Bretonneau[1] gives a caution with reference to these cases which must not be forgotten, to the effect that in some few instances the disease begins at the nares, and extends thence in a manner so insidious as to escape the notice of all who are not forewarned and on the lookout for the occurrence.

The relation between the amount of deposit on the fauces and the extension of false membrane to the air-passages is by no means constant. A very slight deposit on the soft palate and tonsils, soon disappearing, may yet be succeeded by a very abundant exudation in the larynx and trachea, while, on the other hand, most extensive formations of false membrane at the back of the throat may yet never involve the air-passages. The appearances produced by the extension of the diphtheritic deposit to the air-passages are precisely the same as those observed in cynanche trachealis, in which, without any previous affection of the fauces, the inflammation has attacked the larynx and trachea. It has indeed been suggested by M. Isambert,[2] in a very valuable paper, that the condition of the subjacent mucous membrane furnishes a ground of distinction between the affections; and that while in diphtheria the surface beneath the exudation is often ulcerated, no such erosion of the mucous membrane is met with in genuine croup. My own observation does not, however, altogether bear out this difference; for ulceration of the mucous membrane has come under my notice in primary croup, though less frequently than in cases of the diphtheritic kind; and its presence or absence seems to me mainly dependent on the rate of progress of the disease towards a fatal termination. When false membrane is deposited very extensively, and when death takes place in consequence most speedily, the mucous surfaces have appeared least altered; when the course of the disease is slower and the false membrane limited almost or altogether to the larynx, ulceration has seemed to me most frequent and has in some of these cases amounted to an almost complete erosion of the lining of the larynx. In conformity with this I may add that it is in the diphtheritic croup that succeeds to measles, which is usually the least rapid in its course, that we commonly find the alteration of the mucous membrane the most considerable.[3]

I have come indeed to the conclusion, which I long hesitated to adopt, that what differences soever exist between croup and diphtheria, they must be sought elsewhere than in the pathological changes observable in the respiratory organs. The mere extent of false membrane in the air-passages certainly affords no ground for a distinction between the two affections, though I think it is more common to find the false membrane reaching to the tertiary bronchi in diphtheria than in primary croup. A distinction between the two diseases founded on the greater frequency of bronchitis and pneumonia in primary croup becomes to my mind with every year's added experience less and less

---

[1] Archives Gén. de Médecine, Jan. and Sept. 1855.

[2] Ibid, March and April, 1857.

[3] The results of microscopic examination seem at present scarcely definite enough to furnish a solution of this question. See the observations and remarks on the subject in Uhle and Wagner, Allgemeine Pathologie, 5th ed., 1872, pp. 285–289.

tenable; and when once it has invaded the air-passages, diphtheria seems to produce precisely the same changes, to the same extent, and with at least the same rapidity, as primary croup.

But even though this be so, the sameness of the anatomical changes produced by two diseases does not suffice to establish their identity. The practitioner of midwifery knows that simple puerperal metritis and puerperal fever are diseases which differ widely in their symptoms, their course, their danger, and the degree in which they are amenable to remedies, though in both, when they terminate fatally, precisely the same alterations in the womb are discovered. In the same way, if we extend our inquiry beyond the mere changes wrought in the respiratory organs, the differences between croup and diphtheria at once become apparent; and the affinities of the latter disease are seen to be to the class of blood diseases, rather than to that of purely local inflammations to which croup belongs.

Though probably not embracing all points of difference, nor perhaps always holding absolutely true in every detail, the subjoined table may be of use as embodying the main points of difference between croup and diphtheria.

Croup	Diphtheria
Is influenced by climate and season, is endemic in some localities, but not epidemic nor contagious.	Is independent of climate or season, contagious, and often epidemic.
Is apt to recur, though with diminishing severity, in the same patient.	Has no special tendency to recur, though an attack confers no absolute immunity.
Is almost limited to childhood; of very rare occurrence indeed in the adult.	Though specially frequent in childhood, adult age has no exemption from it.
Usually begins with catarrh and fever, which latter is always proportionate to the severity of the local symptoms. Dysphagia rare, slight, always secondary, and subordinate to the laryngeal affection.	Catarrh rare. Symptoms of constitutional disorder often severe from the very outset. Sore throat and difficult deglutition precede laryngeal affection, which is often slight, and sometimes altogether absent.
Glandular swelling and coryza always absent. False membrane on fauces very rare, and not extensive.	Glandular swelling always, coryza often present; deposit of false membrane on tonsils always occurs at some period, often very extensive.
Constitutional disorder always in proportion to gravity of local mischief. No albumen in urine, nor any sign of general blood disorder.	Constitutional disorder often quite out of proportion to local mischief. Albumen present in the urine, and various evidences of blood disorder.
Death always from apnœa.	Death often from asthenia, and various disorders of nervous system.
Has no sequelæ, complete recovery following cure of local affection.	Has many sequelæ, and specially a peculiar form of paralysis, which may continue for months after the disappearance of every sign of local ailment.

Diphtheria presents itself in two forms,—either as a primary or as a secondary disease. In the former case it is often sporadic, and is then generally mild in character; but occasionally it is epidemic, and then conforms to the general laws of epidemic disease, and manifests on its first attack a degree of severity which passes off as its prevalence declines. When it occurs as a secondary affection, it is as a sequela to one or other of those diseases (especially measles and scarlatina), which are distinguished by the alterations that they bring about in the circulating fluid. With scarlet fever too its relations seem to be peculiarly intimate, for while there is no evidence that the one furnishes any protection from the other, both not infrequently prevail together; and it does occasionally happen that even in the same household some individuals will be attacked by diphtheria, and others by well-marked scarlet fever.

Until within the past few years, diphtheria had not been observed in London or its vicinity, within the memory of the present generation, except either as a sequela of measles, or else in that sporadic form which derives all its importance from the extension of false membrane to the larynx and trachea, and the consequent production of croupal symptoms. Recently, however, the disease has assumed a more formidable type, and its *symptoms* have resembled those which it often displays in France, though to the best of my knowledge that disposition to the formation of exudation on abraded surfaces, and at the outlet of all mucous canals, which is by no means unusual there, has occurred much more rarely in this country.

In its less severe forms the disease is ushered in by mild febrile symptoms accompanied with slight sore throat—the most remarkable feature of the case being generally that the depression of the patient is out of proportion to the severity of the local ailment. Examination of the throat shows a slight degree of swelling, and redness not usually very vivid, and at first confined to one tonsil. In the course of a few hours white specks are observed on the tonsil, chiefly on its inner surface, and before long the other tonsil becomes similarly affected, while, in some instances, though by no means constantly, a slight deposit appears on the velum and uvula. One or two applications of caustics or astringents to the part are usually sufficient to clear away the deposit, or it may disappear spontaneously, and not be reproduced, and in two or three days the patient is pretty well again, though strength is in general regained less quickly than might have been expected from the comparative mildness of the attack.

In cases so slight it is no easy matter to recognize the features of a highly dangerous disease; for there is no coryza, no swelling of the submaxillary glands, no increased secretion of saliva, no offensive odor of the breath, nor any disorder of the respiratory functions. Still, out of forerunners as trivial as these, croupal symptoms may be developed, and as the deposit on the fauces, when slight, is often not persistent, no trace of it may be perceptible when the signs of the affection of the larynx first attract attention. Whether croup comes on as a primary or as a secondary disease, its signs are always much the same, and I need not therefore occupy your time in repeating the description of them; but it must not be forgotten that its advances are often most insidious when it succeeds to diphtheritic deposit on the fauces. The cough, in these circumstances, may present but little of the loud clangor of ordinary croup, and the respiration may have little of the characteristic stridor; but grave apprehensions may be all at once excited (and this especially in infants and young children) by the breathing suddenly becoming sibilant and interrupted by paroxysms of urgent dyspnœa, the evidence of the already complete formation of false membrane, and the herald of death, which may not delay four-and-twenty hours from the first sign of serious danger.

But, much though it imports us to be on the lookout for this class of symptoms, they are not the expression of the special severity of the disease, but rather of the accidental extension of its consequences to the air-passages. It is true that to this accident much of the danger of diphtheria is due, and true too that in the worst forms of the disease it is more frequent than in its slighter manifestations; but while we must be always on the lookout for croupal symptoms, they do not constitute the disease: they are by no means the only source of its dangers, nor is it in their occurrence that the most characteristic features of diphtheria are to be sought.

Even in the more serious cases, the course of the disease, in its early stages, is usually slow and often insidious. For a day or two there is perhaps much febrile disturbance and a heat of skin which raises the suspicion that scarlatina is about to appear, of which the painful swelling of the submaxillary glands seems to be a still further indication. No rash, however, makes its appearance; the heat of skin often subsides completely, so that the surface becomes even cooler than natural; while the absence of the red and prominent papillæ which beset the tongue in scarlatina, belies the evidence of the sore throat. The fauces are red and swollen, sometimes very much so, but the redness is not vivid, and there is not in general that difficulty in opening the mouth which is experienced in scarlet fever when the sore throat is at all severe. The false membrane appears almost simultaneously on both tonsils; and soon after on the soft palate and uvula, and the latter is generally much swollen, and contributes a good deal to obstruct the channel of the fauces. Accompanying this state of the throat, there is often a discharge from the nares, resembling the coryza of scarlet fever, and as has already been mentioned, false membrane is occasionally deposited there, whence it may travel to the posterior nares, and so to the throat and air-passages. When the deposit is considerable the appearance of the tongue is peculiar. It is usually red at the tip, but thickly coated with white fur, which on the dorsum and towards the root of the tongue is almost membraniform. It is not usual for the inside of the mouth to be affected, but now and then the gums are red, soft, and spongy, and covered here and there, as well as the inside of the cheek, with patches of false membrane, beneath which the tissue appears red and shining. When the mouth is thus affected the secretion of saliva is considerably increased; but I have never seen that profuse dribbling of it which takes place in stomatitis, nor have I observed that complication of stomatitis with diphtheria of which M. Bretonneau speaks, and which led him to regard the two diseases as closely related to each other. It is after the false membrane has been formed somewhat abundantly for two or three days that it undergoes those changes which impart to the breath its peculiarly offensive [illegible] and give to the fauces that appearance of being the seat of [illegible] ulceration, whence arose the old names of angina maligna, grænosa. Even when the affection of the throat is most considerable, deglutition can still almost always be performed, not easily indeed, but yet in general without that extreme difficulty which one often observes in the sore throat of scarlet fever, and of common quinsy.

The voice is often hoarse and indistinct, independently of actual affection of the larynx; and a short spasmodic, slightly ringing cough, is frequently heard, due to the irritation of the larynx by the mischief in its vicinity. But, though these symptoms do not necessarily imply that the air-passages are actually involved in the disease, they should keep us most anxiously on the watch, since very few tokens indicate this event, and they are often of a kind to escape the notice of the unobservant.

In proportion to the severity of the case is usually the shortness of the premonitory fever, which sometimes does not exceed twelve hours in its duration, and at other times scarcely occurs at all, the child being struck down at once by the disease; false membrane being deposited extensively on the fauces in the course of a few hours, and the coryza, which usually does not appear before the third day, showing itself almost from the first. The mode in which such cases tend to a fatal issue is very various. As a general rule it may, I think, be said that the laryngeal affection, which is so grave a source of peril, does not so frequently occur in cases where the constitutional symptoms of diphtheria are most severe, as in those in which they wear a milder form. At the same time, however, no guarantee is furnished against its supervention by the gravity of the disease in other respects, while, when the larynx becomes involved in severe diphtheria, the case must be regarded as at once utterly hopeless.

Setting aside these cases, we find that the evidence of general constitutional disorder becomes more marked day by day, and this even without an invariable aggravation of the local malady. Of these evidences one of the most important is furnished by the presence of albumen in the urine. I believe that albumen is rarely absent in cases of other than the very mildest diphtheria; though the amount is strangely fluctuating, varying even on successive days; and these fluctuations are by no means constantly associated with any corresponding modifications in the other symptoms of the disease. When the albumen, however, is very abundant, the urine is invariably scanty, and there is perhaps no single symptom of worse omen than the extremely scanty secretion of urine. In cases of average severity the albumen seldom makes its appearance within the first four or five days; and then, according to the subsequent progress, it either goes on increasing, or lessens with the gradual improvement in the patient's condition. The complete suppression of urine is an almost invariably fatal symptom, and I do not know of any instance in which the patient has recovered after the urinary secretion has been suspended for twenty-four hours. In these circumstances, and even in cases where the urinary secretion, though not absolutely suspended, is unusually scanty, uræmic convulsions are likely to occur and suddenly to carry off the patient.

But even where the urinary secretion continues in tolerable quantity, and the albumen is not excessive, the symptoms that attend the progress of the disease are invariably those of depression, and of depression which, like that attendant on the worst forms of puerperal fever, is by no means constantly proportionate to the apparent local mischief. The child, feeble yesterday, becomes still feebler to-day, and often, without any actual increase of deposit, sometimes even in spite of its diminution, and of the absence of any apparent cause for difficult deglutition, his repugnance to take food goes on increasing, until at length he positively refuses all nourishment. This refusal of food, whether in childhood or in adult age, is a very unfavorable occurrence. It is sometimes associated with vomiting, and may then be dependent on the presence of false membrane in the stomach, though this is by no means always the case; but whether it be so or not it tends to reduce the patient's strength very much, and if persistent for any considerable time almost invariably occasions fatal depression. It is not always easy to realize the degree of peril, for the intellect is generally clear, and the muscular powers are not inconsiderable, while at the same time the extremities are cold, and the pulse is either extremely frequent or else very feeble or irregular in its beat. For two or three days together, this condition may continue, the pulse growing feebler, the signs of failing power more manifest, and this in spite of stimulants being administered lavishly, and taken readily, until at length either the signs of the last stage of croup suddenly appear, showing that the local mischief has been extending silently and unperceived, or else an attack of syncope follows on some sudden and violent action of the bowels, or causeless convulsions come on, and in the subsequent coma the patient dies. This depression too, as already mentioned, is by no means constantly proportionate to the extent of the false membrane, nor is the danger of it past even when the local mischief, as far at least as the eye can reach, has altogether disappeared; for I have known frequently recurring syncope take place even when no traces of false membrane remained on the fauces; and fatal convulsions come on when the local mischief was so slight that nothing but the previous death of a member of the family from well-marked diphtheria had called attention to the throat, and had led me to watch with painful solicitude a local ailment which owed all its importance to its being an evidence of grave constitutional disease.

The simultaneous or successive affection of different and distant parts, is one of the great evidences on which we are wont to rely, in proof that a disease belongs to that great class of *blood diseases* whose importance and whose distinctive characters modern pathology has done so much to elucidate. The more closely we study diphtheria, the stronger will its claims appear to be referred to this category. The false membrane, whose most usual seat is on the fauces, whence it extends into the air-passages, is not limited to those situations, but occasionally invades other parts, and is deposited behind the ears, upon the vulva, or on abraded surfaces; while, in the albuminuria which generally accompanies its severer forms, another point of resemblance exists[1] between diphtheria and other maladies which result from pura-

[1] Bouchut and Empis, Gaz. Hebdom., Nov. 12, 1858.

lent infection. In some epidemics of diphtheria the formation of false membrane on different parts has been a frequent occurrence. Thus Bard,[1] describing the disease as it prevailed nearly a century ago in America, speaks of the formation of ulcers behind the ears, covered in some places with sloughs resembling those on the tonsils; and Starr, in his description of the epidemic at Liskeard,[2] notices "a rotten membranous body, or slough, generated on the skin of a patient, on the neck and arm, where blisters had been applied;" and says that the part presented "a white surface which had the aspect of an oversoaked membrane." Such a deposit I saw take place on the neck of a little girl, around whose throat, before the diphtheritic deposit had been recognized on the fauces, a stimulating liniment had been applied to relieve her swollen glands. But besides the formation of false membrane on abraded surfaces, the mucous membrane of the vulva seems often to be the seat of a similar deposit; and in some rare cases the prepuce is affected in the same manner, or small superficial ulcers break out on different parts of the body, and become speedily covered with false membrane. Once, too, I saw in consultation with Mr. Alford, of Haverstock Hill, twin boys, eight months old, in each of whom a small abrasion formed on the raphe of the perineum, and became covered with false membrane. This membrane extended, though unaccompanied with other local symptoms of diphtheria, to the margin of the anus, and to just within the external sphincter. Both children died within a week from the commencement of their illness, sinking as under some grave constitutional disease, with troublesome diarrhœa and exhaustion, which stimulants failed to remove. The identity of the disease in these circumstances with ordinary diphtheria is established beyond doubt by facts such as those observed by M. Trousseau[3] in a village in the neighborhood of Orleans, where diphtheria prevailed, presenting in some persons its ordinary features; manifesting itself in others by deposits of false membrane on the vulva, on the mamma, on blistered surfaces, or on ulcers, and proving fatal in some cases without the throat being at all involved in the disease.

Among the sequelæ of diphtheria we shall presently have to notice peculiar paralytic symptoms, which sometimes affect the extremities; or the pharynx, soft palate, and other parts that have been more immediately involved in the disease. But besides these, which belong rather to the remote phenomena of diphtheria, we sometimes meet with even a graver form of disordered innervation, occurring in its earliest stage, and leading, by affection of the vital centres, to a speedily and often to a suddenly fatal issue. Disordered innervation of the heart is perhaps the most frequent, and betrays itself by a remarkable diminution, sometimes for two or three days, in the frequency of the pulse, which may even sink, as in the case of a little girl, related by Sir W. Jenner, to sixteen beats in the minute. This occurrence indeed is by no means constant, and death may take place by sudden failure of the heart without this forewarning. When observed, however, its import

[1] Loc. cit., p. 892. [2] Idem, p. 440.
[3] De la Diphthérite cutanée, in Arch. de Méd., Juillet, 1830, p. 383.

is always serious, and you may augur ill of any case in which, be the local symptoms what they may, the heart's pulsations fall much below their natural standard.

But there are other cases in which the disordered innervation seems to affect the muscles of respiration rather than the heart itself; the breathing, without any extension of the false membrane to the larynx, and without any notable mischief in the lungs, becoming by degrees more and more labored, and the patient dying at the end of some four-and-twenty hours from asphyxia, for which a post-mortem examination discovers no adequate cause.

It seems then that death may take place in the acute stage of diphtheria, either—

1st. From blood-poisoning, as in cases of malignant fever.

2d. From extension of the local mischief to the larynx.

3d. From progressive exhaustion aggravated by the difficulty in deglutition.

4th. From uræmia and uræmic convulsions.

5th. From various forms of affection of the nervous system, as—

a. Sudden syncope.

b. Disordered innervation of the heart.

c. Disordered innervation of the organs of respiration.

d. General disorder of innervation, accompanied with affection of the stomach, and uncontrollable vomiting.

It is not easy to fix the *duration*[1] of a malady whose course is not infrequently so anomalous, and which, as we shall see hereafter, not seldom leaves sequelæ in its train such as are themselves only fresh manifestations of the workings of the original morbid poison. Of 53 fatal cases, 27 terminated within the first 7 days; and after the termination of the second week death may be regarded as a decidedly unusual and exceptional occurrence; though it is not easy, perhaps even not possible, to fix any date before convalescence is perfectly established at which some of the remote sequelæ of diphtheria may not unexpect-

[1] In 26 cases in which death took place from causes other than the affection of the larynx,

The child died	on the	2d day in	2
"	"	3d "	2
"	"	4th "	3
"	"	5th "	2
"	"	6th "	2
"	"	7th "	2
"	"	9th "	1
"	"	10th "	1
"	"	12th "	3
"	"	14th "	1
"	"	15th "	1
"	"	18th "	2
"	"	20th "	1
"	"	28th "	1
"	"	50th "	1
"	in 2 months in		1
			26

In 27 cases in which death took place chiefly from the affection of the larynx,

The child died	on the	2d day in	1
"	"	3d "	4
"	"	4th "	1
"	"	5th "	4
"	"	6th "	3
"	"	7th "	1
"	"	8th "	1
"	"	9th "	1
"	"	10th "	1
"	"	11th "	1
"	"	12th "	1
"	"	13th "	[illegible]
"	"	14th "	[illegible]
"	"	[illegible]	[illegible]
"	"	21st "	[illegible]
"	"	[illegible]	[illegible]

edly come on and endanger life. The most rapidly fatal cases are those in which death depends on affection of the larynx, and in them death sometimes takes place in from twenty-four to thirty-six hours from the apparent commencement of the attack; the local symptoms throwing the signs of constitutional disorder completely into the shade, sometimes rendering it almost impossible to determine whether a case should be classed with diphtheria or with simple cynanche trachealis.

Reference has already been made to the occasional death of patients in whom the local affection had throughout been so inconsiderable as to produce but few symptoms, or has even altogether disappeared before the fatal issue took place. But other cases are sometimes observed where long-continued illness remains, or where even death takes place not from the disease itself nor from any of its immediate effects, but from its remote sequelæ, from a sort of accidental consequences. These remote results of diphtheria have been noticed both by Bretonneau and Trousseau, and some of them have probably come under the observation of most persons who have had even a very limited experience of the disease. Thus, for instance, I saw a child, between three and four years old, whose infant brother had died of diphtheria, and who herself had had very slight deposit of false membrane on her fauces, attacked by causeless convulsions when apparently convalescent, and when more than a week had elapsed since the throat presented any unnatural condition; and these convulsions terminated in fatal coma within less than twenty-four hours. A lady whose child (aged three years) had died of diphtheria extending to the air-passages, and who herself had suffered from very slight sore throat with a trace of false membrane on the tonsils, was attacked by sudden faintness, almost amounting to syncope, with extreme feebleness of pulse and a sense of impending dissolution, which for more than twenty-four hours was scarcely kept in check by the almost incessant administration of stimulants. Cases of a similar kind might no doubt be multiplied; but besides these earlier sequelæ there is a peculiar form of temporary paralysis, which occurs by no means rarely as a remote consequence of the disease, and which is yet both important in itself and also as furnishing an additional distinction between diphtheria and any simply inflammatory affection.

Both MM. Bretonneau and Trousseau have referred to this peculiar condition; and incidental mention of it is to be found a century ago in the writings of physicians who have noticed the so-called malignant sore throat, by which name diphtheria was then described.[1] It is to M. Faure,[2] however, that we are indebted for the first complete account of it, derived partly from his own observation, partly from facts detailed by others. He describes it as "a state characterized by a gradually increasing loss of power, showing itself especially in all functions connected with muscular movement. In some instances, several sets of organs are affected, in others only one; while, again, in others the whole system is involved in the general debility. But, whatever are the

[1] M. Maingault's valuable essay, De la Paralysie Diphthérique, 8vo., Paris, 1860, contains an interesting historical sketch of the early notices of this affection.

[2] L'Union Médicale de Paris, Février, 1857; and J. f. Kinderkr., Jan. 1858.

variations in this respect, there is no definite relation between the severity of the primary symptoms of diphtheria and that of the sequelæ. The primary symptoms, though very formidable, yet by no means of necessity prove fatal; while, on the other hand, the comparative mildness of the attack will not justify an absolutely favorable prognosis, since death sometimes follows where everything had seemed to warrant the most confident expectation of recovery."

Several cases are related by M. Faure, in illustration of the different phases of this condition, and he then proceeds to sum up the general results as follows: "Some time after an attack of diphtheria, from which the patient had so completely recovered that no trace of false membrane is left behind, the skin grows causelessly more and more colorless, so that at length it assumes an almost livid pallor. Severe pains begin at the same time to be felt in the joints, the patient loses power over his limbs, and soon sinks into a state of indescribable weakness. At the same time, the disorders that appear in different functions show that the various organs which should minister to them are involved, so far as they are dependent upon muscular power. In this respect, however, the phenomena are not constant, for sometimes it is one set of organs, and sometimes another, which suffers most from this weakness.

"Very generally, in consequence of the want of muscular power, or, more strictly speaking, in consequence of its complete abolition, the patient becomes unable to sit upright, or does so with great difficulty; while the legs cannot bear the weight of the body, the arms become nerveless and cease to obey the will, and all the movements grow uncertain, tottering, hesitating, and apparently purposeless. Very remarkable disorders show themselves also within the throat; for the velum is completely paralyzed, and hangs down like a flaccid lifeless curtain, which interferes with speech and deglutition. All the muscles of the jaw, those too of the neck and chest, are partially paralyzed, in consequence of which mastication is rendered difficult, and the food can neither be easily moved about in the mouth nor readily swallowed. From the same cause too it is not infrequently regurgitated, and the laborious deglutition often induces spasm of the respiratory apparatus. Vision is impaired, one or other pupil often remains widely dilated, even in the strongest light, and squinting is not unusual. The sensibility of the skin is much diminished; in the limbs it is sometimes completely lost, though morbid sensations—such, for instance, as formication—are sometimes experienced. Œdema of various parts often occurs, while, though less commonly, parts here and there lose their vitality, and become gangrenous. No general reaction occurs, fever is rare. The skin usually has a certain degree of moisture. The features grow duller and more and more expressionless, though a foolish smile sometimes crosses them, or now and then a ray of intelligence appears. Some patients have frequent fainting fits. As the condition goes on from bad to worse, the weakness becomes extreme; and death at length either follows some fainting fit, or takes place when exhaustion has reached its uttermost—life as it were quietly, almost imperceptibly, passing away."

This fatal termination is, however, an exceptional occurr[illegible] indeed, the symptoms of diphtheritic paralysis are not usually by any means so severe as the above description implies. My own impression too (though I have not statistical data sufficient to warrant a positive statement on the subject) is that diphtheritic paralysis is far rarer in this country than on the Continent, or at least than in Paris. I have not seen in the Children's Hospital any of the graver forms of the affection succeed to diphtheria for which the patient was admitted when in its acute stage; and, further, the number of children received on account of paralytic symptoms at all has been but small, and the cases not severe. Even in private practice, while a large number of diphtheritic patients have come under my observation, the instances of paralysis succeeding have been so few, that I may, I think, feel sure that in London, paralysis does not follow diphtheria with anything like the frequency with which it is stated on the best authority to occur in Paris.[1]

The form in which diphtheritic paralysis most frequently shows itself, is that in which the soft palate is affected, producing nasal voice and occasional difficulty in deglutition. Next in frequency, I have observed impaired power over the limbs, the lower being affected oftener and to a greater degree than the upper; and with this there was associated, in many instances, indistinct articulation, with strabismus, dilated pupils, and imperfect vision. Once I saw a child on whom tracheotomy had been successfully performed on account of diphtheria affecting the larynx, and from whose windpipe the canula had been removed early, attacked some days after the wound had healed completely, by such difficulty in breathing from paralysis of the muscles of the larynx, as to raise in the mind of the medical attendant the question whether fresh disease had not come on. I have also seen death occur in two children three years old—in the one ten and in the other seven weeks after the invasion of diphtheria—and who had both appeared to have completely recovered from the disease. The paralytic symptoms supervened in both these cases on slight catarrh, which, however, was unattended by bronchitis. In both cases the little patients objected to take food; and in one, any attempt at deglutition, especially of fluids, brought on most distressing cough. No râles were heard in the chest, but mucus collected in the windpipe, which the children made fruitless efforts to expectorate; while the pupils became dilated, the lips livid, and the surface cold and clammy, during the attempt to get rid of the obstacle to the entrance of air. At length the power of coughing

---

[1] M. Roger, in his valuable paper on this subject, estimates the frequency of paralysis at a third of the cases in which life was prolonged sufficiently to allow of its occurrence. See his "Recherches sur la Paralysie Diphthéritique," in Archives de Médecine, 1862, vol. i, p. 1. It can scarcely be necessary to observe that as the characters of the same disease vary at different periods in the same country, so may they also differ in different countries at one time; and that discrepancies between the statements of observers in France and England do not of necessity imply error on the part of either. It so chances that in the whole course of my practice I have only four times met with cutaneous diphtheria—once affecting the vulva, twice the anus, and once attacking an abraded surface. Judging by the statements of French physicians, my experience would have been widely different if the scene of my observations had been on the other side of the Channel instead of in England.

ceased, and then the children died—one seven days, the other five days, from the first interruption of their convalescence.

These paralytic symptoms vary in the date of their occurrence as well as in their severity. I have already referred to the failure of the power of the heart, and to the paralysis of the respiratory muscles, as sometimes carrying off patients during the acute stage of diphtheria. The more remote results, however—with the exception of the paralysis of the soft palate, which sometimes persists from the first attack of the disease—do not come on until after a distinct interval of apparent convalescence, marked by nothing but that state of general weakness which might be expected to succeed to the previous illness. They bear no necessary relation to the severity of the previous attack, nor to the quantity of albumen which had been present in the urine; and I remember to have seen them in a very marked form in a little boy, in whom the previous diphtheria was so light as to have been unrecognized, and who was supposed to have suffered only from influenza with a little sore throat. I do not know after how long a period from the attack paralytic symptoms may come on, and to the best of my belief we are not as yet furnished with data sufficient to form a positive opinion on the subject, though the two cases I have related above prove that a lapse even of several weeks furnishes no positive guarantee against their occurrence.

It has been alleged[1] that these paralytic affections have in them nothing of a specific character—that, so far from belonging exclusively to diphtheria, they are occasionally met with, presenting the same essential features, after many acute diseases; or that, in other words, diphtheritic paralyses are but a particular example of a very general rule.

Now I do not believe this; for though, as I have already stated, diphtheritic paralysis has appeared to me to be of far less frequent occurrence in this country than on the Continent, I yet have met with paralysis after diphtheria far more frequently than after any other acute affection of early life. In some very rare instances, indeed, I have known paralytic symptoms succeed to measles and typhoid fever; but even in these cases it has assumed a form similar to that of the so-called essential paralysis of childhood, has affected the same parts from the outset, and has presented nothing of that progressive character which one observes in diphtheritic paralysis. In France—where this paralysis, as I have already mentioned, has occurred in as many as a third of all cases of diphtheria in which the patients have survived the urgent dangers of the acute stage of the disease—there is even stronger ground than my own experience would furnish for regarding it as one of the ordinary sequelæ of the disease, and for looking on it as having as much of a special character as belongs to that form of dropsy which we look upon as one of the peculiar incidents of the desquamative stage of scarlatina.

---

[1] See the most elaborate series of papers by Dr. Gubler, devoted to the support of this paradox, in the Archives de Médecine, 1860. Vol. i, pp. 257, 402, 584, 696; vol. ii, pp. 187, 718; and 1861, vol. i, p. 306.

This disposition to the occurrence of paralysis as its most frequent sequela, is also not without interest as bearing on a question more debated a few years since than it is at the present day—namely, that of the exact *relation* subsisting *between diphtheria and scarlatina.* Of late, indeed, the question seems to have been nearly set at rest by the unanimous recognition of the essential differences between the two diseases.

It may, however, be worth while to sum up briefly the majority of those differences, which I think justify us in the assertion that diphtheria and scarlatina, however allied in some of their characters, are yet diseases essentially distinct from each other:

1st. In all epidemics of scarlatina the anomalous cases, in which the characteristic rash is absent, form but a very small minority. In epidemics of diphtheria, however, the existence of a rash, even though most partial and evanescent, is but rarely noticed, and in the majority of epidemics is not at all observed.

2d. In cases of malignant scarlet fever terminating fatally, and without the appearance of any rash, death usually occurs very early, and is preceded by very marked cerebral disturbance, by violent delirium, or by profound insensibility; while, on the other hand, the fatal issue in diphtheria is generally far less speedy in its approach, and the disease, even in its worst forms, is usually remarkable for the perfect clearness of the intellect almost to the very last.

3d. The characters of the tongue in diphtheria differ entirely from those which it presents in scarlatina; and even the rash, on the occasional appearance of which so much stress has been laid, is in many respects dissimilar from the scarlatinoid eruption. It is for the most part a uniform blush of erythematous redness, unattended by the peculiar punctated appearance which marks the scarlatinoid rash. It appears suddenly in patches, is vivid from the very first, not deepening gradually in intensity like the rash of scarlet fever; while its sudden and speedy disappearance is not followed by any change in the other symptoms, nor by any increase in their severity. I may add, still further, that the appearance of any rash at all is a purely exceptional occurrence.

4th. The œdema of the surface, which is occasionally present, comes on during the acute stage of diphtheria, not during its decline; it is inconsiderable in degree, is unaccompanied by serous effusion into the cavities of the chest or abdomen, and is by no means of necessity associated with albuminuria. The presence of albumen in the urine is not accompanied with any other change in its character, such as would be obvious on a cursory examination; for, though lessened in quantity, it still continues pale in color and acid in its reaction, and I have not met with any instance in which blood was present in it. The albumen seems also often to disappear at a very early period of the disease—its disappearance takes place suddenly; and though its presence is almost invariably observed in cases where the disease is severe, yet there does not seem to be any necessary connection between the urine becoming non-albuminous and the disease assuming a milder type.

5th. The whole train of the sequelæ of the two affections is different; and while, on the one hand, the convalescence f theria presents none of the formidable dropsical symptoms which so often succeed to scarlet fever, the peculiar loss of nervous power, and the temporary muscular paralysis which frequently follow diphtheria, have no analogy to any of the sequelæ of scarlet fever.

6th. Scarlet fever does not protect from diphtheria, nor, on the other hand, does diphtheria defend from scarlet fever. To both of these facts universal experience bears testimony, and it would scarcely be justifiable to assume that every instance, or even the majority of instances, of the succession of diphtheria to scarlet fever, or the opposite, are illustrations of a secondary attack of scarlet fever. An example which puts this in a very strong light was recently communicated to me. In a school in the neighborhood of London diphtheria broke out; many of the lads were affected by it, and one or two died. Several of those who were convalescent from the disease were sent to the seacoast for the more speedy recovery of their strength, and while there some were attacked by scarlet fever; and this also, in one or two cases, proved fatal. Still stronger, however, is the evidence supplied by cases in the Children's Hospital, where patients recovering from scarlatina have been attacked by diphtheria; and the reverse, in which children convalescent from diphtheria have been attacked by scarlatina; showing that the one disease exerts no more preservative influence from the other than does measles or typhoid fever, each of which may follow diphtheria, or be followed by it.

Two main points are involved in the *treatment* of this disease,—the one the control of the local mischief, the other the support of the constitutional powers. All the various measures which have been employed are directed to one or other of these objects; and there is at the present day a degree of unanimity as to the means to be resorted to, such as is of rare occurrence in questions of therapeutics. Depletion, antiphlogistics of all kinds, blisters, and all counter-irritants by which the surface may be abraded, though used at one time, under what are believed to have been mistaken views as to the nature of this affection, are now by common consent altogether discontinued; and the only points debated among practitioners regard the comparative merit of this or that local application, or of this or that tonic medicine.

I do not believe that there is any remedy, either local or general, which exercises a specific influence over diphtheria—such, for instance, as the chlorate of potass seems to possess in controlling stomatitis, or as quinine displays in cutting short an attack of ague. There is, however, usually a very marked connection between the early arrest of the deposit, however affected, and the speedy recovery of the patient, although it sometimes happens that the constitutional symptoms of the disease have a fatal issue after all trace of false membrane has disappeared from the fauces. In illustration of the connection between the arrest of the deposit and the cutting short of the disease, M. Trousseau relates the story of the epidemic prevalence of diphtheria in a village where all the cases treated by the medical men, who confined themselves to the employment of constitutional remedies, proved fatally; while the only cures were wrought by an old woman, who despised the doctors and their remedies, and applied indiscriminately to everybody's throat a rough and rather violent escharotic.

The practice, however, which this story seems to inculcate—and which I, in common with many others, was at one time accustomed to adopt—has come of late years to be regarded as of more than doubtful expediency. The application of a strong solution of nitrate of silver, as two scruples to an ounce of distilled water, or of equal parts of hydrochloric acid and honey, by means of a soft camel's-hair brush, on the first discovery of the deposit, sometimes seems to arrest its extension. At the same time I am fully satisfied that often-repeated cauterization, in the hope of thereby overtaking the spread of the disease, not merely fails of this result, but often produces an increase of swelling and greater difficulty of deglutition.

But, though the repetition of the stronger caustics is injurious, benefit may often be derived from some of the milder local applications. Thus, for instance, a gargle of half an ounce of the solution of chloride of soda to six ounces of water, or a similar application made to the back of the throat with a soft camel's-hair brush, or the syringing the mouth with it every three or four hours, often relieves the local mischief, and at the same time promotes the patient's comfort, by freeing the mouth from the ropy mucus and the other secretions which are apt to accumulate in it. The ingenious apparatus too, now so generally used in one form or other for the diffusion of spray, either for producing local anæsthesia, for applying lotions to the eye, or for perfuming a room—and the idea of which, I believe, we owe to Dr. B. Richardson—is extremely useful in these cases. By means of it we can apply a solution of tannin in glycerin, and mixed with water; or a solution of carbolic acid; or the sulphurous acid diluted with eight times the quantity of water, with much relief and with much real benefit. The mere gargling with iced water, or the frequent swallowing of small pieces of ice, is also of much service in many instances, when the swelling and the difficulty in deglutition are considerable; but, unfortunately, it is almost impossible to induce children to carry out any of these measures with perseverance.

The discharge from the nostrils, which is a very frequent and very troublesome complication, may generally be checked by the injection, twice in the twenty-four hours, of a solution of one or two grains of nitrate of silver to an ounce of water; and the swelling of the submaxillary glands may often be diminished by warm fomentations, or by the application of spongio-piline, or of a linseed-meal poultice to the neck.

Something too may be done to promote the patient's comfort, and to lessen the danger of affection of the air-passages, by providing (as was suggested when I spoke of croup) for the presence of a warm and moist atmosphere in the room; and, in the early stage of the affection, by the inhalation, if the child is old enough to employ it, of the steam of warm water, or of warm vinegar and water.

While the above local measures are had recourse to, the constitutional treatment must be pursued no less diligently. In this it is important to bear in mind that the feverish condition, which is often observed at the outset of diphtheria, must not mislead us into withholding nourishment, or into resorting to any strenuously antiphlogistic treatment. If, indeed, there is much heat of skin at the onset of the attack, if the tongue is coated, and the bowels are constipated, an ipecacuanha emetic may be given, followed by a few grains of grey powder, and a mild saline aperient, as the sulphate of magnesia, or its effervescing citrate. A simple saline, as the citrate of potass, may afterwards be continued every three or four hours, to each dose of which four or five grains of the chlorate of potass should be added. All this time, too, the child should be kept in bed, since it is of the greatest moment to avoid all needless expenditure of the strength; while, though wine may at first be unnecessary, beef tea must be given from the very first, and stimulants can seldom be long delayed. The softness and feebleness of the pulse, indeed, almost always give, in spite of the temporary heat of surface, plain intimation of the course which we shall have to pursue; and very often a shorter time than twenty-four hours suffices to dissipate entirely the febrile symptoms with which the disease set in, and to show it in its real characters.

I have already expressed my disbelief in the existence of any specific remedy for diphtheria, though I have given, and am accustomed to give, the tincture of the perchloride of iron in a large proportion of cases. It has seemed to me to be a valuable medicine, but no more; and in my hands it has never vindicated its claims to those special virtues for which some practitioners give it credit. I generally employ it in combination with the chlorate of potass, giving about four grains of that salt and eight minims of the tincture every four hours, to a child five years old. I have never seen reason for believing that where ordinary doses of a remedy fail, extraordinary doses will succeed; and when one physician talks of giving fifteen minims every quarter of an hour, day and night, for seventy-two hours, I do not know whether to marvel more at the endurance of the patient or the hardihood of the doctor.[1] Iron has seemed to me in some instances to indispose the patient for taking food, or to incapacitate the stomach for bearing it; and sometimes on this account, sometimes simply from its failing to produce any good effect, I have discontinued it and had recourse instead to quinine, with hydrochloric acid and tincture of bark; and this again has succeeded in some instances, and not succeeded in others.

In the great majority of instances, it must be confessed that the employment of medicine has seemed of importance altogether subordinate to the administration of food and stimulants; and children of four years old have taken six ounces of port wine and one or two ounces of brandy, for several days together, not only with manifest advantage, but apparently as the only means by which life could be maintained. When deglutition has been very difficult, or when, without any absolute difficulty in swallowing, the patient has refused nourishment, or the stomach has rejected it, I have had recourse to

[1] Dr. Aubrun, in a communication to the Académie des Sciences at Paris, Nov. 20, 1860: reported in the Journal f. Kinderkrankheiten, Jan. 1861, vol. xxxvi, p. 141.

beef tea enemata with temporary advantage; though in no instance did a patient ultimately recover in whom vomiting, or indisposition to take food, was other than a very transitory symptom.

Mention has been made of the scanty secretion of urine in some cases of diphtheria, and of the excessive quantity of albumen which it is then found to contain, as one of the gravest symptoms of the disease. Dr. Wade[1] of Birmingham—to whom we are indebted for pointing out the structural changes in the kidneys which are found associated with this condition of the urine, and which are in many instances apparent even within the first three or four days from the commencement of diphtheria—insists on the employment of the iodide and chlorate of potass almost from the first, and on the administration of large quantities of fluid, as infallible preventives of this danger, and indeed of every other. There can be no doubt but that the quantity of the urinary secretion may be greatly increased by drinking large quantities of water, and that, in many instances, the absolute (not the merely proportionate) quantity of albumen is simultaneously diminished to a very considerable extent. It is, however, a very different thing to induce a child of three years old, suffering from scarlatinal dropsy, to drink a quart of water daily, from what it is to force upon it large quantities of fluid, at a time when every attempt at deglutition produces intense pain, and when it taxes the attendants to the utmost to induce the patient to swallow enough to maintain the flagging powers of life. It is during the early stage of the disease, when deglutition is commonly most difficult, and dangers from other sources are most pressing, that the troubles of the urinary secretion are commonly encountered in their gravest forms. I have given the iodide of potassium in these cases, just as I have given it in combination with other salines in scarlatinal dropsy. I believe the remedy to be a serviceable one: but I must at the same time add, that there seem to me to be few things more injurious to the advancement of medical knowledge, than the aphoristic dogmatism which enunciates a certain mode of treatment as one in which "no instance of a fatal termination" is met with "where it has been carried out."

Now and then a single dose of ipecacuanha, in the earlier stages of the disease, has relieved the difficulty of deglutition where that was troublesome; but I have not observed any internal remedy check the advance of croupal symptoms coming on in the course of diphtheria for which tonic and stimulant measures had already been necessary. In those instances in which the disease has announced itself almost from the outset by croupal symptoms, I believe that the presence of false membrane on the fauces should not betray us into any wide deviation from that course of treatment which we should adopt in cases of primary cynanche trachealis; and the administration of emetics (though not of antimonials) and the steady employment of mercurials, though the patient may at the same time stand in need of support and stimulants, have seemed to me of great moment. In these cases, however, even

---

[1] In his essay, "Observations on Diphtheria," 8vo., London, 1858; and a subsequent paper "On Diphtheria," printed at Birmingham in 1863.

more than in those of inflammatory croup, the early performance of tracheotomy has appeared to me to be indicated, so soon as remedies ceased to tell on the symptoms of disordered respiration.

I do not know that there is any specific treatment which we can recommend for the removal of the paralytic symptoms that succeed to diphtheria. First of all, it is to be borne in mind that they have a tendency to spontaneous subsidence with the lapse of time; in the next place, the longer the interval between the acute stage of diphtheria and the supervention of the paralytic symptoms, the less is in general their gravity; and thirdly, so long as the impaired power is limited to the extremities, and to the muscles of deglutition, we are warranted in entertaining a favorable view of the case, which, however, is no longer justified when either the muscles of respiration are involved, or the action of the heart is disturbed. As a general rule, tonic remedies are indicated; and I have been accustomed to employ preparations of iron, in combination with nux vomica, or strychnine. I have frequently observed recovery to take place, slowly but steadily, under the use of these means: I do not, however, know of any case in which the improvement was so marked as to justify me in saying, that the remedies, independent of the influence of time and of general hygienic measures, had had an important share in producing it.

There is another form of disease, allied to diphtheria by many of its characters, allied to cynanche laryngea by others, which presents itself to us as *a most dangerous complication of some other affection, almost always of measles*. I was familiar with this, and described[1] it, at a time when my acquaintance with genuine idiopathic diphtheria was very slight and imperfect; and I reproduce my account of it here, because in a few respects—as for instance in the ulcerative stomatitis, with which it was associated—it differed from those forms of diphtheria with which I have since become conversant.

This variety of croup seldom begins until the eruption of measles is on the decline, or till the process of desquamation has commenced. Its occurrence is most frequent from the third to the sixth day from the appearance of the eruption, but it oftener occurs at a later than at an earlier period. It is sometimes attended with well-marked symptoms from the very first; but it often happens that the character of the disease is masked and its course insidious, and that the degree of suffering during life affords no correct index to the amount of mischief which may be revealed by a dissection after death. Of itself it is highly dangerous, and its hazard is increased by the frequent coexistence with it of inflammation of the lungs, which serves moreover to throw the symptoms of croup into the shade. When the laryngeal affection comes on three or four days after the appearance of measles, its presence is usually betokened by much more obvious symptoms than when it occurs after the lapse of a longer period from the febrile attack. Sometimes, however, it develops itself unnoticed simultaneously with the measles, and causes a fatal issue when the medical attendant is least prepared to expect it. The child in such cases is evidently more seriously ill than can be accounted for by the

[1] Medical Gazette, Aug. 25, 1848.

mere existence of measles; but he makes no definite complaint, neither are there any obvious indications of the special suffering of any particular organ. There are considerable drowsiness, disinclination to swallow, and reluctance to speak; but the cough may be very slight, and the respiration free from distinct croupy stridor, while the child speaks in so low a tone that it is almost impossible to appreciate any alteration of the voice. In such circumstances, the most careful observation is needed to avoid error. The loss of voice should of itself direct attention to the state of the larynx; the cry should be listened to attentively, pressure should be made on the larynx, to ascertain whether much tenderness exists, and examination of the fauces should never be neglected.

But little less obscure, and of much more frequent occurrence, are those instances in which the laryngeal affection attends the process of desquamation. Recovery up to a certain point has probably gone on well, when sometimes with, sometimes without an increase of the cough and morbillous catarrh, the febrile symptoms become exacerbated and the child droops again apparently without any adequate cause. Sometimes a loud sonorous cough, succeeded or accompanied by alteration of the respiratory sounds, betrays the nature of the disease; but at other times there are no symptoms besides unusual drowsiness, reluctance to speak, or alteration in the tone of the voice, with disinclination to swallow, or difficulty in the act of deglutition. In many instances deglutition is scarcely at all impeded; and I remember only one case in which the difficulty of swallowing was so great that fluids returned by the nose. But even though these symptoms be but slight, it will usually be observed, on examining the mouth, that the gums have a spongy appearance, or are actually ulcerated, that the tongue is preternaturally red and raw, and that small aphthous ulcers have formed upon its edges and on the lining membrane of the mouth. The soft palate will usually be seen to be red and swollen, and specks of false membrane will be observed on the velum or tonsils. In such a case, if it terminates fatally, the duration of life is very variable; though the disease, for the most part, runs a somewhat chronic course. The child's strength declines daily, and emaciation makes rapid progress; yet no acute symptoms appear. There is great restlessness, and no posture seems easy to the child; or else it sits constantly upright in bed, distress and dyspnœa following any attempt to place it in the recumbent position. The alteration of the voice is succeeded by complete aphonia; the frequent hacking cough, which had previously caused much annoyance, ceases altogether; and, although evidently thirsty, the child often refuses drink, or swallows with difficulty. Diarrhœa, or pneumonia, usually supervenes, and hastens death; though in some instances exacerbation of the croupal symptoms, coupled with the increasing weakness of the child, are the only causes of the fatal termination.

On examining after death the bodies of children who have died of this affection, not only is the mucous membrane of the mouth found inflamed and ulcerated, but the soft palate, fauces, epiglottis, and the upper part of the pharynx are seen to be more or less intensely congested, and coated more or less extensively with false membrane. The epiglottis is often ulcerated on both its surfaces, and partially coated with false membrane; and the mucous membrane of the larynx is generally eroded by numerous small ulcerations, as well as covered with a similar deposit. I have in no instance observed false membrane extending below the larynx; and although the trachea is usually congested, sometimes intensely so, yet this is by no means of invariable occurrence. Bronchitis and pneumonia, especially the latter, are frequent complications of this affection.

The peculiar sound that characterizes the cough of croup, the stridor of the respiration, and the urgent dyspnœa which attend the progress of the disease, result, as I scarcely need remind you almost entirely from the spasmodic action of the muscles of the larynx, and not from the mechanical obstacle which the presence of false membrane offers to the free admission or exit of air. We have seen that these symptoms are, on the whole, less marked in cases where croup appears as a secondary affection, and the larynx becomes involved by the extension to it of disease beginning in the throat, than in those where the air-passages themselves are primarily affected. Still they vary much, both in the period of their occurrence and the degree of their severity, even in those cases that most resemble each other; and they bear no certain relation to the intensity of the inflammation any more than to the amount of the deposit of false membrane. The diversities in this respect depend on constitutional peculiarity rather than on any essential differences in the nature of the disease.

This view, indeed, is not taken by all writers, but some observers of deservedly high repute—such, for instance, as M. Guersant[1]—have conceived that there are differences sufficient to warrant our placing in a separate category those cases of croup which are marked by the predominance of spasmodic symptoms. They have proposed to designate this form of the disease by the name of *laryngitis stridula*, to distinguish it from ordinary croup, the laryngitis pseudo-membranacea. It was doubtless the observation of some cases of this kind that led Dr. Millar[2] more than a century ago, to describe under the name of the "acute asthma" a disease resembling croup in many respects, but presenting a mixture of spasmodic and inflammatory symptoms—the former predominating at the commencement of the disease, the latter towards its close. Dr. Millar appears, indeed, in some measure to have confounded two very different affections,—the true spasmodic croup, or laryngismus stridulus, with the inflammatory croup, or cynanche trachealis, under the idea that they constituted the two stages of one disease. But nevertheless, cases are sometimes observed that bear a very close resemblance to Millar's description, though no advantage seems to me likely to arise from constituting a new species of croup out of a modification in its symptoms produced by the idiosyncrasy of the patient.

In some children there is a greater tendency to spasmodic affections

[1] In the article "Croup," in vol. ix of the 2d edition of the Dictionnaire de Médecine, &c. Paris, 1835.

[2] Observations on the Asthma and on the Hooping-cough, 8vo., London, 1769.

than in others: in such the laryngeal nerves will take the alarm at the very outset of the disease, and the paroxysms of dyspnœa will consequently commence at an early stage, and will soon attain great intensity, but may become masked by the permanent distress of breathing to which the disease in its progress gives rise. In other instances, the symptoms of inflammatory disease, and those of spasmodic disturbance, may be so commingled, or may so alternate with each other, as to render it hard to tell from which the child suffers most. This was the case with a little boy, ten months old, who some years since came under my care, suffering from what seemed at first to be ordinary inflammatory croup. The symptoms, though not very urgent, were plainly marked, and the active employment of antimony soon dissipated them. During the whole course of the disease, however, the child, who seemed highly nervous and excitable, suffered from fits of dyspnœa far more severe than could have been anticipated from the general mildness of the attack, or than would have been supposed to exist by any one who had seen the child only in the intervals of the paroxysm. The cough and respiration had for forty-eight hours entirely lost all croupy character, and nothing but catarrh seemed left behind; when the child was suddenly seized with extreme difficulty of breathing, attended with slight croupy noise, and lay stiff in his nurse's arms with his thumbs drawn into the palms of his hands, and his great toe separated from the others. Four-and-twenty hours had elapsed from the supervention of these new symptoms before I was able to visit the child. He was then extremely restless; his face was flushed, his thumbs were drawn into the palms of his hands and his feet were forcibly extended; his breathing was labored, and attended with a hoarse croupy sound, which became still more distinct whenever the child coughed. The bowels had not acted for a couple of days; but an hour after my visit some purgative medicine, of which large doses had been given during the previous six or eight hours, began to act, and produced three very copious evacuations, with perfect relief to all his symptoms. The carpopedal contractions disappeared, the respiration became easy, and the face ceased to be flushed or anxious. The child slept well through the night, was cheerful on the following day, and slight hoarseness attending his occasional cough was the only remaining symptom. In a day or two that also disappeared, and the child perfectly recovered.

The influence of that spasmodic element which enters so largely into the production of the symptoms of cynanche trachealis, is seen in many cases in the long persistence of a croupy sound with the cough, and in its subsequent recurrence when a patient who has once had croup catches cold. In these cases the nerves have doubtless not thoroughly recovered from the effects of the previous inflammation.

Before closing this lecture, one or two additional illustrations may be adduced of *spasmodic affection of the larynx* in connection with disease seated elsewhere;[1] though the remarks made at an early period of the course, on spasm of the glottis as a frequent attendant on the con-

[1] See Lecture xiii, p. 163.

vulsive affections of infancy, must have made you thoroughly familiar with its occurrence.[1]

MM. Rilliet and Barthez have described a spasmodic cough that returns in paroxysms, is loud, attended with an imperfect hoop, and may be easily taken for hooping-cough by the inattentive observer. It is, however, a symptom of bronchial phthisis, due to the extension to the larynx of irritation seated in a distant part of the respiratory organs.

Intestinal irritation is a frequent cause of nervous cough in childhood. It is sometimes a loud, solitary, ringing cough—the tussis ovilla, tussis ferina of medical writers; at other times it is a short dry cough, attended with no particular inconvenience, but teasing from its frequency. Both of these forms appear to result in many instances from the presence of worms, and speedily cease under the judicious employment of purgative medicines.

Lastly, I may once more remind you of the cough which is occasionally heard in the early stage of inflammatory affections of the brain. It is a very short, hoarse cough, which sometimes continues for a few minutes almost incessantly, then ceases for a time, and then, after a pause, returns again. The disturbance of the brain is sympathized with by the larynx, and the depletion which relieves the former organ removes the irritation of the latter.

---

[1] There is a form of spasmodic affection of the larynx, which, under the name of Thymic Asthma, has attracted considerable attention among Continental writers, though my own experience concerning it is confined to a single case which I observed many years ago. The spasm of the glottis, which is the most prominent symptom in this affection, is supposed to be due to the pressure of the hypertrophied thymus on the larynx, and the consequent irritation of its nerves.

The essay of Haugsted—Thymi in homine, etc.: descriptio anatomica, pathologica et physiologica, 8vo., Hafniæ, 1832—may be consulted with advantage by any one desirous of becoming thoroughly acquainted with the subject I owe to Professor Gairdner, of Glasgow, the obligation of his having directed my attention, in a note at p. 263 of his Lectures on Clinical Medicine, by which he has left all members of our profession largely his debtors; to the memoir by Dr. Hood, of Kilmarnock, on Spasm of the Glottis from enlarged Thymus, published in the Edinburgh Medical Journal for January, 1827. He "who proves, discovers," is an old adage, but a true one; I am glad that it should find a fresh verification, as in Dr. Hood's case, among our northern countrymen.

LECTURE XXVI.

Hooping-Cough.—Course of the disease in its simplest form—Subject to great variations in its mode of onset and degree of severity—Signification of the hoop—Course of the disease when declining—Its danger depends on its complications—Complication with bronchitis—At its outset, or when it has continued for some time—Complication with disorder of the nervous system—Sometimes exists from the first, and causes death even before characters of disease are fully developed—But may come on at any period—Various forms assumed by disorder of nervous system—Great danger when paroxysms of cough terminate in convulsions—Caution as to nervous character of dyspnœa in many cases, and as to danger of overtreating it—Tubercular meningitis rare as a complication.

We pass next to the study of one of the most common disorders of childhood. Few persons attain to adult age without having experienced an attack of hooping-cough, and still fewer of those who escape it when children suffer from it in after-life.

Hooping-cough, then, claims our notice as being essentially a disease of early life; but as it is one which almost every old woman professes to cure, we might fairly expect not to be detained long with its study. We find, however, that in this metropolis it ranks fourth among the causes of death under five years of age; inflammation of the lungs, convulsions, and tubercular meningitis being the only more fatal ailments. Nor do these facts adequately represent its importance; for it is alleged to be the most fatal of all the diseases of early infancy; while 68 per cent. of the total deaths which it occasions take place in children under the age of two years.[1] A cursory inquiry will not suffice to make us thoroughly acquainted with all points of importance in the history of a disease that has so many victims.

The affection in its simplest form consists of a cough of spasmodic character, that usually succeeds to catarrhal symptoms, and having recurred at intervals for a few weeks, ceases without having occasioned any serious disturbance of the general health, or having required any active medical treatment. In its graver forms it is one of the most fearful diseases that we ever have to encounter, often keeping the life of the patient for days or weeks together in almost constant jeopardy, liable to be exaggerated by the most trivial cause, or rendered fatal by the slightest error in treatment; while the highest effort of our art is limited to mitigating the severity and warding off the urgent danger of symptoms which we are unable wholly to subdue, and which we must trust to time and nature thoroughly to cure.

Such great differences in the course of the disease in different cases have given rise to many ingenious theories as to its nature and seat, framed with the view of explaining that which cannot but strike all

[1] Dr. E. Smith, in Reynolds's System of Medicine, vol. i, 2d ed., 1870, p. 53.

observers as so enigmatical in its character. None of these speculations, however, have led to any useful practical result, and we shall be better employed than in their study, if we confine ourselves to the simple observation of *the phenomena of the disease*. In doing this, we will begin with those cases in which it is most simple and least perilous, and will then examine in succession the different modes in which its course becomes complicated and dangerous.

An attack of hooping-cough usually begins with catarrh, and presents at first little or nothing to distinguish it from a common cold, except that at sometimes the cough is attended almost from the outset with a peculiar ringing sound. By degrees the catarrhal symptoms abate, and the slight disturbance of the child's health altogether ceases, but nevertheless the cough continues; it grows louder and lasts longer than before, and assumes something of a suffocative character, in all of which respects a tendency to exacerbation towards night becomes early apparent. As the cough grows severer, its peculiarities become more and more manifest; during each paroxysm the child turns red in the face, and its whole frame is shaken with the violence of the cough. Each fit of coughing is now made up of a number of short, hurried expirations, so forcible, and succeeding each other with such rapidity, that the lungs are emptied, to a great degree, of air, and the child is brought by their continuance into a condition of impending suffocation. At length the child draws breath with a long, loud, sonorous inspiration—the *hoop* from which the disease derives its name—and the attack sometimes terminates. More often, however, the hoop is followed by but a momentary pause, and the hurried expiratory efforts begin again, and are again arrested by the loud inspiration—perhaps only to recommence; until, after the abundant expectoration of glairy mucus, or retching, or actual vomiting, free inspiration takes place, and quiet breathing by degrees returns. If you listen to the chest during a fit of hooping-cough you will hear no sound whatever in the lungs; but when the hoop occurs, you will once more perceive air entering, though not penetrating into the minuter bronchi. It is not till the fit is over, and respiration once more goes on quietly, that the air reaches the pulmonary cells again; but then you will hear vesicular murmur as clear as if nothing ailed the child, or at most interrupted only by a little rhonchus, or by slight mucous râle. If the cough is severe, quiet breathing does not return, nor the vesicular murmur become audible, till some time after the paroxysm is over; and occasionally, short and laborious respiration ushers in each fit of coughing. The child then seems to have a presentiment of the coming seizure; its face grows anxious, it looks up at its mother, and clings more closely to her; or, if old enough to run about, you may observe it, even before its breathing has become manifestly affected, throw down its playthings, and hasten to seize hold of a chair, or of some article of furniture, for support during the approaching fit of coughing.

If the case is uncomplicated, even though the attack be severe, the child's health continues good, and little or nothing ails it during the intervals of the cough. Its appetite is not impaired, but after throwing up the contents of the stomach in a fit of coughing, it asks for food almost immediately. It sleeps soundly, except when roused by the cough; the bowels act regularly, or are perhaps a little constipated, and slight complaint of headache or languor, with loss of the usual cheerfulness, are often all the permanent ill effects to be discerned between the seizures.

After the hoop has been heard, the disease goes on for about a week to increase in severity, the cough becoming more frequent, its paroxysms severer and more suffocating, and attended with more frequent hoop. After remaining stationary for ten days or a fortnight, it begins to decline; and one of the first indications of this is usually afforded by a diminution in the severity of the nocturnal exacerbations. We next find, either that the fits of coughing are less frequent, or, though they should occur as often as before, yet they are less severe and sometimes cease without the occurrence of a hoop. When on the decline, however, exposure to cold, neglect of the state of the bowels, or mental excitement, will suffice in many cases to bring back the hoop, and to increase the previously diminished severity of the attack. For the most part, the cough loses its spasmodic character for many days before it ceases altogether; and you may even find a child, otherwise in good health, who, some six weeks after an attack of hooping-cough, still has occasional returns of cough, which a slight cause would once more convert into an ailment with all the characters of fully developed pertussis.

Such is the ordinary course of the disease in those cases in which it is unattended by any complication, and does not give rise to any formidable symptom, but issues in the complete recovery of the patient. But even in favorable cases its course is often variously modified, while these modifications derive additional importance from frequently betokening or accompanying some of those serious complications to which the danger of the disease is almost exclusively due.

The average *duration of the catarrhal stage* of hooping-cough, as deduced from a comparison of fifty-five cases, in which the date of the occurrence of the first distinct hoop was ascertained, was 12.7 days. In nineteen of these cases the first hoop was heard within seven days from the commencement of the catarrhal symptoms, and in nineteen more cases during the succeeding seven days; but the extreme limits of the duration of the premonitory stage are very wide apart, since on one occasion it lasted only two days, and on another thirty-five days.

But there are many other respects in which the mode of onset of hooping-cough varies, as is clearly shown by the following facts:

In fifty-five cases the average duration of the catarrhal stage was 12.7 days; the extremes being 2 and 35 days. In eighteen cases the catarrhal stage lasted on the average only 8.3 days, when the cough assumed a distinctly paroxysmal character; but no hoop occurred till the fifteenth day. In four cases, after the catarrhal stage had lasted on the average 11.5 days, the cough became paroxysmal, but no hoop occurred during the whole course of the affection. In one case the cough had a distinctly paroxysmal character from the first, but no hoop occurred during the whole course of the affection. In six cases the cough was paroxysmal from the outset, and continued so on the average 9.3 days, at the end of which time distinct hoop accompanied it.

In three cases a distinct hoop attended the cough from the very commencement.

Some of these may be merely accidental differences, but I believe that most of them are by no means unimportant, and that they depend on causes with which a little observation will make you acquainted. My excuse, indeed, for bringing before you such dry detail with reference to hooping-cough, is, that there is scarcely any other disease of early life concerning which we are so much in want of definite facts. Its general features are so obvious, that persons have not observed with equal care those less striking characters which yet are of much moment, as affording sure grounds for prognosis, and trustworthy indications for the guidance of treatment.

Unusual protraction of the catarrhal stage of hooping-cough is, I believe, usually met with either at the commencement of an epidemic of the disease, or towards its close. Epidemic hooping-cough very frequently succeeds to epidemic catarrh; the former disease becoming gradually developed out of the latter, and the pesistence of cough in several cases, long after the decline of all other indications of catarrh, is often one of the first signs of the commencement of an epidemic of hooping-cough. The characters of hooping-cough, like those of other epidemic diseases, often become less marked towards the decline of its prevalence, and we then meet with cases in which catarrhal symptoms continue long, while the paroxysms of cough are slight, and the hoop occurs very seldom and not severely. It may be laid down as a general rule, that those cases in which the catarrhal stage is of long continuance seldom become severe during their subsequent progress, and the same holds good with reference to the majority of those cases in which the hoop does not come on until after the cough has for some time assumed a paroxysmal character. There are, however, some instances, which we shall hereafter have to notice, where the long duration of the paroxysmal and suffocative character of the cough, unattended by any hoop, is a sign of the peculiar intensity of the disease, rather than of its mildness; on the other hand, the preternatural shortness of the catarrhal stage, or its total absence, is not of itself any proof that the disease will be more than usually severe. It is usually observed in very young children, who, as I have already told you, are but little liable to catarrhal affections, and who are not so often attacked by hooping-cough as those who are older. Sometimes, however, when other children in the same family are suffering from it, they contract the disease apparently by contagion, and in that case it frequently happens that no purely catarrhal symptoms precede it, but that the cough from the first presents a paroxysmal character, and soon becomes attended with a distinct hoop.

Instead of coming on with catarrh of moderate intensity, hooping-cough sometimes sets in with great fever, dyspncea, and many symptoms of severe bronchitis; though the results of auscultation do not indicate such serious disease as, judging from the amount of constitutional disturbance, we should expect to discover. In such [illegible] only on the subsidence of the acute symptoms, which usually [illegible] speedily under treatment, that the real nature of the disease [illegible] apparent. We then observe, however, that while the child in all other respects improves, the cough continues unabated, that it soon grows more severe, returning in paroxysms, and being attended before long by the characteristic hoop. Besides these cases there are others, though much less common, in which, though the catarrhal symptoms are not unusually severe, the child yet has paroxysms of dyspnœa, which generally come on at night, and may excite much apprehension on the part of the parents. The attacks do not appear to be induced by any previous fit of coughing, and after lasting from half an hour to an hour they pass off of their own accord, leaving the child free for many hours together, and probably not returning until the following night. While the child continues subject to them, auscultation discovers no sign of serious mischief in the lungs; but in proportion as the paroxysms of the cough increase in distinctness, and the hoop becomes established, the fits of dyspnœa diminish, and in the course of a few days entirely disappear.

Some days usually elapse after the general characters of the disease have become well marked, before it reaches its *acme*, and during this time its nocturnal paroxysms generally increase in a greater ratio, both as to frequency and severity, than those which occur by day. Such, at least, was the course of the disease in thirty-eight out of forty-seven cases in which this point was especially noticed. The nocturnal exacerbation is sometimes so marked, that the fits of coughing are not only severer, but are actually more numerous by night-time than by day. In very mild cases of hooping-cough there is but little difference between the frequency and severity of the paroxysms at night-time and by day; and in other instances, while the child rests quietly through the greater part of the night, there is yet a marked aggravation of the cough on first lying down at night, and on first waking in the morning. When the exacerbations occur at those two periods, the evening exacerbation is often induced by the child being removed to a bed-room less warm than the apartment in which it spends the day, while the morning attack results from the accumulation of mucus in the bronchi during the hours of sleep.

Neither of these causes, however, is the sole occasion of the increased severity of the disease at night, nor is the occurrence peculiar to hooping-cough, but is observed also in asthma, and in many other affections of the respiratory organs in adults. The severity of the nocturnal paroxysms is often a very good criterion of the general severity of the disease; and any exacerbation of the disease is usually attended with special increase of the nocturnal paroxysms, and not merely by more frequent coughing and hooping, but likewise by a marked increase of dyspnœa. On the other hand, a diminution of the nocturnal exacerbations is one of the most frequent indications that the disease has begun to lose something of its previous severity, and the cough often ceases entirely at night for some time before it disappears completely during the daytime.

Cough, preceded by catarrhal symptoms, aggravated in paroxysms, assuming a suffocative character, and attended with a peculiar sonorous inspiration called a hoop, were said to be the characteristics of this disease. The last two of these phenomena are the special results of the nervous element which goes to make up the very compound character of hooping-cough. Hence, in those cases which are very mild, there is so little spasm of the glottis, that air enters freely when the child draws breath after a fit of coughing, and the hoop is occasional and faint, while it is still more seldom that the cough displays that suffocative character which, when severe, constitutes one of its most formidable peculiarities.

None of the phenomena of this disease call for such close observation as *the hoop* from which it derives its name. Its occurrence indicates on the one hand the existence of spasm of the glottis; and hence in those cases which are very slight it takes place but seldom, while it hardly ever comes on until the disease has lasted a certain time, and acquired a certain degree of intensity. It shows, however, on the other hand, that air does enter when the child endeavors to inspire, and, therefore, in cases of severe hooping-cough, a loud, long-drawn, sonorous hoop, instead of adding to our apprehension, tends rather to quiet it, for it assures us that the spasm does not amount to actual closure of the glottis, and that, for this time at least, the child will not choke in the fit of coughing. I have already mentioned to you that the nocturnal dyspnœa which excites anxiety in some cases while hooping-cough is coming on, may disappear altogether when the disease has assumed its regular type, and the hoop has become loud and distinct. Just in the same way, the violent suffocative character of the paroxysm often abates, the fits of coughing become fewer, and the dyspnœa grows less urgent, after the hoop has become developed.

But, if the disease should increase in severity, cough comes on more frequently, and the paroxysms are of longer continuance, so that the face grows quite livid before they pass away, the lips become purple, the eyes seem starting from their sockets, as in a person who is being strangled. Some of the small vessels give way, and ecchymosis more or less extensive takes place beneath the conjunctivæ; or blood bursts forth from the back of the throat, or tinges the mucus which at last is expectorated from the air-tubes, or is rejected by vomiting from the stomach. The pauses in the fit are now no longer marked by the sonorous hoop, but after a momentary cessation, the cough recommences; and though when at length the attack passes off a hoop is heard, it is more stridulous than it used to be, though not so loud. Each paroxysm of cough is now preceded and followed by marked dyspnœa, and the child has scarcely recovered from one attack before another comes on. The hoop now sometimes disappears altogether, or is very occasional, very short, and suppressed; and then the cough itself loses its former character; the child dreads its approach much and tries to suppress it, but in vain; the whole frame labors with the convulsive efforts, but no sound is produced; the larynx is now completely closed; violent, but fruitless, expiratory efforts are made, as in some of the worst cases of spasmodic croup, till general convulsions come on; or at length the spasmodic constriction yields, and the attempt at expiration is successful. The spasm over, the child once more draws breath, but it is left quite exhausted by the violence of the struggle; while sometimes [illegible] it has recovered from this seizure, another, and then another, succeeds, till one at length proves fatal.

When the disease has approached to this degree of intensity, we should rejoice to hear the loud, long hoop again, which would be a sure token of some diminution in the suffocative character of the cough. We should next find that as the hoop regained its former character, those more numerous but less distinct efforts, which the child had made before, would be merged in the single prolonged inspiration. The dyspnœa would next diminish, and then the severity of each paroxysm would grow less; and then they would not recur so often, and the hoop would be less loud and the night attacks less frequent. If amendment were to continue, the attacks would become more brief, and they would sometimes pass off without any hoop, while the mucous expectoration would become more copious; next the hoop would altogether cease, but the cough would continue to recur in paroxysms, and to present something of its old suffocative character; and then this too would cease, though cough might still continue for a time longer.

The variations in the course of hooping-cough which I have now described, depend for the most part either on the greater or less intensity of the disease, or on some idiosyncrasy of the patient, or on some peculiarity in the epidemic constitution of the year. There are, however, other, and some of them much more important changes in its symptoms and its course, which result from hooping-cough becoming complicated with another disease. Of these *complications*, by far the most frequent and most perilous are those which it presents with bronchitis and pneumonia on the one hand; and with convulsions, congestion of the brain, or tubercular meningitis, on the other. Their importance, too, is greatly increased by there being no period of the disease to which we can look as bringing with it any immunity from either; but, from the commencement of the cough to its complete disappearance, we are at any moment exposed to the risk of disease, either of the lungs or of the brain, converting a trivial into a most formidable affection.[1]

---

[1] Of 35 children who died of hooping-cough under my care, 17 perished in consequence of the supervention of bronchitis or pneumonia; 18 from congestion of the brain, from convulsions coming on in a fit of coughing, or from tubercular meningitis.

Reckoning the commencement of the disease from the first distinct hoop, or first appearance of a well-marked paroxysmal character of the cough, it appears that of 31 cases in which this point was noted—

Dying through the lungs.	Dying through the brain.	Total.	Dying within
0	1	1	7 days.
2	4	6	14 "
2	3	5	21 "
0	2	2	28 "
1	1	2	5 weeks.
2	0	2	6 "
3	3	6	7 "
1	1	2	8 "
4	1	5	from 8 weeks to 3 months.
15	16	31	

The circumstances in which *hooping-cough becomes associated with other affections of the respiratory organs* are very various. Sometimes, as I have already mentioned, rather severe bronchitic symptoms, frequent short cough, and considerable dyspnœa, precede the full development of the disease. This occurrence is oftenest met with at the commencement of epidemics of hooping-cough, or in children the mucous membrane of whose air-tubes may be supposed to have acquired a peculiar susceptibility from many previous bronchitic seizures. On the whole, however, these are not the cases which need excite our greatest solicitude, for the constitutional symptoms, which are generally out of all proportion to the amount of the local mischief, usually subside in the course of a few days, just as we often observe to be the case with epidemic influenza in the adult; and as the characteristic cough and hoop come on, all cause for anxiety disappears.

Those cases are in general much more serious in which the symptoms of bronchitis or pneumonia come on after the cough has assumed the characters of hooping-cough. This complication sometimes occurs very early in the course of the disease, and then the bronchitis and hooping-cough appear to be developed almost simultaneously. For a day or two, perhaps, a hoop has been heard accompanying the cough at intervals, and nothing has appeared to indicate that the attack will be unusually severe, when all the symptoms suddenly become very much aggravated; the skin grows hot; the respiration and pulse become very much hurried, and this increase in their frequency is permanent, though much greater at one time than at another. The cough at the same time becomes more frequent and more severe, and the hoop is more violent, but the cough is almost entirely unattended with expectoration, or if a little mucus is spit up it is almost always streaked with blood. Though very violent, the fits of coughing are not very long, and they seldom or never end with vomiting. The ear detects mucous râle through nearly the whole of both lungs: on a deep inspiration still smaller sounds are heard, for inflammation has attacked the minuter air-tubes; and the case is one of hooping-cough complicated with capillary bronchitis.

Supposing the disease to continue, the cough will often in a day or two lose its characteristic hoop, an occurrence which you will likewise observe in the course of many other intercurrent febrile or inflammatory affections that may supervene during an attack of hooping-cough. The cough, too, may become less frequent, or may lose its paroxysmal character, though it will still appear to cause much suffering. The respiration will increase in frequency, the child constantly laboring for breath, and being distressed by the slightest movement, since that adds to its dyspnœa. In one little child two years old, the inspirations two days before her death were 130 in the minute, and then on the following day they sank to 80: but her feet were now cold, her face was livid, and her pulse very feeble. It was she of whose lungs I showed the drawing some days since, illustrative of vesicular bronchitis: and her case might be taken as a type of those in which acute bronchitis comes on at an early stage of hooping-cough.

Death takes place more speedily in cases of this kind than [illegible] any other form of affection of the lungs which comes on in the course of hooping-cough. I have seen a child die on the sixth day from the first appearance of any indication that the disease was other than a very mild attack of hooping-cough. It will not surprise you that the fatal event should take place so speedily, if you bear in mind that after death we discover either intense injection, even of the smaller bronchi, with copious effusion of pus into their cavities, or very extensive vesicular bronchitis, or both conditions together.

But it is not only at the outset of an attack of hooping-cough that we encounter the danger of its becoming complicated with other disease of the lungs. Exposure to cold, or damp, may at almost any time induce an exacerbation of the cough, or a distinct attack of bronchitis. If, however, the disease has already lasted for some ten days or a fortnight, without having presented any grave features, such intercurrent bronchitic seizures are usually very tractable.

As a general rule, those cases have appeared to me to be far more serious in which bronchitic symptoms become developed of their own accord out of severe hooping-cough. In such cases there has usually been a gradual increase in the child's sufferings; the cough growing more frequent, and, though not more violent, yet evidently occasioning the child greater suffering while the hoop is unchanged in its character. At the same time the child seems overwhelmed by the disease; its face is anxious and puffed, the eyes are much suffused, the skin usually dry and hot; dyspnœa is no longer confined to the periods just before and just after a fit of coughing, but the respiration is habitually wheezing, hurried, and rather irregular. The ear, at the same time, detects mucous or subcrepitant râle through the whole of both lungs. Such cases are seldom very rapid in their course. The symptoms, after exciting our solicitude for a week, ten days, or a fortnight, may gradually abate in severity, and the disease may run the remainder of its course slowly, but safely. If the case should have an unfavorable issue, this sometimes takes place speedily, owing to the supervention of cerebral symptoms; and the child then dies during a paroxysm of coughing. Or the minute bronchi may become involved in the inflammatory mischief; the case may assume the characters of pneumonia, and bronchial breathing and dulness on percussion may reveal during the patient's lifetime the nature of the mischief which will be disclosed on an examination after death.

In a still more numerous class of cases, the disease retains its chronic character to the last, and presents little or no variation from day to day. The violence of the cough, and the frequency of its return, sometimes continue unabated, though often they undergo a marked diminution. The respiration grows more hurried than before, the fever becomes exacerbated, and the emaciation extreme; while the child's strength is still more enfeebled by the supervention of a troublesome diarrhœa, which no remedies are adequate to restrain. Death at length takes place, sometimes from pure exhaustion; and the transition from sleep to death is so gentle as to be almost imperceptible. At other times an increase of the symptoms of bronchitis or pneumonia becomes apparent for two or three days previously; or in other cases the child dies exhausted in a fit of coughing, or convulsions take place a few hours before death, and the patient dies convulsed or comatose.

The *complication of hooping-cough with serious disorder of the nervous system* is almost as frequent as its association with grave mischief in the lungs and air-tubes, and even more dangerous and perplexing. Hazard from this source attends alike the onset of the disease, its acme, and decline; and the mode in which the danger presents itself is no less variable than are the seasons of its occurrence. The nervous system sometimes suffers so severely from the very first, that death takes place almost before the disease has had time to assume its usual characters. At other times hooping-cough comes on naturally; its two elements, the bronchitic and the nervous (if I may be allowed the expression), increase daily in intensity, till all at once the symptoms of the former recede, and are almost lost in those of the latter, which in a day or two bring on the fatal termination of the case. Or, lastly, no symptoms referable to the nervous system call for our solicitude until after the hooping-cough has continued many weeks; but then the long continuance of the disease seems to excite mischief in the brain, and death overtakes the patient when we had already begun to hope that nothing more than time was needed to perfect his cure.

Danger from this cause sometimes assumes the form of simple congestion of the brain; drowsiness is followed by convulsions, and these are succeeded by fatal coma. In other instances the spinal system of nerves becomes excited to more tumultuous reaction; and carpopedal contractions, and attacks of spasm of the glottis, are superadded to frequently recurring general convulsions; while in some cases the long continuance of hooping-cough gives rise to the development of tubercular meningitis. The time will not be lost that we may spend in the examination of each of these various modes in which hooping-cough becomes complicated with disorder of the nervous system.

In very young children, and in those in whom the process of dentition is still going on at the time of their becoming affected with hooping-cough, the symptoms of disturbance of the nervous system are sometimes formidable even from the outset. In such cases the preliminary catarrh is usually of short duration, and the cough, though not very frequent, yet assumes a paroxysmal character almost from the first. Each fit of coughing is extremely violent and suffocative; it lasts for several minutes, is not attended by any distinct hoop, nor followed by vomiting, but ceases apparently from the child being too exhausted to make any further effort. In the intervals of the cough the face is flushed, the eyes are suffused, and the child is very drowsy, and averse to being disturbed—a condition which is manifestly increased by each paroxysm of coughing. When the cough comes on, the flush of the face deepens to a livid hue, the pupils become dilated, convulsions seem impending and at length come on, and though but of short continuance, yet they often leave the child in a state of profound stupor. This condition seldom lasts long: sometimes the effort at coughing brings on a fatal convulsive seizure, at other times the cough does not return, but convulsions recur independently of it, and in twenty-four or thirty-six hours from their first occurrence the child dies.

No cases of hooping-cough run so surely or so speedily as these to a fatal termination, which even the most judicious treatment will often fail to prevent. I have seen death take place in less than a week from the commencement of the cough, and have known several instances of its occurrence long before the lapse of a fortnight.

The fact that the cough has run its course naturally up to a certain point affords, however, no guarantee against the supervention of a danger similar to that which we have just been contemplating. It is indeed but seldom that any case which for the first ten days or fortnight has been mild in character, afterwards presents these alarming symptoms of cerebral disturbance; for in most instances the cough will have been severe from the commencement, the paroxysms frequent and of long continuance, the hoop loud, each attack terminating with vomiting, and the return of each being much dreaded by the child. In all this, however, there is nothing to direct special attention to the head, and the approach of the new danger is not always very obvious. Sometimes the first indication that the head suffers is afforded by the increased irritability of the stomach, which becomes almost unable to retain food or drink. And here let me urge upon you the importance of duly estimating the signification of this symptom. Vomiting, independent of the fits of coughing, if it persists for above twenty-four hours, and is not referable to the remedies you are employing, nor connected with obvious gastric disorder, should always excite your solicitude, and direct your attention most anxiously to the head.

At other times, either in connection with this irritability of the stomach, or even independently of it, the child is observed to become daily more heavy and drowsy, and averse to movement; complaining of headache if able to talk, and appearing overwhelmed by the disease to a greater degree than can be accounted for either by the severity of the paroxysms or by the frequency of their recurrence. This condition is generally succeeded by aggravation of the dyspnœa both before and after each fit of coughing, the respiration sometimes not regaining its proper frequency during the interval between their return, though auscultation fails to detect any adequate cause for this hurried breathing. In some instances the hoop still continues as loud as before; but if that be the case, the cough grows harder, and hardly any mucus is expectorated; while streaks of blood are seen in the matters rejected by vomiting. It happens more frequently, however, that these symptoms are associated with a more or less complete suppression of the hoop; the cough losing something of its distinctly paroxysmal character, but becoming more suffocative; the child, on each occasion of its return, vainly striving to suppress it. A convulsive seizure now, in some cases, supervenes on an effort to cough, and in this the child expires; or the fatal convulsion may come on to all appearance causelessly; or, more frequently, the first convulsion does not occasion death, but it leaves the child in a comatose condition, which is interrupted by the frequent return of convulsions, one of which at length proves fatal.

It happens sometimes that children who are laboring under severe hooping-cough are suddenly seized, during a paroxysm of coughing, with a fit of convulsions; and they may die in this fit, even though they had not previously seemed to suffer from any serious disorder of the nervous system. Death in such cases takes place as the result of spasmodic closure of the larynx, and consequent congestion of the brain; you watch for a few moments the fruitless expiratory efforts of the child, and then all is over, just as in many fatal cases of spasmodic croup. The relation between hooping-cough and spasmodic croup, indeed, is sometimes very apparent; and you may observe, after some unusually violent fit of coughing, the thumbs drawn into the palms, the hand flexed upon the wrist, or the great toe drawn apart from the others. At first, probably, the symptoms will be slight, and will soon pass away; but their import is most serious. You will expect soon to see other and graver indications of the disturbance of the nervous system—if, indeed, they are not already present. It is especially in cases of this sort that you will observe a degree of dyspnœa which you cannot explain; and that the child will seem to make the most violent efforts to suppress the cough—efforts which are really involuntary, and are the result of the spasmodic closure of the glottis, which is sure, if complete and long continued, to be followed by an attack of convulsions. If treatment fail, the carpopedal contractions will become permanent, the eyes will close but partially, the breathing will grow extremely unequal and irregular, as well as hurried, the hoop will no longer be heard, and the cough itself will yield only a kind of smothered sound. The surface will grow quite livid, in consequence of the extremely imperfect performance of the respiratory function; the child will sink into a state of stupor, in which it will lie with dilated pupils and constant twitching of the muscles of its face, till a great effort to cough comes on, and passes almost at once into a convulsive paroxysm. The fits at length occur independent of any attempt at coughing, and once I saw a considerable degree of stiffness of the whole spinal column precede for twelve hours the death of a little boy, who fell a victim to hooping-cough thus sadly complicated with disorder of the nervous system.

It would be only by the recital of cases that I could bring before your notice each minute variation in the characters of these formidable complications of hooping-cough; and for such details our time is insufficient. There are two points, however, bearing on this subject, which I am most anxious to impress on your memory. One is, that the supervention of dyspnœa, or the sudden aggravation of difficulty of breathing which had existed previously, is often one of the earliest indications of serious affection of the nervous system. The other point, on which I shall have to dwell at our next lecture, is, that if, mistaking the import of this nervous dyspnœa, you direct your treatment to some imagined mischief in the chest, and make free use of antimony and other depressing medicines, you will aggravate, instead of relieving the difficulty of breathing; and—the irritability of the nervous system increasing in proportion as the respiration becomes impaired—you will hasten the occurrence of convulsions, and of that formidable train of symptoms which we have just been contemplating.

I mentioned that *tubercular meningitis* is now and then met with a complication of hooping-cough. Fortunately it is not of frequent occurrence, though the danger of its supervention should never be forgotten in the case of weakly children who have long suffered from severe hooping-cough. A few instances of it have come under my observation; and I have notes of two cases of it. In one of these cases the cerebral disease was associated with such a large amount of mischief in the chest as would of itself have sufficed to destroy the child. The other case was of much importance, as showing the insidious manner in which fatal disease may steal on, presenting little to excite serious apprehension till long after the possibility of doing good has passed away. The patient, a boy five years old, of a phthisical family on his mother's side, was attacked by hooping-cough, from which he suffered severely. The disease was attended by great dyspnœa, with general œdema and great lividity of the surface. No auscultatory signs of serious mischief in the lungs existed at any time; but the oppression of breathing was so considerable, and the child seemed so completely overwhelmed by the disorder, that I feared he would not recover. After he had suffered from the cough for about five weeks, and three weeks before his death, matters seemed to take a more favorable turn; his cough diminished greatly both in frequency and severity, and his strength returned under a tonic plan of treatment. He still, however, continued low-spirited, and very much disposed to sleep; and this condition of depression progressively increased, until, about a week before his death, he sank into a state of complete stupor; but no convulsions occurred either as precursors of the stupor or during its continuance. He lay on his back, either sleeping, or in a state of stupor, from which, however, he could be partially roused, when his pupils, before contracted, would become suddenly dilated to the full, and he would stare wildly about for a few moments; the pupils would then oscillate for a short time between dilatation and contraction, but soon revert to their former contracted condition. The bowels were not constipated at any time, neither did vomiting occur, and the pulse continued frequent till within a day or two of his death. Strabismus came on in a day or two before he died, and two days before his death deglutition became difficult, and he began to make slight automatic movements with his hands and arms. Paroxysms of cough continued to recur to the very last; they were suffocative in character, but unattended by hoop. At the end of the eighth week from the commencement of his cough, the child, who was extremely emaciated, died quietly.

After death, the membranes of the brain were found much congested; there was a large quantity of fluid in the ventricles; the central parts of the brain were diffluent, and its lower parts were likewise considerably softened. The membranes at the base of the brain presented an opalescent appearance, and were bestudded with numerous minute granules, while about the optic nerves they were greatly thickened and infiltrated with that hyaline matter to which I have often called your attention.

There was much congestion of the bronchi and pulmonary substance. The lungs contained a good deal of tubercle, mostly in the state of gray granulations, and a small cavity occupied the lower part of the left lower lobe.

Many points of importance connected with the history of hooping-cough remain for our examination before we can proceed to consider its treatment: but all of these must be reserved till our next meeting.

LECTURE XXVII.

Hooping-Cough continued.—Complications with diarrhœa and intestinal disorder—With great irritability of the stomach—With measles and varicella—Duration of the disease—Relapses—Influence of age, sex, season, &c., in its production—Post-mortem appearances.

Treatment.—No real specific for hooping-cough—Treatment of first and second stages—Utility of hydrocyanic acid—Of counter-irritation—Of attention to temperature—Danger of overtreating the bronchitis of hooping-cough—Treatment of third stage of disease.

It is a peculiarity of the affection which we are now studying, that much of the suffering, and almost all the danger that attend it, are the result, not of the disorder itself, but of some complication that supervenes during its course. We have already examined the two most frequent and most formidable sources of danger to patients laboring under hooping-cough, but others remain, against which it behooves us to be no less sedulously on our guard.

Some days ago I mentioned to you that a state of extreme irritability of the lining of the air-tubes is one of the characteristics of early childhood. To this are due the attacks of catarrh which children often experience while teething, and the cough which, wholly independent of exposure to cold, comes on as the result of sympathy with irritation in some distant viscus. This high degree of susceptibility, however, is not confined to the bronchi, but is possessed in the young subject by the whole tract of mucous membranes: diarrhœa often accompanies catarrh, or alternates with it, and in the course of inflammation of the lungs, the patient's life is sometimes jeopardized, or his death hastened, by the supervention of an intractable looseness of the bowels.

Diarrhœa, though comparatively seldom fatal, is frequently a very troublesome complication of hooping-cough, and if it continues, it greatly reduces the strength of a child, and interferes with the employment of some of those means to which otherwise we might have recourse. It sometimes sets in with the preliminary catarrh, and abates as that subsides, but in other cases it harasses the patient at intervals during the whole course of the affection. It is, however, when it comes on in the course of an attack of hooping-cough which has already attained considerable severity, that it should excite our chief solicitude. It does not, indeed, in the majority of instances, betoken the supervention of disease in the intestines, but it is one of the forms of constitutional disturbance that attend upon a congested state of the brain, or it indicates the advance of serious mischief in the lungs. I have, indeed, seen diarrhœa become the most prominent symptom in a case of severe hooping-cough, the bowels being for days so irritable that their action was excited by the slightest article of food or drink, while the abdomen was exquisitely tender; and yet, when death at length took place, unusual redness and prominence of the Peyerian glands were the only morbid appearances in the intestines, while the signs of intense bronchitis, and inflammation, which in some parts had advanced to suppuration, were discovered in the lungs.

An *irritable state of the stomach*, with occasional *vomiting*, are symptoms almost constantly observed at some period or other in the course of hooping-cough. In cases of a mild character, they usually occur only when the cough has reached its acme, and vomiting succeeds to none but the severest fits of coughing, while it is one of the earliest symptoms to cease as the severity of the disease declines. Sometimes, however, very distressing nausea harasses the patient, and efforts to vomit not only follow the paroxysms of coughing, but are excited by food or by the blandest fluid. I have already warned you of the serious import of this symptom in many instances, and have called your attention to it as being frequently one of the earliest indications of cerebral mischief. In some few instances I have observed it come on very early in the disease, and subside by degrees as the cough assumed a distinctly paroxysmal character; just as is the case sometimes with that nervous dyspnœa of which I spoke in my last lecture. Sometimes it continues to be a troublesome though almost a solitary symptom of disturbance of the nervous system, the cough not being severe, nor the child's health at all seriously impaired; and in two instances that I met with, it appeared to be the result of a state of extreme irritability about the fauces, so that the cough, which hardly ever occurred at other times, was immediately excited by any attempt at deglutition, and the effort to cough terminated almost directly in vomiting. Nausea and vomiting are sometimes associated with general intestinal disorder and diarrhœa; at other times there is equal evidence of disorder of the digestive organs in a constipated state of the bowels, a red tongue, with perhaps numerous small aphthous ulcers about the mouth, or in the large quantity of frothy mucus rejected by the stomach at each effort to vomit.

Before leaving the subject of the complications of hooping-cough, I must notice the relation that appears to exist between it and two of the *eruptive fevers*, namely, *measles* and *chicken-pox*. It has been thought, indeed, by some writers, that there is no connection between these diseases other than that of their accidental association; but my own experience would lead me to incline to an opposite opinion, which is likewise entertained by several high authorities. I am not, indeed, able to adduce a number of observations bearing on this point sufficient to establish the fact beyond doubt; but my belief is, that the occurrence of any one of these diseases during the epidemic prevalence of another, increases the liability of the child to become affected by that which is epidemic, and that an exacerbation of the fever of hooping-cough, and the appearance of more serious illness than the local symptoms account for, is very likely to be due to the approach either of measles or of varicella. Like other intercurrent febrile and inflammatory affections, both measles and chicken-pox often produce some temporary abatement of the paroxysms of hooping-cough, and sometimes cure the disease altogether. In this, however, there is nothing constant, for hooping-cough often appears not to be in the least modified in its character by the supervention of the other malady; while in some cases the complication adds to the mischief in the chest, and increases the patient's suffering and danger.

Although there are many important points of analogy between hooping-cough and some of the exanthemata, yet in nothing is the difference between these affections more apparent than in the uncertain duration of the former, in the exacerbations which take place during its course, either causelessly or from very slight occasions, and in the actual relapses that sometimes occur after apparent cure. It is a matter of considerable difficulty, in the case of a disease so protracted in its course as hooping-cough, to make even an approximation to a correct estimate of its *duration*. In twenty-five cases, however, I had the opportunity of watching the patients from the time when the cough first assumed a paroxysmal character, or the hoop first became audible, until the final cessation of all cough. From this small number of observations I should be disposed to estimate the average duration of hooping-cough at ten weeks; of which period nearly two weeks[1] would be occupied by the preliminary catarrh, for four weeks the cough would present the characteristic hoop, and the cough would continue for about the same period to occur occasionally, gradually losing its paroxysmal character; though exposure to cold, or any trivial cause, would suffice to bring back the hoop, and to restore to the paroxysms of the cough all their former intensity. So long as any cough continues, even though very occasional in its occurrence, and though the hoop have entirely ceased for many weeks, the patient cannot be regarded as well; while the neglect of proper hygienic precautions may protract the duration of the cough for between three and four months—an occurrence by no means unusual among the poor. I have on several occasions treated children for hooping-cough during the spring, in whom the hoop has disappeared, and the cough almost ceased, in the warm months of summer; but on the approach of autumn has returned with nearly its former intensity. In other cases, hooping-cough contracted in the early part of autumn has returned during the prevalence of cold March winds; or a casual catarrhal seizure has been followed by a recurrence of all the signs of the disease in a severe form. These relapses of hooping-cough frequently set in with considerable severity, the paroxysms of cough being very frequent, and the hoop loud and often repeated; but, if treated

---

[1] The estimate of the duration of the catarrhal stage is deduced from the observations of 55 cases, and the exact period of its continuance was 12.7 days. Of the 25 in which the total duration of the cough from the occurrence of the first hoop was noted, 11, or nearly half, showed a duration of eight weeks; and the duration of the remaining 14 cases varied from four to twelve weeks.

judiciously, they are much more amenable to remedies than is the first attack of the disease.

A true *recurrence of hooping-cough*, after the disease has been perfectly cured, is at least as unusual as the occurrence of measles or small-pox twice in the same subject. Only one instance of hooping-cough affecting the same patient more than once has come under my notice. In that case the patient was a girl aged seven years, who, when three years old, had very severe hooping-cough, which lasted for several weeks, the paroxysms of cough being frequent and the hoop loud and often repeated. In March, 1845, hooping-cough being then epidemic, she experienced a return of the disease in a very severe form, and continued to suffer from it until the end of June.

But little more remains to complete the history of the disease, except that we notice briefly the *circumstances in which it comes on.* It is essentially an affection of childhood, few children escaping from it, while more than half the cases of it occur before the completion of the third year. After the age of five years its frequency rapidly diminishes, and after ten it becomes so extremely rare that, out of 1367 cases in which I noticed the patient's age, I find but eleven in which it exceeded ten years.[1] The occurrence of the disease appears to be influenced to a considerable degree by sex as well as age; and, as is the case with a large number of the non-inflammatory disorders of the nervous system, females suffer from it in a considerably larger proportion than males. Of 100 cases of hooping-cough at the Children's Infirmary, 55.3 per cent. occurred in females, only 44.7 per cent. in males; although the total number of female children to the total number of males among my patients at that institution was only as 50.2 to 49.8.

Age and sex exert an evident influence on the mortality of the disease as well as on its prevalence, both being greatest in early childhood, though hooping-cough does not seem to be so formidable before the commencement of dentition as it is while that process is going on.

---

[1] Of the above 1367 cases—

41.2	per cent. occurred	during	the first	2	years of life.
56.7	"	"	"	3	"
82 9	"	"	"	5	"
98.4	"	"	"	10	"

The subjoined table shows the proportion borne by these hooping-cough cases to 14,440 cases of all diseases at the same ages, which occurred during the same period at the Children's Infirmary. Cases of hooping-cough constituted—

8.4	per cent.	of all cases	occurring	under the age of 6 months.			
10 4	"	"	"	from 6	months	to 12	months.
10.8	"	"	"	" 12	"	18	"
9.8	"	"	"	" 18	"	2	years.
12.2	"	"	"	" 2	years to	3	"
14.6	"	"	"	" 3	"	4	"
13.2	"	"	"	" 4	"	5	"
11.2	"	"	"	under		5	"
7.2	"	"	"	from 5		10	"
.8	"	"	"	" 10	"	15	"

Female children are not only more liable to the affection, but it proves more fatal to them than to boys in the proportion of about 3 to 2.[1]

Hooping-cough is a disease of all climates, and though more frequent in the cold than in the warm months of the year, yet its epidemics break out at almost all seasons. The epidemic of 1841–2 reached its acme in the months of December and January; while in 1845, cases of hooping-cough were by far more numerous in the months of June and July than during any other part of the year. Though little influenced by the season of the year, the outbreak of an epidemic of hooping-cough seldom, if ever, takes place suddenly, and altogether without warning. Sometimes, as already mentioned, it succeeds to an epidemic of measles, but still more frequently it follows an unusual prevalence of catarrh, in which the cough gradually becomes paroxysmal, and at length puts on the characters of hooping-cough. In a similar way, epidemic hooping-cough sometimes resolves itself into simple catarrh: the signs of disturbance of the nervous system by degrees disappearing, and the cases presenting the indications of mere bronchial irritation.

The question whether hooping-cough is a contagious disease, has long since been set at rest by a general answer in the affirmative. How long it retains this character is an inquiry to which it is not possible to return any very precise reply; but so long as a child who has suffered from hooping-cough continues to cough at all, even though only once or twice a day, I should be unwilling to restore him to the society of children who have not already had the disease. All children are not equally susceptible of the contagion, and infants under six months old appear to be especially indisposed to receive it, either by association with other children, or as the result of atmospheric influence. If carefully kept from contact with other children, infants of tender age will very often escape during the general prevalence of hooping-cough; and in nearly half of the cases of hooping-cough that I have met with in infants under six months old, other children in the family had suffered from it for a week or ten days before the infants showed any symptom of it.

You may expect, perhaps, that before I pass to the consideration

---

[1] The subjoined table shows the age at which death took place in 35 fatal cases of hooping-cough:

0 under 6 months.	6 between 4 years and 5 years.
5 between 6 months and 1 year.	1 " 5 " 6 "
6 " 1 year and 2 years.	8 " 6 " 7 "
8 " 2 " 3 "	1 " 7 " 8 "
4 " 3 " 4 "	1 " 10 " 11 "

This result tallies very closely with that afforded by the Fifth Report of the Registrar-General, from which it appears that the deaths from hooping-cough in London were to the deaths from all causes in the proportion of—

5.6 per cent. under 1 year old.	5.0 per cent. between 5 and 10 years.
10.6 " between 1 and 3 years.	.8 " " 10 " 15 "
10.2 " " 3 " 5 "	

Of the 35 cases that came under my notice, 21 occurred in female, and only 14 in male children; and the mortality under ten years of age from hooping-cough is to the total mortality at that age in London in the proportion of 8.9 per cent. among female and 6.1 per cent. among male children.

of the treatment of hooping-cough, I should say something about the *morbid appearances* to which it gives rise, and about the essential nature of the affection. I know, however, of no morbid appearances peculiar to this disease, nor do I think that much would be gained by a disquisition on its seat, or on the occult cause of its symptoms. It is through the medium of the lungs or of the brain, that death takes place in nearly every instance of fatal hooping-cough; and almost all the structural lesions of importance are found in one or other of those organs. The vessels of the brain and its membranes are often found overfilled with blood, though even in cases where death has taken place in convulsions, or has been preceded by a comatose condition, these appearances are sometimes much less marked than might have been expected, and occasionally are altogether absent. Softening of the cerebral substance, or other indications of inflammatory action, are very seldom met with; increased vascularity of the organ, with perhaps a small quantity of fluid in the ventricles, being almost the only morbid appearances in the encephalon.

It is but seldom that the lungs are found free from disease, though they present no structural changes that can be regarded as characteristic of hooping-cough. The mucous membrane of the bronchi is generally injected; sometimes it is intensely red; while an abundant secretion of thick mucus occupies the cavities of the air-tubes, and their calibre is much increased. This dilatation of the bronchi, which sometimes is very remarkable, arises from inflammation of the air-tubes, just as it does in ordinary bronchitis, and is not due, as has been erroneously supposed, to the violence of the child's inspiratory efforts. The emphysematous condition of the lung, which is likewise observed in many cases of fatal hooping-cough, has also been referred to the same forcible attempts at inspiration. MM. Rilliet and Barthez,[1] however, have observed, that the supposed violence of the inspiratory efforts during hooping-cough is altogether a mistaken assumption; for the efforts made during a paroxysm of coughing are expiratory, the lungs during a severe seizure being almost emptied of air; while in the inspiratory efforts that succeed, the air at first does not penetrate beyond the larger bronchi, and is long before it again freely permeates the pulmonary vesicles. The objection raised by these gentlemen to the *inspiratory* theory as explaining the production of emphysema in cases of uncomplicated hooping-cough, is, I believe, quite unanswerable. The fact, however, still remains that the condition is met with, and sometimes in an extreme degree, in the lungs of children who have died of hooping-cough unassociated with other diseases of the respiratory organs. To such cases the *expiratory* theory[2] applies preeminently; for, during the violent expiratory efforts with a closed glottis which characterize a paroxysm of the cough, the air is driven forcibly towards the upper part, and the circumference of the lungs; in other words, towards just those parts which are the least compressed,

---

[1] Lib. cit, vol. ii, 2d ed., p. 631.

[2] See Sir W. Jenner's exposition of it in vol. xl of the Medico-Chirurgical Transactions.

and which observation shows to be the favorite seats of emphysema. In those other cases of hooping-cough in which extensive collapse of the lungs takes place, the emphysema is produced by just the opposite means; on which indeed I need not dwell now, since I explained them fully in a former lecture.[1] I may, however, just observe, that the forcible expiratory efforts which are so characteristic of hooping-cough, as they tend in one way to the production of emphysema, so in another they exercise a powerful influence in occasioning collapse of the lung; and few cases of hooping-cough terminate fatally in which you will not find after death a more or less considerable portion of lung in this condition. It may be simply collapsed, resuming its natural appearance readily when inflated; or the bronchial tubes may have been the seat of inflammation, and be more or less filled with puriform mucus, when the characters of vesicular bronchitis will be superadded to those of mere collapse or carnification, and air will permeate the organ very imperfectly, or not at all. It cannot be necessary to describe again those other changes which may take place in carnified lung, and which end in the infiltration of pus into its tissue, or in the formation of vomicæ, since I have already done so very minutely.[2]

I do not dwell upon other appearances in the chest, such as pleurisy and lobar pneumonia, which are much less often met with, and which have none other than a perfectly casual connection with hooping-cough; but I must notice one morbid condition alleged to have been frequently observed, and which is of the more importance, since it has served as the foundation of a theory of the disease. The pneumogastric nerves have been discovered by various observers redder than natural, and in some cases swollen and softened—appearances which have been regarded as indicating that they had been the seat of inflammation. Even those observers, however, who have noticed this condition, appear to have met with it but seldom, while others have sought for it in vain in a

---

[1] Lecture xx, p. 271.

[2] It would be unjust to leave this subject without calling the reader's attention to the excellent account of collapse or carnification of the lung contained in Sir J. Alderson's paper on the Pathology of Hooping-Cough, published in the year 1830, in vol. xvi of the Medico-Chirurgical Transactions. In this paper he not only describes very correctly the anatomical characters of this condition, which had merely been indicated by previous observers, and speaks of it as a state different from pneumonia, which MM. Rufz and Gerhard did four years later, but he also suggests an explanation of its occurrence, which the recent researches of MM. Bailly and Legendre prove not to have been far from the truth.

It may be well to quote two passages from this paper: "In many other [cases] I have invariably found the same appearances, uncomplicated with any evidence of pleuritic inflammation. In the lower and posterior portions of the lungs, the structure was rendered very firm and dense; the portions which were the subjects of this change were exactly defined by the septa; of a dull red color, devoid of air, sinking instantly in water, and thin slices undergoing no change by ablution. The individual lobules were more dense than in hepatized lungs; and the cellular membrane between them retaining its natural structure, conveyed to the touch the same sensation that is felt on touching the pancreas. . . . . I apprehend that the appearances detailed differ from those found in peripneumony. In hooping-cough, the lung is always dense and *contracted*, as if the air had been expelled, and from the throwing out of adhesive matter, the sides of the air-cells had been agglutinated together: while in hepatization the lung is less dense than in hooping-cough, and is rendered more voluminous than in its natural state" (pp. 90–91).

large number of cases. Professor Albers, of Bonn,[1] states that, having examined the bodies of 47 children who died of hooping-cough, he found the nervi vagi perfectly healthy in 43. In 3 the vagus of the right side, and in 1 that of the left side, was slightly reddened; but this redness corresponded to the side towards which the body had been inclined, and in no respect differed from what is observed in the bodies of plethoric persons, and of patients who have died of typhus fever. Out of 24 examinations of the bodies of children who have died of hooping-cough, it has only once happened to me to observe any alteration in the appearance of the vagus, though my attention has been directed to it on every occasion. In that instance both nerves seemed to be of a decidedly redder color than natural, although they were not otherwise altered. We are, I think, warranted in concluding that an appearance so frequently absent, cannot be one of much moment, that it is probably a post-mortem alteration, and that certainly it cannot be adduced in support of any particular hypothesis as to the nature of the disease.

I have endeavored to describe to you the symptoms of this affection, to make you acquainted with the circumstances in which it occurs, with the course that it usually follows, and with the chief dangers that threaten a child while suffering from it. It now remains to examine the *treatment* which may be best calculated to mitigate its severity, and to ward off or overcome the dangers that attend it.

There are few diseases for the cure of which specifics have been more eagerly sought after, or more earnestly recommended, than for that of hooping-cough; neither is there anything unreasonable in the expectation that a remedy may some day or other be discovered which shall cut short its course with as much certainty as quinine arrests an intermittent fever, or which shall render the constitution insusceptible to its poison as generally as vaccination preserves from variola. At present, however, no such remedy has been discovered; and though the severity of an attack of hooping-cough, or its duration, varies greatly in different individuals, during different epidemics, or at different seasons of the year, yet we are unable by any medicinal agents to produce effects such as in these cases flow from causes quite beyond our control.

For the present, then, the treatment of hooping-cough must be conducted in accordance with the ordinary principles of therapeutics, and we shall study their application best by examining in succession the course which, in each stage of the disease, it will be our duty to pursue. The *first stage* of hooping-cough is distinguished, as you know, by catarrhal symptoms, with some degree of febrile disturbance, and a cough which gradually assumes more and more of a paroxysmal character, until at length it returns in well-marked fits, and is attended by a distinct hoop. In the majority of cases the treatment of this first stage of hooping-cough must be just that of an ordinary catarrh. The child must remain in the house, and it is desirable that it should be confined to its own apartments, both of which should be maintained at a tempera-

[1] Quoted by Aberle, De Tussi Convulsivâ, 8vo., p. 45. Vindobonæ, 1843.

ture of 60°, so that when it leaves the day for the night nursery, it may not, as is too commonly the case, enter a colder atmosphere, and thus have the irritability of the bronchi increased and the severity of the cough aggravated. If these precautions are carefully observed, and the diet is light and unstimulating, there is but little need of medicine beyond what may be required to keep the bowels regularly open. If the cough is at all troublesome, a mixture may be given, containing small doses of the ipecacuanha and antimonial wines, with a few drops of laudanum or of the compound tincture of camphor[1]—medicines that I should advise you always to use in preference to the syrup of poppies, the strength of which is very variable, and its action uncertain. If, as is sometimes the case, the child should wheeze a good deal, this symptom will be much relieved by the administration of an emetic of ipecacuanha every evening, or more frequently if necessary. It is not always, indeed, that either much care or much medicine is needed; and if hooping-cough comes on in a perfectly healthy child, in whom the process of dentition is completed, and during the warm months of summer, strict confinement to the house may not be necessary. Usually, however, care in this stage is very important, and will do much towards mitigating the severity of the subsequent course of the disease, while no precautionary measure is of so much moment as the preservation of the child from fluctuations of temperature, and from damp as well as cold.

When the first stage of hooping-cough has passed into the *second*, in which the disease assumes its characteristic features, the condition of the patient must still determine whether any remedies are to be employed, and must likewise influence their selection. It sometimes happens that the cough and hoop are very slight, and the paroxysms but few in the course of the day; and, in such circumstances, medicine can well be dispensed with. If the paroxysmal character of the cough is well marked, and the fits are of frequent occurrence, but the child in other respects ails little, much benefit will accrue from the use of the hydrocyanic acid. I usually begin with a dose of half a minim of the acid of the London Pharmacopœia every four hours for a child nine months old; and so in proportion for older children. The specific influence of the remedy is, I think, both more safely and also more efficiently exerted by increasing the frequency of its administration, than by adding to the dose, and I should therefore prefer to give half a dose every two hours rather than to double the dose without increasing the frequency of its repetition.[2] This remedy sometimes exerts an almost magical influence on the cough, diminishing the frequency and severity of its paroxysms almost immediately; while in other cases it seems perfectly inert; and again, in others, without at all diminishing the severity of

[1] See Formula No. 9, p. 263.

[2] (No. 15.)

℞. Acid. Hydrocy. dil., ♏iv.
Syrupi simplicis, ʒj.
Aquæ distill, ℥vij. M. A teaspoonful to be taken every six hours.

(No. 16.)

℞. Acid. Hydrocy. dil., ♏iv.
Mist. Amygdalæ, ℥j. M. A teaspoonful to be taken every six hours.

For a child 9 months old.

the cough, it manifests its peculiar poisonous action on the system, so as to render its discontinuance advisable. I have never but once, however, seen really alarming symptoms follow its use, though I have employed it in many hundreds of cases. In that instance I gave one minim of dilute hydrocyanic acid every four hours to a little boy two years and a half old. He had hooped for four days before he came under my care, and was then suffering from rather severe cough, and considerable dyspnœa. He took the acid for four days without any effect being produced either on his system generally or on the cough; but at the end of that time, after taking each dose, he uttered a cry, became quite faint, and would have fallen if not supported. This result having followed three or four times, the child's mother discontinued the medicine, and, of course I did not resume its employment. Similar though less severe symptoms were produced by the same medicine in the sister of this child, a little girl of five years of age; but in neither instance was the severity of the cough in the least mitigated by it. Though no other instances of the kind have come under my notice, I always give a caution to the parents to diminish the dose of the medicine, or even entirely to discontinue it, if the child appears faint or dizzy, or bewildered, after its administration; and I never persevere with the use of the acid unless it gives a very decided earnest of good within three or four days after its first exhibition.

In many instances, although the severity of the cough may be greatly relieved by the hydrocyanic acid, it yet does not enable us entirely to dispense with other remedies. If there is much wheezing at the chest, an emetic of ipecacuanha should be given once or twice a day, in order to free the air-passages from the mucus which collects in them, often in very considerable quantity, and thus tends by the obstruction it offers to the free admission of air, to favor the occurrence of collapse of the lung. The degree to which the child suffers from the accumulation of phlegm in the bronchi must determine whether the emetic shall be given once or oftener during the day. If it is given but once, the evening should be the time selected for its administration; and, after the air-tubes have been thus relieved, the child will often rest well, instead of passing as it otherwise would do a restless night, disturbed by dyspnœa and frequent fits of coughing. In other instances the cough is unattended by much secretion, the child scarcely wheezes at all, and even after a severe paroxysm rarely vomits, and never rejects more than a small quantity of phlegm; but when night comes on, the cough grows very distressing by its frequent return, even more than by the severity of the paroxysms. When this is the case, a small dose of Dover's powder, or of Dover's powder and the extract of hemlock,[1] often soothes this irritability of the air-tubes, and diminishes the frequency of the cough. The same effect, too, follows the use of belladonna, the dose of

---

[1] (No. 17.)

℞. Pulv. Ipecac. co., gr. ss.
Pulv. Extracti Conii, gr. j.
Pulv. Cinnamomi, gr. ij.
Sacchari albi, gr. iv. M.

The powder to be taken at bedtime. For a child of two years old.

which medicine, small at first, may afterwards be by degrees increased, and that very largely, with less risk or inconvenience than attends the employment in increasing doses of any sedative into the composition of which opium enters. I always give the tincture as the handiest preparation; and should begin with two minims every four hours for a child of a year old. If there is a good deal of febrile disturbance, if the cough is hard as well as violent, if it seems to occasion pain, and is unattended by expectoration, while, in the intervals of the paroxysms, a frequent, short, hacking cough distresses the child, and generally diffused rhonchus is heard throughout the lungs, the hydrocyanic acid may be advantageously combined with small doses of tartar emetic or of the Vinum Ipecacuanhæ. In other cases, if the existence of drowsiness, with a flushed face, becoming livid during the fit of coughing, and the suppression of the previously distinct hoop, betoken the presence of cerebral congestion, the application of a few leeches to the head will not only greatly relieve these symptoms but will also diminish both the frequency and severity of the cough, and prepare the way for the more effective employment of the hydrocyanic acid.

There are two proceedings which demand a special notice, as having of late years been recommended almost as specifics in hooping-cough. One of them consists in the inhalation of chloroform on the approach of each paroxysm, as a means of cutting it short, or even of entirely preventing its occurrence. There can be no doubt but that just as chloroform sometimes controls convulsions or relieves spasm of the glottis, so it is equally capable of diminishing, or even of arresting, the violence of fits of hooping-cough. I have found it of great service in some of those cases of the disease in which the return of each paroxysm of coughing was the signal for the occurrence of general convulsions; but it scarcely need be added that its efficient employment in these circumstances requires the constant presence in the house of some one conversant with its administration. In those almost desperate cases, too, there is the drawback from its use arising from the fact that inasmuch as death may take place during any of the convulsive seizures, so its occurrence at the time when the chloroform was being administered would almost certainly leave the impression on the mind of the friends that death was due to its employment. If, however, warning is given beforehand of the possibility of this accident, the chloroform may be resorted to as an agent of great power, though, as in other instances where it is employed at short intervals, tolerance of it is soon established, and it will cease in the course of twenty-four or forty-eight hours to produce any effect whatever. In mild cases of the disease, the results which one commonly attains are not remarkable; for the sense of suffocation which precedes and accompanies a fit of coughing, renders young children intolerant of anything being held near their mouth; while the sense of nausea which the inhalation of chloroform produces, so disgusts those who are older, that in spite of the relief which it may yield, I have on several occasions seen older children, who at first had had ready recourse to the chloroform, after a few trials discontinue it, preferring even the unmitigated cough to the nauseating effects of the remedy. Still, with due precaution, its trial is free from any objection, and in the course of a chronic ailment there is often an advantage in being provided with means which, though they may be of slight service to the patient, at any rate convince the friends that we are not indifferent to his sufferings, nor indisposed to try all means for their alleviation.

The other measure consists in the local application to the back of the fauces, or directly to the larynx itself, of a solution of nitrate of silver, of a strength varying from gr. xv to ℈ij of the salt to an ounce of distilled water, by means of a probang, such as that employed by Dr. Horace Green for the introduction of medicated solutions into the interior of the glottis. This proceeding was first advocated by Dr. Ebenezer Watson, in a paper published in the year 1849,[1] and afterwards dwelt on by him more fully in a book which appeared five years afterwards, and in which he complains of his suggestions having been passed over without notice.[2] Before the appearance of his book I had made a few trials of his plan, and have subsequently resorted to it sufficiently often to be able to form a fair opinion of its value. I have no doubt but that in very many instances the sponge of the probang is actually passed within the glottis; and also that by this manipulation, whether completely successful or not, the violence of the paroxysms of the cough is sometimes lessened, and their frequency diminished. This result, however, was by no means constant; the milder cases were those in which the benefits of the proceeding were most apparent; while, as perhaps might not unnaturally be expected, in those in which there was abiding dyspnœa, or in which any bronchitic complication existed, little if any good was obtained.

The great practical difficulty, however, and one which I am convinced will prevent any frequent resort to the proceeding in the case of children, arises from their extreme repugnance to it, and their dread of its repetition. Sometimes by coaxing and promises I succeeded in it daily for three or four days; but no persuasion enabled me to carry its employment further, while on several occasions I saw paroxysms of cough brought on by the mere fear that the solution was about to be applied. There are very few proceedings, indeed, which are so surely and largely beneficial as to repay us for adopting them at the cost of a passion of tears, or agony of terror, and this is certainly not one of them.

Counter-irritation to the chest and spine is a popular remedy for hooping-cough, in which many non-professional persons place great confidence, while they employ it through all the stages of the disease. I do not think that you will in general gain much by the employment of counter-irritation until the disease has begun to decline, though it is then often of much service. There are, however, some circumstances in which counter-irritation may be advantageously resorted to, even before the affection has attained its greatest degree of severity. The attacks of dyspnœa which sometimes occur during the increase of the disease, are often much relieved by a mustard-poultice to the chest; and if, as occasionally happens, these attacks return, though with

---

[1] Edinburgh Monthly Journal, Dec. 1849.

[2] On the Topical Medication of the Larynx, &c., 8vo. London, 1854. See p. 123.

varying severity, almost every night for several nights together, the application of a mustard-poultice to the chest, and the immersion of the lower part of the body in a hot bath, on three or four successive evenings, may be of service. In cases of this kind, too, the daily friction of the chest and spine with an embrocation of soap liniment and the Tinctura *Lyttæ*, so as to keep up a slight degree of redness of the surface, is often beneficial; or that popular remedy, Roche's embrocation, may be used, if the parents of the child fancy, as they often do, that it is possessed of some specific virtue.

As a general rule, blisters to the chest are not desirable remedies in young children; but if the cough should be frequent, hard, and painful, or if, in connection with the evidences of congestion of the brain, the cough is suffocative and the hoop suppressed, much good often results from their application. They must not, however, be allowed to remain above four hours upon the skin; neither is it desirable to attempt to keep them discharging, on account of the very troublesome sores which they sometimes produce. For the same reason, too, I do not advise you to employ inunction of the tartar emetic ointment, although this proceeding was once highly recommended, and very generally adopted, as a remedy for hooping-cough.

Attention to maintain a warm and equable temperature around the child, to prevent the stomach becoming disordered by unsuitable food, and to avoid constipation, will in many instances suffice to conduct a child in safety through the second stage of hooping-cough. If the severity of the cough, or the condition of the child in other respects, seems to call for more decided interference, your motto in the selection and employment of remedies must be, "*ne quid nimis*;" and especially must this be your rule in the management of those complications which often render hooping-cough so dangerous a disease.

In no case is it of more importance to bear in mind this caution as to the danger of overtreating a patient who suffers from hooping-cough, than when, at the commencement of the second stage of the disease, a sudden increase of fever, and the supervention of a state of permanent dyspnœa, seem to announce to you that active inflammation has attacked the lungs or air-tubes. It is quite possible that such may be the import of the symptoms, but it is at least as likely that they result from disturbance of the nervous system. In such a case, then, I would advise you to allow nothing but the positive evidence of auscultation to lead you to resort to free depletion and the use of large doses of tartar emetic;—remedies to which you might feel disposed at once to have recourse. If you feel in doubt, remain for some time with the child, watch it carefully, auscultate it more than once during your visit, and repeat your visit every two or three hours,[1] rather than resort at

[1] I cannot refrain from directing the attention of junior practitioners to the anecdote which Dr. Cheyne relates (at page xvii of the Introduction to his work on Hydrocephalus), of the very different results that followed the practice of two army surgeons, one of whom visited his patients, during the prevalence of an epidemic disease twice, the other four or five times daily. The moral which Dr. Cheyne drew from the tale, though obvious enough, is not sufficiently borne in mind by many who undertake the treatment of children's diseases.

once to measures which, powerful either for evil or for good, may, if unwisely employed, destroy the life they were intended to save.

Example teaches louder than precept, and you may learn a useful practical lesson from the following history:

A little boy, about two years old, had had slight catarrh for a fortnight, and towards the end of this time it was thought he had hooped once or twice, though very slightly. He ailed but little, and had had none other than domestic remedies during this period; but one night, without any apparent cause, he became very feverish, his cough grew worse, and his respiration very hurried. On this account he was depleted very freely by leeches, and calomel and antimony were given in large doses for two days, though without any considerable diminution of the dyspnœa. When this treatment was first adopted, it was thought that air entered one lung but scantily; but on the evening of the second day both lungs admitted air equally well, although a good deal of mucous râle attended the respiration. On the morning of the third day, the child's face was flushed, and he looked much oppressed; his lips were rather livid, his respiration was extremely hurried and irregular; he coughed little, but his cough had a suffocative character, and was not attended by a distinct hoop. The hurried respiration was supposed to indicate the continuance of graver mischief in the lungs than was apparent on auscultation, and antimony was accordingly given in emetic doses. It did not produce much sickness, and the respiration diminished but little in frequency during its employment. On the fourth day the child still breathed very hurriedly, and his inspirations varied from 40 to 60 in a minute, without there being any obvious cause for these great changes in their frequency. On the fifth day the breathing increased in rapidity, while the pulse began to lose power; and not only had the antimony ceased to exert any emetic action, but squills and ipecacuanha failed to induce vomiting. Active measures were suspended towards the evening of this day, and a grain of Dover's powder, given every six hours, somewhat diminished the hurry of the breathing; but it was discontinued after the third dose, on account of the gradually deepening drowsiness of the child. The child, however, still continued heavy and oppressed, the cough became more frequent and more suffocative, the breathing more rapid and more irregular. On the morning of the seventh day, a fit of coughing terminated in convulsions; and from that time until the morning of the eighth day, when the child died, they were extremely violent, frequent in their return, followed by carpopedal contractions, which did not subside in the intervals between them; while after each convulsion the respiration became most distressingly hurried and irregular. After a time the breathing grew constantly labored, the face became of a deep livid color, the hands were clenched, and the wrists bent upon the forearm; the spine was drawn slightly backwards, and sensation was quite abolished. At length a slight convulsive movement passed across the face, and the limbs relaxed in death. Permission was not obtained to make a post-mortem examination.

Other cases have come under my notice, in some of which I fell into the error against which I have just tried to warn you: in some I saw the patient too late to rectify the mistake which others had committed, while in some the right course of treatment adopted from the first was followed by success. In a case such as I have related, the want of correspondence between the general symptoms and the auscultatory signs should have deterred from the copious depletion and the free use of calomel and antimony in the first instance, while it still further contra-indicated the employment of antimony in emetic doses subsequently. Two or three leeches to the head, when the serious symptoms first came on, would probably have relieved the congested brain; the tepid bath would have soothed the irritability and diminished the fever; and hydrocyanic acid would, most likely, have been of service in quieting the hurried breathing. If much febrile disturbance had still continued small doses of ipecacuanha, antimony, and hyoscyamus, might have been tried, the antimonial not being given in such doses as to exert any very considerable depressing influence on the system. A stimulating liniment to the chest and spine should have been used several times in the course of the day, and any sudden access of hurried breathing should have been met by the application of a mustard-poultice to the chest.

The difficulties of diagnosis are sometimes rendered smaller, and the right course of treatment more obvious, by the occurrence of occasional carpopedal contractions, or of momentary strabismus from the very commencement of this nervous dyspnœa; or in other cases by the absence of any auscultatory signs of mischief in the chest, such as could for a moment lead you to refer the hurried breathing to disease going on in the lungs.

Even when acute bronchitis really exists, you must not forget the peculiar impress which hooping-cough stamps upon it. You must bear in mind the impediment to the due aeration of the blood which each fit of coughing occasions, and the influence on the nervous system generally of the imperfect decarbonization of the circulating fluid; how it heightens the irritability of the spinal system, thus exciting the hurried and irregular breathing, and rendering the child peculiarly liable to convulsive seizures. If active interference, therefore, be necessary, you would abstract blood very cautiously, while you would employ nitre, ipecacuanha, and James's powder in small doses, as febrifuges and expectorants, rather than to attempt to bring the child rapidly under the influence of antimony. At the same time, the peculiar tendency to obstruction of the air-tubes, and consequent collapse of the lungs, which characterizes hooping-cough, would lead you to endeavor to keep the bronchi free, by the administration once or twice a day of an emetic of ipecacuanha. You would employ liniments, mustard-poultices, or blisters to the chest, to combat any exacerbation of dyspnœa; and if the paroxysms of cough were severe, you would combine hydrocyanic acid with your other remedies. If the powers appear to be on the decline, and the child neither expectorated with the cough, nor rejected much phlegm by vomiting although the bronchi were loaded with mucus, you would at once discontinue antiphlogistic measures, and have recourse to the decoction of senega, with ammonia and squills,[1] while you endeavored by a nutritious diet to support your patient's strength.

[1] See Formula No. 12, p. 279.

The time allotted to this lecture will not enable me to do more than just indicate the main points to which your attention should be directed; and I must now pass on to notice briefly your conduct in the *third stage* of the disease. It is now that the cough diminishes in frequency and severity, that the hoop grows less loud and less constant, and that any signs of constitutional disturbance that had existed before by degrees disappear. When the disorder runs this favorable course no medicine is needed, and but few restrictions, beyond such as the avoidance of damp and cold requires. Change of air generally expedites the cure; and if the opportunity offers, and the season of the year is favorable, it should never be neglected. There are many instances, however, in which medical treatment in the decline of hooping-cough is of very considerable service. It sometimes happens that the bronchi continue loaded with secretion, which is either expectorated, or rejected by vomiting in very considerable quantities after each fit of coughing, while the skin is cold, the tongue moist, and the pulse soft and rather deficient in power. In this condition, alum,[1] long a popular remedy in hooping-cough, is often of much service, diminishing the secretion, arresting the sickness, and rendering the cough much less frequent. It may be given in doses of three or four grains every four or six hours to a child of a year and a half to two years old. This remedy, indeed, may sometimes be used with advantage, even before the disorder has begun to decline, if the condition be such as I have just referred to, namely, fever being absent, and the bronchial secretion very abundant, even though the cough is violent. In other cases, in which the cough continues violent after the other symptoms have abated, and in which, though there is no superabundance of secretion in the air-tubes, yet the attacks of cough often end with the rejection of a considerable quantity of mucus from the stomach, and loss of appetite and general dyspeptic symptoms are present, the hydrochloric acid is often of much service. It has been recommended as a specific against hooping-cough, in doses of from two to six drachms daily;[2] but I have never employed it in other than moderate doses, such as one would prescribe in other circumstances.[3]

---

[1] (No. 18.)
℞. Alum Sulphat., gr. xxiv.
Acid. Sulph. dil., ♏xij.
Syr. Rhœados, ʒiv.
Aquæ puræ, ℥ijss. M.
A dessertspoonful every six hours.

[2] I have made a few trials of the nitric acid in large doses, as recommended by Dr. Arnoldi, and by Dr. Gibb in his treatise on Hooping-Cough. Post 8vo., London, 1854, p. 341; but cannot at all subscribe to Dr. Gibb's statement that "it shortens the disease almost as effectually as quinine does intermittent fever." The nitric acid has, within the past six years, fallen into comparative oblivion, and the last new specific, vaunted as loudly as if its advocates had not extolled other remedies before as equally infallible, is the bromide of ammonium. It has been employed among the out-patients of the Children's Hospital on a scale large enough to demonstrate its worthlessness.

[3] (No. 19.)
℞. Acid. Hydrochlor. dil., ♏xxxij.
Tinct. Opii, ♏iv.
Syr. Mori, ʒiv.
Aquæ puræ, ℥ijss. M.
A dessertspoonful three times a day.

Another mode of treatment which has been vaunted as almost a specific consists[1] in the administration of the sulphate of zinc and the extract of belladonna, in doses gradually increased until the quantity given is at last far larger than could have been employed at first without the production of poisonous effects. I believe that, when, on the subsidence of the bronchitic symptoms which attend the first stage of hooping-cough, the nervous element still persists, giving rise to frequent, violent, spasmodic fits of coughing, a combination of zinc and belladonna is often of much service. I believe that these remedies are useful just as other tonics and antispasmodics are useful, but my own experience would not lead me to think that two scruples of sulphate of zinc, and six grains of belladonna, could be given to children of eight years of age, with advantage, or even with safety.

If the cough continues frequent, and the hoop loud, while the only signs of constitutional disturbance are those of mere weakness, iron will generally put a stop to it sooner than any other remedy.[2] If, however, there should be a degree of feverishness, or of gastro-intestinal disorder, which for the present contraindicates the use of iron, Battley's liquor cinchonæ may be given with great advantage, in combination with small doses of hydrocyanic acid;[3] while every attention must of course be paid, by mild alteratives and other appropriate means, to improve the condition of the digestive organs.

It is probably unnecessary to enter into further details, to specify minutely the diet that a convalescent requires, or to refer to the utility of liniments to the chest, or the occasional benefit of anodynes at night. Of all the means, indeed, which promote recovery from hooping-cough, or from the feeble health that it often leaves behind, there is none to compare with the salutary influence of change of air, and especially of a change to the seacoast.

There still remain numerous remedies that have a more or less well-merited reputation in cases of hooping-cough. I must content myself with having pointed out to you the kind of weapons that, in different circumstances, must be employed; and must leave to you the selection of the one whose form and size may, on different occasions, seem to you most fitting. The armory is large enough to yield you an ample choice.

---

[1] Dr. Fuller, on Diseases of the Chest. 8vo. London, 1862, p. 336.

[2] (No. 20.)

℞. Mist. Ferri co., ℥iv.
Tinct. Scillæ, ♏xvj.
Tinct. Conii, ♏xl.
Mist. Amygdalæ, ℥ij ʒiij. M.

A dessertspoonful three times a day.

[3] (No. 21.)

℞. Acid. Hydrocy. dil., ♏viij.
Liq. Cinchonæ, ʒiss.
Syr. Aurant., ʒiss.
Aquæ Flor. Aurant., ʒiij.
Aquæ destil., ℥vj. M.

ʒij two teaspoonfuls three times a day.

All the above are suited for children of two years old.

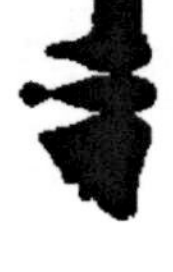

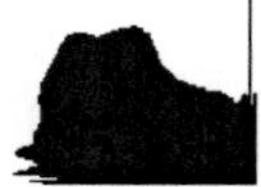

LECTURE XXVIII.

PULMONARY PHTHISIS.—Differences exist between the tuberculous cachexia in the child and in the adult—Statistical table illustrating its peculiarities in early life—Anatomical characteristics of pulmonary phthisis in the child—Frequency of miliary tubercle and of gray granulations in the lung, independent of each other, and of other forms of tubercle—Frequency of tubercular infiltration—Rarity of cavities—Frequent affection of bronchial glands—Description of each of these peculiarities—Changes in tuberculous bronchial glands—Perforation of bronchi, and elimination of tubercular matter.

Symptoms of phthisis.—Their differences from those of the disease in the adult—Danger of overlooking its early stages, or of mistaking it for remittent fever, &c.—Peculiarities of its subsequent course.

Bronchial phthisis.—Its characteristics—Remarkable fluctuations in its course—Occasional unexpected recovery—Case of its occurrence attended with expectoration of tubercular matter—Its fatal termination usually preceded by merging of its symptoms in those of general pulmonary phthisis—Occasional fatal hæmoptysis, but this accident not limited to cases of bronchial phthisis.

Phthisis in very early infancy.—Pulmonary symptoms often obscured by signs of generally defective nutrition.

WE enter to-day on the examination of one of the most painfully interesting diseases with which we have to do. It is a disease that we not only often see in hospitals, or in the dwellings of the poor, but which has brought grief into the habitations of many among us, and has robbed us of those whom we most dearly loved; while the very mention of its name gives rise to a feeling of utter hopelessness as to its issue. I need hardly say that I propose to-day to call your attention to *Pulmonary Consumption* or *Phthisis*,—a malady that attacks persons of all ages, of both sexes, and of every rank, and which, under every variety of condition, medicine seems to be equally unable to cure.

It may, however, occur to some of you that, important though this affection is, yet in speaking of it I am transgressing the bounds that I set myself, when I proposed to treat only of those maladies which are either limited in their occurrence to the period of childhood, or on which the early years of the patient impress some well-marked peculiarity. It is true, indeed, that at whatever age phthisis comes on, it presents the same grand features, it works the same kind of changes, and tends to the same fatal result. But yet the disease in the young subject displays differences from its character in the old sufficient to attract the notice of the observant; nor are these differences merely curious, but they influence our prognosis and modify our treatment—and hence it is fitting that we devote some time to their examination.

"That great constitutional malady, of which pulmonary consumption is only a fragment, plays its part," in childhood as well as in adult age, "most conspicuously in the lungs." In the adult, however, the lungs are so almost invariably the seat of tubercular deposit that out of 123 cases, M. Louis found but one exception to the rule th

exists in any viscus, it will be discovered also in the lungs. In the child, though the lungs are still the most frequent seat of tubercle, yet M. Louis' law no longer holds good, for MM. Rilliet and Barthez found 47 exceptions to it out of 312 instances in which tubercle was discovered in some one or more organs of the body.

The first great difference, then, between the tubercular cachexia in childhood and in adult age, consists in the same organs not being equally liable to it at the two periods of life.

The following table will place this difference clearly before you. It shows the proportion per cent. in which different viscera were the seat of tubercle in children and in adults. The figures in the first column are deduced from 312 cases which form the basis of MM. Rilliet and Barthez's essay on the tuberculous cachexia; those in the second, from the 123 cases on which M. Louis' work on phthisis is founded; and the third contains the results arrived at by Lombard on an examination of 100 adults.

Of 100 instances in which tubercle was deposited in some of the viscera it was present in—

	Children from 1 to 15 years.	Adults from 20 years and upwards.	
	According to Rilliet and Barthez	According to Louis.	According to Lombard.
In the lungs, ...	84	100	100
" bronchial glands, ...	79	28	9
" mesenteric, "	46	83	19
" small intestines, ...	42	83	0
" spleen, ...	40	13	6
" pleura, ...	34	2	1
" peritoneum, ...	27	0	0
" liver, ...	22	0	1
" large intestines, ...	19	10	0
" membranes of the brain, . .	16	0	2
" kidneys, ...	15	2	1
" brain, ...	11	0.8	2
" stomach, ...	6	0	0
" heart and pericardium, . .	8	0	0

This table shows not only that the liability of certain organs to become the seat of tubercle is different in childhood from what it is in the adult, but also that tubercle is simultaneously deposited in a greater number of organs in the young than in the old. This greater intensity of the tuberculous cachexia in early life is a fact of much importance. It explains how it happens that death sometimes takes place in the child before tubercle has anywhere undergone those changes which seem almost always to precede the fatal event in the adult.[1]

These, however, are not the only peculiarities of the disease in early life, but the *anatomical characters of tubercle in the lungs* (and of this I am now more particularly speaking) differ in some respects *in the child* from those which are observed in the grown person.

[1] I have thrown together in the following note some details with reference to phthisis in early life, which, though far too few to warrant the deduction of any

The *first* of these peculiarities consists in the frequency with which gray granulations and crude miliary tubercles exist in the lungs independent of each other, and of any other form of tubercular deposit. In the adult, M. Louis[1] discovered miliary tubercles alone only in 2 out of 123 cases of phthisis ; and gray granulations alone only in 5 more. In

---

positive conclusions, may not be without value as furnishing materials for comparison with the results obtained by other observers.

Table of 497 Cases, showing influence of Sex and Age in predisposing to Pulmonary Phthisis.

	Under 1 year.		From 1-2.		From 2-3.		From 3-5.		From 5-10.		From 10-15.		TOTAL.		
	M.	F.	M.	F.	M.	F.	M.	F.	M.	F.	M.	F.	M.	F.	TOTAL
TOTAL EXAMINATIONS,	29	17	34	38	47	33	58	55	83	75	13	15	264	233	497
Tubercle present in chest,	8	8	8	11	17	11	23	30	40	38	5	6	101	104	205
" not " "	21	9	26	28	30	22	35	25	43	37	8	9	163	129	292

The degree of the tubercular deposit is not the same in all cases, but was stated to have been slight in 60, moderate in 53, considerable in 92, which were thus distributed:

	Under 1 year.		From 1-2.		From 2-3.		From 3-5.		From 5-10.		From 10-15.		TOTAL.		
	M.	F.	M.	F.	M.	F.	M.	F.	M.	F.	M.	F.	M.	F.	TOTAL
Slight, ...	...		2	0	4	1	7	13	15	18	4	1	32	28	60
Moderate, ...	1	2	1	5	5	8	6	7	9	13		1	22	31	53
Considerable, ...	7	6	5	6	8	7	10	10	16	12	1	4	47	45	92
													101	104	205

In 182 of the above cases, the forms assumed by the tubercular deposit were as follows:

	Gray Granulations.	Yellow Tubercle.	Yellow Tubercle softened.	Yellow Tubercle in cretaceous state.	Tubercular Infiltration.	Small Vomicæ.	Large cavities.	Tubercle of Bronchial Glands.
Gray granulations, ...	63	40	7	1	12	5	4	44
Yellow tubercle, ...	40	74	10	—	21	11	4	71
" " softened, ...	7	11	13	—	31	8	—	13
" " in cretaceous state,	2	—	—	7	—	—	—	1
Tubercular infiltration, ...	12	21	3	—	30	8	8	30
Small vomicæ, ...	5	11	8	—	8	18	4	19
Large cavities, ...	4	4	1	—	8	3	12	6
Tubercle of bronchial glands, . .	44	65	13	1	30	18	11	119

In 21 of the 119 cases in which the bronchial glands were the seat of tubercle the pulmonary tissue was unaffected ; and this although thrice the deposit in the glands was universal, and in one of the three cases had gone on to softening.

The tubercle of the glands was incipient in 25
" " " general in 54
" " " ed the stage of softening in 21
" " able, cheesy state in 9
" taceous change in 10

[1] Recherches s

the child, MM. Rilliet and Barthez[1] found miliary tubercles [illegible] 107, and gray granulations alone in 36 out of 265 cases; [illegible] aminations made by myself, or in my presence, yield 34 [illegible] the presence of miliary tubercles alone, and 23 of the presence of [illegible] granulations alone in the tissue of the lungs.[2]

The great rapidity with which the deposit and development of tubercle often take place in early life, is doubtless one chief [illegible] this peculiarity. If we examine the lungs of an adult affected with the tuberculous cachexia, we shall often observe their lower lobes containing gray semitransparent granulations; as we advance higher, we shall probably find that the granulations have lost much of their transparency, and that they present a yellowish spot in their centre, while near to the apex of the lung the deposit exists in no other form than that of bodies presenting the whitish-yellow color and friable texture characteristic of crude tubercle. These appearances seem to [illegible] that the deposit of tubercle has taken place slowly and at successive periods, so that those tubercles which occupy the apex of the lung are already approaching maturity at a time when the disease is just beginning to invade the lower lobes. In the child, however, it not seldom happens that all the lobes of both lungs present a nearly equal amount of tuberculous deposit, and that this is seen to be nearly equally advanced in all. Thus we may find the gray granulations diffused in about the same abundance through all parts of the lungs, and all equally transparent; or we may observe each granulation presenting a yellow spot in its centre; or the change may be complete, and crude yellow tubercle may be everywhere present.

This same fact, of the acute course of tuberculization of the lungs in children, receives a further illustration from the *second* anatomical peculiarity of the disease; namely, the great frequency with which yellow infiltration of tubercle is observed in early life; MM. Rilliet and Barthez having met with it in 88 out of 265 children, or in 33 per cent.; and I, in 30 out of 132, or in 22.7 per cent. It is a form of degeneration of the lung which seldom exists alone, but is almost invariably associated with gray granulations or yellow tubercle, and usually coexists with a state of very far advanced tuberculization of the bronchial glands. It is often limited to one lobe, generally the upper: or sometimes the middle lobe in those cases in which the right lung is the seat of the disease. Those portions of the lung which are affected by it become converted into a firm solid mass, having [illegible] both of the color and consistence of cheese, presenting a smooth [illegible] when cut, and by its solidity compressing the bronchial tubes [illegible] traverse it, so as considerably to reduce their calibre. If the [illegible] life is prolonged, a process of softening generally takes place; the [illegible] breaks down, and a cavity is the result, the parietes of which are [illegible] by solid tubercle. At other times, especially if the disease [illegible]

[1] Op. cit., vol. iii, pp. 221 and 227.

[2] Of late years the pressure of other duties has interfered with my [illegible] ence at post-mortem examinations. I have therefore not included the [illegible] last seven years, not because I in any measure doubt their correctness, [illegible] I cannot personally vouch for their accuracy.

course with great rapidity, the lung thus infiltrated seems to undergo a different kind of softening, which does not lead to the formation of a central cavity, but pervades its tissue throughout, which then presents a reddish-yellow, or rose-colored tint, and breaks down easily into a kind of putrilage, as if the changes produced were the result of a mixture of true pneumonic hepatization, and of tubercular degeneration. Cases of this sort go far towards substantiating the correctness of M. Rokitansky's theory with reference to the nature of this tubercular infiltration, as compared with the ordinary form of tubercular deposit. He conceives that the deposit of tubercle in the form of gray or yellow granulations takes place in the interstitial cellular tissue of the lung; while in the case of tubercular infiltration the matter poured out into the interior of the pulmonary vesicles during an attack of pneumonia becomes converted into tubercle under the influence of the tubercular cachexia.

A *third* peculiarity of phthisis in the child, as contrasted with the same disease in the adult, consists in the greater rarity of cavities in the lungs during early life. Of 123 cases which form the basis of M. Louis' work on phthisis, cavities were present in by far the majority of instances; and though the numbers are not exactly stated, the exceptions would seem to have been but very few. Out of 265 cases, however, that came under the notice of MM. Rilliet and Barthez, only 76, or 28.6 per cent., presented cavities in the lungs; and they existed in only 22.7 per cent. or in 30 of the 132 cases which came under my own observation. These cavities sometimes resemble those which we usually meet with in the adult; and this is especially the case with children above six years of age, in whom, indeed, the general characters of phthisis approximate closely to those of the same disease in the grown person. In other instances, they are not so much caverns, as very small excavations (*vacuôles*, as the French call them), produced by the softening of small tubercular deposits. Such excavations communicate with the bronchi and with each other, and are sometimes exceedingly numerous, but do not occasion such a destruction of the pulmonary tissue as to produce anywhere a cavity of considerable dimensions. Besides these two forms of cavity, there is a third, to which I have already referred, namely, that produced by softening of the yellow tubercular infiltration, which is more commonly met with in very early life than subsequently. Cavities of this kind sometimes form with great rapidity, and attain a considerable size. The whole of one lobe of the lung may even become converted into a sac, which is often almost quite empty, while its parietes are formed by little besides the pleura and the fibrous capsule of the lung, with a very thin lining of dense tubercular matter. It is far from unusual to meet with cavities of this kind in the bodies of infants only a few months old, who have never thriven, but have presented few signs of phthisis, with the exception of progressive loss of flesh and strength, and somewhat hurried respiration.

The *last* anatomical peculiarity of [illegible] and childhood to which I shall direct your a[illegible] deposit of *tubercle in the bronchial* [illegible] deposit gives rise. Even in the adult, tubercle is deposited in the bronchial glands in about a fourth of all cases of phthisis; but the deposit there is subsidiary to its deposit in the lungs. In the child, however, this is far from being always the case; but the disease of the glands is often as important as that in the lungs, sometimes much more considerable.

The tubercular deposit does not appear to begin simultaneously in all the glands, nor to advance in all with the same rapidity; but those about the bifurcation of the trachea, and close to the primary bronchi, are usually the first affected; and the disease in them often attains a more advanced stage than elsewhere. The state in which the glands are most frequently met with is one of tubercular infiltration, the whole of their substance being converted into a firm, resistant texture, resembling a portion of lung which has been the seat of tubercular infiltration; and this even although the number of affected glands may be but small, and though the lungs be but little or not at all involved in the disease. Sometimes, however, we may meet with the affection in an incipient state, and it is then usual to find the glands which it has attacked somewhat enlarged and injected, and their tissue infiltrated with fluid, and less firm than natural. The tubercular deposit does not proceed invariably from the centre to the circumference, but frequently two or three small deposits may be discerned at different parts of the same gland; or the tubercular matter may be accumulated entirely at one end of the gland, while its other extremity is merely softened and injected. Even when the disease starts from several points, it is not often that the deposit assumes the distinctly circumscribed form of miliary tubercle, and still less often that of gray granulation; but it generally presents the character of tubercular infiltration which had taken place at the same time in two or three different situations. Sometimes it is impossible to distinguish any one spot as that from which the disease commenced, but the whole tissue of the gland has a whitish hue, which appears due to the general infiltration of tuberculous matter. Whatever may have been the mode in which the deposit of tubercle began, the tendency of the advance of the disease is to convert the entire substance of the gland into firm tuberculous matter, in which no trace of the original tissue can be detected. The metamorphosis of the gland is attended with considerable increase of its size; the enlargement, however, being much greater in the case of those glands which are situated externally to the lungs, than of those which are imbedded in the pulmonary substance. The enlargement of the glands is not attended, as might have been anticipated beforehand, with a thinning of their originally delicate cellular envelope, but it increases in density and firmness, and at the same time acquires a very considerable thickness. Most of the glands which have become converted into tubercle are inclosed within a cyst a line or more in thickness, and extremely resistant; its inner surface being smooth, of a [illegible] rose tint, and sometimes presenting a considerable degree of vascularity.

In a large proportion of cases in which tubercle is found in the bronchial glands, it has not passed beyond the crude stage; but if it is not cut short by the advance of phthisis in the lungs, a pro-

softening next commences; and the softening usually, though not invariably, begins at the centre of the glands, and extends towards their circumference. The softening is seldom found equally advanced in all the glands; but in some, a small central cavity containing liquid tubercle is surrounded by a thick wall of solid matter; while in others the whole substance has been softened, and the gland is no longer anything else than a cyst containing a quantity of puriform fluid. When tubercle deposited in the lung has undergone the process of softening, an effort is made by nature to get rid of the morbid matter, which is expectorated; and the cavity, thus emptied of its contents, now and then cicatrizes, and the patient is cured. The cases of cure, indeed, bear but a very small proportion to those in which death takes place, for, in general, fresh deposits of tubercle successively undergo this softening, until but a comparatively small portion of the lung remains unaffected by the disease; or the abundant secretion from the bronchial tubes exhausts the patient, or death ensues from the degree to which other organs are implicated in the tuberculous cachexia. When the bronchial glands are the seat of the disease, a similar effort is made to eliminate the morbid matter from the system; and many circumstances concur to render this a more hopeful task than it is when the pulmonary substance itself is the seat of the disease.

The means by which this is effected deserve to be examined. When tuberculization of the bronchial glands has attained an advanced stage, we generally observe a process of thickening and infiltration to have commenced in the cellular tissue around each gland, by no means unlike that which takes place in the pia mater at the base of the brain in cases of tubercular meningitis. This cellular tissue often assumes a grayish semi-transparent aspect, and presents a number of minute granules of tubercle diffused through it. By a process of combined inflammation and tuberculization, the connection between the gland and the adjacent bronchial tube becomes extremely intimate. The cellular tissue in the intervals between the bronchial rings becomes next infiltrated with tubercle, and is then the first part of the wall of the bronchial tube which disappears during a process of absorption that advances from without inwards. The cellular tissue sometimes becomes quite removed before the cartilages of the bronchi are much affected; but in process of time they too become absorbed, and the perforation of the tube is then complete; the tuberculated gland, however, blocking up the aperture in its walls, and projecting into its cavity. The next step consists in the thinning of the envelope of the gland, and the next is the discharge of its contents into the tube: and the cyst then in all probability collapses, and becomes applied to the outside of the bronchus, so as to form a part of its parietes. But we are still in want of some exact observations as to this last stage in the cure of bronchial phthisis.

This process does not take place with equal frequency in all the bronchial glands; for those which are situated around the trachea, and wholly external to the lung, meeting with no obstacle to their increase in size, often attain a great magnitude without at all compromising the integrity of the trachea. Those, however, which are in contact with the secondary and tertiary bronchi, and are imbedded [illegible] monary substance (which prevents their attaining any considerable [illegible] not infrequently perforate the tube in the manner above described [illegible] and this not only after they have become softened, but even [illegible] tubercle they contain is still in the crude state.

Although the progress of the tubercular degeneration is most [illegible] in those glands which are situated near to the larger air-tubes, [illegible] by no means limited to them, but is in many instances [illegible] in the pulmonary glands that are imbedded in different parts of the substance of the lungs. They do not, however, become inclosed [illegible] a cyst as dense and resisting as that which surrounds the [illegible] bronchial glands: while in a great number of instances the pulmonary substance for a short distance around them presents a far more [illegible] dant tubercular deposit than is apparent in any other part of the lung. If a tuberculous gland, thus imbedded in the tissue of the lung, [illegible] become softened, the excavation thereby produced may easily be mis- taken for a cavity in the lung itself. A pulmonary cavity of [illegible] small dimensions, however, is hardly ever solitary, unless it proceeds from the softening of tubercular infiltration; but the deposit of tubercle which takes place in the neighborhood of a diseased pulmonary gland is always in the form of distinct deposits—not of tubercular infiltration.

Tuberculization of the glands does not occasion perforation [illegible] of the bronchial tubes, but in some rare instances the œsophagus, tra- chea, and pulmonary artery have been perforated by the same process as is usually limited to the air-tubes.

In some cases in which tuberculization has never advanced [illegible] comes to a standstill, and the tubercle itself undergoes the cretaceous change. This, however, is a rare occurrence, for it has come under my notice only in 10 out of 119 cases; though, on the other hand, it is more frequent than in the lung, in which it has come under my notice in the child only in 7 out of 132 instances. In 9 other instances, the contents of the bronchial glands, though not actually cretaceous, were very dry and friable, as if the more fluid constituents of the tubercle had been removed, and the cretaceous change were about to commence. This change has never come under my notice as having taken place in any gland which had attained considerable size in consequence of the deposit of tubercle in it, nor have I ever seen it when the tuberculiza- tion of the glands was general, or when the lungs showed evidence of general, or of advanced phthisical disease.

It is now more than five-and-twenty years since these peculiarities first attracted my attention, and were insisted on by me in my [illegible] The researches of morbid anatomists, aided by the microscope, [illegible] thrown abundant light on many questions then obscure; they [illegible] shown that the so-called gray granulation is the one original [illegible] all tubercular deposit, and that the change from gray to yellow [illegible] the result of the natural metamorphosis of such deposit; [illegible] as it has been termed. They have further given its true [illegible] to the yellow infiltration, and have established as fact wh[illegible] since was but plausible theory—that the appearance is [illegible] tion (I beg pardon for the word, which is not of my [illegible]

products of inflammation, not to any change in tubercle originally deposited; that it is the evidence of a bygone pneumonia, though of a change at the same time which attests the scrofulous character of the patient in whom it has occurred.

Our deeper insight into the meaning of the facts does not alter the facts themselves. The rapid change of gray into yellow tubercle illustrates still more forcibly the acute course which the disease sometimes runs, than did the older views, according to which the two conditions, though allied, were yet supposed to be distinct. The tendency to the so-called tubercular infiltration illustrates the importance as it does the frequency of bronchio-pneumonia in early life; but explains at the same time the fact that there is more hope of the eventual clearing up of the signs of phthisis in early life when they have succeeded to acute symptoms, than when they have come on by slow degrees.

The *symptoms of phthisis in early life* resemble in many respects those which characterize the disease in adult age, while the points of difference become fewer and fewer in proportion as the child grows older, until they cease altogether at the period of puberty. During childhood, however, even those cases which run a course most similar to that of ordinary phthisis in the adult are in general distinguished by the absence of hæmoptysis at any stage of the affection,—the absence of expectoration, or its very rare occurrence,—the comparative slightness of the cough, and the rarity of those colliquative sweats which so much exhaust the grown person. In many instances the child droops, loses its appetite and flesh and strength, and complains of vague pain in the chest and abdomen for many weeks before the occurrence of cough excites any apprehension that the lungs are the seat of disease. When the cough does come on, it is slight, short, and dry, and attracts attention by its frequency, rather than by the discomfort which it occasions the child. Its usual amusements cease to occupy the child, who sits about, listless and fretful in the daytime, while the skin often grows hot and dry, and the lips become parched as night approaches; but there is so little that is definite in these symptoms, that they are not infrequently supposed to indicate the existence of typhoid fever, or to be due to the presence of worms in the intestines.

It is important to bear in mind that strumous dyspepsia, as it has been called by many writers, is of more frequent occurrence in childhood than in adult age, and that its symptoms may be all that marks the advance of phthisis in the lungs until within a month or two of the patient's death. A definite commencement can almost always be assigned to an attack of typhoid fever; and the great heat of skin, the very rapid pulse, the thirst, and the delirium at night, which attend it even in its less severe forms, are symptoms which, if borne in mind, would prevent our mistaking for it those slighter and more vague ailments that are experienced during the first stage of phthisis, in all except the rare instances in which the disease runs a very acute course. The referring the symptoms of incipient consumption to the presence of worms in the intestinal canal, is a mistake even less excusable; the natural temperature of the skin, and natural frequency of the respiration,—the appetite at one time as ravenous as it is deficient at another,—the tongue either clean and moist, or else thickly coated,—the condition [illegible] bowels, which is generally one of constipation—and the [illegible] that almost always follows the action of purgatives, are indi[illegible] the presence of worms sufficiently characteristic to guard the [illegible] observer from error.[1]

Fluctuations take place in the child's condition, and a [illegible] of bronchitis often seems to be the exciting cause of that aggravation of the pulmonary symptoms which is observed before long. The respiration now becomes habitually quicker than natural, instead of [illegible] being easily accelerated, and is often accompanied with considerable wheezing: the cough grows more frequent and lasts longer, but is still in most instances unattended by expectoration, owing to the fact that the child almost always swallows those matters which the adult would spit up. The loss of flesh, and the decay of strength, advance [illegible] more rapidly than the signs of pulmonary disease. Well-marked hectic, however, is infrequent; and if night-sweats occur, they are often limited to the head and face. Towards the close of the disease the mouth often becomes aphthous, especially in infants; but though diarrhœa sometimes occurs, it does not often seem to contribute so much to the exhaustion of the child as to that of the adult, and that alternation of diarrhœa and hectic sweats, which is so frequent in the grown person, is seldom or never observed in the child. When death at length takes place, it either occurs from exhaustion, or succeeds to some intercurrent attack of bronchitis or pneumonia; or follows the gradual supervention of symptoms of tubercular meningitis; a mode of termination of the disease more frequent in children under the age of three years, than in those who are older.

In those cases in which tubercle has been deposited in great abundance in the bronchial glands, constituting what is called *bronchial phthisis*, the symptoms deviate still more from those which are usually observed in the adult. Bronchial phthisis occurs in its best-marked form between the ages of two and six years, although, as it is scarcely necessary to observe, tuberculization of the glands is by no means limited to that age. Its symptoms in many instances first become distinctly evident after some severe bronchitic seizure, which either accompanied measles or came on without any apparent exciting cause. In other cases, although the commencement of the affection is not clearly traceable to a single attack of severe bronchitis, yet the patients in whom it occurs had in all probability been subject to frequent returns of catarrh or bronchitis, which, though not alarming in their symptoms, yet left behind them a cough that never entirely subsided. By degrees the cough becomes severer: it returns in paroxysms not unlike those of pertussis: it sometimes induces efforts to vomit, and can scarcely be distinguished from the cough of the earlier stages of hooping-cough. The respiration grows habitually oppressed and wheezing, the [illegible]

[1] The observations of Dr. Ringer and others, which held forth the hope that the thermometer would furnish the earliest and most trustworthy information of the coming on of phthisis, before the disease manifests itself by local symptoms, do not appear to have received adequate confirmation. They are dissented from [illegible] Roger, a most competent and unprejudiced authority. Op. cit., p. 371.

becomes puffed and swollen, the veins of the neck distended just as in patients with heart disease, and the superficial vessels of the thorax become enlarged, just as those of the abdomen do in cases of ascites, or of mesenteric disease.

The great fluctuations which take place in the condition of the patient constitute one of the most striking characteristics of this form of phthisis. Attacks of bronchitis sometimes come on, during which the respiration is painfully accelerated and oppressed, and the paroxysmal cough is merged for a time in a constant hacking, or in suppressed attempts at coughing. These bronchitic symptoms, which often seem to threaten life, and sometimes actually destroy it, clear up by degrees in the majority of cases, but leave the child with a severer cough and a more hurried respiration than before, while it loses flesh rapidly, and not infrequently sweats a good deal about the head and upper part of the trunk. Accommodation of posture, too, in many instances becomes necessary to the comfort of the little patient, who perhaps can breathe only when supported in its mother's lap, or when much propped up in bed. It is seldom, when the disease has reached this degree of severity, that there is not also so large a measure of tuberculous affection of the lungs and other viscera as to render recovery quite hopeless, and the characteristic signs of bronchial phthisis become lost by degrees in those of ordinary consumption. Sometimes, however, a long pause takes place in the progress of the disease, even though thus far advanced: the cough, which had acquired fresh intensity, gradually abates,—the respiration is no longer habitually wheezing,—the patient can repose in any attitude,—the flesh lost is regained,—and, were it not that cough still continues, though less frequent and less severe, that the breathing is more hurried than natural, and that auscultation contributes still further to undeceive us,—we might fancy that all ground for anxiety was passing away, and that the child was on the highroad towards recovery. In some cases, too, in which symptoms such as have been described are observed, recovery does eventually take place. It is seldom possible to say in any case by what means this recovery is brought about; sometimes, no doubt, the tubercular matter makes its way into the air-tubes, and is got rid of by expectoration. Once I observed the disappearance of most well-marked general signs of consumption, in the case of a girl eight years old, during the copious expectoration of a tenacious mucus, in which were small quantities of a substance like broken-down cheese, or grains of boiled rice, and which alternated with an expectoration of thick, puriform matter more or less tinged with blood. In the case of this child an attack of measles, while in her seventh year, had been succeeded by cough, the formation of abscesses in her neck, and a frequent puriform and sanguineous discharge from her nose. The abscesses had not been long healed when her mother's alarm was excited by her expectorating blood mixed with the phlegm which she brought up when coughing. Though not much emaciated, the child looked unhealthy; her pulse was very feeble, and there were many small petechiæ on her extremities. The lungs, however, were tolerably free from disease; for [illegible] heard during auscultation than a good deal of moist sounds, which were most evident at the upper part of the chest. Expectoration such as I have described continued for nearly three months, in the course of which time the child by degrees lost her cough, and gained strength under the use of steel and other tonics. Two years afterwards no auscultatory signs of disease were perceptible, except a little creaking under both clavicles; and at the end of five years even this had disappeared.

The fatal termination of bronchial phthisis usually takes place in consequence of the lungs becoming seriously involved in the tubercular disease, though life is sometimes suddenly cut off by hæmoptysis, owing to the perforation of one of the larger vessels of the thorax by a tuberculated bronchial gland. It must not, however, be supposed that this is the only means by which fatal hemorrhage is produced, for it takes place in other instances in precisely the same circumstances as in the adult. Seven cases of fatal hæmoptysis have come under my notice in children; but in four no examination was made after death. In the fifth case, which was that of a boy between five and six years old, who died at the end of nine months' illness, blood pouring in abundance from his nose and mouth, the amount of disease, both of the lungs and bronchial glands, was very considerable; but no large vessel had been perforated, and it was not possible satisfactorily to determine the source of the hemorrhage. In the sixth case, that of a little boy five years old, in whom symptoms of pneumonia had supervened upon previous signs of phthisis, the source of the bleeding in the single and fatal attack of hæmoptysis, which took place at a time when he seemed recovering, likewise eluded the most careful anatomical investigation. In the seventh case, there was a cavity in the upper part of the right lower lobe. This cavity was traversed by a vessel on which an aneurism had formed, of the size of a hazelnut. The sudden rupture of this aneurism was the occasion of the patient's death.

A very considerable degree of tuberculization of the bronchial glands is by no means uncommon even in very early infancy; but it then generally forms only a part of such extensive tubercular disease that its special symptoms are lost in those of the general malady. In such cases, too, it frequently occurs that the signs of thoracic disease are almost entirely merged in those of generally defective nutrition. The existence even of a large cavity in the lung may be announced in early infancy by nothing more serious than some acceleration of the breathing and an occasional short cough; while the frequent vomiting,—the irregular, often relaxed, condition of the bowels,—the unhealthy evacuations,—the red tongue and the aphthous state of the mouth,—may direct the attention almost exclusively to the condition of the digestive organs.

Many points still remain for our investigation, but we must postpone their consideration, and the study of the auscultatory phenomena of the disease, to the next lecture.

LECTURE XXIX.

Phthisis, continued —Peculiarities of its auscultatory signs in early life—Some of less value than in the adult—Influence of tuberculous bronchial glands in exaggerating the signs of disease of the lung—Difficulty in appreciating some signs which are well marked in the adult—Sign peculiar to early life.

Different forms of phthisis.—Acute phthisis; illustrative case—Tuberculous pneumonia—Bronchitis grafted on phthisis may lead to an overestimate of the tuberculous disease.

Duration of phthisis; its course sometimes very acute, at others extremely chronic.—Cases in illustration—Modes of death in phthisis—Head symptoms sometimes precede death independent of cerebral disease.

Prophylaxis, and treatment of phthisis.

It would be little better than a waste of your time to enter into a minute description of all the modifications of the respiratory sounds to which the presence of tubercle in the lungs of children may give occasion: our time will be better spent than in such detail, if we direct our attention to those respects in which the *auscultatory signs of phthisis in childhood* differ from those which betoken its existence in the adult, or in which the same auscultatory phenomena require a different interpretation at the one period of life, from that which is justly applied to them at the other.

The grand difference, indeed, is to be sought in the latter rather than in the former of these respects. Tubercle, at whatever age it is developed in the lungs, gives rise to much the same auscultatory phenomena; but many of those modifications of the respiratory sound which would warrant us in pronouncing positively that phthisis existed in the adult, cannot be relied on with the same certainty in the child: still less can they be regarded as proving the existence of so large an amount of disease in the latter case as in the former. It may be stated, then, that

1st. *Many of the auscultatory signs of phthisis deserve less reliance, or have a less grave import, in the child than in the adult.*

One of the earliest signs of tubercular deposit in the lungs of the grown person is furnished by that peculiar modification of the respiratory sound to which the name of coarse breathing has been applied; and this acquires still greater importance when associated, as it often is, with dry rhonchus and creaking sounds. Much of the value of this sign depends on its being limited to the infra-clavicular regions, or, at least, on its being heard there with much greater distinctness than elsewhere. Since, however, the deposit of tubercle in the lungs of children is more uniform, and more generally diffused than in the adult, the additional value which the localization of these signs furnishes is lost; and it becomes impossible to determine whether the bronchial irritation that they betoken is induced by the presence of tubercle in the lungs, or by some other cause.

Prolongation of the expiratory sound beneath the clavicle, and interrupted respiration,—the *respiration saccadée* of French authors,—which are two of the earliest and most important indications of phthisis in the grown person, are, on the whole, of less value in the child. Their occurrence, indeed, should always excite suspicion as to the existence of phthisis, but they are not infrequently very well marked in cases where but slight disorder of the respiratory organs is present; and where the perfect recovery of the child, and its subsequent sound health, prove that tubercular disease either was altogether absent, or at any rate was extremely slight.

The exaggeration of these two signs is probably, in some measure, due to a cause which adds greatly to the intensity of some other of those auscultatory phenomena that usually betoken far-advanced phthisis. MM. Rilliet and Barthez were, I believe, the first who pointed out the fact that the bronchial glands, when enlarged by the deposit of tubercle, and thus brought into contact with the walls of the chest, which they do not touch in the healthy state, conduct to the ear of the auscultator sounds that in other circumstances are imperceptible. The air passing through the larger bronchi is now heard, on applying the stethoscope to the walls of the chest, in the supra-scapular, and less often in the infra-clavicular region, and can scarcely be distinguished from bronchial breathing produced by solidification of the pulmonary tissue itself. The sounds which are caused by the presence of mucus in the larger air-tubes are in the same way conducted to the ear in other situations than those,—such as the root of the lung, where alone they would be heard if the glands were not enlarged. The auscultator may thus be betrayed into the error of supposing that hopeless phthisis exists in cases where yet the amount of disease in the lung is but small, and where life may be prolonged for many years. Morbid sounds, too, produced in one lung, may thus be conducted to the walls of the chest on the opposite side, and the extent of disease may, in consequence, be overrated; or the sounds which, when perceived in the front of the chest, may arise from real disease in that situation, being transmitted to the back through the medium of the glands, may thus give rise to the conclusion that far more serious mischief exists than is really the case. The means of avoiding error from this cause consist in the careful comparison of the results of auscultation with those of percussion, and of those of auscultation on one day with those which it yields a few days afterwards. If the sounds proceed from solidification of the lung, or from cavities in its substance, the results of auscultation will be as invariable as those of percussion; but if they are merely sounds transmitted from the larger air-tubes, they will be found to vary much on different occasions; while the dulness on percussion in certain parts will continue unchanged, inasmuch as it proceeds from the presence of the enlarged glands. This variability in the results of auscultation is one of the most important indications of bronchial phthisis. It depends not merely on the accidental variations in the sounds produced in the larger air-tubes, but also on the changes which the varying degree of compression of the bronchi, produced by the increase or diminution in the size of the glands, may occasion, and on the variations in the irritation of the air-tubes which this pressure produces. The risk in cases of bronchial phthisis is not so much that of forming an altogether erroneous diagnosis, as of expressing a prognosis far more unfavorable than the nature of the case actually justifies. In cases where a considerable measure of bronchitis is associated with tuberculization of the glands, we are especially likely to fall into this error, and can avoid it only by much caution, and by frequently repeated auscultation.

There are differences of another kind, however, between the results of auscultation in cases of phthisis in the young and old, and which depend—

2d. *On the absence, or difficult appreciation, of some auscultatory phenomena in the child, to which much value is attached in the case of the adult.*

To this head belong the differences resulting from the loss in the child of almost all that information which, in older persons, is afforded by the different modifications of the vocal resonance. The shrill voice of the child, the small power of modulating it that is possessed in early life, and the consequent difficulty of inducing the patient to utter a few sentences, or even a few words, in the same key, even when fear does not reduce the voice to a mere whisper, take away almost all value from the modifications of the voice-sound in young subjects.

The extreme excitability of children tends, as it does also in the female subject, to reduce very low the value of mere inequality of breathing between the two lungs; for it is by no means a rare occurrence for the lung which on one day seemed to admit but little air, to yield the sounds of well-marked puerile respiration on the next day, and for the feeble respiration to have changed sides. Before, therefore, any conclusion can be drawn from the feebleness of the respiration in either lung, its situation, degree, and extent must be confirmed by repeated observation.

The finer variations in the sonoriety of the chest are not so easily distinguished in childhood as in more advanced age. The main cause of this appears to be furnished by the extreme resonance of the chest in early childhood, which will admit of very considerable reduction before percussion elicits a sound that the ear would recognize as at all dull. Extremely gentle percussion is much more likely to bring out the more delicate variations of sound, than those smart taps on the chest, which, in the grown person, will often answer the purpose sufficiently well.

A last source of difference may be mentioned as arising—

3d. *From the occurrence of some physical signs peculiar to the form which phthisis assumes in early life.*

The only sign that comes with propriety into this category, is that dulness between the scapulæ which is not infrequently produced by the presence of tuberculous glands, and which, when it coexists with tolerable resonance over the upper part of the lungs, and moderately good respiration in those situations, may be regarded as pathognomonic of bronchial phthisis. The absence of dulness in this situation, however, does not of itself warrant the inference that the glands are free from disease, but merely that they have not yet attained any very considerable degree of enlargement.

It may perhaps be useful, before we proceed to the study of some other peculiarities of phthisis in childhood, briefly to recapitulate the *general characteristics of the disease in early life.* The chief of these are—

1st. The frequent latency of the thoracic symptoms during its early stages.

2d. The almost invariable absence of hæmoptysis at the commencement of the disease, and its comparatively rare occurrence during its subsequent progress.

3d. The partial or complete absence of expectoration.

4th. The rarity of profuse general sweats; and the ill-marked character of the hectic symptoms.

5th. The frequency with which death takes place from intercurrent bronchitis or pneumonia.

Bronchial phthisis is characterized by—

1st. The frequent development of its symptoms out of one or more attacks of bronchitis.

2d. The peculiar paroxsymal cough which attends it, resembling that of incipient pertussis.

3d. The great and frequent fluctuations in the patient's condition, and the occasional apparently causeless aggravation both of the cough and dyspnœa.

In very early infancy, phthisis is remarkable for the very frequent latency of the chest symptoms, which, through its entire course, are often entirely merged in the signs of impaired nutrition.

The most important peculiarities in the auscultatory phenomena of consumption in the child are—

1st. The smaller value of coarse respiration, prolonged expiration, and interrupted breathing, owing to their general diffusion over the chest, and to their occasional existence independent of phthisis.

2d. The apparent, and to some extent the real, exaggeration of the signs both of early and far-advanced disease of the lungs, in some cases of bronchial phthisis.

3d. The loss of that information which the phenomena of the voice furnish in the case of the adult.

4th. The small value of inequality of breathing in the two lungs.

5th. The difficulty of detecting minute variations in the sonority of the chest; and

6th. The existence of dulness in the interscapular region, together with moderate resonance of the upper part of the chest, and tolerably good respiration there, which are characteristic of the presence of enlarged bronchial glands.

Hitherto we have been occupied with the study of the more common forms of phthisis in childhood; but *deviations* are occasionally met with *from the ordinary course of the disease*, with which it behooves us to make ourselves acquainted. *Phthisis occasionally runs a course so extremely rapid* that many of its most characteristic symptoms have not time to manifest themselves. In such cases we are exposed to considerable risk of error, for the history of the patient's indisposition goes back only to a few weeks or days; the evidence of impaired nutrition is almost or altogether wanting, and the *symptoms* appear to be those of an acute malady coming on suddenly, rather than those of a slow and wasting disease.

A remarkable instance of this came under my notice some years ago, in the case of a little boy, nine months old, who was fat and ruddy, and had always had perfectly good health until the 10th of April. On that day he was taken with symptoms which his mother supposed to be those of a bad cold. On account of this he was kept in the house, and various domestic remedies were employed, though without any improvement, and on April 24th he came under my notice. There did not then appear to be any urgent symptom, though the child seemed much oppressed at the chest. The case appeared to be one of rather severe catarrh, occurring during the period of dentition. The gums were lanced, and a mixture containing the vinum ipecacuanhæ was ordered, to which, finding the symptoms did not abate, small doses of antimonial wine were added on the 27th. On the 30th I was informed that the child was much worse, that his dyspnœa was greatly increased, and that his hands and feet had been swollen for the previous forty-eight hours. I found the little boy breathing fifty times in the minute, with great oppression at the chest, the face much flushed, the skin dry, the trunk hot, the limbs cool, and the hands and feet much swollen. Auscultation detected generally diffused small crepitation through both lungs, with indistinct bronchial breathing at the upper and back part of the left side. Three hours after this visit, the child died without a struggle on being lifted out of bed for his mother to apply some leeches to his chest.

On examining the body after death, a very thick layer of fat was found everywhere beneath the integuments. The lungs presented an extreme degree of tubercular degeneration and many of the bronchial glands were enlarged by the morbid deposit to the size of a pigeon's egg. None of the tubercle in the lungs was softened, but it existed both in the form of yellow miliary tubercle, of tubercular infiltration, and of masses of crude tubercle formed by the agglomeration of many separate deposits. The pulmonary substance in the intervals between the tubercular deposits was of a bright red color, in the first stage of pneumonia, and in many parts bordering on the second stage, and there was very considerable injection of the bronchial tubes. The various abdominal viscera contained tubercle, but it was not far advanced in the mesenteric glands.

This case represents a class in which there is much hazar

an erroneous diagnosis. It shows the possibility of tubercular [illegible] taking place to a very great extent without at all interfering [illegible] general nutrition of the body, and without giving rise to any [illegible] so serious as to attract the notice of a very careful and [illegible] mother. It illustrates also the mode in which the fatal termination [illegible] many cases of phthisis in children is brought about, and suggests [illegible] inquiry whether there are any means of distinguishing between [illegible] *culous pneumonia*, and pneumonia which occurs uncomplicated [illegible] phthisical disease of the lungs.

Pneumonia often complicates phthisis in early life, in circumstances where no diagnostic difficulty occurs; but it is of much importance to detect the consumptive element in cases which to the superficial observer present no other symptoms than those of acute inflammation of the lungs. The existence of a considerable amount of tubercular deposit in the lungs may be suspected in those cases in which the degree of oppression of the chest has, from the very commencement of the illness, been altogether out of proportion to the severity of the catarrhal or bronchitic symptoms with which the disease set in. A further evidence of its nature is afforded, if the skin, though very dry, presents a less considerable or a less pungent heat than attends simple pneumonia, while the pulse from the very outset is less developed. Suspicion would be strengthened if the frequency of respiration very greatly exceeded the amount of mischief disclosed by auscultation, and especially if the rapidity of the breathing, though so great that it would excite the most serious alarm if the case were one of pneumonia, should yet continue the same for days together without marked deterioration in the patient's condition. Auscultation also would throw much light on the nature of the case, for the sounds detected in the chest would be the subcrepitant and mucous râles, rather than the small crepitation of pneumonia; while, though the [illegible] sounds would be discovered at the lower part of the chest, the greatest dulness on percussion would generally be detected at the upper part, and bronchial breathing would very likely be perceived more or less distinctly in the same situation.

The importance of distinguishing those cases in which inflammation supervenes in a lung already the seat of tubercular deposit, from others in which the organ had been previously healthy, is by no means confined to cases of the severest kind, in which life is immediately threatened. In every instance of pneumonia in early life, both your prognosis and your treatment would be greatly modified if there were good grounds for believing that tubercular disease had for some time previously affected the lungs. Hence follows the necessity for that very minute inquiry as to the previous health of the patient, and of the other members of the family, on which so much stress was laid at the commencement of this course of lectures. If you learned that several children in the [illegible] had already died of phthisis or of some other affection—such as tubercular meningitis—which you knew to be most intimately associated with the tuberculous diathesis, the possibility of the same complication existing in the patient under your care would at once occur [illegible]. This complication would be rendered highly probable, if you [illegible] ascertain that the child had been particularly liable to catch cold, [illegible] for some months been seldom free from cough for many days together, or had suffered from cough every winter, for two or three years, and had already experienced two or three attacks similar to that which you are called on to treat, and which, though severe, had yet subsided by degrees, without the employment of very active measures. The probability would be raised almost to certainty if there existed that want of correspondence between the general symptoms and physical signs, or between the results of auscultation and percussion, to which reference has already been made; or if the history of the present illness went back to a period anterior to that which you would be disposed to assign to it, if the affection had been simple pneumonia.

You would carefully abstain from all rigorous antiphlogistic measures in the management of a case of tuberculous pneumonia. Bearing in mind the influence of enlarged bronchial glands in rendering parts of the chest dull on percussion, and in exaggerating in some respects the morbid sounds, you would not overestimate the degree or extent of the inflammatory mischief. At the same time you would not allow even a considerable measure of improvement to lead you to speak too decidedly of the ultimate recovery of your patient; since you would not forget that, if inflammation do not originate tuberculous disease, it may yet communicate increased activity to its progress.

The overlooking the more serious malady, owing to its symptoms being thrown into the shade by those of the other more curable affection, is not the only error to which you are exposed in cases of infantile phthisis. The degree of *irritation of the bronchi* that exists in different instances, varies exceedingly; sometimes it is so considerable that when the child is placed under your care its respiration is wheezing, difficult, and very hurried, its cough violent and exhausting; while such is the general anxiety of the countenance, and so great is the depression of the vital powers, that the struggle seems as if it could not be long protracted. Percussion detects dulness at the upper part of the chest; the bronchi are so laden with phlegm that air scarcely penetrates beyond the larger tubes, and mucous râle is heard throughout the whole of the lungs, while at the upper part it is so large as to amount almost to gurgling. You regard the case as one of far-advanced phthisis, and suppose that softened tubercle is diffused through the whole of both lungs, and that cavities exist at their apex. You form the most gloomy prognosis, and entertain, very probably express, the conviction that a few weeks at furthest will be the period of your patient's life. By degrees, however, the most urgent symptoms subside, and some signs of returning health appear; the respiration grows slower and more tranquil, the cough abates, perhaps almost ceases. The signs of a cavity grow less and less distinct, in proportion as the secretion in the bronchi diminishes; and after some months, while the patient's general condition deviates but little from a state of health, a little dulness at the upper and back part of the chest, unequal breathing, prolonged expiration, or morbid sounds equally slight, are the only auscultatory evidence that the most careful examination can discover of pulmonary disease.

Non-professional persons are apt to imagine the mi

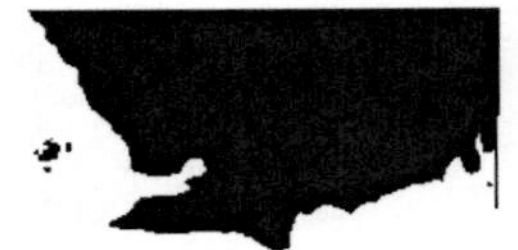

of this kind to have been greater than it really was. The error is one as to the degree of the malady rather than as to its kind. In cases that present these symptoms, phthisis has in reality existed, but the chief tubercular deposit has probably been seated in the bronchial glands, and their enlargement gave rise to much of the dulness on percussion, and exaggerated the morbid sounds at the upper part of the chest. From some accidental cause, such as cold or damp, or from the mucous membrane of the bronchi sympathising with disorder of the digestive organs, or from inappropriate treatment, which aggravated the evil it should have relieved, or even without any cause that we can assign, it had come to pass that the air-tubes were in a state of great irritation. The due regulation of temperature, appropriate general treatment, and nature's own healing power, improved the health and diminished the irritability of the bronchi; while very probably the diseased glands emptied themselves, at least in part, into the air-tubes, and the tubercle was thus eliminated from the system. You should, therefore, always express your opinion very guardedly with reference to the condition of a child suffering from phthisis, until you have confirmed the results of auscultation by its frequent repetition, and till you have had the opportunity of determining how large a portion of the physical signs is due to the morbid deposit, and how much to that irritation of the bronchi which you may fairly hope to mitigate, if not to remove.

The average *duration of phthisis* in childhood is estimated by MM. Rilliet and Barthez at from three to seven months, though, as they justly observe, its extreme limits vary from two months in unusually rapid cases, to two years and upwards in other instances, in which the course of the disease is very protracted. It is my impression, indeed, that the ordinary duration of phthisis in childhood is less brief even among the poor than the observations of these gentlemen, made among the children in the Hôpital des Enfans, at Paris, have led them to believe. I am certain too that in the wealthier classes of society, phthisis, when not congenital, or when not coming on within the first months of infancy, runs a much slower course, though it is not possible to state in figures the conclusions drawn from private practice, in which the number of observations has to make up for the imperfect and fragmentary character of each. The difference in duration, indeed, between the two extremes of phthisis is very wide; a few weeks limiting it in some cases, while in others the disease has continued for two, three, four, and nearly five years, before it terminated fatally.

That form of *acute phthisis* in which the patient dies as the result of the constitutional malady rather than of local mischief going on in some one organ, is much oftener met with as a sequela of some other disease, such as measles, hooping-cough, or typhoid fever, than as an idiopathic affection. It follows sometimes on the decline of one or other of those disorders, and develops itself out of the convalescence from it, the fever not entirely subsiding, the appetite not returning, the strength not being regained, but the amendment which yesterday seemed to promise, being belied by the deterioration of to-day; and in such circumstances, a month or five weeks will sometimes bring the

child to the grave, all its functions suffering so equally, that we feel at a loss as to the one to which we should endeavor chiefly to minister.

But though less frequent, the cases are of greater moment, because they are more likely to be misinterpreted, in which this acute tuberculosis develops itself out of a condition of previous health, though that health is oftener valetudinarianism than vigor. Causelessly, the child loses flesh, and strength, and appetite, and cheerfulness; it frets about everything, but says it has no pain, that it ails nothing; nor is anything observable save that the pulse is habitually quicker, and the skin often hotter than natural. The nights are restless, though the child frequently wants to lie down in the daytime, and sometimes delirium comes on towards bedtime; while when awake there is a remarkable degree of nervousness, the manner is frightened, almost hysterical. Often this condition gradually passes away as symptoms of tubercular meningitis come on, and the case loses its peculiarities as its hopeless nature becomes apparent; though not infrequently, if we examine the body after death, we shall be surprised at finding the evidence of cerebral disease slighter than we had expected, and a little fluid in the ventricles, a little opacity of the arachnoid and a few granulations at the base of the brain, may be all the alterations discoverable. In other instances the symptoms put on more and more the character of fever; the delirium becomes more frequent, and at last constant; the prostration extreme, the tongue dry and tremulous, the teeth covered with sordes, and the abdomen full, tender, tympanitic, so that the distinction between the case and one of typhoid fever is almost impossible; and, indeed, the previous history of the patient, and the longer duration of the ailment, constitute almost the only means by which we can discriminate between them. This course of phthisis, too, is not limited to any age, but may even be observed in infants at the breast: and the extreme rarity of typhoid fever at so early an age would in them still further raise the presumption that the symptoms were due to the rapid development of tubercle.

So little notice has been taken of the *chronic form of phthisis* in children, that it may be well to relate a few examples of it. In March, 1842, I saw a little girl, six years old, whose father had died of phthisis, and who had had a cough ever since she suffered from measles two and a half years before. Her mother's anxiety had been excited by the increase of this cough, and by the child's losing flesh during the few weeks previous to her coming to me. Auscultation at this time discovered that air entered the lung in the left infra-clavicular region more scantily than in the right, and that the respiration was coarse, and attended with much creaking at the upper part of both lungs. In May, the general symptoms were much improved, and the creaking sounds were no longer heard. For many months the child continued to appear tolerably well, though her cough never ceased entirely; but in the early part of the winter of 1844 her health completely failed. Examination of the chest in the beginning of December elicited great deficiency of resonance at the upper part of the left lung, both in front and behind. Bronchial breathing, intermixed with large mucous râle, was heard in the left suprascapular region, and

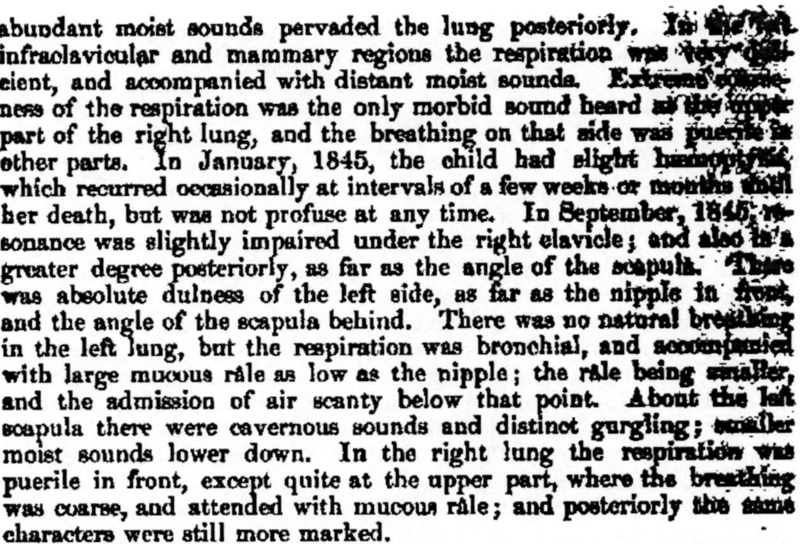

abundant moist sounds pervaded the lung posteriorly. In the left infraclavicular and mammary regions the respiration was very deficient, and accompanied with distant moist sounds. Extreme [illegible]ness of the respiration was the only morbid sound heard at the upper part of the right lung, and the breathing on that side was puerile in other parts. In January, 1845, the child had slight hæmoptysis, which recurred occasionally at intervals of a few weeks or months until her death, but was not profuse at any time. In September, 1845, resonance was slightly impaired under the right clavicle; and also in a greater degree posteriorly, as far as the angle of the scapula. There was absolute dulness of the left side, as far as the nipple in front, and the angle of the scapula behind. There was no natural breathing in the left lung, but the respiration was bronchial, and accompanied with large mucous râle as low as the nipple; the râle being smaller, and the admission of air scanty below that point. About the left scapula there were cavernous sounds and distinct gurgling; smaller moist sounds lower down. In the right lung the respiration was puerile in front, except quite at the upper part, where the breathing was coarse, and attended with mucous râle; and posteriorly the same characters were still more marked.

It cannot be necessary to detail the results of the subsequent examinations of the chest, which showed that disease advanced slowly in the right lung, though there was at no time proof of the existence of a cavity there. The child's condition fluctuated; sometimes she seemed almost dying under an aggravation of all the symptoms, and then again she rallied, and was able to walk about, and seemed tolerably comfortable. Life was prolonged until June 1st, 1847; and she had seemed almost as well as usual until a very few days before her death. Unfortunately, permission to examine the body could not be obtained; but the stethoscopic signs enable us to trace back the phthisical disease for more than five years, while the evidence of a large cavity in the left lung was distinct twenty-one months before death took place.

Nor is this a solitary case, but if time allowed I could give many other illustrations of the slow progress of phthisis, terminating sometimes in imperfect convalescence; but oftener in gradual decline and tardy death. Often, indeed, it is useless to speculate on the issue of a case of chronic phthisis, or on its possible duration; for it is by no means unlikely that the child may live, with but little deterioration in its condition, until measles or hooping-cough imparts a fresh stimulus to the consumptive disease, or excites some fatal attack of bronchitis or pneumonia. I used to see occasionally a little boy, who was aged only three years when he first came under my notice, and whom I had the opportunity of watching till he was eleven years old. When first brought to me he had been suffering from cough ever since an attack of what his mother called inflammation of the lungs, when he was sixteen months old; his cervical glands had recently suppurated; he had unusually well-marked hectic fever, and profuse night-sweats; and a month before I saw him had spit blood once. His right side yielded throughout a dull sound on percussion; breathing in that lung was scanty, and attended by large moist sounds. The child [illegible]

Devonshire to pass the winter, and, as I expected, to die there of phthisis; but he returned in better health; he grew tall, and played about like other children, though he seldom passed more than a few months without attacks of a pleuritic character, the pain of which he used to refer to his right side, and which usually subsided in the course of a few days, without any treatment more severe than a mustard poultice, and some diaphoretic medicine. His cough never left him entirely; but both that and the quantity and character of his expectoration varied, and sometimes he spat a little blood. In October, 1844, the auscultatory signs were as follows: The left lung yielded, as it had constantly done, the sounds of puerile breathing in front; posteriorly, the breathing in the lung was also good, except that there were some moist sounds in the infrascapular region, and that the breathing had a coarse and almost tubular character about the upper angle of the scapula. In the right lung, in front, the respiration was puerile, with now and then a little distant crepitus as low down as the lower edge of the second rib, at which point the moist sounds became larger. Posteriorly there were large moist sounds intermixed with puerile breathing in the suprascapular region; gurgling, cavernous breathing, and bronchial voice about the scapula; and lower down there was very little respiration, and that of a bronchial character, becoming quite inaudible in the lateral region. In the axillary region the respiration was coarse, accompanied with large mucous râles. In March, 1849, I saw him for the last time. He had then continued for more than eighteen months free from any serious pleuritic attack, and from hæmoptysis. His respiration was still hurried, but he had gained flesh, and sometimes had walked five or six miles in a day without inconvenience. Auscultation showed, too, that his disease had been stationary for the previous five years—if, indeed, it had not actually improved. The moist sounds about the left scapula were smaller, and heard over a smaller surface. The indications of a cavity in the back part of the right lung continued unchanged, but not increased; while in other respects auscultation gave exactly the same results as before. Other cases of a similar kind have come under my observation, in which the history of phthisis went back for several years, and in which the signs of caverns in the lungs were unmistakable; the children continuing to lead a sort of valetudinarian existence, improving in health, and gaining flesh and strength in the summer, but losing ground again with the return of winter.

In the present condition of our knowledge, it is not possible to state with certainty either the anatomical characters of phthisical cavities of long standing, or the signs which, during the patient's lifetime, would warrant the expectation that the disease will run a tardy course; but it is well to bear in mind, that such cases are by no means very rare; that the powers of repair are far greater in the child than in the adult. We must now, therefore, pass on to notice briefly the treatment of the disease, after glancing for a moment at the *different modes in which it brings about a fatal issue.*

In a very large proportion of cases of phthisis, the functions of all the organs of the body become at length so much disturbed, and nutrition generally is so impaired, that the patient dies, because the whole machine is worn out. But though this is the case in many instances, yet it often happens even when the powers have long seemed utterly exhausted, and when the body is wasted almost to a skeleton, that death is far from tranquil, but is preceded by hours of severe agony, for which it is not easy to account. In many cases, and especially in those where the disease runs a rapid course, the fatal termination is due to an attack of intercurrent bronchitis or pneumonia, which is sometimes supposed to have been the patient's only disease, until a post-mortem examination reveals the tubercular degeneration of the lungs, to which the inflammatory affection was but secondary. Death from hæmoptysis is rare, and still rarer is the perforation of the lung by the walls of the cavity giving way at some point, and thus producing pneumothorax. The abdominal symptoms sometimes mask the thoracic, and the patient, who, had life been prolonged, would have sunk eventually under pulmonary phthisis, dies of tubercular peritonitis. Many children, in whom the signs of incipient phthisis have appeared, die of tubercular meningitis, excited by the membranes of the brain having become the seat of tubercular deposit; and some, in whom the disease has attained a more advanced stage, are suddenly carried off by head symptoms, the cause of which is explained by the discovery of large masses of tubercle in the cerebral substance. Convulsions, however, sometimes precede death for several hours, or head symptoms of greater or less intensity constitute the most striking feature in the patient's history for some days before death takes place; and yet an examination of the body throws no light upon the cause of their occurrence. Sometimes, too, the symptoms that precede death are those of fever of a typhoid character, rather than of serious mischief in the chest; though it will generally be found in such cases that acute inflammation of the tubercular lung, how little soever betrayed by local signs, has been the occasion of the patient's symptoms, and the cause of his death.

Though the study of phthisis, in its effects and its symptoms, has occupied us during almost the whole of two lectures, yet there need be but little said with reference to its *treatment*. The main principles by which we are to be guided in its treatment are the same at every age; nor do the differences in the patient's years bring with them many or important modifications in the means by which these principles are to be carried into action.

Among the prophylactic measures adapted to early life, none is of more importance than the keeping the infant at the breast for the first twelve or eighteen months of its existence, by which time it will have passed through some at least of the dangers incidental to the period of teething. The task of thus nursing the infant, however, ought not to be undertaken by a mother who has shown any tendency to consumption, or in whose family consumptive disease has been prevalent, but ought at once to be intrusted to a healthy wet-nurse. This rule does not rest on mere theoretical grounds; but actual observation has shown that under some morbid states of the system the milk undergoes great changes, and loses much of its nutritive properties. In the case of the cow, these changes have been ascertained by Dr. Klencke, of Leipsic, to be very remarkable; and analogical reasoning would warrant the belief that the scrofulous taint in the human subject may give rise to alterations of a similar kind. Dr. Klencke[1] confirmed the observation of Sir Robert Carswell and others, that stall-fed cows are very liable to become tuberculous; and found, moreover, that in these circumstances their milk loses much or the whole of its sugar; that the butter and casein diminish, while albumen is found sometimes in as high a proportion as 15 per cent., and elain in the proportion of 1.4 per cent., and that in some cases lactic acid is likewise present. Even if we set aside the assumption of scrofulous disease being actually transmitted through the medium of the milk, of which there is perhaps no clear evidence, it is yet apparent that a very slight degree of such an alteration in its constituents as has just been mentioned, must render it very unfit for the nutriment of a delicate infant.

It is needless to dwell here on the general rules for feeding and clothing children as they grow older, or to insist on the necessity for the bed-rooms being airy and well ventilated. When the damp and cold weather of winter approaches, removal to a warm climate, in which exercise in the open air may still be continued, is much to be preferred to keeping the child for weeks together a prisoner to the house; and as a general rule more is gained by change of climate in early life than in adult age. In children who are old enough to be taught to wear it, I have sometimes seen the respirator of much service, in enabling them to continue to take exercise in the open air at a season when, in previous years, exposure to the external air had always induced or greatly aggravated the signs of bronchial irritation. Whenever catarrhal symptoms appear, no care can be too great to bestow on the attempt speedily to remove them. In doing so, however, and in the management of all ailments that come on in children who have shown a disposition to consumptive disease, much caution must be used, in order to avoid over-treating them. On this account it is of extreme importance to encounter them at their very commencement, when mild measures will suffice for their cure; and, for the same reason, the child should be defended with the most punctilious care from the contagion of hooping-cough and of the eruptive fevers—diseases in the course of which serious thoracic complications are so apt to supervene.

In carrying out this plan of unwearied watchfulness, and of attention to minute detail continued for months and years, you will have brighter hopes with children for your patients, than if you were called on to exercise similar precautions in the case of persons more advanced in life. Without raising baseless expectations, too, you may communicate something of hope to the parents, and thus lighten for them their anxious task; nor will the appearance even of decided physical signs of tubercular deposit, nor the evidence that in some parts that tubercle is softened, warrant an absolutely hopeless prognosis. Cases such as have been related show how long life may be prolonged in circumstances the most inauspicious; and, where speedy death has been expected, an unlimited reprieve seems almost a pardon.

---

[1] Ueber die Ansteckung und Verbreitung der Scrofelkrankheit bei Menschen durch den Genuss der Kuhmilch, 16mo., Leipzig, 1846. See especially chapter iii, pp. 21–61.

It may suffice to have said thus much about the management of phthisis in childhood; for when the disease is actually developed, we have the same indications as in the adult, and these must be met by similar means. Iron, quinine, and the mineral acids are the most important of our tonic remedies; and for these the extract of bark and the extract of logwood may be substituted, if much tendency exists to a relaxed state of the bowels. In cases where the glands of the neck are affected, and where there seems to be reason for supposing that the disease approximates to bronchial phthisis, the syrup of the iodide of iron may be employed with advantage. Such cases, too, have seemed to me to profit most by the cod-liver oil; though I must confess that my own experience of it does not altogether bear out the high encomiums which have been bestowed upon it by some practitioners. Sometimes I have known it excite diarrhœa; at other times it completely spoils the appetite; while, as a general rule, I think it is not borne well in cases where dyspeptic symptoms are, as is so often the case, at all a prominent feature in the disease. Sometimes, too, the child's repugnance to the remedy is unconquerable; though this does not often occur. If given in a little orange wine, or orange juice, sweetened with syrup of orange-peel if necessary, its taste is in general perfectly disguised; while sometimes, nauseous though the oil is, children become really fond of its flavor. In some cases, where children either cannot bear, or will not take, cod-liver oil, I have employed glycerin, and in others the so-called pancreatic emulsion—a compound which, in spite of the mistaken physiological hypothesis of its advocates, is a serviceable nutriment. I do not know, however, that either it or glycerin answers any higher purpose than that of food; or that in this respect either is superior to cream. The sickness and the paroxysmal cough are best relieved by the hydrocyanic acid, with which the liquor cinchonæ of Mr. Battley may be combined,[1] in cases where we are afraid to venture on any but the mildest tonics. Among local measures, the use of stimulating liniments to the chest is even more valuable in early life than in the adult; and sometimes the application of a blister, about the size of a shilling, under one or other clavicle, and its frequent repetition, is followed by a very great amendment in the patient's condition, and by a marked improvement in the physical signs furnished by the subjacent lung.

I have very rarely employed local depletion, except in the treatment of the pneumonia which so often attacks the phthisical patient; but it

---

[1] See Formula No. 21, p. 400.

Another very useful formula in these cases, and one which has the further advantage of forming a very agreeable vehicle for the cod-liver oil, is the following:

(No. 22.)

℞. Acid. Nitr. dil., ♏xvj.
Acid. Hydrochlor. dil., ♏xxiv.
Acid. Hydrocy. dil., ♏viij.
Spiritus Chloroformi, ♏xl.
Træ. Aurantii, ʒiss.
Syrupi simplicis, ʒij.
Aquæ destillatæ, ad ℥iv. M.

A tablespoonful every six hours. For a child four years old.

has then seemed sometimes to be of great service; and it will probably be safer to trust to a moderate abstraction of blood by leeches, followed by small doses of antimonials, rather than to administer mercury, or to give antimony in larger doses without previous depletion. The habitual cough of phthisis requires small doses of ipecacuanha wine, combined or not with antimony, and laudanum or compound tincture of camphor in small doses,—remedies which, on account of their strength being definite, are always to be preferred, in the management of the affections of childhood, to a preparation so variable as the syrup of poppies. Opiates in various forms, and for various purposes, may be needed to check diarrhœa, or to relieve suffering; and you must not allow any preconceived notion of the danger of employing opium in infantile diseases to prevent your having recourse to so valuable a medicine.

We must here leave this subject, so full of painful interest, and proceed at our next lecture to the study of diseases of the heart in early life.

LECTURE XXX.

DISEASES OF THE HEART.—Rarer in childhood than in the adult, and why—But rarity formerly exaggerated—Causes of disease of the heart in chilhood, rheumatism the most frequent—Heart sometimes affected when rheumatic symptoms are very slight—Both endocarditis and pericarditis may come on independently of rheumatism—As sequelæ of scarlatina or other fevers—As consequences of congenital defects—As complications of pleurisy—Or as purely idiopathic affections—Cases illustrative of pericarditis in different circumstances.

Endocarditis.—Symptoms not always well marked—Advance of valvular disease sometimes very gradual—Doubt as to whether valvular disease is not sometimes independent of previous inflammation.

Prognosis in valvular disease.—Less unfavorable in child than in adult—Power of growing heart to adapt itself to effects of disease and to repair its evils—Such favorable cases still exceptional—Importance of presence or absence of dilatation in determining issue of case—Illustrative cases of dilatation without valvular disease—Anæmic bruits much rarer in early life, but disordered action of heart occurs at all ages—Summary of conclusions.

AMONG the many causes of suffering and death to which persons in adult age or advancing years are exposed, *diseases of the heart* and great vessels occupy a very prominent place. The frequency of these affections is, indeed, but very imperfectly shown by our tables of mortality, which represent them as occasioning less than one and a half per cent. of the total deaths at all ages in the metropolis: but we know that in a large proportion of cases of rl bronchitis, and dropsy, the real cause of the fat the cardiac mischief with which those mal

In childhood, however, many of the most influential causes of heart disease are of comparatively rare occurrence; rheumatism is popularly regarded as an affection almost confined to youth and early manhood, as granular degeneration of the kidney is to adult and declining age; while all those forms of atheromatous deposit in the coats of arteries, or in the substance of the valves of the heart, which are a fertile source of suffering, and in their consequences a frequent cause of death, belong essentially to the processes of decay which accompany the decline of life. Hence, probably it came to pass that being rarely looked for, it was seldom found; so that, thirty years ago, the subject of heart disease was entirely unnoticed in one of the two standard works on children's diseases in our language, and was dismissed with a notice of six lines in the other. It must almost provoke a smile now for me to refer to the publication of a few cases of endocarditis in childhood by myself in 1843 (soon after the appearance of MM. Rilliet and Barthez's classical treatise, in which it had also been described, and cases of it recorded), as having made a positive addition to medical knowledge. I refer to it, however, for the illustration it affords of the slow steps by which all progress is made, as well as of the evil done by allowing inferential reasoning to interfere with actual observation. It was inferred that heart disease must be very rare in childhood; and therefore it was not looked for. Rilliet and Barthez inquired for, and found it; and in a smaller field, and less skilled to search, I too did the same.

The advance of knowledge, brings with it now every year some fresh illustration of the occurrence of heart disease in early life, in circumstances where it once would not have been expected. Rheumatism, if less frequent than in the adult, is yet associated with affection of the heart in a greater proportionate number of instances in the child.[1] The state of the circulating fluid which attends and follows scarlatina seems to predispose to inflammation of the lining or investing membrane of the heart in childhood, in the same manner, though not to the same extent, as does the state which accompanies Bright's disease in the adult. In themselves, too, and in their complications congenital malformations constitute a large class of affections of the heart peculiar to early life; while the microscope has already taught us that fatty degeneration of the heart may occur in the infant of some months old, as well as in the man of sixty years. Not many years since it would have been necessary to adduce statistical evidence in support of the assertion that disease of the heart was far from being of infrequent occurrence in early life. This, however, is no longer requisite, for the

---

[1] The carefully compiled statistics of St. Bartholomew's Hospital show for the three years 1869–71 a total of 819 cases of acute rheumatism at all ages. Of these cases 76 occurred between the ages of 5 and 15, 748 above that age. In 61.8 per cent. of the former, and in only 88 1 per cent. of the latter, it was complicated with heart affection. In the Hospital for Sick Children younger children are admitted, and probably less severe cases of rheumatism than would be received into St. Bartholomew's Hospital; and the law as to the special liability to heart disease as a complication of rheumatism in early life is found expressed there far more strongly. In 64 out of 100 cases of acute rheumatism in children between the age of 2 and 12 of which I have a record, the heart was affected, and in 62 out of the 64 this affection was permanent.

fact is universally admitted; and I may add that the 122 cases of disease of the heart, on which the following observations are founded, are but a few of the total number that, during the past thirty years, have come under my notice.

Of the above-mentioned 122 cases, 44 were instances of pericarditis, either alone or associated with inflammation of the endocardium, 71 were cases of endocarditis, and 7 of dilatation or hypertrophy of the heart, uncombined with valvular disease. I have purposely excluded from consideration cases of mere malformation of the heart, since, interesting though that subject is, it yet is one on which it would be foreign to my purpose to enter.

It would, I conceive, answer no useful end to occupy time with a minute detail of those characters, either of pericarditis or of inflammation of the endocardium, which are common to all ages, while at the same time it may be of some advantage to point out to you any special difficulties which you may encounter in detecting those affections in early life, and any special circumstances which should make you anxiously watch for their occurrence.

In 5 cases of pericarditis, in 48 of endocarditis, and in 22 in which both the pericardium and endocardium were involved,—making a total of 75 out of 122 cases, or in 60.1 per cent.,—rheumatism was either certainly known, or alleged on good grounds, to have been the starting-point of the mischief. Warned by what is known of the tendency of rheumatism to involve the heart, you are not likely to overlook the symptoms of cardiac affection, when fever, and pain, and swelling of the joints announce the child's illness to be of a rheumatic character, and you will be inexcusable if, in such circumstances, pericarditis or endocarditis should escape your observation. But if you will always avoid this error, you must bear in mind that, in the child, the heart is sometimes affected, even in cases where the extreme mildness of the general rheumatic symptoms would, if your patient were an adult, leave no room for the least apprehension on that score; and that the comparatively slight degree of fever, the small amount of pain in the limbs, and the almost complete absence of swelling of the joints, afford no guarantee that the heart may not become the seat of serious disease. It happens, too, less rarely in the case of children than of the adult, that the general indications of rheumatism follow the heart affection, instead of preceding it; so that fever, with hurried circulation and distinct friction-sound, or endocardial murmur, may exist for two or three days, or even longer, before the occurrence of pain, and the appearance of swelling of the joints, show that the disease of the heart is only a part of the great malady which has attacked the whole system.

Every threatening of rheumatism, therefore, is to be watched with the most anxious solicitude in the young subject, since so serious a complication as disease of the heart may accompany extremely slight general symptoms. Nor must auscultation be neglected in cases of what may seem to be simple fever, since rheumatic inflammation may attack the heart before any other signs of rheumatism have manifested themselves.

In 3 cases of pericarditis, in 10 of endocarditis, and in 2 where both peri- and endocarditis were associated, or in 15 out of 122 instances, the disease of the heart was traced to an attack of scarlet fever; the cardiac symptoms did not manifest themselves in the acute stage of the affection, but during the progress of desquamation. They were accompanied by fever and anasarca, which, however, did not exceed mere puffiness of the face and extremities, until, in two of the instances of pericarditis, both of which ran a chronic course, dropsy came on as the consequence of the heart disease.

Acute endocarditis supervened in one instance on the decline of the eruption of measles, and was associated with pneumonia, of which the patient died. In two other cases of chronic valvular disease, the symptoms of heart affection developed themselves gradually after convalescence from measles in one instance, after recovery from typhoid fever in the other; and these, as well as the cases in which disease of the heart supervened during the course of scarlatina, are doubtless to be referred to the category of cardiac disease dependent on an altered state of the circulating fluid, and suggest an additional ground for carefully watching your patients during their convalescence from any form of fever.

Congenital malformation of the heart seems to have an important, though not perhaps an easily explicable, influence in predisposing to inflammation of its valves, or of its investing membrane. Thus, in one case of acute pericarditis, in one of chronic pericarditis with affection of the endocardium, and in two others of old-standing valvular disease, there was some malformation of the heart which must have existed from birth, though in two instances the symptoms did not appear till long afterwards. In one of these two cases they came on gradually, rather more than two months before the death of the child at 8 years old; in the other, they were first observed at 3 years old, and death took place at the age of 15 years. It is well, then, in cases of heart disease the origin of which is obscure, to bear in mind this possible cause of the affection, and the rather since this consideration may control our treatment, and keep us back from the employment of overactive measures against an ailment which may owe its origin to some cause utterly beyond the power of medicine to remove.

Five cases of pericarditis appeared to depend on the extension to the pericardium of inflammation beginning in the pleura; an occurrence which, though not peculiar to early life, is, I believe, more frequent then than at a later period, and also oftener overlooked, from the child's restlessness and distress rendering all attempts at careful auscultation of the front of its chest impracticable. To be aware of the possibility of this occurrence will do much towards preventing you from overlooking it.

Three cases of simple pericarditis, one of pericarditis coupled with inflammation of the endocardium, and eight of endocarditis, were not clearly traceable to any exciting cause. Knowing, however, how slight an attack of rheumatism is often accompanied by heart affection, I hesitate much more than I should once have done to pronounce them idiopathic. In 3 out of the 7 cases, also, of dilated or hypertrophied heart, unconnected with valvular disease, the symptoms supervened gradually, and were not preceded by acute illness of any kind; once the symptoms of dilated heart came on during the course of very severe chorea, and continued after its cessation, and once they followed a violent blow on the chest.

I do not know of any *special symptom* of acute inflammation of the pericardium in early life, but I am sure that it is often overlooked when present; and this, partly from the child's restlessness, partly from its being masked in many instances by the signs of other disease in the chest. To this latter cause it was probably due that I did not detect pericarditis complicating pleurisy of the left side, in a boy six years old, though on his death, two years afterwards, I found a patch of old lymph on the left ventricle, near the apex of the heart, and a good deal of old white lymph coating the right auricle, and white spots at several points about the base of the heart, showing that the pericardium had been the seat of extensive inflammation. The affection of the pericardium was doubtless here, and is probably, in most of these cases, secondary to that of the pleura, since the products of a far more advanced inflammation are in general found in the latter cavity than in the former. In some instances the two serous membranes would seem to have become affected simultaneously, while in others the indications of pericarditis are perceptible before those of pleurisy appear. In one case, which terminated fatally, the patient, a little girl aged sixteen months, was almost moribund when she came under my notice: convulsions came on in two or three hours, and she died after they had continued for twelve hours. In this instance the attack had commenced eight days previously, with violent sickness followed by severe febrile disturbance and great dyspnœa, though by but little cough. In a second case, that of a little girl aged three and a half years, slight cough and febrile symptoms had existed for nearly a fortnight, when they suddenly, and without any obvious cause, became greatly aggravated; the cough grew constant, short and hacking; the respiration rose to 72, the pulse to 156 in the minute. The child became extremely restless, appeared to suffer much, made frequent efforts to vomit, and often crammed her hand down her throat, as though to pull something away which obstructed her breathing. In neither of these cases was the existence of pericarditis suspected. In the last-mentioned case the restlessness of the child precluded careful auscultation; but dulness on percussion, and bronchial breathing, were perceived through the whole of the posterior part of the left side of the chest, and small crepitation was heard on the right side. In a third case, a little boy, seven months old, died in extreme distress at the end of four days, during which his restlessness was extreme, and his cries were constant. Auscultation was almost impossible, owing to his extreme disquiet, but after death the lungs were found free from disease; but recent lymph was deposited on both layers of the pericardium, and its sac contained sero-purulent fluid. It was interesting also to observe, on removing the recent lymph from the heart's surface, that the visceral layer of the pericardium was opaque and thickened, and of a dead white color, the evidence of a former attack, which probably took place wl was three months old, at which time he was alleged to have had pneumonia.

There is little danger, in cases which set in with symptoms so severe as those just described, of our falling into serious error, either of diagnosis or of treatment. Everything will point to most serious mischief in the chest; and even should the tender age of the child and its extreme restlessness prevent careful auscultation, or should the signs of heart disease be masked by those of mischief in the lung or pleura, enough will yet be discovered to show the necessity for immediate and active interference; while, if we bear in mind the possibility of such a complication, that will go far towards preventing us from overlooking its occurrence.

I have seen other instances in which pericarditis secondary to pleurisy supervened in the course of scarlatinal dropsy; and if from these I could deduce any additional sign to guard you against overlooking the pericarditis it would be that furnished by very marked orthopnœa. In one case—that of a little boy aged one year and eleven months—this was especially remarkable; for while in other respects his condition varied much and frequently, and the signs of thoracic mischief differed greatly in their urgency, he constantly maintained the sitting posture, and always most strenuously resisted any attempt to lay him down. This peculiarity continued during an illness of many weeks, and did not cease till his powers completely failed with the approach of death.

Concerning rheumatic pericarditis I have no additional remark to make; but on account of its rarity it may be worth while to relate to you a case in which acute inflammation of the pericardium occurred in a little boy who was four months old at his death, and in whom free communication existed between the two sides of the heart. He did not come under my observation until the day on which he died; but the history which I heard of him was, that he was very livid at birth, that respiration was established with difficulty, and that the dark hue of his surface never went off completely. At times he seemed cheerful, and used to breathe pretty well, but at other times he was attacked, without apparent cause, by difficult respiration, during which he became very cold and quite purple, made a grunting noise, and frothed at the mouth. These attacks never came on while he was sucking; they were preceded by crying, though usually he was very quiet.

On October 19, 1848, an attack came on similar to the previous seizures, though more severe, lasting between one and two hours, and not being preceded by crying. On the 20th a similar attack came on, and lasted from four to half-past seven P.M., and another returned on the morning of the 24th, at noon of which day he was brought to me. His surface was then generally very pale, but with a marked livid hue of the lips and fingers, and around the mouth. His skin was cool; almost cold, his respiration irregular and very frequent, and his pulse extremely feeble. Auscultation detected no unnatural sound with the heart's action.

As he was being carried home a fresh seizure came on, and proved fatal in half an hour.

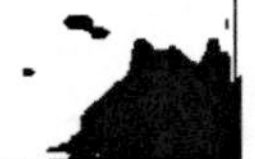

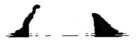

The lungs and pleuræ generally were healthy.

The pleura where it is in contact with the pericardium, and that membrane itself, were of a bright red color, with the vessels minutely injected. The sac of the pericardium contained ℥j of a dirty yellowish, sero-purulent fluid, in which little granules of lymph, like minute grains of rice, were floating. It did not anywhere adhere to the heart, but its parietal layer, which was intensely red, and beset with numerous little ecchymoses, was lined through a great extent by a thin layer of lymph. This layer was thicker on the right than on the left half of the pericardium, and especially so about the right auricle. Lymph was also deposited between the left auricle and the root of the pulmonary artery.

The pericardium investing the heart was intensely red, and numerous small flocculi of lymph covered its surface. Besides this there was an old white spot, half an inch long by a quarter of an inch broad, at the apex of the left ventricle, having just the character of the white spots of old pericarditis; and there was another small spot on the posterior surface of the right auricle.

The foramen ovale was wide open, so as to admit the finger with ease; the pulmonary artery was very small; the ductus arteriosus wide open, and the septum of the ventricle very imperfect; the ductus venosus was closed.

Reference has already been made to the occasional occurrence of inflammation of the investing or of the lining membrane of the heart independent of any other disease, and unassociated with inflammation of the lungs or pleura. In such cases the indications of disturbance of the respiration are either altogether absent, or comparatively slight, and if auscultation is neglected, or but carelessly performed, disease may, in such circumstances, go on unchecked till it has disorganized the heart, and doomed the patient to a life of remediless suffering.

A striking instance of this *idiopathic inflammation of the pericardium* and lining membrane of the heart came under my notice many years since, in the person of a healthy boy, eleven years old, who, on May 8, 1843, complained of feeling cold, and began to cough. The chilliness was succeeded by fever, and he continued gradually getting worse till the 13th, when I visited him for the first time. He had had no other medicine than a purgative powder. On May 13, I found him lying in bed; his face dusky and rather anxious, his eyes heavy, and his respiration slightly accelerated; coughing frequently, but without expectoration; skin burning hot; pulse frequent and hard. He made no complaint, except of slight uneasiness about the left breast. On examining the chest there was found to be very extended dulness over the heart, with slight tenderness on pressure. A very loud and prolonged rasping sound was heard in the place of the first sound, loudest a little below the nipple, though very audible over the whole left side of the chest, and also distinguishable, though less clearly, for a considerable distance to the right of the sternum. The second sound was heard clearly just over the aortic valves, but was not distinct elsewhere, being obscured by the loudness of the bruit. Respiration was good in both lungs.

The child was cupped to six ounces between the left scapula and the spine; and a grain of calomel, with the same quantity of Dover's powder, was given every four hours.

On the following day it was found that the sense of discomfort in the chest had been relieved by the cupping, and that the child had slept well in the night. He looked less anxious, though his eyes were still heavy and suffused, and his skin was less hot and less dusky. The pulse was 114, thrilling, but not full. There was now slight prominence of the cardiac region, and the heart's sounds were obscurer and more distant than on the previous day. The bruit was now manifestly a friction-sound louder at the base than at the apex of the heart, and altogether obscuring the first sound; while the second sound could be heard over the aortic valves. Six more leeches were applied over the heart, and the hemorrhage from their bites was so profuse as to occasion some faintness. Mercurial inunction was now superadded to the treatment previously employed, and the child's condition continued through the 15th to be much the same as it had been on the previous day. On May 16th, there was some improvement in the general symptoms, and the pulse was softer. The friction-sound was now no longer audible, but a loud rasping sound was heard in the place of the first sound. The second sound was now distinguishable at the apex of the heart, as well as over the aortic valves, and its characters were quite natural. On the 19th the child's mouth was slightly sore, and the dose of the remedies was diminished. On the 22d the soreness of the mouth was considerable, and all active treatment was discontinued on that day. The child gradually regained his strength, but the bruit accompanying the first sound continued, and was heard a month afterwards, with no other change than being rather softer and more prolonged. Four years afterwards I saw him again. He had continued well in the interval, and had never suffered from palpitation of the heart, nor from any other ailment referable to the chest; but his pulse was small, jerking, and not always equal in force; and the natural character of the first sound was altogether lost in a loud prolonged bruit.

In such cases as this the occurrence of the heart disease is not easy of explanation. No sign of rheumatism appeared during the whole course of the affection, nor was it associated with any other disorder, such as scarlatina, which by the alterations that it induces in the composition of the circulating fluid, could be supposed to favor the supervention of inflammation of the heart or other viscera.[1] The organs of respiration were unaffected throughout, so that the case could not for a moment be conceived to be one in which the heart disease was secondary, and produced by the extension of the inflammation beyond the limits by which it was originally circumscribed. But though the cardiac affection came on independently of those conditions, which we regard, and with justice, as usually essential to its production, it ran as acute a-

[1] As Bright's disease, for instance, in the adult favors the occurrence of pericarditis, according to the elaborate researches of Dr. Taylor, in vol. xxviii of the Medico-Chirurgical Transactions.

course and produced injury as extensive, as if it had been excited by any of its ordinary causes.

Idiopathic pericarditis, uncomplicated with pleurisy, and sufficiently severe to give rise to symptoms appreciable during the lifetime of the patient, is certainly a very rare occurrence. I cannot speak with accuracy as to the frequency in early life of those white spots on the surface of the pericardium, which were pointed out by M. Bizot and Sir J. Paget[1] as being of such common occurrence in the adult, and which were rightly regarded as of much moment so long as they were supposed to be the invariable indications of a bygone inflammation. In some instances they are no doubt due to that cause, and probably whenever met with towards the base of the heart we shall not be wrong in regarding them as the results of inflammation. When found in their more common seat in childhood, near the apex of the left ventricle, the true explanation of their presence is furnished by the so-called attrition theory, which refers them to the friction of the heart against the resisting chest-wall.[2] This theory, while it explains the presence of these patches, deprives them at the same time of most of their pathological importance.

The total number of cases in which *endocarditis*, either acute or chronic, was present, was 105. In 30 of these its symptoms were masked more or less completely, by complication with pericarditis; while in the remaining 75 instances the affection of the endocardium existed alone. Of the 75 cases of uncomplicated endocarditis, 30 were attended with acute symptoms, while in the others the affection presented itself in a chronic form. In some of these cases the signs of heart affection manifested themselves with considerable severity, and consisted in uneasiness about the heart, palpitation, increase of its impulse, with inequality of its pulsations on one occasion, irregularity of its action on another; dyspnœa and occasional orthopnœa. Symptoms so marked as these compelled attention to the condition of the chest, and auscultation at once detected the loud bruit of endocardial inflammation. In others, however, just as in the adult, the stethoscope alone gave information of the commencement of mischief, which otherwise would have been unsuspected.

In the case in which endocarditis accompanied measles its symptoms were masked by those of the pneumonia with which it was associated, and in the instance where it succeeded to convalescence from that disease, no urgent symptoms appeared. In some of the cases of endocarditis which came on without obvious exciting cause, though there was much heat of skin, some acceleration of breathing, and some increase of the heart's action, yet neither the general nor the local symptoms

---

[1] Mémoires de la Société Méd. d'Observation, tome i, p. 350; and Medico-Chirurgical Transactions, vol. xxiii.

[2] Sir W. Jenner, in his Lectures on Rickets, already referred to, Med. Gazette, April 7, 1860, p. 334, points out how it is that, owing to the deformity of the chest-walls in rickets, the apex of the heart comes into close contact with the left rib just where it projects or knuckles inwards, and thus occasions the white patches to be seated near the left apex instead of about the centre of the anterior part of the right ventricle, which is their common situation in the adult.

were at all more urgent than are constantly observed in attacks of simple fever, or of influenza in childhood. In other instances, where the patient did not come under my notice till after the evil had reached a chronic stage, there was so little history of any acute attack of illness preceding it, as to render it impossible to fix the exact date at which it began. It seems, then, that just as in rheumatic endocarditis, the symptoms may vary in degree, and be in one case so severe as to force themselves upon our notice, and in another so slight as almost to elude our observation, so it is in cases where the endocarditis is or appears to be idiopathic. In cases of acute rheumatism you are aware of this danger; you do not wait till the patient's sufferings inform you that the mischief has been done, but you are on the watch against the first threatenings of its approach, and your sense of hearing gives you earlier information, and surer information, concerning this, than all the other signs together. But if the same evil, against which you guard thus studiously in cases of rheumatism, may occur independently of it, and may scarcely give warning of its approach, until it is almost or altogether too late to cure, a measure at least of the same precaution should be observed at all times; and in no instance of febrile disturbance in early life, how simple soever the case may seem, should you consider the examination of the patient complete, until after auscultation. With all your care, there will probably still be cases in which the commencement of the heart affection will escape your notice; in which you will accidentally make the discovery of its existence when auscultating the chest for some other purpose, or in which the gradual supervention of the signs of valvular disease will call your attention to it long after the ailment has become chronic.

The early detection of the disease is of the more importance, since its gradual approach affords no assurance that it may not go on to ruin the health, and at length to destroy the life of the sufferer. Nothing could be more gradual than the advance of the early stages of the disease of the heart, in the case of a little girl ten years old, who came under my notice in the month of March, some years ago. Her mother stated, that, though not robust, she had never had any definite illness, but that for the previous year she had been growing thinner, and had suffered from palpitation of the heart, which had by degrees become more and more distressing, and that for the past three months she had likewise been troubled with cough. The child when brought to me was greatly emaciated; her face was anxious and distressed; her breath short, so that it was with difficulty that she walked even a short distance; she had frequent short cough, without expectoration, and she suffered much from palpitation of the heart, and a sense of discomfort at the chest. The heart's action was violent; dulness in the præcordial region was extended; a very loud, harsh, rasping sound accompanied the first sound of the heart, loudest towards and to the left of the nipple, but heard over the whole of the chest, both before and behind. Varying remedies brought slight temporary relief to her sufferings, but nevertheless she grew worse every month. She became more and more emaciated; the distress at the chest and the palpitation of the heart increased, her cough became more violent, and once she had an attack of hæmoptysis;

For about a month before her death the cough altogether ceased, but she was now unable to leave her bed, from increasing weakness; the palpitation continued unmitigated, and her extremities became slightly anasarcous. During the last week of her life her respiration was extremely difficult, and became increasingly slow, till she died on October 10. The lungs were very emphysematous, and much congested, but not otherwise diseased. The heart was extremely large, but its right cavities did not exceed the natural size; the pulmonary valves were healthy; the edges of the tricuspid valve were slightly thickened; the left auricle was enormously dilated, but its walls were not at all attenuated; the pulmonary veins were much dilated; the left ventricle was dilated, its walls were thickened; the chordæ tendineæ of the mitral valve were greatly shortened, so that the valve could not close; the valve itself was shrunken, thickened, and cartilaginous; and there existed likewise slight thickening of the edges of the semilunar valves of the aorta.

The symptoms in this case, from the earliest period to which the patient's history goes back, were those of chronic valvular disease, with hypertrophy and dilatation of the heart; but no clue is afforded us by which we can guess when the inflammation of the endocardium, probably the first in this train of evils, attacked the heart. The constitutional disturbance which attended it was so slight as to escape the mother's notice, and to call for no special complaint from the child; but it is likely that more watchful care would have taken the alarm at some comparatively slight feverish seizure; that auscultation would have discovered the disease at its commencement; and that treatment would have diminished, though it might not have altogether prevented, the subsequent disorganization of the heart.

I have referred to endocarditis as having been, though undiscovered, still the probable cause of the disease of the heart in this instance. But yet there is another explanation of the mischief, and one which some other cases of chronic valvular disease that I have either watched during life or examined after death would admit of, namely, that the mischief has been produced by some other than an inflammatory process. We know that this may be the case in the adult; and equally so, I apprehend, in the child; nor is the fact of less practical moment in the one case than in the other. In each instance it influences our treatment, and warns us not to be too active in the use of antiphlogistic measures, nor too pertinacious in their continuance, and suggests the probability that what we discover is only the sign of some long-past mischief.[1]

It is true, indeed, that in very many instances the disease of the valves goes on, as in the poor child whose case I have just related, from bad to worse; inflammation in some instances recurring at intervals, and adding something each time to the previous mischief; or the disorganization of the heart advancing slowly but with uninterrupted course.

[1] This supposition, which clears up what otherwise would be very obscure with reference to the cause of some cases of chronic valvular disease, is, as probably scarcely need be stated, propounded by Sir W. Stokes in his work on Diseases of the Heart, 8vo., Dublin, 1854. See page 146 and following pages.

But, nevertheless, one meets sometimes with exceptions to this rule, and observes instances in which the signs of cardiac mischief remain stationary, and the sufferings of the child grow less with its increasing years. Nor is it, probably, that in these cases the disease simply does not advance, but many things seem to show that there is, as Dr. Latham suggests, "a certain *protective* power possibly inherent in the growing heart, whereby it can accommodate its form and manner of increase to material accidents, and so repress or counteract their evil tendencies."

Dr. Latham,[1]—whose name I cannot mention without the expression of respect and gratitude due to one to whose instructions I owe so much,—relates, in illustration of this fact, the history of two young ladies in whom the auscultatory signs of valvular imperfection existed from early childhood, but who never suffered any important disturbance of the general health that could be attributed to it. Instances still more striking have come under my own observation, in which, not only were the signs of heart disease present, without the evil results that might be apprehended from it, but in which the suffering lessened with advancing years; though auscultation still gave assurance that its cause persisted. A little girl, six years old, whose health had never been robust, and who had suffered much from measles and scarlatina, the latter of which left her liable to attacks of what was said to be inflammation of the chest, came under my notice at the end of April, 1846. She was then laboring under urgent dyspnœa, with symptoms of acute bronchitis, and, in the course of auscultation, a systolic murmur was heard at the apex of the heart. The bronchitic symptoms by degrees subsided, but dyspnœa continued; the child was wholly unable to rest, except when propped nearly upright; she was distressed by palpitation; her cough was frequent, and, when worse than usual, she expectorated with it small quantities of florid blood. Her face was pale, but with a livid flush on either cheek; the carotids pulsated visibly, and the jugular veins were distended, while her heart beat at the rate of 150 in the minute. The heart's impulse was increased, and dulness in the præcordial region extended far beyond its proper limits. It was next noted that the smallness of the pulse corresponded ill with the laboring of the heart; and a distinct sense of *frémissement*, when the hand was laid upon the præcordial region, completed the signs of great contraction of the mitral orifice, with hypertrophy and dilatation of the heart. From time to time the child suffered much since then with a return of her old symptoms; and, after the lapse of twenty months, the bruit still continued: the hand placed upon the cardiac region was still sensible of a distinct purring tremor, and the pulse was exceedingly small and feeble. But the heart no longer labored as it used to do; its pulsations did not exceed 110 in the minute; and though the child was still unable to lie flat in bed, the distressing orthopnœa had ceased for many months. Her eyelids were no longer puffy, nor her limbs anasarcous, as they were before; her cough troubled her but little, and hæmoptysis was very rare. She had gained flesh, was cheerful, and played, though not so boisterously as other children might do,

[1] On Diseases of the Heart, vol. i, pp. 241–8.

yet with such heartiness that I could scarcely believe her to be the little suffering thing for whom, a year before, one would have chosen speedy death as the happiest lot that could befall her.

Nor was this gradual recovery of the heart from serious injury less striking in the case of the boy whose history I related to you as an instance of idiopathic pericarditis and endocarditis. Not only did he continue well four years after his recovery, but I saw him again ten years after it, he being then twenty-one years old. The heart's impulse was still considerable; the sound continued long and loud and rough, but the young man had no other ailment than occasional palpitation, and sometimes slight sense of discomfort at the chest: and this, although he was leading a loose kind of life—strolling over the country as a ballad-singer, often getting wet, and walking long distances of twenty miles and upwards in a day, and this, as he said, without fatigue.

Other cases of a similar kind, though less remarkable than these two, have come under my notice—cases which would warrant, I think, a more hopeful prognosis in cases of valvular disease of the heart in childhood than we should be justified in entertaining if our patient were an adult. But consolatory as it is to know that time helps in some instances to repair the damage done to the heart in childhood, yet these fortunate cases are after all but exceptional ones. These exceptions, too, are not by any means proportionate to the number of instances in which the original inflammatory attack has been slight, or in which it has not recurred; but of two cases whose early history has been identical, the progress of the one will be by slow degrees of improvement towards comparative health, of the other by slow deterioration to a painful death. In the latter case, too, a post-mortem examination may often fail to discover any such large extent of valvular disease as might be expected from the nature of the symptoms during life.

On what, then, it may be asked, does the difference between the two sets of cases depend? I believe that the presence or absence of dilatation of the heart, or the degree in which that condition exists, governs the severity of the symptoms, and determines the issue of the case in a very large number of instances.

In enumerating the cases on which the remarks in these lectures are based, I referred to seven instances in which dilatation of the heart existed unaccompanied by disease of the valves. In these cases the absence of valvular disease was the more unexpected since a systolic murmur was audible in all of them during life.

The first of these cases, and one of the most remarkable, came under my notice in 1849. The patient was a little girl 7¾ years old, who had been liable to palpitation of the heart since an attack of scarlatina two years before. For some months previous to her coming under my notice, her health had been indifferent; but an attack of catarrh from which she had suffered about a month, appeared to have called all her symptoms into activity. I found her at the end of this time laboring under generally diffused bronchitis, her face flushed, her respiration hurried and irregular, varying from 60 to 80 in the minute; her heart beating at the rate of 130; and its pulsations attended with a loud systolic bruit at the apex. Her condition deteriorated, the cough grew harder and more distressing, and the respiration rose habitually to between 80 and 90; while the child took a posture on her face, in which she remained almost habitually, and never obtained any sleep except in that attitude. I saw her for the first time on April 1. She died on the morning of the 5th, quite quietly, having had an anodyne of four minims of laudanum the previous night, which procured her some rest, but no profound sleep.

There were three patches of pulmonary apoplexy, each of about the size of a walnut, in the right lung; and one in the left, somewhat smaller; the languette of the left upper lobe was in a state of collapse, the air-tubes much congested, and containing a good deal of tenacious mucus. The pericardium contained an ounce of transparent serum. The heart was almost as large as two fists, and of a rounded form; its increase of size being due apparently rather to enlargement of the right than of the left half of the organ; though the left cavities of the heart also were unusually large. Both the left auricle and ventricle contained a good deal of black coagulum. The enormously dilated right auricle was filled with firm parti-colored coagulum; and there was a good deal of black coagulum in the right ventricle. The whole of the right ventricle was enormously dilated; but the dilatation was most remarkable at that part from which the pulmonary artery springs, and which formed behind the pillars of the tricuspid valve almost a second ventricle, so large was it. All the valves were carefully examined, and presented no trace of disease, and the foramen ovale was closed.

A boy, 10 years old, came into the Children's Hospital to die. No history of his previous illness was obtained; but he was very anasarcous, and had a large quantity of fluid in his abdomen, though his urine was free from albumen. The pericardium was found universally adherent, and the endocardium throughout presented a remarkable degree of opacity, though there was no thickening of any of the valves. The heart was very much enlarged owing to dilatation of both its sides; though the left was the more affected. The left ventricle alone was as large as the whole heart of a child 9½ years old, whose body was in the dead-house at the same time, though its walls were scarcely thicker, nor was the aortic orifice larger.

A little girl, when six years old, had an attack of rheumatism, not very severe, since she was scarcely confined to bed at all by it. A month afterwards she first complained of pain in her heart, which for some weeks beat very much. Six months afterwards she began to swell about her face; the limbs afterwards became anasarcous, but the degree of the anasarca had varied much. Nine months after the rheumatic attack she was admitted into the hospital, being then 7½ years old. There was some œdema of the legs and of the lower part of the back, as well as of the abdominal integuments; no ascites, but considerable enlargement of the liver. There was obvious bulging of the left side of the chest. The heart's impulse was visible in the 4th, 5th, and 6th interspaces. Apex beat in sixth interspace, 1¼ inch outside nipple line, and 1¾ inch in oblique line below nipple. Impulse somewhat heaving; thrill and impulse in left costal angle.

Upper dulness limit	3d rib.
Right " "	a finger's breadth to right of sternum.
Oblique diameter of heart	5¾ inches.
Transverse " "	5 "
Longitudinal " "	3¾ "

At apex a prolonged systolic murmur was heard, which diminished rapidly in loudness as one passed upwards, though still audible over whole heart's region. No second sound heard.

Rest and treatment relieved the child, who, having been admitted on February 26, was able to return home on April 16. Her health, however, soon failed again, when she lost the care and comforts of the hospital. She was readmitted on May 6, complaining of constant præcordial pain, probably connected with the supervention of pericarditis, for a friction-sound was now for a time audible. Once more she improved, and left the hospital on August 13. Dr. Gee, at that time the able and unwearied registrar of the hospital, now my much-valued colleague, whose notes I have already quoted, found that the

Upper dulness limit had now extended to the second rib.	
Right " " " " "	two inches to right of sternum, and half an inch to left of right nipple.

It had, however, already reached this limit on May 22. The heart's impulse was less extensive than in February; the friction-sound had completely disappeared, but a systolic murmur was audible over the whole præcordial region; and scarcely any second sound was to be heard.

Since she left the hospital I have not seen this little one; but there can be no doubt but that if she has not already found a resting-place and a grave within the walls of some other institution, she will come again to seek such small mitigation of her sufferings as is all that medicine has to offer her. I have related her case not because I assume that it is an instance of dilatation of the heart, independent of valvular disease, but because it is the dilatation which is the cause of her suffering and the source of her danger; and because I have now seen many instances which seem to show that in early life the occurrence of this condition is the one great danger to guard against, since, when it has occurred to any considerable extent, nature seems unable to exert that power of repair and readjustment which, in other cases, she sometimes puts forth so beneficially.[1]

But how to guard against the danger? By rest—rest as complete as can be given to an organ which is in perpetual activity, whose repose

[1] I have not entered on the question of the mode of production of dilatation of the heart in the young subject. I have no doubt but that muscular weakness has a large share in its production, as the observance of extreme quiet after any attack of endocardial inflammation or of exhausting disease has in its prevention. Dr. Bristowe, in his able paper on Mitral Regurgitation, independently of Organic Disease of the Heart, published in British and Foreign Medico-Chirurgical Review for July, 1861, discusses the subject most fully, and with thorough mastery of all the questions involved in its elucidation.

is but momentary and partial; one half quiescent for a fraction of a minute, while its other half is powerfully contracting—an alternating ebb and flow which ceases only with life itself. Such rest as we can give then is rather diminution of labor; calling on the heart for as few pulsations to the minute, and those as little vigorous as possible. I suppose that in early life changes in the muscular substance of the heart, whether for better or for worse, take place more readily than in the grown person; that therefore the heart's cavities after inflammation dilate more readily, and mischief is thus done, which subsequent hypertrophy atones for as best it can—how ill, and with how much suffering, a few visits to the Children's Hospital will tell far better than many words of mine. To avoid all this, our only means, and those by no means ineffectual, consist in long-continued absolute rest in the recumbent posture for many weeks; and then for many months more none but the gentlest movements; for a year or more the being carried up and down stairs; and for several years more no violent exertion, no running, no dancing. I have known the strict observance of these precautions followed by disappearance of the signs of valvular insufficiency, by the lessening of the area of dulness, and by the complete cessation of the morbid sound which had accompanied the heart's action. The difficulty in carrying out these precautions rests not with the children, but with their parents, who will seldom take the trouble to understand the grounds for restrictions, or to listen to our unwelcome tale of the agonies which their neglect will entail upon the little ones in after years. Unfortunately, the doctor, who professes to be no more than Nature's minister, holds but too often in the public esteem a far inferior position to that of the bold empiric who pretends to be her master.

One more caution may not be out of place with reference to cardiac disease in early life, namely, that the presence of a bruit with the heart's sounds in the child depends more invariably on organic disease than in the adult; inasmuch as those endocardial, arterial, or venous murmurs which are produced by an impoverished state of the blood are very rarely indeed heard in children under seven years old, and are by no means common until that age is attained at which the changes that take place as puberty approaches have commenced, or are on the eve of beginning. I think that I can speak with confidence as to the rarity of such murmurs in childhood, though I cannot venture to assign a reason for it; since the very slight difference between the composition of the blood in early life and in after years can scarcely be alleged as affording an adequate explanation of the fact.

At the same time, however, that we should be most keenly alive to the importance of every sign of heart disease in early life, we should bear in mind that the friends of our patients not infrequently take causeless alarm at the occurrence of occasional palpitation and dyspnœa on exertion, especially if accompanied with irregularity of the pulse. Mere deranged action of the heart is by no means uncommon in children of all ages, though rarer before seven years old than subsequently. It is most frequently observed in fragile, excitable children, and is not readily amenable to direct treatment, though it subsides in the course of time under a system of general management calculated to improve the health, and of exercise judiciously regulated, and always kept within such limits as not to occasion fatigue.

In conclusion, let me sum up in a few sentences the most important facts concerning disease of the heart in childhood, which I have endeavored to bring before your notice:

1st. While disease of the heart is less common in childhood than in the adult, there is no absolute immunity in early life from any of those affections to which the organ in after years is liable.

2d. Of all the causes of heart affection, inflammation is the most frequent; and while all blood diseases predispose to its occurrence, none exert so powerful an influence in exciting it as rheumatism.

3d. While inflammation is by far the most frequent cause of valvular disease, there is, nevertheless, reason to believe that it is not the sole cause, but that the valves may become disorganized quite independently of previous endocarditis; and a knowledge of this fact ought to govern our treatment in all cases where the history of the commencement of the affection is at all obscure.

4th. The disposition of valvular disease to increase is not only liable to more frequent exceptions in the child than in the adult, but there is also in early life a special power of repair and of self-adjustment in the heart which warrants our expressing a more cheerful prognosis than would be justifiable in cases of cardiac disease occurring in the grown person.

5th. At the same time, however, the feebleness of the heart in early life, the liability of the child to cachectic conditions and exhausting diseases, the rapidity of the circulation, and the facility with which it may be excited by very slight causes, all tend to favor the occurrence of dilatation of the heart whenever a slight amount of valvular obstruction exists, or even altogether independent of it. Hence it becomes of even more importance in the child than in the adult to insist on long-continued rest, and on the avoidance of all causes which could tend to excite the circulation, not only after attacks of rheumatism, but also after typhoid or scarlet fever, or of any of those more chronic diseases,—such, for instance, as chorea,—which are not only associated with disturbance of the circulation, but also with disorder of the circulating fluid itself.

LECTURE XXXI.

DISEASES OF THE ORGANS OF DIGESTION AND ASSIMILATION.—Peculiarities of the digestive organs—They require a peculiar kind of food, the milk—Composition of that fluid, its adaptation for the nutriment of the infant—Changes in the digestive organs as the child grows older—These changes take place more slowly in the human subject than in animals.

Evils of giving other food than the mother's milk until the infant is old enough to bear it.—Shown by the increased mortality it produces—Different modes in which such food acts injuriously—Appearances found in bodies of children who have died from imperfect nutrition.

Great importance of infants being suckled, even for a short time.—Difficulty of analysis of the milk—Suggestions for determining fitness of a person for duties of a wet-nurse—Rules for management of children who are brought up without the breast—Substitute for mother's milk—Caution with reference to occasional unhealthy condition of cow's milk.

WE prefaced our investigation of the diseases of the nervous and respiratory systems with an inquiry into the peculiarities of structure and of function which characterize those organs in early life. A similar inquiry will not be out of place now, as preliminary to the study of the *diseases of the organs of digestion and assimilation, and their dependencies.*

Man, when he has attained to maturity, is able to support his life, and to preserve his health, upon food of various kinds; and the structure of his organs is such as to enable him to live upon an exclusively animal diet, or upon food furnished entirely by the vegetable kingdom. We know that in either case the ultimate elements from which the body is nourished are the same; but that while in the former instance they are furnished as it were ready to hand, they have in the latter to be eliminated by nature's chemistry, through a process which occupies much time, and which requires considerable complexity in the apparatus that effects it.

Those powers, however, of which the adult is possessed, belong in but comparatively small measure to the infant. The growing animal, indeed, needs proportionally more food than the adult; for not merely is the daily waste to be repaired, and that constant reproduction of the tissues to be provided for which is essential to the maintenance of vitality, in all parts of the body, but each day is to bring with it an increase in size and stature. But though in early life an ample supply of food is so necessary, yet the organs by which it is to be assimilated, like those which have other offices to perform, are at that time frail and delicate, and must not be overworked. Their development is incomplete; and even those animals whose digestive apparatus becomes eventually most complex, are fitted at first for subsisting only on the simplest food. Thus, for instance, the peculiarities which characterize the digestive process in ruminants do not begin till some time after birth: the fourth stomach is the only one called into use; the others are little more than indicated in the new-born animal. Preparations, however, for their future mode of subsistence are early discernible in the herbivora, whose dentition has already commenced at birth, and advances with rapidity to attain its completeness. In the infant, on the other hand, the jaws which long remain edentulous, the non-developed cæcum, and the salivary glands, whose functions seem scarcely to commence for the first few months of life,[1] sufficiently indicate that it is intended to subsist longer than the young of most animals on food which shall require few changes to be wrought in it. The food, soon converted in the stomach passes rapidly out of it, and the infant speedily seeks for more, requiring, as every one knows, to be fed far more frequently than the adult; while digestion being perfected at once, and no necessity existing for those supplementary processes which the cæcum in after life effects, the peristaltic action of the bowels is more rapid, excrementitious matters are quickly expelled, and the healthy infant passes two or three evacuations in the twenty-four hours.[2]

But while the digestive organs are thus adapted to insure the rapid performance of their functions, and to provide for the quick as well as for the complete nutrition of the body, the question naturally suggests itself, where shall that food be found which, while it yields the necessary sustenance, is yet so easily assimilated as not to require powers of which the delicate organs of the young are destitute? We should search in vain through the animal and vegetable kingdom for any substance completely fulfilling these conditions; but nature has supplied the want, and given to almost every mother the means of herself nourishing her young.

Milk, the proper aliment of the young, expressly prepared for it within its mother's organism, contains, ready combined, all those elements which are necessary, whether for its growth or for the maintenance of its proper temperature, by serving as materials for respiration. The mean of 89 analyses of human milk, by MM. Vernois and Becquerel[3]

---

[1] See the observations of Bidder and Schmidt, on the absence of secretion from the salivary glands of young animals, at p. 22 of their work, Die Verdauungs-Säfte und der Stoffwechsel, 8vo. Mitau und Leipzig, 1852.

[2] I am indebted to my friend, Professor Rolleston, of Oxford, for demonstrating to me the incorrectness of some of the statements adopted in the first three editions of this work from Schultz's Essay, Ueber den Akt des Erbrechens, &c., in the Analekten über Kinderkrankheiten, vol. ii, Heft vi, p. 62, with reference to the peculiarities in the form and position of the stomach during fœtal and early infantile life. Dr. Brinton, in a note at p. 818 of the Article "Stomach," in the Cyclopædia of Anatomy and Physiology, also notices some exaggeration in Schultz's statements. I cannot, however, mention in seeming disparagement the name of one whose scientific career has long since been run, without adding, that in spite of failing health which conducted him to an early grave, Schultz was a most laborious pioneer in those investigations into the process of digestion which have yielded to others who have followed him such an abundant harvest.

[3] The statements with reference to the chemistry of the milk are taken from Scherer's article "Milch," in Wagner's Handwörterbuch der Physiologie, vol. ii, p. 448; and from the elaborate work of MM. Vernois and A. Becquerel, Du Lait chez la Femme, &c., 8vo., Paris, 1858. See their analy[illegible]alyses of former observers, in the table at p. 15 of their work.

yields the following result. It has a specific gravity of 103[illegible] is composed of

Water,	889.08
Solid matters,	110.92

These solid constituents are made up of

Sugar,	43.64
Casein and extractive matter,	39.24
Butter,	26.66
Incombustible salts,	1.38
	110.92

How small must be the effort needed to effect the assimilation of this fluid! The chief of its solid constituents, the casein, differs little, if at all, from the albumen of the blood, while in combination with it is a considerable quantity of the phosphate of lime—a salt that enters largely into the composition of the bones. Among its other components we find butter and sugar, the former of which probably in part contributes to the formation of the fat that is so abundantly deposited in the healthy infant, while the remainder of it supplies materials for the generation of heat, by being resolved, together with the saccharine matter, into its ultimate elements of carbonic acid and water. This food, too, is not merely suitable for the infant soon after birth, but it continues to be the aliment most proper for it for many months; the casein increasing in quantity as the infant grows older, and the demand for materials to maintain its growth increases.

By degrees the stomach alters in form; its muscularity increases; the powers of the digestive organs become greater, and the child grows able to derive support from food in which the nutritive principles are not presented in so simple a form as in the milk. At the ninth month teeth begin to appear—the first clear evidence of those changes which nature is working in the organism, and the indication that before very long the child will be able entirely to dispense with that elaborately prepared nourishment which it has hitherto derived from its mother. In the human subject the process of dentition not only begins late, but it goes on slowly; the first molar tooth is seldom cut before the commencement of the second year: dentition is not concluded till its end. Nature's object in the laws by which she governs the brute creation, appears to be, to fit the young animals as soon as possible to provide for themselves, and to shorten the period during which they must depend for sustenance on their mother; and, therefore, they begin to cut their teeth much sooner, and the process is completed within a much shorter time, than in the infant. Young rabbits are always provided with ten teeth when born, and the others make their appearance within ten days. In the different ruminants, the teeth have either begun to appear before birth, or they show themselves a few days afterwards; and in either case dentition is completed within the first month, and in dogs and cats during the first ten weeks of existence.

For the difference in this respect between the lower animals and man, it seems to me that a moral reason, not altogether visionary, may be assigned. The young animal has to learn nothing more than how to apply those instincts with which Almighty power has endowed it for its own support and the perpetuation of its species. But the infant is to be trained to become a man: its moral as well as its physical nature is to be cultivated: parental influence is to be the means of doing this; and Providence may have wisely determined that the infant shall for months be dependent on its mother for support, in order that her instinctive feelings may lay the firm foundation of the love that causes her to cling to her little one with a fondness that surpasses all other affection, and which gives her the patience, the gentleness, the untiring energy, that make her the child's best guardian, friend, and teacher, during its early years.

But whether it is right or wrong to seek in something higher than the material, for the reasons of this physical law, it yet is a law, and one which cannot be violated with impunity. The infant whose mother refuses to perform towards it a mother't part, or who, by accident, disease, or death, is deprived of the food that nature destined for it, too often languishes and dies. Such children you may often see, with no fat to give plumpness to their limbs,—no red particles in their blood to impart a healthy hue to their skin,—their face wearing in infancy the lineaments of age,—their voice a constant wail,—their whole aspect an embodiment of woe. But give to such children the food that nature destined for them, and if the remedy do not come all too late to save them, the mournful cry will cease, the face will assume a look of content, by degrees the features of infancy will disclose themselves, the limbs will grow round, the skin pure red and white; and when, at length, we hear the merry laugh of babyhood, it seems almost as if the little sufferer of some weeks before must have been a changeling, and this the real child brought back from fairy-land.

Much care, much patience, judicious management in all respects, may, indeed counteract the otherwise inevitable evils that result from the attempt to bring up infants by hand. The statement, however, just made with reference to the hazard of such an experiment, and to the evil consequences that almost of necessity attend it, is by no means overcharged. M. Villermé, one of the most distinguished statisticians of France, has compared the results of the two systems as followed in three of the principal foundling hospitals in that country.[1] At Lyons, at the time when he wrote, each infant on its reception, was given into the charge of a wet-nurse, and its stay in the hospice did not exceed a very few days, after which it was sent to be nursed in the country. At Rheims, the stay of the infant in the hospice was equally short; but neither while there, nor afterwards when at nurse in the country, was it brought up at the breast. At Paris, the stay of the children in the hospice was often very much longer; but they were usually, though

[1] De la Mortalité des Enfans Trouvés, in the Annales d'Hygiène, vol. xix, p. 47. Further information on this and other allied subjects will be found in a review of the works of Terme, Monfalcon, and others, on the Foundling Hospitals of France, published by the author in the British and Foreign Medical Review for April, 1842.

not invariably, suckled by wet-nurses. The mortality under [illegible] the children admitted into these institutions was

At Lyons, ...	33.7 per cent.
" Paris, ...	60.3 "
" Rheims, ...	63.9 "

These results need no comment, and render it almost unnecessary to adduce any further evidence of the dangers that are inseparable from the attempt to bring up infants on artificial food. One more illustration of the fact, however, may be adduced from the work of a benevolent ecclesiastic, M. Gaillard, on the foundling hospitals of France. He observes:

"At Parthenay, in the department of Deux-Sèvres, of 153 foundlings 54 died between the ages of one day and twelve months, or 35 per cent., which is a higher proportion than that presented at Poitiers. At X——, of 244 new-born infants, 197, or 80 per cent., had died by the end of the first year. Struck by the enormous difference between this rate of mortality and that afforded by the hospices at Poitiers and Parthenay, I determined to investigate its cause. I ascertained that in this hospice as much attention is paid to the children, and the nurses are under as strict oversight, as at Poitiers and Parthenay. But at X—— none of the children are suckled, but all are fed; and the reason assigned for so doing, is the fear of infecting the nurses with syphilis. Be this as it may, I have been assured by many persons connected with the institution, that the fearful mortality just mentioned can be attributed to no other cause than the practice of not suckling the children. The officers of the hospice have tried all means to remedy this evil, but neither their own efforts, nor those of some most excellent female assistants, have been of the slightest service; and the only measure by which they could reduce the mortality, was the having recourse to suckling the children by wet-nurses."[1]

It can hardly be necessary to say, that these statements are not to be taken as representing the ordinary mortality among infants brought up by hand, since many causes will suggest themselves as concurring to render the life of foundlings especially precarious. Neither, indeed, is the whole of the mortality among other children who have been deprived of the mother's milk, to be attributed to the food which is substituted for it; but in many cases, if the mother does not suckle her infant, she delegates to another the performance of her other maternal duties, and the baby is left to languish in the house of a stranger. That this cause is very influential in producing a high rate of mortality among infants, appears from the fact mentioned by M. Benoiston de Chateauneuf,[2] that while among children suckled by their mothers only 18.36 per cent. die within a year after their birth, 29 per cent. of those put out to wet-nurse die during the same period.

It is not enough, however, for us to know that food other than the mother's milk is injurious to the young infant; but it behooves us, both

[1] Recherches sur les Enfans Trouvés, &c., par l'Abbé A. H. Gaillard, 8vo., p. [illegible] Paris, 1837.

[2] Considérations sur les Enfans Trouvés, 8vo., p. 57. Paris, 1824.

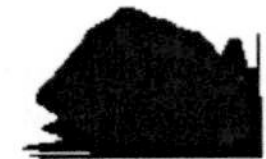

as physiologists and as physicians, to push our inquiries further,—to ascertain as far as possible the means by which this injurious effect is produced, and to determine what organs of the body suffer most severely, and the mode in which they are affected. Unfortunately, the information which I am able to give you on these points is much less definite than I could wish; for the evils that result from improper food in infancy do not, like some diseases, arrest attention by their alarming symptoms, or by their rapidly fatal result, and hence they have received less than their due share of notice.

If *improper food* is given to an infant, the contractions of the stomach are in general speedily excited, and the food is rejected. This eructation of a portion of its food may indeed be noticed even in infants at the breast, who have either sucked more than their stomach can conveniently hold, or whose digestive powers are temporarily weakened by some trivial ailment. But the hint which nature gives is too often thrown away on those who have the charge of the infant. Food of the same kind is given again perhaps in smaller quantity, or with some slight difference in its mode of preparation; and part, or the whole of it, is now retained for a time, though not long enough for its complete assimilation; but if not rejected by vomiting, it passes the pylorus while digestion is but half completed. Unfortunately, the farinaceous articles of food which are so often selected, on account of their supposed lightness, as fit to form the almost exclusive diet of infants, belong to the class of substances that are assimilated with difficulty; so that a large proportion of the contents of the stomach, in the young child brought up by hand, enter the duodenum in a state wholly unfit to be acted on by the bile. The intestines become irritated by these undigested matters; and, in the effort to get rid of them, diarrhœa is excited; while, if not speedily expelled, they pass into a state of fermentation or putrefaction, and thus produce those horribly offensive evacuations which are frequently voided by children in these circumstances.

It would be natural to expect that a child should lose flesh and strength, even if the food given to it were no otherwise objectionable than as being difficultly digested. But not only are the sago, arrowroot, or gruel, with which the child is fed, in themselves less easy of digestion than the milk, which is its proper aliment; they, moreover, when reduced to their ultimate elements, present essential differences from it, and differences by which they are rendered so much the more inapt to nourish the body during the period of its most active development and growth. It would be out of place to enter here into minute details with reference to the physiology of digestion, or the composition of different articles of food, in order to illustrate this subject; neither, indeed, is it necessary to do so. You are aware that physiological and chemical research have proved that food has to answer two distinct purposes in the organism; the one to furnish materials for the growth of the body; the other to afford matter for the maintenance of its temperature; and that life cannot long be supported, except on a diet in which the elements of nutrition and the elements of respiration bear a certain proportion to each other. Now, in milk, the proper food of infants, the elements of the former are to those of the latter, [illegible] to the approximative estimate of an English chemist,[1] in [illegible] tion of 1 to 2; while in arrowroot, sago, and tapioca, they [illegible] 1 to 26, and even in wheaten flour only as 1 to 7. If to [illegible] the absence in these substances of the oleaginous matters which the milk contributes to supply the body with fat (and which can be [illegible] nated from farinaceous substances only by a conversion of [illegible] ments, to which the feeble powers of digestion in early life [illegible] equal), and the smaller quantity, and, to a certain extent, the [illegible] kind of the salts which they contain, it becomes at once apparent that by such a diet the health, if not the life, of the infant must almost inevitably be sacrificed. The body wastes most rapidly; for it is forced from its own tissues to supply the nitrogenous elements essential to the maintenance of life, and which its food contains in far too scanty a proportion. Every organ in the body contributes to the general support, and life is thus prolonged, if no kind disease curtail it, until each member has furnished all that it can spare, and then death takes place from starvation; its approach, indeed, having been slower, but the suffering which preceded it not therefore less, than if all food had been withheld.

I have dwelt at length upon this, which is the most frequent cause of the *atrophy of new-born children;* but similar effects are produced when, from any other reason, an infant is imperfectly nourished, whether, as sometimes occurs, the mother's milk is so deteriorated as to be unsuitable for its support; or, whether, as often happens, the child having been weaned prematurely, its digestive organs are unequal to the task of assimilating the food that has been substituted for the mother's milk. In both cases the abdominal viscera become disordered, nutrition is ill performed, and the child falls into a state of atrophy.

On examining after death the bodies of children who have died in these circumstances, the complete absorption of all the fat, and the removal of much even of the cellular tissue, is the point that first attracts our notice. The thoracic viscera present no unnatural appearance, unless it be that large portions of the lungs are sometimes found in a state of collapse. There is also seldom anything unnatural in the condition of the liver, except the congested state of the organ, the vessels of which, being often loaded with venous blood, form a marked contrast to the generally anæmic appearance of the other viscera. The gall-bladder is usually full of bile,—probably because, as in the case of persons who have died of inanition, the empty stomach has long ceased to stimulate it to contraction by its movements. The stomach and small intestines are in general nearly empty; the fundus of the stomach is sometimes found more or less softened,—a condition the occurrence of which after death is probably favored by the tendency of those kinds of food that are usually given in early life, to pass [illegible] state of fermentation, in the course of which an acid is produced [illegible] is capable of dissolving the animal tissues. In some instances [illegible]

[1] Dr. R. D. Thomson, On the Relation between the Constituents of [illegible] the Systems of Animals, in vol. xxix of the Medico-Chirurgical Trans[illegible]

children have been fed on an exclusively farinaceous diet, the mucous membrane, even low down in the intestines, has been found covered with a thin coating of starch, which presented the characteristic blue color when tested with iodine.[1] The intestines are generally pale, though with patches intermingled of a red or dark-gray color; besides which, small circumscribed spots of bright vascularity are sometimes interspersed through the small intestines, being especially evident at their upper part. Peyer's glands usually appear much more prominent than is natural; sometimes they are of a brighter red than the surrounding intestine, and somewhat swollen, and sometimes they are of a dark-gray tint, and present a singular punctated appearance. In the large intestines there is also sometimes a remarkable development of the solitary glands, the dark orifice of which renders them very evident; and in a few instances they become still more apparent from the mucous membrane immediately around each presenting a dark-gray color. The appearances, in short, are those of general inanition, coupled with the signs of irritation or inflammation of the whole secreting apparatus of the intestinal canal.[2]

The full consideration of every question connected with the imperfect nutrition of infants would require little else than a complete treatise on *the dietetics of early life*. In these Lectures I can aim at nothing more than to bring before your notice a few points of the greatest importance.

Although it is very desirable that for the first six months of their

---

[1] According to some experiments by M. Guillot, of Paris, referred to by Dr. Stewart, of New York, in a paper, republished from an American journal, in the Dublin Medical Journal, March, 1845.

[2] This account of the post-mortem appearances observed in infants who have been imperfectly nourished, is not merely borne out by the very interesting paper of MM. Friedleben and Flesch, in vol v of the Zeitschrift für rationelle Medicin, Heidelberg, 1846, but receives a remarkable illustration in the more recent work of M. Bednar, Physician to the Foundling Hospital at Vienna. The observations of the former gentlemen are founded on the examination of fifteen infants, all of whom were under one year old, who were brought up, either exclusively or in great measure, on artificial food, and who died, after long-continued illness, in a state of atrophy, or else sank rapidly under profuse watery diarrhœa. In cases of the former class, a condition regarded by the writers as the result of chronic inflammation of Peyer's glands was the chief morbid appearance; while in those instances where death took place rapidly swelling and congestion of the same bodies,—betokening, as they believe, their recent inflammation,—were almost always present. They found, too, that in all these cases the disease of the colon was comparatively slight, and evidently secondary to the more serious changes in the small intestine. Dr. Bednar's patients were all under three months,—many only a few days old,—partly suckled by women each of whom had several nurslings, partly fed on artificial food. As might be anticipated, the mortality is high; and of such almost uniform occurrence is swelling of the mesenteric and Peyerian glands, and even of the solitary glands of the large intestines, that, when treating of diarrhœa, he speaks of this state of the glands as being a condition of no sort of importance; and even expresses the opinion that in the large intestines it is to be regarded as a physiological rather than a pathological occurrence. No more striking comment could be written on the mischiefs and the dangers of artificial feeding of infants. See pp. 37 and 38 of Bednar's Krankheiten der Neugebornen, &c., 1st ed., 8vo. Wien, 1850. The same facts, too, are still further illustrated by the more recent observations of Hervieux on the changes in Peyer's and the solitary glands in new-born infants, published in the Gazette Medicale, févr. 17, 1856; and several following numbers.

existence children should derive their support entirely [illegible] mother, and that until they are a year or at least nine months [illegible] mother's milk should form the chief part of their food, yet [illegible] cumstances may occur to render the full adoption of this plan [illegible] cable. In some women the supply of milk, although at first [illegible], yet in the course of a few weeks undergoes so considerable a diminution as to become altogether insufficient for the child's support; while in other cases, although its quantity continues undiminished, yet from some defect in its quality it does not furnish the infant with proper nutriment. Cases of the former kind are not unusual in young, tolerably healthy, but not robust women; while instances of the latter are met with chiefly among those who have given birth to several children, whose health is bad, or whose powers are enfeebled by hard living or hard work. The children in the former case thrive well enough for the first six weeks or two months; but then obtaining the milk in too small a quantity to meet the demands of their rapidly growing organism, they pine and fret, they lose both flesh and strength, and unless the food given to supply their wants be judiciously selected, their stomach and bowels become disordered, and nutrition, instead of being aided, is more seriously impaired. If, however, a healthy wet-nurse is employed to supply the mother's inability to nourish her child, its health will soon return; and by the sacrifice of the infant of the poor woman, the offspring of the wealthy will be preserved. But many circumstances besides those moral considerations which should never be forgotten before the determination is formed to employ a wet-nurse, may put this expedient out of the question; and it becomes, therefore, our duty to inquire what course a mother should pursue, who has learned by experience that she is unable to suckle her child for more than a very short period.

Knowing the attempt to rear her child entirely at the breast to be vain, the mother may in such a case naturally be tempted to bring it up by hand from the very first. But, how short soever the period may be during which the mother is able to suckle her child, it is very desirable that she should nurse it during that period, and also, that her milk should then constitute its only food. For the first four or five days after the infant's birth the milk possesses peculiar qualities, and not merely abounds in fatty and saccharine matters, but presents its casein in a more easily assimilable form than subsequently.[1] It afterwards loses these characteristics; but still, during the first few weeks of [illegible] it contains casein in smaller quantities than enter into its composition at a later period. The secretion, in short, is especially adapted [illegible] feeble powers of the digestive organs soon after birth; and [illegible] difficulty of providing any good substitute for it is greater in [illegible] tion to the tender age of the infant, while art often imitates [illegible] gradual increase of the casein, by which the main [illegible]

[1] See on this subject a very interesting paper by Dr. Moore, of Dublin [illegible] Coagulability of Human Milk," in Dublin Journal of Medical Science [illegible] 1849.

infant's sustenance is made to bear a constant proportion to the demands of its daily growth.[1]

The same course of conduct would be proper in the case of women whose milk is of so poor a quality that their infants do not thrive upon it, since, though its deficiency in casein may render it unfit for the permanent support of the child, yet that circumstance will not prove prejudicial to it during the first few weeks of its existence.

Unfortunately we are not possessed of any ready means by which we can determine, in the majority of instances, that a woman's milk is ill suited for the nourishment of her child; and, in practice, the infant's not thriving is often the first indication that we have of the propriety of a change. Certain qualities, indeed, which healthy milk ought to have, are readily ascertainable. Thus, for instance, it should have a specific gravity of about 1.032, and an alkaline reaction; and, after the first month, should be free from colostrum corpuscles; while the oil-globules, which should be present in great number, ought to be of tolerably equal size, and each distinct from the other. In spite of presenting all these characters, however, the milk may have undergone very important changes, though of a kind which dexterous chemical analysis will alone discover. An increase in the quantity of the fatty matters in the milk seems, according to the observations of M. Becquerel, to be an almost constant attendant upon all diseases, whether acute or chronic, syphilis and far-advanced phthisis alone excepted; while acute diseases are attended by a notable increase, and chronic ailments by a still more remarkable diminution of the casein. Such changes in its composition cannot but modify very greatly its suitability as an aliment for the child; while the difficulty of ascertaining the existence of any of these alterations may at least teach us that the apparently healthy character of the milk is but a very imperfect guarantee of its real excellence.

Still, even though the difficulties of a complete analysis of the milk will generally render the attempt to make it impracticable, and though conclusions drawn from a partial examination will almost certainly be erroneous, there are, fortunately, some general rules fairly deducible from chemical analysis and clinical observation combined, which will generally suffice to guide us aright in the choice of a person to undertake the duties of wet-nurse to an infant whose mother, either from necessity or choice, fails to perform the duty of suckling it herself. The apparently good health of the woman and her child is of all evidence the most conclusive in favor of her fitness; but M. Becquerel

[1] Though I have allowed the above paragraph to stand unaltered in this edition, yet it must be observed that the elaborate researches of MM. Vernois and Becquerel do not altogether bear out its accuracy. They deny, on the strength of twenty-six observations on the milk of different women within a fortnight after delivery, that any such excess of sugar, and feeble proportion of casein, then characterize it, as is stated above, on the authority of the late Professor Simon, of Berlin. They admit the existence of a larger quantity of butter, which, however, continues only so long as the colostrum corpuscles are still present. It is, however, much to be regretted that they did not institute a series of comparative observations, with reference to this point, on the milk of the cow, since the question involved in the accuracy of one or the other of the opposing statements is of very great practical importance.

found the nearest approach to a perfectly physiological state of the milk in women from twenty to twenty-five years old, multiparæ, of strong constitution, previously well-nourished, brunettes, with small mammæ but an abundant secretion of milk, from three to five months after delivery, and in whom the menstrual discharge was suspended.

The question, however, which we often have to answer, and to answer, too, sometimes very soon after the infant's birth, is not as to the goodness of a wet-nurse, but as to *the best substitute for the mother's milk*. Now it is obvious that the more nearly the substitute we select approaches to the character of the mother's milk, the greater will be the prospect of the attempt to rear the infant upon it proving successful. Discarding, therefore, all those preparations of arrowroot, flour, or biscuit-powder, in which the vulgar repose such confidence, we shall not need any labored argument to convince us that in the milk of some other animal we shall be likely to find the infant's most appropriate food. You will perceive, however, by the subjoined table, that there are many important differences between the milk of all the domestic animals and of the human female; both in the actual quantities of its constituents, and in their relative proportion to each other.

Table showing the Composition of the Milk in Man and in various Animals.[1]

	Specific Gravity.	1000 parts contain		The solid constituents are composed of			
		Fluid.	Solids.	Sugar.	Butter.	Casein and Extractive Matters.	Incombustible Salts.
In Man, . .	1032 67	889.08	110.92	43.64	26 66	39.24	1 38
In the Cow,	1033 38	864.06	135 94	38.03	36.12	55.15	6 64
In the Ass,	1034.57	890 12	109.88	50 46	18.53	35.65	5.24
In the Goat,	1033.53	844.90	155 10	36 91	56.87	55.14	6.18
In the Ewe,	1040.98	832.32	167.68	39.43	54.31	69.78	7.16

The above table shows you that it is only in the milk of the ass that the solid constituents are arranged in the same order as in the human subject; casein preponderating in the milk of the cow and ewe, and butter in that of the goat. On this account, therefore, asses' milk is regarded, and with propriety, as the best substitute for the child's natural food. Unfortunately, however, expense is very frequently a bar to its employment, and compels us to have recourse to cows' milk, as being so much more readily procured. But though the cost may be a valid objection to the permanent employment of asses' milk, it is yet very desirable, when a young infant cannot have the breast, that it should be supplied with asses' milk for the first four or five weeks, until the first dangers of the experiment of bringing it up by hand have been surmounted. The deficiency of asses' milk in oily matter may, as has been suggested,[2] be very much rectified by the addition to it of about a twentieth part of cream. The laxative property which it

[1] Vernois and Becquerel, op. cit., p. 167.
[2] By Dr. Moore, of Dublin, in his paper already referred to.

possesses is not so easily counteracted; and though Sir Henry Marsh's recommendation of heating it to 212° sometimes removes this quality, yet the experiment has not in my hands been by any means invariably successful. In such cases, however, the addition of about a fourth part of lime-water to the milk will generally suffice to control all tendency to diarrhœa.

When cows' milk is given, it must be borne in mind that it contains more casein than human milk, and less sugar; and that it is therefore necessary that it should be given in a diluted state, and slightly sweetened. The degree of dilution must vary according to the infant's age; at first, the milk may be mixed with an equal quantity of water, but as the child grows older the proportion of water may be reduced to one-third. Attention must be paid to the temperature of the food when given to the infant, which ought to be as nearly as possible the same as that of the mother's milk, namely, from 90° to 95° Fahrenheit; and in all cases in which care is needed, a thermometer should be employed, in order to insure the food being always given at the same temperature. Human milk is alkaline; and even if kept for a considerable time it shows but little tendency to become sour. The milk of animals in perfect health likewise invariably presents an alkaline reaction, and that of cows when at grass forms no exception to this rule. Comparatively slight causes, however, exert a marked influence upon the milk of the cow in all respects; even in the most favorable circumstances, if the animal is shut up in a city and stall-fed, all the solid constituents of its milk suffer a remarkable diminution; while the secretion further has a great tendency to become acid, or to undergo even more serious deterioration.[1] There is evidently no occasion, then, to assume any intentional adulteration of the milk, in order to account for the symptoms of gastric and intestinal disorder so often produced by it in the case of children brought up in large towns. Whenever, therefore, the attempt is made to rear an infant by hand, in circumstances which render it impossible to obtain the milk of cows that are at pasture, it is desirable that the milk should be daily tested, and that any acidity should be neutralized by the addition of lime-water, or of prepared chalk, in quantity just sufficient to impart to it a slightly alkaline reaction. If the bowels are disposed to be constipated, carbonate of magnesia may be substituted for the chalk. Unfortunately, there seem, as I stated a day or two ago, to be good reasons for believing that the milk of stall-fed cows often undergoes a deterioration much more serious than the merely becoming ascescent; and that changes not infrequently take place in it such as must render it wholly unfit for an infant's food, and calculated only to promote disease. The possibility of their occurrence shows the necessity, when an infant who is brought up by hand fails in health, for making a careful inquiry

[1] See the analysis of Vernois and Becquerel, op. cit., p. 131, and the results of Dr. Mayer's observations on cows in Berlin and its neighborhood, in a valuable paper on the Artificial Feeding of Infants, in the first volume of the Verhandlungen der Gesellschaft für Geburtshülfe in Berlin, 8vo., p. 56, Berlin, 1846; and also two papers by Dr. Peddie in the London and Edinburgh Monthly Journal for 1848; and the observations of Dr. Klencke, of Leipsic, already referred to at p. 424.

into the source of the milk with which it is fed; and for examining the fluid, if possible, both chemically and under the microscope, before proceeding to prescribe remedies for ailments which may be caused entirely by the unwholesome nature of its food.

The quantity of food proper to be given to an infant at one time, and the total amount which it may be supposed to require in the twenty-four hours, though questions of most obvious importance, have hitherto scarcely received any attempt at solution. The only observations bearing on the subject, with which I am acquainted, were made some years ago by M. Guillot[1] at the Foundling Hospital in Paris. He weighed children both immediately before and immediately after suckling, and found that the increase of weight varied from about two to five ounces in children under a month old; and concludes that a thousand grammes, or about two pounds and a quarter avoirdupois, is the smallest quantity of milk that would suffice for the daily nourishment of a healthy infant during the first month of its existence. The number of children, however, on whom his observations were made, as well as the number of observations on each child, were both far too few to yield more than a very rough approximation to the truth with reference to this subject.

It may suffice for to-day, thus to have brought before you the main principles by which you must be guided in the attempt to rear a young infant by hand. Details as to the general dietetic management of infancy or childhood would not only carry us beyond the period allotted for this lecture, but would be a departure from our special object,—of investigating the *diseases* of early life.

LECTURE XXXII.

Atrophy of Young Children.—Not a special disease, but a condition that may be induced by various causes.

Thrush, a peculiar affection of the mouth, generally associated with impaired nutrition.—Its characters, different opinions as to its nature—General state of children in whom it occurs. Microscopic researches as to its nature, the deposit produced by a cryptogamic vegetation—Conditions that favor its development—Inferences as to its treatment.

Dentition.—High rate of mortality while it is going on—Erroneous views with reference to the cause of this, and to the nature of the process—Physiology of dentition—Order of appearance of the teeth—Pauses in their evolution—Frequently attended with local suffering—Various morbid conditions of mucous membrane of the mouth excited by it.

Management of children when teething.—Circumstances in which lancing the gums is likely to be useful—Dietetic and medical management—Treatment of affections of the mouth—Caution with reference to cure of cutaneous eruptions during the time of teething.

At our last meeting we were occupied with various prelim[illegible] quiries, of importance to the thorough understanding of the [illegible]

[1] Journal für Kinderkrankheiten, July, 1852, vol. xix, p. [illegible]

the digestive organs in early life, on the study of which we are now about to enter. We examined the structural and functional peculiarities of those organs in the young, and endeavored to ascertain wherein consists the special fitness of the mother's milk for the nutriment of her infant. We further tried to discover the mode in which other food acts injuriously on the infant, and sought from the knowledge thus acquired to deduce rules for our guidance, whenever it should become necessary to provide a young child with a substitute for that sustenance which nature intended that it should receive.

These considerations naturally brought under our notice the symptoms which betoken that the process of nutrition is imperfectly carried on, and the appearances which, when death takes place from this cause, are revealed on an examination of the body. It may seem to you, however, that the *atrophy of young children* calls for a more elaborate study than ours of yesterday, and for a more minute account of its symptoms. But to attempt this would be to enter upon almost endless details, which would leave upon your memory no clear impression. Whether all food is withheld from an infant, or whether it is supplied with food which it cannot assimilate, or whether disease prevents it from digesting food on which a healthy infant would thrive, the main result is the same, and the child dies of inanition. Various accidents may abridge the infant's life, or may make it sink in one case, in circumstances somewhat different from those which precede its death in another. Sometimes the vital powers grow so feeble that the inspiratory efforts no longer suffice to fill the lungs with air; sometimes the irritable stomach rejects all food, while at other times diarrhœa comes on which no medicine can check. But in these symptoms there is nothing characteristic of one special cause—they may occur alike in the infant who, though healthy when born, was early deprived of its mother's milk, or in the child who is the subject of general tuberculous disease, or whose strength has been exhausted and its digestive powers impaired by dysentery. The symptoms, then, that accompany the atrophy of new-born children must be expected to vary much in different cases; while the considerations brought before you in the last lecture will, I think, furnish you with a clue to the complete understanding of them all.

Before we pass, however, to the special study of the diseases of the digestive organs and their appendages, I wish to call your attention to that *peculiar condition of the mucous membrane of the mouth*, popularly known as the *thrush*, which is so frequently met with in connection with the artificial feeding of young infants—so almost invariably associated with the evidences of their impaired nutrition, that the present seems to be the best place for noticing it.

If you examine the mouth of a young infant on whom the attempt is being made to bring it up without the mother's milk, you will often observe its mucous membrane to be beset with numerous small white spots, that look like little bits of curd lying upon its surface, but which on a more attentive examination are found to be so firmly adherent to it as not to be removed without some difficulty, when the subjacent membrane is left of a deep red color and often bleeding slightly. These specks appear upon the inner surface of the lips, especially near the

angles of the mouth or the inside of the cheeks; and upon the tongue, where they are more numerous at the tip and edges than towards the centre. They are likewise seen upon the gums, though less frequently and in smaller number. When they first appear they are in general of a circular form, scarcely larger than a small pin's head; but after having existed for a day or two some of the spots become three or four times as large, while at the same time they in general lose something of their circular form. By degrees these small white crusts fall off of their own accord, usually leaving the mucous membrane where they were seated redder than before—a color which gradually subsides as the mouth returns to its natural condition; or the white specks are reproduced and again detached several times before the membrane resumes its healthy aspect. In some cases these specks coalesce, or the deposit, from its first appearance, presents more of the character of a false membrane, and the mouth is then seen to be extensively coated with it; though even then, if the deposit is carefully removed, the mucous membrane beneath will be found neither bleeding nor abraded, but merely redder than natural. In these circumstances the deposit generally loses something of the dead white color characteristic of the smaller spots, and presents a slightly yellowish tint. On the Continent, where the severer form of the affection is not infrequently seen, it was supposed, though the opinion is now with propriety abandoned, to be an essentially different ailment from the slighter forms of the disease, in which the points of deposit are distinct, while further confusion was introduced into the subject by the employment of the term *aphthæ*[1] to designate both this affection, and another of a perfectly different nature (which I shall speak of hereafter), characterized by inflammation and ulceration of the mucous follicles of the mouth. The term *aphthæ* will be most properly employed as a synonym for this follicular stomatitis; while I prefer to restrict the use of the word *thrush*[2]—of which the French *muguet*, the old English term *millet*, are synonyms—to the ailment some of whose characters I have just described, and for which there is at present no correct designation in scientific terminology.

Children in whom either form of this deposit exists in any considerable degree usually appear out of health; and it will generally be found on inquiry that this indisposition had preceded for some days the eruption in the mouth. For the most part such children are emaciated, and present those symptoms that attend upon imperfect nutrition, while the bowels are in general relaxed, and the evacuations of a green color, and very sour. The acridity of the motions sometimes irritates and inflames the margins of the anus, and a blush of erythematous redness not infrequently extends over the nates and buttocks, while in some instances a deposit of a similar kind to that in the mouth occupies

[1] The use of the word ἄφθαι by Hippocrates, and its application by him to ulcerations of the uterus, plainly shows that in his mind the idea of a breach of surface was always associated with it; though it is very probable that under a mistaken belief of its nature he may also have used the same word to designate true thrush. See Foesius, Œconomia Hippocratis, *sub voce*.

[2] A word the etymology of which is uncertain; as is that of its Swedish synonym Torsk, and the Danish and Norwegian Trödske.

the edges of the intestine. In spite, however, of the popular notion with reference to this point, the appearance of the deposit at the margin of the anus is of extremely rare occurrence, though redness and soreness at the edge of the bowel are very frequent. The deposit in the mouth sometimes renders sucking very difficult, and may even impair deglutition, while the child, thus obtaining but little food, lies in a state of torpor and drowsiness, the result of its debility.

In its more serious form this affection was said to prove fatal to a large number of the inmates of the different foundling hospitals on the Continent. Observation has shown, however, that although the deposit exists in the mouth of very many children who die in those institutions, yet their death is due not to the local affection, but to the constitutional disease, of which that is only one out of many evidences.

In spite of the exaggerated importance that was long attached to the local affection of the mouth, which was erroneously imagined to be the cause of all the symptoms of disordered health, of which it is in reality merely the accompaniment, much uncertainty existed as to its real nature, though it was generally imagined to be a variety of pseudo-membranous inflammation, not unlike that of croup or diphtheria. This hypothesis, however, which left many peculiarities of the disease unexplained, has been conclusively set aside, and the real nature of this, as of so many other ailments, has been made quite clear by microscopic research.

In the year 1842 Professsor Berg, of Stockholm, physician to the Foundling Hospital in that city, communicated to the Swedish Society of Medicine his discovery of a cryptogamic vegetation in the deposit of thrush; and a German observer, M. Gruby, confirmed M. Berg's researches in a paper addressed in the same year to the Royal Academy of Sciences at Paris, though his views differed in some points from those of M. Berg. From the time of this discovery two opposing views of the nature of the affection have till recently been maintained. According to the one opinion, the parasitic growth, like the muscardine on the silk-worm, or the confervæ developed on other living animals, itself constitutes the essential part of the disease; while according to the other, the white substance in the mouth is in reality an inflammatory exudation, in which, though confervæ may be developed, yet their presence is accidental, and subject to many exceptions.

The correctness of the former opinion, which was maintained by M. Berg, and substantiated in great measure by his researches, has now been so generally admitted that I need not further occupy your time with details of the controversy, but will describe as briefly as possible the nature of the affection as it has been ascertained by means of the microscope; and as it is described by one of the most recent observers, M. Robin.[1]

---

1. Not to incumber this lecture with the citation of authorities, it may suffice to refer to the valuable essay of Dr. Berg, of Stockholm, analyzed in the Journal für Kinderkrankheiten for September and October, 1847, and since translated into German, under the title Ueber die Schwämmchen der Kinder, 8vo., Bremen, 1848, as a most able defence of the first-mentioned opinion; and to the papers by Dr. Kronenberg, of Moscow, in that journal for February and September of the same year,

In connection with various disorders of the digestive apparatus in children, and also in the course of some exhausting disease in the adult, the mucous membrane of the mouth, and sometimes also that of the pharynx and œsophagus, becomes the seat of inflammation, which, though by no means severe, is yet attended with a change of the secretion from alkaline to acid, and with an abundant production of epithelium. This state of the mucous membrane, though not absolutely essential, is yet in the highest degree favorable to the development on its surface of a fungus, the *Oidium albicans*, the sporules of which in these circumstances increase with great rapidity, and elongate into fibrils, by whose multiplication and accumulation, together with the abundant epithelial scales, a thick white layer is formed upon the dorsal surface of the tongue, the palate, the velum, the interior of the cheeks, the lips, and even in some cases the pharynx and œsophagus. It appears, too, that during the first weeks of infancy[1] the mucous membrane of the mouth yields, even in a state of health, and wholly independently of whether or no the child is brought up at the breast, an acid reaction, a circumstance which accounts for the far greater liability of infants than of adults to this affection, so that in the former case a very slight disorder will lead to its development, while in the latter it is the sign and the consequence of very serious disease.

This account of the affection explains many points previously inexplicable concerning it. It furnishes a reason for the prevalence of thrush in foundling hospitals, and institutions of a similar kind, where the same cups, spoons, &c., are used in common by the children, and often without sufficient attention to cleanliness. That the disease may be produced by the actual transplantation of the sporules from one child to another was conclusively established by M. Berg,[2] who tried the experiment in four instances, and found that on each occasion the deposit of the sporules on the mucous membrane of the mouth of a healthy infant was succeeded by the development of the conferva, and the occurrence of thrush.

The conditions, then, which generally coincide in the production of thrush are—1st, certain ailments of the digestive organs, dependent on impaired nutrition; 2d, consequent inflammation of the mucous membrane of the mouth, associated with an increase in the acidity of its secretion, and an unusually abundant formation of epithelium; and 3d, the development on the surface of a cryptogamic vegetation, which is not the cause, but rather the result of the child's illness. It follows, then, that in the *treatment* of this affection the removal of the constitutional disturbance is of at least as much importance as the ministering

---

for observations and arguments tending to support the opposite view. The elaborate essay of M. Seux, in his Recherches sur les Maladies des Enfants, 8vo., Paris, 1855, also claims mention here, for in it every question connected with this affection is treated of with an almost painful minuteness. With reference to the production of confervæ on the mucous surfaces of the human body in disease, the fullest account has been given by Hannover, in Müller's Archiv. for 1842, p. 281; and by M. Robin in his Histoire naturelle des Végétaux parasites qui croissent sur l'Homme et sur les Animaux vivants, 8vo., Paris, 1853.

[1] Seux, op. cit., pp. 18–21.

[2] Seux, op. cit., pp. 76–80.

to the local malady. Two facts, indeed,[1] will serve, without further comment, to place this matter in a very strong light; one is, that in 21 out of 26 examinations of the bodies of children who had died of thrush the small intestines presented morbid appearances, which, though of various kinds, were all analogous to those referred to in the last lecture as dependent on imperfect nutrition and artificial feeding. The other is, that while in the Foundling Hospital at Marseilles the mortality of children affected with thrush is only 5 in 100, in that at Paris it has been stated by different observers as 9 in 10, 109 in 140, 22 in 24, and 25 in 48. Of the two institutions, that at Paris is the more salubrious; but there the appearance of the affection of the mouth is the signal for the immediate withdrawal of the child from the breast; while at Marseilles the opposite plan is pursued, and a child, even though previously fed artificially, is at once given to a wet-nurse on the first sign of thrush being discovered. The extreme rarity, too, with which in private practice the thrush in a young infant assumes the characters of a serious affection furnishes further proof, if it were wanting, that the local ailment is of little moment apart from the complications which impart to it its gravity. It will, therefore, be inexpedient to dwell here on anything more than the local treatment of the case, since its general management must vary as widely as the causes to which the affection of the mouth is due. One point of considerable moment, and to which less care than it deserves is usually paid, is the removing from the mouth, after each time that the infant has fed, all remains of the milk or other food that it has taken. For this purpose, whenever the least sign of thrush appears, the mouth should be carefully wiped out with a piece of soft rag, dipped in a little warm water, every time after food had been given. Supposing the attack to be but slight, this precaution will of itself suffice in many instances to remove all traces of the affection in two or three days. If, however, there be much redness of the mucous membrane of the mouth, or if the aphthous spots be numerous, some medicated topical application is useful. Various detergents have been recommended, among which the mel boracis, and a mixture of the Armenian bole with honey, are very frequently employed. An objection, however, has been raised, and I think on good grounds, to any application into the composition of which honey or other saccharine matters enter, on the ground that the tendency of those substances to pass into a state of fermentation will make them favor, rather than prevent, the formation of confervæ in the interior of the mouth. It is my custom to dissolve half a drachm of borax with one drachm of glycerin in an ounce of water, and to direct that after the mouth had been carefully cleansed with warm water this lotion should be applied to it on a piece of lint or soft linen. In the milder forms of the affection the borax lotion usually answers every purpose. Should it, however, appear insufficient, a solution of two grains of the nitrate of silver in an ounce of distilled water may be employed in the same way twice a day, while at other times the solution of borax may be used in the manner just directed.

[1] Op. cit., pp. 147 and 218–220.

The close connection that subsists between this local affection and the condition of generally impaired nutrition, which engaged our attention yesterday, induced me to bring the subject now under your notice. I do not know, however, that any better plan can be adopted, in studying the diseases of the organs of digestion and assimilation, than chiefly to follow an anatomical arrangement, and to consider, first, the diseases of the mouth, then those of the stomach, then those of the intestines, and lastly those of the other abdominal viscera.

It may, perchance, seem to you that, according to this plan, it is not proposed to assign any place of importance to the disorders of dentition, though in our tables of mortality we find teething registered as having occasioned the death of nearly 5 (4.8) per cent. of all children who died in this metropolis under one year old, and of 7.3 per cent. of those who died between the age of twelve months and three years. Many other circumstances, too, tend to increase the impression which this fact naturally makes; for not only do nurses attribute to teething the most varied forms of constitutional disturbance, and mothers express anxious apprehensions as the period of dentition approaches, but medical men hold forth to anxious parents the expectation that their child will have better health when it has cut all its teeth. The time of teething, truly, is in reality one of more than ordinary peril to the child; though why it should be so is not always rightly understood. It is a time of most active development of the organism—a time of transition from one state of being to another, in respect of all those important functions by whose due performance the body is nourished and built up. Statistics, embracing the largest numbers, prove the dangers of this period, and warrant us in regarding the completion of the process of teething as a fair subject for congratulation.

The error which has been committed with reference to this matter, not merely by the vulgar, but by members of our own profession also, consists, not in overrating the hazards of the time when changes so important are being accomplished, but in regarding only one of the manifestations—though that, indeed, is the most striking one—of the many important ends which nature is then laboring to bring about. A child in perfect health usually cuts its teeth at a certain time and in a certain order, just as a girl at a certain age presents the various signs of approaching puberty, and at length begins to menstruate. In the latter case we do not fix our attention solely on the menstrual flux; nor, should it fail to appear, do we have recourse to the empirical employment of emmenagogue medicines. We examine into the cause of its absence, try to ascertain whether it depends on the state of the health in general, or of the uterine system in particular, and regulate accordingly our attempts at cure. The epoch of dentition is to be looked at just in the same way as that in which we regard the epoch of puberty. Constitutional disturbance is more common, and serious disease more frequent at those times than at others; but their causes lie deeper than the [illegible]

[1] See, for instance, the table of mortality at different months, at p. [illegible] Quetelet et Smits, Recherches sur la Réproduction et la Mortalité, [illegible] Bruxelles, 1842.

which irritates the gum that it has not yet pierced in the one case, or than the womb which has not yielded the due discharge of blood in the other. You might produce hemorrhage from the uterine vessels in the latter instance, or might cut through the gum which inclosed the teeth in the former, with no other effect than that of aggravating the condition of your patient.

In speaking of the diseases of the nervous and respiratory systems, your attention has on several occasions been drawn to the greater frequency of some of those affections just at the time when the process of teething is going on; and you will have to remark a similar fact with reference to some of the disorders of the abdominal viscera. These maladies, however, are not peculiar to the time of teething, nor, when they occur at that period, do they present symptoms different from those which characterize them in other circumstances, while it often happens that the changes which mark the transition from infancy to childhood are accomplished so quietly as to be attended with no notable disturbance of the general health.

The great changes which Nature is constantly bringing about around us and within us are the result of laws operating silently but unceasingly; and hence it is that in her works we see little of the failure which often disappoints human endeavors, or of the dangers which often attend on their accomplishment. Thus, when Nature's object is to render the child no longer dependent on the mother for its food, she begins to prepare for this long beforehand. The first indication of it is furnished by the greatly increased activity of the salivary glands; organs whose function, as I told you in the last lecture, seems for some little time after birth to be wholly in abeyance. If you look into the mouth of a young infant you will be struck by the very small amount of saliva that moistens its surface—a fact that explains in great measure the tendency to dryness which the tongue then presents under the influence of very trivial ailments. About the fourth or fifth month, however, this condition undergoes a marked alteration; the mouth is now found constantly full of saliva, and the child is continually driveling; but no other indication appears of the approach of the teeth to the surface, except that the ridge of the gums sometimes becomes broader than it was before. No further change may take place for many weeks; and it is generally near the end of the seventh month, oftener later than earlier, before the first teeth make their appearance. The middle incisors of the lower jaw are generally the first to pierce the gum; next in order appear the middle incisors of the upper jaw; then usually the lateral incisors of the lower, and last of all the lateral of the upper. This, however, is not quite invariable, for sometimes all the upper incisors are cut before the lower lateral incisors make their appearance. The first four molars next succeed, and often without any very definite order as to whether those of the upper or of the lower jaw are first visible, though in the majority of cases the lower molars are the first to appear. The four canine teeth follow; and lastly, the four posterior molars—making, in all, the number of twenty deciduous teeth.

We must not, however, picture to ourselves this process as going on uninterruptedly until completed—a mistake into which parents often fall, whose anxiety respecting their children is consequently excited by observing that, after several teeth have appeared in rapid succession, dentition appears to come to a standstill. Nature has so ordered it that the process of dentition, beginning at the seventh or eighth month, shall not be completed until the twenty-fourth or thirtieth; and has doubtless done so in some measure with the view of diminishing the risk of constitutional disturbance which might be incurred if the evolution of the teeth went on without a pause. A little observation will show you that, while the irruption of the lower central incisors is generally completed in a week, an interval of six weeks or two months often takes place before the upper incisors make their appearance, which then are in general quickly followed by the lateral incisors. A pause of three or four months now frequently occurs before we see the first molar teeth, another of equal length previous to the appearance of the canine teeth, and then another still longer before the last molars are cut.

Though a perfectly natural process, dentition is yet almost always attended with some degree of suffering. Many of us, no doubt, can remember feeling much pain when we cut our wisdom teeth, and children probably experience the same kind of annoyance. This, however, is not always the case; for sometimes we discover that an infant has cut a tooth, who had yet shown no sign of discomfort, nor any indication that dentition was commencing, with the exception of an increased flow of saliva. More frequently, indeed, the mouth becomes hot, and the gums look tumid, tense, and shining, while the exact position of each tooth is marked for some time before its appearance, by the prominence of the gum; or the eruption of the teeth is preceded or accompanied by a somewhat different condition of the mouth, in which there are much heat, and intense redness of the mucous membrane, an extremely copious flow of thin saliva, and a disposition to the formation of small aphthous ulcerations on the tongue, at the outer surface of the alveolæ, or at the duplicature of the lip, though the gums themselves may not be particularly swollen or painful. Either of these states is usually attended with some degree of febrile disturbance, and apparently with considerable suffering to the infant, who is constantly fretful and peevish, or cries out occasionally as if in pain. A third morbid condition of the mouth is sometimes seen, which is usually ushered in or attended by very considerable fever and disorder of the chylopoietic viscera. The gums then become extremely hot and swollen, and unusually tender, especially over some tooth or other in particular, and in that situation we find the gum swollen up into a kind of little tumor. Small unhealthy ulcerations, with a sloughy appearance, often form upon the summit of the gum, and especially around any tooth which has partly pierced through it. To this affection, which is often very painful, and often difficult of cure, the name of *Odontitis Infantum* has been applied by some continental writers.

In considering the rules by which you must direct the *management of children when teething*, it can scarcely be necessary to caution you against regarding all diseases that may come on during dentition as of necessity connected with that process, or with the general changes then going on in the organism: still less need I warn you against looking upon all ailments at that time as symptomatic of the local uneasiness which the child suffers in its mouth. Some persons, indeed, act as if they held both these notions to their fullest extent; and, following up in practice this coarsely mechanical theory, they lance the gums of every child who has not yet cut all its teeth, almost or altogether irrespective of the nature of the affection from which it suffers. Such a proceeding is nothing better than a piece of barbarous empiricism, which causes the infant much pain, and is useless or mischievous in a dozen instances for one in which it affords relief. Still less is the gum-lancet to be employed, merely with the view of expediting the process that nature is engaged in. The gradual protrusion of the teeth occasions the slow absorption of the superjacent gum, and for this process the division of the gum by a scalpel forms at best but a clumsy substitute.

The circumstances in which the use of the gum-lancet is really indicated are comparatively few. You may employ it when a tooth is so nearly through that you can feel sure it will burst the gum in a day or two at latest; for then, by making an incision through the very thin gum, you may certainly spare the infant much suffering. Or you may lance the gums if they are red, and swollen, and tense, and injected; but then you scarify them in order that they may bleed, and that their congested vessels may be thus relieved: you do not divide them to let out the imprisoned tooth. In such circumstances it may be necessary to repeat your scarification several times with the same object; and it is therefore well to explain beforehand to the mother the reasons of your proceeding, lest she should expect to see the tooth at once make its appearance. There are, besides, cases in which the general constitutional disturbance that often attends dentition continues for several days, or even weeks, while yet the condition of the swollen gum remains unaltered, and the tooth does not seem to approach nearer to the surface. In such a case you may try the experiment of lancing the gums, or you may try it in the case of a child in whom you have already observed that catarrh, or fever, or diarrhœa has been excited by the approach of each tooth to the surface, and has ceased immediately that the tooth has pierced the gum. Lastly, in the cases of sudden and apparently causeless convulsions, which are occasionally met with in children, you will be justified in lancing the gums if you find that the process of dentition is going on with activity; but you would do no good if you lanced the gums during one of those periods of repose which you will remember interrupt from time to time the evolution of the teeth. You must therefore inquire not merely what teeth the child has cut, but also when the last made their appearance; and must seek for some evidence either that the process is still going on, or that its activity is once more recommencing, before you would have ground for supposing the source of irritation of the nervous system to be such as your gum-lancet would relieve.

If the process of teething is going on perfectly naturally no interference, medical or other, is either necessary or proper. The special liability of children to illness at this time must indeed be borne in mind, and care must be taken not to make any alteration in the infant's food while it is actually cutting its teeth, but rather to choose the opportunity of some one of those pauses to which reference has been made, as occurring between the dates of appearance of the successive teeth, for any such change. Should the child at any time appear very feverish some simple febrifuge medicine may be given; as, for instance, a mixture of the bicarbonate of potash not quite neutralized with citric acid, to each dose of which two or three minims of the tincture of hyoscyamus may be added if the child is very restless and fretful.[1] The diet must be carefully regulated; and as the heat of the mouth may induce the child to suck too often, in order to obtain the grateful relief of moisture, and by so doing to overload its stomach, water or barley-water should be freely given to it; and the mother should be cautious not to put it too frequently to the breast. If the child has been weaned still greater care will be required, for it will often be found that it is no longer able to digest its ordinary food, which either is at once rejected by the stomach, or else passes through the intestines undigested. Very thin arrowroot, made with water, with the addition of one-third of milk, will suit in many cases; or you may occasionally substitute for this equal parts of milk and water, thickened by dissolving isinglass in it till its consistence equals that of thick barley-water; or may employ the white decoction of Sydenham, with the addition of one part of milk. If the bowels are disordered, half a grain of Dover's powder night and morning will often restrain their overaction; while the child may take during the day a mucilaginous mixture,[2] containing small doses of the vinum ipecacuanhæ and of some alkali, as the bicarbonate of potash or the liquor potassæ. The dysuria from which infants sometimes suffer when teething is relieved by a similar plan of treatment, with the addition of small doses of castor-oil if the bowels do not act regularly; while the tepid bath is often extremely serviceable in diminishing that great heat of skin which exists in many of these cases.

That state of the mouth in which small aphthous ulcers appear upon the tongue and about the alveolæ is usually connected with disorder of the digestive organs, to the relief of which our treatment must be chiefly directed. It is seldom necessary to do more locally than to pay great attention to cleanse the mouth every time after the child has sucked or taken food, and afterwards to apply to it a solution of borax, in the manner I pointed out to you at the commencement of this lecture. Now and then the submaxillary glands become swollen and tender while the infant is cutting some of its teeth; but this condition generally subsides of its own accord. Sometimes, however, the irrita-

---

[1] See Formula No. 8, p. 68.

[2] (No. 23.)

℞. Misturæ Acaciæ, ℥vj.
Liquoris Potassæ, ♏xxx.
Vin. Ipecacuanhæ, ♏xxiv.
Syrupi Althææ, ℥iv.
Aquæ puræ, ℥xiij. M.

A dessertspoonful every six hours. For a child from 12 to 18 [illegible]

tion extends to some of the absorbent glands beneath the jaw or near its angle; and in scrofulous subjects they occasionally inflame and suppurate. In such children, too, strumous ophthalmia and otorrhœa are not infrequently excited by dentition.

That severe form of inflammation of the gums to which the name of *Odontitis* has been given sometimes occasions great suffering, and may even endanger the child's life, though no instance has come under my own notice in which it proved actually fatal. The gum-lancet will here do no good whatever, its employment would be intensely painful, and that unhealthy ulceration which attends the inflammation of the gums would attack the edges of the cut, and thus aggravate, instead of relieving, the child's sufferings. Local depletion by leeches, however, is extremely useful in such cases. Some writers have suggested that the leeches should be applied to the gum itself; but I have always contented myself with the much easier plan of applying them to the angle of the jaw, and have seldom been disappointed in obtaining very marked relief of all the symptoms. The diet must be most carefully regulated, the state of the bowels attended to, and a mildly antiphlogistic plan of treatment adopted, while the borax lotion may be used locally with advantage. There is, however, one remedy which acts in the various forms of stomatitis almost like a charm, and which proves exceedingly useful even when inflammation of the mouth is associated with the process of teething. This remedy, for the introduction of which into practice in cases of stomatitis the profession is indebted to Dr. Hunt,[1] is the chlorate of potash, which may be given dissolved in water and sweetened, in the dose of four grains every four hours to a child a year old, with almost a certainty of effecting a cure in the course of four or five days.

Two or three exceptions, however, to the ordinary course of even severe odontitis have come under my notice, in which the affection of the gums became chronic, and so continued during the whole period of dentition. The gum in these cases was spongy and livid, like that of a person suffering from scurvy, and so swollen that the teeth were almost hidden by it, while an unhealthy ulceration of its edges surrounded each tooth. In one instance this condition lasted during the whole period of cutting the incisor teeth; but the gum got well during the pause which ensued before the molar teeth made their appearance; while in another scarcely any improvement was apparent until, at the age of two years and four months, the first dentition was completed. The children in both of these cases were weakly, and in one of them an eruption of purpura, which appeared at the age of fifteen months, served to assimilate the characters of the ailment even more closely to scurvy, while the only treatment which was beneficial consisted in the employment of acids, quinine, and wine in small quantities. I refer to these cases on account of their singularity; and their occurrence was, indeed, the more remarkable, since they were met with in the children of persons in the upper ranks of society, and resident in healthy situations in the country.

---

[1] Medico-Chirurgical Transactions, vol. xxvi, p. 142.

In conclusion, I may just refer to those *eczematous and* [illegible] *eruptions* of the face and scalp which often occur in teething [illegible] The old prejudice which regards diseases of the skin [illegible] time as having in them something salutary, and that [illegible] not desirable to attempt their cure, is not destitute of a [illegible] tion in fact. Instances of the sudden disappearance of [illegible] the scalp during the period of dentition being followed by [illegible] pairment of the general health, by convulsions, or by other [illegible] mischief in the brain, are far from uncommon. Their [illegible] fore, must never be attempted, except by the gentlest [illegible] every threatening of the supervention of cerebral congestion, [illegible] more serious disease of the brain, must be most closely watched [illegible] most vigorously combated. Sometimes too it will be found [illegible] ever the cutaneous affection has made a certain advance [illegible] the signs of other disease invariably appear. In such a case it [illegible] to content yourselves with keeping the local ailment in check [illegible] than, by persevering in the attempt to cure it, to endanger in [illegible] serious respects the welfare of the child.

LECTURE XXXIII.

INFLAMMATION OF THE MOUTH, OR STOMATITIS.—Its three varieties.

Follicular stomatitis.—Often a secondary affection—Most frequent before [illegible] is completed—Its symptoms—Character of the aphthæ, or ulceration [illegible] mouth—Not a serious disorder—Its treatment.

Ulcerative stomatitis.—Principally affects the gums—Its course usually [illegible] Has very little tendency to degenerate into gangrene—Its treatment [illegible] chlorate of potash almost a specific for it.

Gangrenous stomatitis.—Extremely rare, but very fatal—Essential [illegible] tween it and the other forms of stomatitis—Dependent on alterations [illegible] blood, such as occur in fevers—Its mode of commencement, symptoms [illegible] course—State of the gangrenous parts on dissection.

Treatment.—Importance of efficient cauterization—What caustics are to [illegible] and how they are to be applied.

The disease does not depend on the administration of mercury.

CYNANCHE TONSILLARIS.—Unusual in young children—Its symptoms not [illegible]

HYPERTROPHY OF THE TONSILS.—Its frequency and importance in [illegible] symptoms—Extreme dyspnœa sometimes produced by it—Modification [illegible] duces in form of mouth and nose—Deformity of chest resulting from [illegible] produced—Treatment—Frequent necessity for excision of tonsils.

RETRO-PHARYNGEAL ABSCESS.—An affection of great rarity, not confined [illegible] hood—Sometimes idiopathic, sometimes succeeds to fevers—Its [illegible] Illustrative cases—Occasional difficulty in its diagnosis—Treatment [illegible]

CYNANCHE PAROTIDEA.—Most common near period of puberty—[illegible] contagious—Its symptoms—Metastasis of inflammation rare—Treatment [illegible]

AMONG the local accidents which complicate dentition [illegible] condition of the mucous membrane of the mouth, which, [illegible] attended by serious danger, is often the source of much suffering to the patient.

Inflammation of the mouth, however, is an occurrence by no means confined to the period of teething, but it comes on in children of all ages, assumes very different forms, and leads to very different results in one case from those which characterize it in another. The mucous follicles of the mouth are the chief seat of the disease in one case, the substance of the gum in another, that of the cheek in a third. In the first the affection issues in the formation of several small ulcers, which heal eventually of their own accord; in the second an unhealthy process of ulceration destroys the gums and denudes the teeth, but it is tardy in its advance, and tends to a spontaneous cure; while in the last mortification involves all the tissues of the cheek, and spreads with a rapidity which remedies generally fail to check, and which is arrested at last only by the patient's death.

Each of these varieties of *stomatitis* requires from us more than a passing notice.

The first—the *follicular stomatitis* of some writers, the *aphthous stomatitis* of others—is met with either as a concomitant or sequela of measles, or as an idiopathic affection. In the former case it depends on the extension to the mouth of a state of inflammation similar to that which gives rise to the eruption on the skin; in the latter it is often associated with obvious gastric or intestinal disorder. Under either of these conditions it is rare after five years of age; and though it often depends on causes quite independent of dentition, yet from the period when teething has commenced, to the end of the third year, is the time of its most common occurrence; while in early infancy *aphthæ* are unusual, though genuine thrush, such as I have described in the last lecture, is a frequent ailment. When it constitutes an idiopathic affection, more or less fever and restlessness, loss of appetite, an unhealthy state of the evacuations, and frequently a relaxed condition of the bowels, precede the local ailment for several days. Attention is generally called to the state of the mouth by the child being observed to suck, or to take food, with manifest pain and difficulty; while at the same time the secretion of saliva is greatly increased, and the submaxillary glands are swollen and tender. The mouth is hot, its mucous membrane generally of a livid red, while a coat of thin mucus covers the centre of the tongue. On the surface of the tongue, especially near its tip; on the inside of the lips, particularly on the lower lip and about its fold; on the inside of the cheek, near the angles of the mouth; and less often in other situations also, may be seen several small isolated transparent vesicles, or the ulcers which, after bursting, they leave behind. The ulcers are small, of a rounded or oval form, not very deep, but having sharply cut edges; and their surface is covered by a yellowish-white, firmly adherent slough
is first directed to the mouth several of these sma
exist, for the vesicular stage of the affection ap
very short, while the ulcers are indolent, and se
many days without showing any disposition to
size. The eruption of a single crop of vesicles, a

vesicles into minute ulcerations, that heal in the course of time, [illegible] complete the history of this affection; for while the mucous membrane in the situation of some of these ulcers at length resumes its natural condition, other vesicles appear, which again degenerate into little ulcers, and thus keep up the ailment, sometimes for weeks together. In some cases, not above five or six of these little ulcers exist at once, or they may even be less numerous, while it is very seldom that more than fifteen or twenty of them are observable at one time. By the successive appearance of fresh ulcerations, and the coalescence of several, an ulcerated strip of considerable extent sometimes forms, especially at the tip of the tongue, or on the lower lip. When the ulcers are healing, no change in their aspect is observable, and they continue to the last covered by the same yellow slough, but by degrees they diminish in size: and seldom or never is any cicatrix observable in the situation which they occupied. In some cases the affection is complicated with a herpetic eruption about the edges of the lips, the vesicles of which degenerate into ulcerations similar to those observed in the interior of the mouth, and by their soreness add very much to the sufferings of the patient.

Even though no remedies should be employed, this affection shows no tendency to rapid increase; it is but very seldom that any cryptogamic formation, such as characterizes thrush, takes place on the surface of the ulcerations, or that any tendency appears to the formation of false membrane in the mouth; while even when most severe it is unattended by any disposition to gangrene. It is sometimes a source of much annoyance to the child, but need never excite any serious solicitude, except when it occurs as a sequela of measles. In that case, however, as was observed in a former lecture,[1] it occasionally becomes associated with diphtheritic deposits on the fauces, and with ulcerative inflammation of the larynx, though our anxiety is then excited less by the affection itself than by its concomitants.

In the *treatment* of this affection our attention must be chiefly directed to correcting the gastric and intestinal disorder by which it is accompanied; and when this object has been attained the local ailment in many cases speedily subsides. The borax lotion mentioned in the last lecture is one of the best local applications that can be used; but if the ulcerations shew no tendency to heal, it may be desirable to touch them once a day with a solution of five grains of nitrate of silver dissolved in an ounce of distilled water.

Between the mild affection we have just been studying, and the *second form of stomatitis*, to the examination of which we are now to pass, there are comparatively few points of resemblance. [illegible] variety of the disease attacks the gums, and sometimes destroys [illegible] extensively, unlike the former ailment, which even though [illegible] continue long, seldom occasions any actual loss of substance. [illegible] process, however, by which the destruction of the gums is [illegible] is one of ulceration, not of mortification—a fact which it is [illegible] tance to bear in mind, lest we should fall into the error of [illegible]

[1] Lecture XXV, p. 368.

servers, who have confounded together, under the name of Cancrum Oris, both this affection and that more formidable malady, true gangrene of the mouth. There can be no doubt, indeed, but that in a few rare instances gangrene has supervened on the long-standing ulceration; though I believe with M. Trousseau that this never occurs except when the affection has already extended to the adjacent surface of the cheek. The affinities of this disease are unquestionably with diphtheria rather than with gangrene, though I am not sure that this affinity amounts to actual identity.[1] It is characterized by ulceration as much as by the deposit of false membrane on the ulcerated surface; it is invariably unaccompanied by any of those signs of constitutional disorder which are so conspicuous in pharyngeal diphtheria, and to the best of my knowledge no increase of its prevalence has been observed to be associated with the more frequent occurrence of diphtheria. But whether the two diseases are the same or only similar, it will probably be convenient to express the resemblance by the term Diphtheritic or Diphtheroid Stomatitis; though I am not prepared at present to discard its old appellations of Noma[2] and of Ulcerative Stomatitis, by which it used formerly to be designated. In any case, however, it will be convenient to restrict the term *Cancrum Oris* to *Gangrenous Stomatitis*, or gangrene of the mouth.

It is by no means a constant occurrence for any special derangement of the general health to precede the attack of *ulcerative stomatitis*, though the children who are affected by it are seldom robust, and in many instances are such as have suffered from deficient food, or from a damp and unhealthy lodging, or from both. In children who are not very carefully tended, the ulceration has sometimes made considerable progress before its existence is suspected, and the profuse flow of the saliva, or the offensive smell of the breath, is the symptom which at length excites attention. Coupled with this, too, there is often considerable swelling of the upper lip, and the submaxillary glands are frequently swollen and painful. On opening the mouth, the gums are seen to be red, and swollen and spongy, and their edge is covered with a dirty white or grayish pultaceous deposit, on removing which their surface is exposed, raw and bleeding. At first, only the front of the gum is thus affected; but as the disease advances, it creeps round between the teeth to their posterior surface, and then, destroying the gum both in front and behind them, leaves them denuded, and very loose in their sockets; but it is not often that they actually fall out. The gums of the incisor teeth are usually first affected: those of the lower jaw more frequently and more extensively than those of the upper; but if the disease is severe, the gums at the side of the mouth become likewise involved, though it is seldom that the two sides suffer equally. Sometimes aphthous ulcers, like those of follicular stomatitis, are seen on the inside of the mouth in connection with this state of the gums; but oftener it exists alone. On those parts of the lips and cheeks, however, which

[1] See, with reference to this question, T [illegible] d., vol. i, p. 383.

[2] From νομαι, used by Hippocrate[illegible] See Foesius, Œconomia Hippocratis[illegible]

are opposite to, and consequently in contact with, the [illegible] irregular ulcerations form, which are covered with a pultaceous [illegible] membranous deposit, similar to that which exists on the gums [illegible] selves. Sometimes, too, deposits of false membrane take place [illegible] parts of the inside of the mouth, the surface beneath being red [illegible] and bleeding, though not distinctly ulcerated. If the disease [illegible] and long-continued, the tongue assumes a sodden appearance [illegible] indented by the teeth; and the cheek, on one or other side, is [illegible] swollen, while the saliva, though rather less abundantly secreted [illegible] at the commencement of the affection, continues horribly fetid [illegible] often streaked with blood, the gums themselves bleeding on the slightest touch. But even if left alone, the affection usually subsides in the course of time, though it may continue almost stationary for days or weeks together, and this notwithstanding that the general [illegible] tolerably good. The termination of this unhealthy ulceration by gan-grene is so rare, that though a very large number of cases of ulcerative stomatitis have come under my notice, I have seen only one [illegible] in which it was succeeded by true gangrene of the mouth. When re-covery has commenced, the disease ceases to spread; the drivelling of fetid saliva diminishes; the white pultaceous deposit on the gums [illegible] on the ulcerations of the cheek or lips, becomes less abundant; [illegible] ulcers themselves grow smaller; and, finally, the gums become [illegible] and their edges of a bright red, though still for a long time [illegible] a disposition to become once more the seat of the ulcerative process, [illegible] continuing for a still longer time to cover the teeth but very imper-fectly.

Various internal remedies and local applications have been at differ-ent times recommended for *the cure of this affection.* Tonics have been much employed, and the supposed analogy between this state of the gums and that which exists in scurvy, has led practitioners to give the preference to remedies reputed to be possessed of antiscorbutic proper-ties. Lotions of alum, or the burnt alum in substance, or the chloride of lime in powder, have all been used locally with more or less benefit. It was my custom also to prescribe these remedies in cases of ulcerative stomatitis; but since I became acquainted with the virtues of the chlo-rate of potash, I have learned to rely upon it almost exclusively. It ap-pears, indeed, almost to deserve the name of a specific in this affection; for a marked improvement seldom fails to be observed in the [illegible] condition after it has been administered for two or three days; and [illegible] week or ten days the cure is generally complete. Three grains [illegible] four hours, dissolved in water, and sweetened, is a sufficient dose [illegible] child three years old; and five grains every four hours appear [illegible] as well as a larger dose for a child of eight or nine. If the bowels [illegible] constipated, a purgative should be previously administered; but [illegible] seems to be no form, nor any stage of the affection, in which [illegible] rate of potash is not useful. The diet should be light but [illegible] and quinine or other tonics are sometimes serviceable if the child [illegible] should continue feeble after the local malady has been cured.

Ulcerative stomatitis is an affection of such frequent occ[illegible] many instance of it come under my notice every year, [illegible] the damp autumnal months; while it is attended with so little danger that the only case which I have known to prove fatal was one in which gangrene of the mouth supervened upon it. *Gangrenous stomatitis*, on the other hand, is a disease so rare, that I have only ten times had the opportunity of witnessing it; but so fatal, that in eight out of those ten cases the patients died. The larger experience of other observers shows an almost equally unfavorable result, since twenty out of twenty-one cases that came under the notice of MM. Rilliet and Barthez had a fatal termination; and a recent French writer,[1] who has collected from different sources 239 cases, which did not all occur in children, states that 176 of the number, or 75 per cent., terminated fatally. The formidable nature of the disease requires that we study it more closely than considering the rarity of its occurrence would otherwise be necessary; and it is the more important to do so, in order that we may avoid the not very uncommon error which confounds this dangerous affection with that comparatively trifling ailment—ulcerative stomatitis.

The constitutional disturbance which often precedes the other two affections of the mouth that we have just been studying, was seen to be generally of a trivial nature, and never so severe as to excite serious anxiety. Gangrene of the mouth, on the other hand, seldom comes on, except in children whose health has been already much impaired by previous disease, and especially by such diseases as are connected with important changes in the circulating fluid. In strict propriety, indeed, I doubt whether we ought not to remove both this and those other allied affections, in which the skin or the genital organs become the seat of gangrene, from among the class of local ailments, and refer them to the category of blood diseases. Of twenty-nine cases of gangrene of the mouth, which MM. Rilliet and Barthez either observed themselves, or of which they found mention in the writings of other physicians, only one appeared to be an instance of the disease in an idiopathic form; while in twelve cases it followed an attack of measles. Of the ten cases which I have observed, and five of which I examined after death, two succeeded to typhoid fever, four to measles; one, which eventually recovered after the application of strong acid to the slough, and with the help of all the comforts of the hospital, appeared to have been induced by want and an unhealthy dwelling; one came on in a child whose health had been completely broken down by ague, one supervened in a tuberculous child, who had been affected for many weeks with ulcerative stomatitis in a severe form; and in the tenth instance the active employment of mercury for the cure of acute encephalitis produced profuse salivation, which was followed by gangrene. Though not confined to any one period of childhood, gangrene of the mouth is more frequent between the ages of two and five than either earlier or later. Of the 10 cases that came under my own observation, 2 were in children between two and three years old, 2 in children aged three, 4 in children between four and five, 1 at six and a quarter, and 1 at eight years of age. Of the 29 cases mentioned by MM. Rilliet and Barthez, 19 occurred between two and five; 10 between six and twelve; and M.

[1] Tourdes, Du Noma, &c., 4to. Thèse de Strasbourg, 1848.

Tourdes'[1] comparison of 102 cases between one and a half [illegible] years, likewise yields the greatest number during the third [illegible] years.

Although all the tissues of the cheek become involved in the [illegible] of this affection, yet difference of opinion has existed with reference to the part in which it commences; some observers conceiving that it usually begins in the substance of the cheek, while others regard the mucous membrane as being the part which is invariably the first attacked. So far as my own observation enables me to judge, I am disposed to regard this latter view, which is that of MM. Rilliet and Barthez, and of M. Baron, and which is moreover supported by the minute researches of Professor Albers,[2] of Bonn, as generally correct. At the same time, however, I must admit that I have had but few opportunities of personally investigating this subject, while a very competent observer, Dr. Löschner,[3] physician to the Children's Hospital at Prague, while he admits the occasional commencement of the affection in either way, believes the former to be the more common. According to his observations, the appearance of a swelling, having a hard central spot or nucleus, surrounded by tense, elastic, but less dense tissue, gradually passing off into the texture of the adjacent parts, is the first step in the process; ulceration of the mucous membrane being secondary to this peculiar infiltration of the cellular tissue of the cheek. It is, indeed, very probable that the gangrene sometimes begins in the one way and sometimes in the other; while any dispute concerning it loses almost all its practical moment, if we regard this and other forms of gangrene as resulting from merely accidental differences in the mode in which the graver deterioration of the circulating fluid manifests itself.

The early stages of the affection are attended by scarcely any suffering, owing to which, as well as to the circumstance that the children in whom it supervenes are almost always laboring under some other disease, or in the course of convalescence from it, it is probably that that the malady is often not discovered until after it has made considerable progress. There may for a day or two have been an unusual fetor of the breath, and a profuse secretion of offensive saliva; but the appearance of swelling of the cheek is frequently the first symptom that leads to a careful examination of the state of the mouth. The characters of the swelling of the cheek are almost pathognomonic of gangrene of the mouth. It is not a mere puffiness of the integument [illegible] unaccompanied by any change of its color, such as is sometimes [illegible] served in ulcerative stomatitis; but the cheek is tense, and [illegible] shining—it looks as if its surface had been besmeared with [illegible] the centre of the swollen part there is generally a spot of [illegible] red than that around. The cheek feels hard, and is often [illegible] ing that the mouth cannot be opened wide enough to get [illegible]

[1] Op. cit., p. 31.

[2] Archiv. f. physiol. Heilkunde, ix, 7–8, 1850; and Schmidt's [illegible] p. 195.

[3] Der Brand im Kindesalter, in the Vierteljahrsschrift für [illegible] vol xv, p. 68.

of its interior. The disease is almost always limited to one side, and generally to one cheek. Sometimes, however, it extends to the lower lip; and occasionally it begins in that situation. The upper lip is now and then reached, by the progress of the disease, but is never its primary seat. Whatever be the situation of the external swelling, there will generally be found within the mouth, at a point corresponding to the bright red central spot, a deep excavated ulcer, with irregular jagged edges, and a surface covered by a dark-brown shreddy slough. The gums opposite to the ulcer are of a dark color, covered with the putrilage from its surface, and in part destroyed, leaving the teeth loose, and the alveolæ denuded. Sometimes, especially if the disease is further advanced, no single spot of ulceration is recognizable, but the whole inside of the cheek is occupied by a dirty putrilage, in the midst of which large shreds of dead mucous membrane hang down. As the disease extends within the cheek, a similar process of destruction goes on upon the gum; the loosened teeth drop out one by one, and the alveolar process of the jaw loses its vitality for a more or less considerable extent, while sometimes a portion of the ramus of the jaw itself becomes necrosed. The saliva continues to be secreted profusely, but shows, by the changes which takes place in its characters, the progress of the disease. At first, though remarkable for its fetor, it is otherwise unaltered; but afterwards it loses its transparency, and receives from the putrefying tissues over which it passes, a dirty greenish or brownish color, and at the same time acquires a still more repulsive odor.

While the gangrene is thus going on inside the mouth, changes no less remarkable are taking place on the exterior of the face. The redness and swelling of the cheek extend, and the deep red central spot grows larger. A black point appears in its midst: at first it is but a speck, but it increases rapidly, still retaining a circular form; it attains the bigness of a sixpence, a shilling, a half-crown, or even a larger size. A ring of intense redness now encircles it, the gangrene ceases to extend, and the slough begins to separate. Death often takes place before the detachment of the eschar is complete, and it is fortunate when it does so, for sloughing usually commences in the parts left behind. The interior of the mouth is now exposed; its mucous membrane and the substance of the cheek hang down in shreds from amidst a blackening mass, and form one of the most loathsome spectacles that can be conceived; while the horrible stench which the mortified parts spread around, makes the task of watching the poor child as repulsive as it is distressing.

Happily it is not often that acute suffering of the child occurs to heighten the distress of the sad scene. Usually the patient has but little pain from the very first, but is generally more drowsy than natural, though sometimes the nights are restless; and in those cases in which gangrene of the mouth supervened in the course of typhoid fever, the delirium which existed before continued unmodified. The pulse grows feebler as the disease advances; but cheerfulness is often undisturbed, and the child will sit up in bed playing as happily with its toys as though it ailed nothing, l [illegible] e of the black eschar on the cheek has shown the case to be all but hopeless; or even after the slough has become detached, and the cavity of the mouth exposed. The desire for food, too, often continues unabated till within a few hours of the child's death, which generally takes place quietly, though sometimes it is preceded by convulsions.

Since gangrene of the mouth occurs in the course of a great variety of diseases, the only morbid appearances characteristic of it are those which result from the local mischief. On three occasions I dissected the gangrenous parts very carefully, and the alterations which presented themselves to my notice were precisely the same as have been described by MM. Rilliet and Barthez. The absorbent glands, both superficial and deepseated, on the affected side, are enlarged, and the cellular tissue of the cheek is infiltrated with serum, which is more abundant the nearer one approaches to the slough. In the substance of the eschar the distinction of parts is no longer easy, but with care the vessels and nerves may still be traced; and the reason why fatal hemorrhage so seldom cuts short the life of patients suffering from this affection is at once explained by the clot which plugs up the vessels for some distance on either side of the gangrenous mass. On one occasion I found the root of the tongue, the tonsils, pharynx, both surfaces of the epiglottis, and about an inch of the œsophagus, completely coated with a moderately firm, yellow false membrane about a line in thickness, easily detached, and leaving the subjacent mucous membrane only a little redder than natural. A few patches of a similar deposit existed in the larynx, but not continuous with that in the pharynx. In this case, great difficulty of deglutition had existed for three days before the death of the child. The association of diphtheria with gangrene of the mouth is, indeed, an accidental complication, and not one of frequent occurrence, but pneumonia is met with in so large a number of instances, that it must be looked on as more than an accidental occurrence, and probably as a result of the general deterioration of the circulating fluid to which the gangrene itself is due, rather than as owing to any cause acting especially on the lungs. It existed in 19 out of 21 cases, which formed the basis of MM. Rilliet and Barthez's[1] observations, and in 4 out of the 5 instances in which I was able to examine the bodies after death. In the 5th case, that of a girl, three years old, who died on the 10th day of cancrum oris, and on the 23d from the appearance of the rash of measles, though there was no pneumonia, yet the evidences of the relation of the affection to the class of blood diseases were most remarkable. The gangrene had been limited to the right side of the face; but in addition to a thrombus in the upper part of the right internal jugular vein, a large black unchanged clot occupied its lower part; and thrombus occupied the left internal jugular at its entrance into the subclavian vein. Both lungs were crepitant, but both were studded with a large number of small resistant nodules, for the most part of the size of a small pea, some of which were solitary, others aggregated, and were especially numerous in the dependent part of the lower lobe, and in its free anterior margin. On section, these nodules were found to be formed of

[1] Maladies des Enfans, vol. ii, p. 379.

form fluid, contained in the parenchyma of the lung, the tissue of which around them was neither inflamed nor condensed.

The arrest of the sloughing is the one point to which in the *treatment* of this affection the attention of all practitioners has been directed. The small amount of success which has attended their efforts is partly attributable to the circumstance that the affection has frequently been overlooked until it has already made considerable progress; in part also to the fact that, when recognized, the local remedies employed in order to check the gangrene have either been too mild, or have been applied with too timorous a hand. Unfortunately, too, there is considerable difficulty in applying any caustic effectually to the interior of the mouth; for the tense and swollen condition of the cheek prevents our obtaining easy access to the gangrenous parts. The use of chloroform, however, happily removes that other great difficulty which the severe pain attendant on the cauterization formerly opposed to its effectual performance. Ineffectual cauterization, indeed, is useless, or worse than useless; and though every endeavor should be made to prevent the needless destruction of healthy parts, yet of the two evils, that of doing too much is unquestionably less than that of doing too little. Of this, indeed, we need have the less fear, since the power of repair after the gangrene has once been arrested is most remarkable; and I saw some years since, in a case which was under the care of my colleague, Mr. Holmes, a perforation of the cheek near the angle of the lower lip contract from the size of a florin to a mere pinhole aperture, which at length closed, leaving a comparatively small amount of puckering of the adjacent parts, and certainly none of that frightful deformity which one would have fancied to be inevitable. It is of importance, moreover, not only that the cauterization should be done effectually, but also that it should be practiced early. M. Baron, indeed, speaks of incising the slough in the cheek, and then applying the actual cautery to the part; but I am not aware of any instance in which this suggestion has been acted on with a good result. When once the mortification has extended through the substance of the cheek, the chances of arresting its progress must be very few. As the sloughing advances from within outwards, it is to the interior of the mouth that our remedies must be applied; and since the advance of the disease is too rapid to allow of our trying mild means at first, and afterwards resorting, if necessary, to such as are more powerful, we must employ an agent sufficiently energetic at once to arrest its progress. Various caustics have been recommended for this purpose, but none appear to be so well fitted to accomplish it as the strong hydrochloric or nitric acid. I am accustomed to employ the latter, applying it by means of a bit of sponge, or of soft lint or tow, fastened to a quill; while I endeavor, by means of a spoon or of a spatula, to guard the tongue, and other healthy parts, as far as possible from the action of the acid. In one of the cases that I saw recover, the arrest of the disease appeared to be entirely owing to this agent; and though the alveolar processes of the left side of the lower jaw, from the first molar tooth backwards, died, and exfoliated, apparently from having been destroyed by the acid, yet it must be owned that life was cheaply saved even at that cost. Some increase of the swelling of the cheek almost invariably follows the application of this agent—a circumstance which may at first occasion unfounded apprehension lest the disease is worse. Twelve hours, however, must not be allowed to elapse without the mouth being carefully examined, in order to ascertain whether the disease has really been checked, or whether there is any appearance of mortification in the parts beyond the yellow eschar left by the first application of the acid. The cauterization may now be repeated if it appears necessary, and even though the disease had seemed completely checked; yet reliance must not be placed on the improvement continuing, but the mouth must be examined every twelve hours, for fear the mortification should spread unobserved. During the whole progress of the case the mouth must be syringed frequently with warm water, or with camomile tea mixed with a small quantity of the solution of chloride of lime, in order to free it from the putrid matters that collect within it, and to diminish as much as possible their offensive odor. Should the case go on well, the frequent repetition of the strong acid will be unnecessary; but the surface may still require its application in a diluted form, or it may suffice to syringe the mouth frequently with a chloride of lime or carbolic acid lotion, or to apply the chloride in powder once or twice a day, according to the suggestion of MM. Rilliet and Barthez. In all of the cases of this affection that have come of late years under my notice, I have likewise employed the chlorate of potash internally, but it has not appeared to exert much influence over it; and valuable though the remedy is in ulcerative stomatitis, yet I should scarcely feel disposed to rely upon it, to the exclusion of local treatment, in true gangrene of the mouth. Two cases, however, of cancrum oris succeeding to fever in children of twelve and thirteen years of age, were treated with most complete success by Dr. Burrows, in St. Bartholomew's Hospital, without the employment of any other local measures than a chloride of soda gargle, but with good diet, wine and chlorate of potash, in doses of ten grains every four hours.

During the whole course of treatment you have another indication to fulfil, namely, to support your patient's strength by nutritious diet, and by the employment of wine and other stimulants, and by the administration of quinine, or of the extract or tincture of bark, or of whatever form of tonic may seem best suited to the peculiarities of the case.

In conclusion, let me remind you that during the whole progress of the case your prognosis must be regulated by the state of the local disease, rather than by the urgency of the general symptoms. So long as the sloughing is unchecked the affection is tending rapidly to a fatal issue, and this even though the pulse is not very feeble, though the appetite is good, and the child still retains its cheerfulness.

It might seem to you to be an omission on my part, if I left the subject of inflammation and gangrene of the mouth, without some notice of the supposed influence of mercury in its production. There can be no doubt but that this preparation, even when given in small doses, has in a few instances produced severe ptyalism, inflammation of the mouth, loss of the teeth, and necrosis, more or less extensive, of the lower jaw. In some cases, too, the inflammation has terminated in gangrene of the cheek, which has presented many of the characters that we have just been noticing; and in such circumstances inquests have sometimes been held, and blame has been attached to the medical attendant for alleged want of caution in the administration of so powerful an agent as mercury. Now, although mercury should never be given without necessity, nor its administration continued without watching its effects most carefully, yet I cannot but regard the supervention of gangrene of the mouth during its use as merely an accidental coincidence, or else as the result of some peculiar idiosyncrasy of the patient, such as has been observed in the adult as well as in the child. Nearly 60,000 children, of all ages, have come under my care, during my connection with the Children's Infirmary and the Children's Hospital, and I have administered mercury to any of them who seemed to require it, but hardly ever saw salivation follow its employment before the completion of the first dentition; and never but once observed that medicine, at any age, to produce an affection of the mouth sufficiently serious to cause me a moment's anxiety. In that one instance, however, the death of the child, a boy aged four years and a half, was, I think, due to the employment of mercury.

An inconvenience—I do not know that it deserves a more serious designation—inseparable from the arrangement of subjects which I have adopted, is that we pass at once from diseases that are very hazardous, to others which are of a comparatively trifling character, or are the sources of discomfort rather than of severe suffering. Of this some of the ailments which remain for our consideration to-day are no inapt illustrations.

Inflammation of the soft palate, tonsils, and fauces, constituting *Cynanche Tonsillaris*, is not strictly limited to any age, nor attended with any special symptoms when it occurs in the child. It is, however, comparatively rare under twelve years of age, and is almost always less severe than at or after puberty, while I scarcely remember to have met with it under five years of age—a circumstance which attaches special importance to sore throat in young children, since it will usually be found to betoken the approach of scarlet fever or of diphtheria rather than the existence of simple inflammation of the tonsils.

But, though acute inflammation of the tonsils is unusual in early childhood, a sort of chronic inflammation of those glands, which leads to their very considerable enlargement, is far from uncommon; and this *hypertrophy of the tonsils*, which, in the adult, is little more than an inconvenience, is, in the child, not infrequently the cause of more serious evils. It is seldom traceable to any acute attack of angina, but usually comes on in children who are out of health, feeble, and strumous; or takes place slowly during the latter stages of the first dentition, the irritation of which appears in some cases to be its only exciting cause.

Unless accidentally discovered, the enlargement of the tonsils has usually become very considerable before it attracts much notice, and hence it is comparatively seldom observed in children under three years old, though M. Robert, a French surgeon,[1] who has written a very excellent paper on the subject, speaks of having noticed it as early as the sixth month.

---

[1] In the Bulletin Général de Thérapeutique, May and July, 1843.

One of the first symptoms that attract attention is the habitually loud snoring of the child during sleep, owing to the enlarged tonsils pressing up the velum, and thus obstructing the passage of air through the posterior nares, while at the same time the voice becomes thick; and both of these symptoms are remarkably aggravated during, and for some time after, even slight attacks of catarrh. An amount of enlargement of the tonsils sufficient to cause these symptoms is by no means uncommon, and if it does not exceed this extent the inconvenience to which it gives rise will in general disappear altogether with the development of the mouth and vocal organs at the period of puberty. Often, however, it is more considerable, and then the tonsils produce a degree of deafness, partly by actual pressure on the Eustachian tubes, partly by the state of habitual congestion which they maintain in the parts in their neighborhood; the respiration, moreover, becomes rather labored, and the child has a constant hacking cough, occasionally aggravated and paroxysmal—two symptoms which I have known to raise in more than one instance an unfounded apprehension of phthisis; and to lead in other cases, where some phthisical disease actually existed, to the expression of a more gloomy prognosis than was warranted by the amount of mischief in the lungs. Now and then the difficulty of respiration from mere enlargement of the tonsils has been so considerable as to threaten life. My friend and former colleague, Mr. Shaw, once had a little boy under his care, who, in addition to constant dyspnœa, suffered from occasional fits of suffocation arising from this cause; and one of these fits was so severe that in order to preserve the child's life it was necessary to perform laryngotomy. Recently, too, I saw a little boy two years old, whose life was in urgent danger from enlargement of the tonsils, which, however, were happily removed, and the otherwise inevitable opening of his windpipe was thus avoided.

The long existence of considerable enlargement of the tonsils, and the consequent almost complete obstruction to the passage of air through the nostrils, give rise to a peculiar alteration in the form of the parts thus thrown out of use. The nostrils become extremely small, narrow, and compressed; and the peculiar character which the physiognomy thus acquires is further increased by the accompanying modification in the development of the upper jaw. The superior dental arch remains very narrow, so as not to allow adequate room for the teeth, which consequently overlap each other very much, while at the same time the palate becomes unusually high and arched. Nor is this the only mode in which due development is interfered with; but it was noticed many years ago by Dupuytren that enlargement of the tonsils and the pigeon-breast very usually go together. The fact was confirmed by others, but I believe that Mr. Shaw[1] was the first person to offer an explanation of it. He pointed out how the obstacle to the free entrance of air into the lungs prevents their being filled at each inspiratory effort; so that a vacuum would be formed between them and the walls of the

---

[1] Medical Gazette, Oct. 23, 1841. See also his remarks in the article 'Thorax,' in the Cyclopædia of Anatomy and Physiology, p. 1039; and also those of M. Robert, in his paper already referred to.

chest, were it not that the pressure of the external air on the yielding parietes of the thorax forces them inwards to occupy the vacant space; and doing so most readily where their resistance is least, namely, at the commencement of the costal cartilages, produces the well-known lateral flattening of the thorax, and prominence of the sternum. The little boy whose case I have just mentioned as necessitating the operation of laryngotomy, gave in his own person a striking illustration of the correctness of the explanation which I have just given you. "On his admission into the hospital," says Mr. Shaw, "and for several weeks afterwards, it was observed that he had the pigeon-breast form of chest; but after his tonsils were excised, and his breathing had been perfectly free for some time, the sternum subsided to its proper level, and the thorax recovered its natural shape."

Enlargement of the tonsils, then, though at first sight it may appear a trivial ailment, is yet one which you must by no means neglect. A weakly child, whose tonsils are but slightly enlarged, will often get rid of his ailment as he gains health and strength, or at puberty will completely outgrow it. Any slight attack of cold, however, is apt to be followed by the increase or the return of the enlargement; and though this may often be kept in check by the application of powdered alum once or twice a day to the tonsils, or by touching them every day or two with the solid nitrate of silver, yet on the whole the tendency is towards the increase rather than the lessening of the evil. In no case, indeed, in which the hypertrophy of the tonsils is considerable, or of long standing, have I found these measures, or the painting the exterior of the throat just above the angle of the jaw with tincture of iodine, of much service, and excision of the tonsils is then the only remedy. Since, too, chloroform can be administered for this operation, as well as for any other, provided the mouth is kept open by a suitable gag, such as Mr. T. Smith has invented for operations on the cleft palate, there is no longer any necessity for waiting until the child is old enough to exercise some self-control. There is one circumstance which would always induce me, independent of other grounds, to advise the immediate excision of enlarged tonsils; namely, the existence of a constant or frequent cough, or the presence of any other symptom warranting a suspicion of phthisical disease in the chest. The enlarged tonsils not only mechanically interfere with the ready entrance of air into the lungs, but they keep up a constant irritation of the air-passages, and thus maintain a condition most unfavorable to the arrest of tubercular disease in the chest; while on more than one occasion I have seen most threatening symptoms disappear with great rapidity after their removal. If, after the tonsils have been removed, the chest is long in regaining its natural form, the use of dumb-bells, and the careful practice of gymnastic exercises, are often of much service. Dupuytren's recommendation, too, to stand the child with its back against a wall, and then placing the hand upon the most prominent part of the sternum, to press firmly upon it during each expiratory effort, remitting the pressure, during inspiration, in order that the child may fill its chest as completely as possible, I have found to be, in spite of its seeming roughness, extremely valuable as an additional means of [illegible] deformity of the pigeon-breast.

In the year 1840, Dr. Fleming, of Dublin,[1] called attention to the occasional occurrence of *abscess behind the pharynx*, which, pressing forward against the trachea, gives rise to urgent dyspnœa and sometimes even produces suffocation. Isolated cases of this accident had, indeed, fallen under the notice of previous observers, but by none, with the exception of Abercrombie,[2] had they been made the subject of special remark; while to Dr. Fleming unquestionably belongs the merit of having laid down distinct rules for its diagnosis, and clear directions for its treatment. Since Dr. Fleming's paper was published, many other instances of the affection have been recorded, especially by M. Mondière[3] and Duparcque,[4] the latter of whom also pointed out certain distinctive differences between cases where the matter accumulates behind the pharynx, and others in which it collects lower down, behind the œsophagus; and by Dr. Allin,[5] an American physician, who in a very able paper has collected the statistics of fifty-eight cases of the affection. Neither form of it is exclusively confined to early life; yet it happens in children with sufficient frequency to entitle it to some notice in a course of Lectures on the Diseases of Childhood.[6]

There are a few cases on record of the formation of retro-pharyngeal abscess as the result of direct injury; or of its occurrence in connec-

[1] Dublin Journal of Medical Science, vol xvii, p 41.
[2] Edinburgh Medical and Surgical Journal, vol. xv, 1819, p. 260.
[3] L'Expérience, Jan. 20, 27, and Février 3, 1842.
[4] Annales d'Obstétrique, Dec. 1842, p. 242.
[5] New York Journal of Medicine, vol. vii, Nov. 1851, p. 307.
[6] M. Mondière states that 11 out of 18 patients whose history he collected had not reached adult age, and that 7 were between 11 weeks and 4½ years old; and M. Duparcque mentions that in 10 out of the 30 cases to which he refers, the age of the patients was less than 4½ years. Unfortunately, however, M. Mondière's references are very incomplete, and M. Duparcque gives none at all. In this respect, Dr. Allin's paper leaves nothing to be desired. In all the instances in which the age is not expressly stated in his tables, it is yet apparent from the context that the patients had reached adult age, or at least had passed the period of puberty. If to the 58 cases that he mentions 11 others be added from different sources, we obtain the following results:

Under six months old,				5
Between six months and one year, or stated to be infants,				8
"	one year and two,			3
"	two	"	three,	2
"	three	"	five,	7
"	five	"	ten,	1
"	ten	"	fifteen,	2
Above			fifteen,	41
				69

Of the eleven additional cases it may be stated that four in the adult are recorded by M Mondière in his paper in L'Expérience; two in the child are recorded by Dr. Abercrombie in the Edinburgh Journal; one in an infant is related by Dr. Nolt in the Deutsche Klinik, and republished in Schmidt's Jahrbücher, vol. [illegible], 1852, p. 288; the remaining four are those which came under my own observation. To all these must be added the laborious compilation of M. Gautier, Des Abcès Rétropharyngiens, 8vo., Genève et Bâle, based on 97 observations, of which 95 are collected from different sources, 2 are original. I do not know, however, that the work suggests any important modification either of opinions or of practice.

tion with disease of the cervical vertebræ, an instance of which has come under my own observation. Leaving, however, these exceptional cases out of consideration, the affection may be said to present itself either as a sequela of fever, or as an idiopathic disease; the latter much more frequently than the former. In either case the characteristic indications of its existence are difficulty in swallowing and in breathing; often accompanied with a peculiar sound in respiration, though not with the stridor of croupy breathing, nor with the loud clangor of croupy cough. These symptoms are aggravated in the recumbent posture, any attempt to assume which is followed by immediate threatening of suffocation; though, in spite of this, the affection often continues with unabated severity, but yet without destroying life, for several days together, and presents in this respect a very important difference from the course of croup. Moreover, a remarkable stiffness of the neck, and retraction with immobility of the head, are present in many instances; while, though the glands are not enlarged, there is often a distinct swelling of the lateral parts of the neck, which is frequently more apparent on one than on the other side. If in these circumstances the finger is carried over the root of the tongue, and down towards the pharynx, a firm, somewhat elastic swelling will be detected, closing more or less completely the canal of the pharynx, and projecting forward over the opening of the glottis, so as to interfere with the access of air to the lungs. Sometimes on opening the mouth and depressing the tongue, the swelling can be distinctly seen almost or quite in the mesial line, pressing forward the velum palati, and obviously encroaching greatly on the entrance of the windpipe; but sometimes the tumor is situated too low down to be brought into view, while in other cases the mouth cannot be opened sufficiently to allow of the back of the throat being seen; and the tumor can then be detected only by the finger.

Four cases of the affection have come under my own observation, of which two were idiopathic, while in the other two the abscess was secondary to disease of the cervical vertebræ. The first patient was an idiot girl, 5½ years old, who was attacked by mild scarlatina on January 24th. During the course of the fever no remarkable symptom presented itself, but on its decline the child complained much of her mouth, frequently put her hand to it, and refused all except liquid food on account of its hurting her: but on looking into her throat, neither redness nor swelling was perceptible.

About February 7, swelling appeared near each angle of the lower jaw, but rather lower down than in the situation of the parotid gland. The swelling on the left side subsided on the application of a few leeches, but that on the right side increased, and at the same time the difficulty in deglutition became more distressing. By February
the dysphagia had become very much increased; the chil
swallow only by gulps, and at each effort she was
for breath; though at other times she lay in a
with labored respiration, and frothing slightly at
16th the child was still worse: her respirat
though not attended by the violent strug

often observed in cases of croup; a dirty-yellowish puriform [illegible] rendered frothy by air, now collected as a sort of foam at her [illegible] and deglutition almost choked her; but still there was no swelling [illegible] the tonsils, and the swelling of the side of the neck was so [illegible] did not think it possible for matter to be anywhere near the [illegible] On the following day she died, apparently as much from [illegible] as from asphyxia; it having for some days been impossible to give her more than a very small quantity of nourishment.

Immediately on dividing the cervical fascia on the right side, a quantity of thick, yellow, healthy pus poured out. This matter had burrowed close to the œsophagus to within little more than an inch of the clavicle; and also in an oblique direction behind the œsophagus, towards the left side, completely detaching it from its connections on the right side, though not on the left. It passed up behind the œsophagus and pharynx quite to the base of the skull, a few shreds of cellular tissue bathed in pus being all that remained of their posterior attachments. The tonsils were not enlarged, and the glottis was neither red nor swollen, but quite natural.

In the other case the affection was idiopathic, and the child a boy only eight months old. He became dull, drooped, and appeared to have a stoppage in his nose which rendered respiration difficult. After these vague symptoms had lasted for a month, the child began to swallow with difficulty, and deglutition sometimes was quite impossible, while his respiration, habitually difficult, became especially so when he was asleep. For five weeks he was treated for some supposed head affection with aperients, cold lotions to the head, &c.; and for another week, his symptoms having increased in severity, his case was regarded by another practitioner as one of bronchitis.

At the end of six weeks from his first indisposition the boy came under my notice. He was lying asleep in his mother's arms, his head rather thrown back, his face very pale and somewhat puffy, his mouth wide open, and his tongue turned up to the roof of his mouth. His breathing was labored, and attended with an extremely loud [illegible] cluck, not at all resembling the stridor of croup. This sound was louder and his breathing was more difficult when asleep than while awake, though both were very marked even then, and the entrance of air into the lungs was imperfect, especially on the left side.

The child sucked moderately well, leaving off to breathe very [illegible] quently, but managing to swallow, and not returning the milk [illegible] through the nose or mouth.

On passing my finger down the throat, I felt a hard body [illegible] root of the tongue, which seemed to occupy the space compl[illegible] on depressing the tongue I saw the uvula and velum forced [illegible] by a body completely occupying the isthmus of the fauces. [illegible] face of this tumor was generally red, but one or two [illegible] appeared on it, as if due to the presence of matter showing [illegible] thin investment; and a sharp-pointed bistoury, the bla[illegible] was defended by plaster, being plunged into it, nearly [illegible] yellow pus escaped, and the tumor immediately collapsed.

Air now entered the chest freely; the child sucked read[illegible] fell asleep, breathing quietly. The same evening, his respiration becoming once more less tranquil, his mother put her finger down his throat, and pressed, as she has been directed, against the side of the abscess, when a little pus escaped, with immediate relief to the child. On the day after the puncture the swelling was the size of a hazelnut, situated almost completely to the left of the mesial line. It felt hard to the touch, but a little pus could be squeezed out of it on pressure; and this continued to be the case for about three days, the swelling itself not entirely disappearing for nearly three weeks, though it produced no further symptom, and the child afterwards continued perfectly well. In one of the two cases which were secondary to disease of the cervical vertebræ, the abscess was not suspected during life, and was discovered only on a post-mortem examination in front of the spinal column, and reaching from the exposed odontoid process down to the apex of the lung. In the other case, the boy, aged 3½ years, with disease and deformity of the cervical spine, was admitted into the hospital on account of dyspnœa so urgent as to raise the question of the necessity for immediate tracheotomy. Happily the prominence at the back of the pharynx was detected; and from 3 to 4 ounces of pus were let out by an opening made at the back of the throat. The dyspnœa ceased at once; and the disease of the bones passed into a quiescent state during the child's stay of a month in the hospital.

Though in the first case the affection was not recognized during life, yet in it no less than in the second the characteristic symptoms of retro-pharyngeal abscess were clearly manifest. Such, too, I believe to be the case in the great majority of instances, though there are circumstances which now and then somewhat obscure the *diagnosis*. In the first place, there does not seem to be any uniformity in the character of the earlier symptoms—fever and cerebral disturbance attending it in some cases, dyspnœa being the prominent symptom in others: so that suspicion as to the real nature of the disease is often lulled to sleep, and the true import of the dysphagia or of the difficult breathing is not apprehended even when it becomes manifest. Moreover, the duration of the earlier symptoms is very various; and while the disease sometimes runs a chronic course, in other cases it attains an extreme degree of severity in two or three days, and even destroys life within that period by the intensity of the cerebral disturbance which sometimes accompanies it. Nor is this all: but dysphagia, though generally insisted on as a pathognomonic symptom of the affection, is sometimes not very remarkable; while now and then, as in one of the cases related by Dr. Abercrombie, and in that detailed by Dr. Peacock, it was altogether absent. In the latter case, too, owing to the peculiar form of the abscess, no tumor was discovered on inspection of the throat, nor was any perceived even on introduction of the finger. This, however, is an extremely unusual occurrence.

M. Duparcque enumerates the following symptoms as peculiar to cases where the abscess has formed behind the [illegible]. 1st. Severe pain, produced even by moderate pressure on [illegible] and upper part of the trachea. 2d. The circumstance that [illegible] produces entire suspension of respiration. 3[illegible] forwards and to the right. I cannot, however, from my own experience, say anything as to the special significance of these symptoms, though they are certainly such as one would anticipate meeting with, when the seat of the abscess is lower than the pharynx.

From the uncertainty of its early signs it is not possible to lay down any definite rules for the *treatment* of the first stage of this affection. In some instances, indeed, as in the case of a child one month old, related by Dr. Fleming, it is probably not recognised at all, but comes to an end by the matter making for itself a way before the more formidable symptoms of dyspnœa and difficult deglutition have manifested themselves, and escaping through the nares.

In the subsequent stages of the affection, when its nature has become clearly obvious, the indication is a very simple one; and there is seldom much difficulty in carrying it out. The abscess is to be punctured, and with the escape of the matter all the formidable symptoms at once disappear. For this purpose a sharp-pointed bistoury, the blade of which is protected by sticking-plaster wrapped round it, answers generally perfectly well; but for cases where the seat of the tumor is very low down, or where there is difficulty in opening the mouth, a trocar and a canula, such as Dr. Fleming employed for the purpose, may be preferable. The only additional caution which I have to offer for the subsequent management of the patient is, that for a day or two pressure be occasionally made with the finger on the tumor, in order to keep the sac of the abscess completely empty, since otherwise the matter may collect again, and give rise to a renewal of the former symptoms.

Inflammation of the parotid gland—the *Cynanche parotidea* of scientific writers, called *mumps* by the vulgar—is an affection met with among children and young persons, concerning which a few words only need be said; and I know of no more suitable place than the present for introducing it, though strictly speaking its affinities would seem to be rather with the exanthemata, and especially with measles. It attacks young persons after seven years of age, much oftener, and with much greater severity, than infants or very young children. Though it sometimes occurs as a sporadic affection, it is more commonly met with as an epidemic: and being likewise propagated by contagion, it not infrequently attacks most of the inmates of a boarding-school, or of any other public institution in which large numbers of the youth of either sex are collected together. Its period of incubation seems to vary extremely, from eight to twenty-one days being the alleged limits and twelve days the most usual time, in which it approximates to the law that governs the incubation period of measles.[2] The seat of the disease is in one or both parotid glands, and in the adjoining cellular tissue; but if the attack is at all severe, the submaxillary and other salivary glands generally become involved during its progress. It generally set in with the ordinary symptoms of slight fever or catarrh, which are followed in about twenty-four hours by

---

[1] Loc. cit., p. 58.

[2] Rilliet and Barthez, op. cit., 2d ed., vol. ii, p. 618; and Wagner, Jahrb. f. Kinderheilk, 1869, p. 335.

stiffness of the neck and pain about the lower jaw, any movement of which, either for the purpose of speaking or of mastication, is obviously attended with considerable suffering. At the same time, too, a swelling makes its appearance about the angle of the lower jaw, sometimes on one side only, at other times on both; and this swelling increasing rapidly in size, occasions great disfigurement of the face. The swelling is usually very tense, but the color of the skin is in general unaltered, except in some cases in which the glands on both sides, being swollen, and pressing much upon the veins, the return of blood from the head is impeded, and the face assumes a flushed appearance. If the swelling is very considerable, deglutition for a short time is rendered so difficult as to be almost impossible, and the tongue becomes dry from the child breathing with its mouth open; but the secretion of saliva is neither morbidly increased nor diminished. If the disease is severe, the child suffers much, is very feverish, and may even be lightheaded; but in the course of forty-eight hours from the appearance of the swelling it reaches its height, and the fever begins to subside and the swelling to diminish. The time of the final disappearance of the swelling is very variable, being five or six days in some cases, ten days or a fortnight in others; while in some instances the glands on one side are affected first, and when the attack is subsiding there, those of the opposite side become affected in a similar way, and the duration of the ailment is thus protracted. The occurrence of suppuration in the neighborhood of the gland is a rare termination of the inflammation; but is, I believe, oftener met with in infants and young children than in those who are approaching the period of puberty. On the other hand, metastasis of the disease from the parotid to the mamma, the testicle, or the brain, of all of which instances are recorded by different writers, appears to be rare in proportion to the tender age of the patient. The most formidable of those metastases, indeed—that to the brain—would seem to be an accident very seldom met with; and neither of it, nor of the translation of the disease to the mamma or the testicle, can I say anything from personal experience.

The *treatment* of this affection is in general very simple, and requires the judicious selection of precautionary measures rather than active interference. Mild antiphlogistic medicines, with the application of warmth locally, are all that is usually needed; and local depletion is neither necessary nor useful. The period during which much distress and much difficulty of deglutition exist is generally very short; so that even in severe cases it will be our wisest course to await the spontaneous subsidence of the swelling. If suppuration should take place in the cellular tissue about the gland, a warm poultice must be substituted for the fomentations previously employed. Even when the gland remains enlarged, as it sometimes does for some time after the subsidence of the febrile symptoms, it is yet in general the best plan to let it alone, since the swelling is sure eventually to disappear of its own accord.

With reference to the management of the metastases of the disease, I have no observations to make, further than that inflammation of the brain, however induced, is not an affection with which we can safely temporize; while a mild and palliative treatment will generally answer every purpose, when either the mamma or the testicle has become the seat of the affection.

LECTURE XXXIV.

DISEASES OF THE STOMACH.—Vomiting often symptomatic of disease elsewhere—Occasionally occurs suddenly in a previously healthy infant without signs of general illness—Its treatment—Is often one out of many symptoms of indigestion—Infantile dyspepsia—Sometimes connected with general debility of the system; at others, dependent on special disorder of the stomach—Its symptoms and treatment.

SOFTENING OF THE STOMACH.—Discovered after death in various degrees—Different theories as to its nature—Great frequency in early infancy—Explanation of this fact.

HÆMATEMESIS AND MELÆNA.—Very rare—Sometimes connected with injury to the child during labor—Their occurrence often difficult of explanation—Illustrative cases—Spurious hæmatemesis.

THE diseases to which the *stomach* is liable in early life are neither numerous nor important, although its functions are more or less disordered in the course of most of the affections of childhood. *Vomiting*, indeed, is more frequent in the infant than in the adult, and the greater irritability of the stomach continues even after the first few months of existence are past, and does not completely cease during the early years of childhood. Hence it happens, as we have already seen, that vomiting is sometimes one of the first symptoms of inflammation of the lungs or pleura; while it frequently ushers in the eruptive fevers, and marks the early stages of cerebral disease. Causes more purely local produce a similar effect, and vomiting often attends upon infantile diarrhœa, and is associated with signs of intestinal disorder, especially when such disorder has been excited by improper food. But besides these cases, in which the disorder of the stomach is either the result of disease seated elsewhere, or in which the disturbance of its function is sufficiently explained by the nature of the ingesta, instances are sometimes observed in which the stomach becomes so irritable as almost always to reject its contents, or in which, though the food taken is not brought up again, the organ is unable to effect its digestion.

It sometimes happens that young infants are suddenly seized with vomiting, which, though violent, and frequently repeated, is attended by few or no indications of general intestinal disorder. The child in such cases seems still anxious for the breast; but so great is the irritability of the stomach, that the milk is either thrown up unchanged immediately after it has been swallowed, or it is retained only for a very few

minutes, and is then rejected in a curdled state; while each application of the child to the breast is followed by the same result. It will generally be found, when this accident takes place in the previously healthy child of a healthy mother, that it has been occasioned by some act of indiscretion on the part of its mother or nurse. She perhaps has been absent from her nursling longer than usual, and, returning tired from a long walk, or from some fatiguing occupation, has at once offered it the breast, and allowed it to suck abundantly; or the infant has been roused from sleep before its customary hour, or it has been overexcited or overwearied at play, or, in hot weather has been carried about in the sun without proper protection from its rays.

The infant in whom, from any of these causes, vomiting has come on, must at once be taken from the breast, and, for a couple of hours, neither food nor medicine should be given to it. It may then be offered a teaspoonful of cold water; and should the stomach retain this, one or two more spoonfuls may be given in the course of the next half-hour. If this is not rejected, a little isinglass may be dissolved in the water, which must still be given by a teaspoonful at a time, frequently repeated; or cold barley-water may be given in the same manner. In eight or ten hours, if no return of vomiting takes place, the experiment may be tried of giving the child its mother's milk, or cow's milk diluted with water, in small quantities, and from a teaspoon. If the food thus given does not occasion sickness, the infant may in from twelve to twenty-four hours be restored to the breast; with the precaution, however, of allowing it to suck only very small quantities at a time, lest the stomach being overloaded, the vomiting should again be produced.

In many instances where the sickness has arisen from some accidental cause, such as those above referred to, the adoption of these precautions will suffice to restore the child's health. If, however, other indications of gastric or intestinal disorder have preceded the sickness, or are associated with it, medicine cannot be wholly dispensed with. According to the age of the child, a quarter, half, or a whole grain of calomel may be laid upon the tongue, while sucking is forbidden, and the plan already recommended is in other respects strictly carried out. If the vomiting has already continued for several hours before the adoption of any treatment, a small mustard poultice may likewise be applied to the epigastrium. In about a couple of hours after the calomel has been given, the child may have a teaspoonful of a mixture containing small doses of the bicarbonate of potash and chloric ether, or of ether and of hydrocyanic acid; and this may be continued every three or four hours so long as any unusual irritability of the stomach remains.

Sickness, however, is not always a solitary symptom, unattended by other indications of gastric disorder, but is sometimes associated with the signs of general impairment of the digestive powers. In its graver forms, *indigestion* is associated with greatly impaired nutrition, and with all those serious results which are characteristic of the atrophy of young children. But it sometimes happens that, though the child does not lose much flesh, yet digestion is ill performed, and various dyspeptic symptoms appear, which would be troublesome rather than alarming, if it were not that they are often connected with the strumous di-

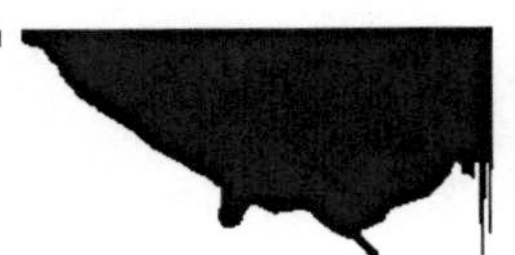

athesis, and are the first indications of a state of constitution in which, after the lapse of a few months, pulmonary phthisis is very apt to supervene.

In some of these cases there is complete anorexia, the infant caring neither for the breast nor for any other food that may be offered it. It loses the look of health, and grows pale and languid, although it may not have any especial disorder either of the stomach or of the bowels. It sucks but seldom, and is soon satisfied; and even of the small quantity taken, a portion is often regurgitated almost immediately. This state of things is sometimes brought on by a mother's overanxious care, who, fearful of her infant taking cold, keeps it in a room too hot or too imperfectly ventilated. It follows, also, in delicate infants, on attacks of catarrh or diarrhœa, but is then for the most part a passing evil which time will cure. In the majority of cases, however, the loss of appetite is associated with evidence of the stomach's inability to digest even the small quantity of food taken, and there exists more or less marked gastric or intestinal disorder. Anorexia, too, is far from being a constant attendant upon infantile dyspepsia; but in still more numerous instances, although the power of assimilating the food is in a great measure lost, yet there is an unnatural craving for it, and the infant never seems so comfortable as when sucking. But though it sucks much, the milk evidently does not sit well upon the stomach; for soon after sucking the child begins to cry, and appears to be in much pain until it has vomited. The rejection of the milk is followed by immediate relief; but at the same time by the desire for more food, and the child can often be pacified only by allowing it to suck again. In other cases, vomiting is of much less frequent occurrence, and there is neither craving desire for food, nor much pain after sucking, but the infant is distressed by frequent acid or offensive eructations; its breath has a sour or nauseous smell, and its evacuations have a most fetid odor. The condition of the bowels that exists in connection with these different forms of dyspepsia is variable. In cases of simple anorexia, the debility of the stomach is participated in by the intestines; their peristaltic action is feeble, and constipation is of frequent occurrence, though the evacuations do not always present any marked deviation from their character in health. Constipation, however, though a frequent, is not an invariable attendant on indigestion, but the bowels in some cases act with due regularity. If the infant is brought up entirely at the breast, the evacuations are usually liquid, of a very pale yellow color, often extremely offensive, and contain shreds of curdled milk, which, having escaped through the pylorus, pass unchanged along the whole tract of the intestines. In many instances, however, the infant having been observed not to thrive at the breast, arrowroot or other farinaceous food is given to it, which the digestive powers are quite unable to assimilate, and which gives to the motions the appearance of putty or pipeclay, besmeared more or less abundantly with intestinal mucus. The evacuations are often parti-colored, and sometimes one or two unhealthy motions are followed by others which appear perfectly natural; while attacks of diarrhœa often come on, and the matters discharged are then watery, of a dark, dirty-green color, and exceedingly offensive odor.

Dyspeptic infants, like dyspeptic adults, often continue to keep up their flesh much better than could be expected, and in many cases eventually grow up to be strong and healthy children. Still, the condition is one that not merely entails considerable suffering upon the child, but, by its continuance, seriously impairs the health, renders the child but little able to bear up against any intercurrent disease, and develops the seeds of latent phthisis.

Within the space that can be allotted to each subject in these lectures, it is not possible to do more than just glance at some of the main points to be borne in mind in the *treatment* of infantile dyspepsia. Those cases, the chief symptom of which consists in the loss of appetite, usually require and are much benefited by a generally tonic plan of treatment. All causes unfavorable to health must be examined into, and, as far as possible, removed. It must be seen that the nursery is well ventilated, and that its temperature is not too high; while it will often be found that no remedy is half so efficacious as change of air. Next, it must not be forgotten that the regurgitation of the food is due in great measure to the weakness and consequent irritability of the stomach; and care must therefore be taken not to overload it. If these two points are attended to, benefit may then be looked for from the administration of tonics. These tonics may either be such as the infusion of orange-peel with a few drops of sulphuric acid and of some tincture;[1] or, should any disposition to diarrhœa have appeared, the extract with the compound tincture of bark will be preferable;[2] or, if the stomach is very irritable, the liquor cinchonæ in combination with small doses of hydrocyanic acid[3] may be given with advantage, when any other medicine would be rejected. As the general health improves, the constipated condition of the bowels so usual in these cases will by degrees disappear. Even if the symptom should call for medical interference, it is not by drastic purgatives that its cure must be attempted. A soap suppository will sometimes excite the bowels to daily action; or friction of the abdomen twice a day with warm oil, or with a liniment composed of one part of Linimentum Saponis, one of olive oil, and two of tincture of aloes, will sometimes have the same effect. Should it become necessary to give aperients internally, the decoction of aloes sweetened with licorice, and mixed with caraway or aniseed water, generally answers the purpose very well;[4] while the employment

---

[1] (No. 24.)

℞. Acid. Sulph. dil., ♏xvj.
Tinct. Aurantii, ʒj.
Syrupi, ʒj.
Inf. Aurantii, ℥j.
Aq. Cinnamomi, ʒij. M.

A teaspoonful three times a day for a child a year old.

[2] See Formula No. 4, p. 57.

[3] See Formula No. 21, p. 400.

[4] (No. 25.)

℞. Decoct. Aloës Co, ʒvj.
Extr. Glycyrrhizæ, ℈j.
Aquæ Anisi, ʒij. M.

One or two teaspoonfuls when required for a child a year old.

of mercurials must be restricted to cases in which there is [illegible] deficiency in the biliary secretion.

A different plan must be adopted in those forms of indigestion which depend on some cause other than mere debility of the system. The rule, indeed, which limits the quantity of food to be taken at one time is no less applicable here, for the rejection of the curdled milk may be the result of nothing more than of an effort which nature makes to reduce the work that the stomach has to do within the powers of that organ. But when, notwithstanding that due attention is paid to this important point, uneasiness is always produced by taking food, and is not relieved till after the lapse of twenty minutes or half an hour, when vomiting takes place or when the infant suffers much from flatulence and from frequent acid or nauseous eructations, it is clear that the symptoms are due to something more than the mere feebleness of the system.

It is not, however, in these cases, the mere fact of the infant vomiting its food, or of the milk so vomited being rejected in a coagulated state, which indicates the stomach to be disordered, but it is the circumstance of firmly coagulated milk being rejected with much pain, and after the lapse of a considerable interval from the time of taking food, which warrants this conclusion.[1] The coagulation of its casein is the first change which the milk of any animal undergoes when introduced into the stomach, though the coagulum formed by human milk is soft, flocculent, and not so thoroughly separated from the other elements of the fluid as the firm hard curd of cow's milk is from the whey in which it floats. In a state of health, the abundantly secreted gastric juice speedily redissolves the chief part of the casein, while the subsequent addition to it of the alkaline bile converts it into an albuminate of soda; and being thus assimilated as nearly as possible to the characters of one of the chief elements of the blood, it is easily absorbed by the lacteals, and passes into the mass of the circulating fluid.

Milk tends, however, to undergo changes spontaneously, which produce its coagulation, and the occurrence of these changes is greatly favored by a moderately high temperature, such as that which exists in the stomach. But the alterations in the fluid which attend upon this spontaneous coagulation are very different from those which are brought about in it by the vital processes of digestion. A free acid becomes developed abundantly within it, and the acid thus generated shows none of the solvent power of gastric juice, but by its presence impedes rather than favors digestion. Every nurse is aware that a very slight acidity of the milk with which the infant is fed will suffice to occasion vomiting, stomach-ache and diarrhœa; and the result, as far as the child is concerned, must be much the same whether the acetous fermentation had begun in the milk before it was swallowed, or whether it commences afterwards, in consequence of the disordered

[1] The physiology and chemistry of the digestion of milk will be found fully treated in the article Milch, in Wagner's Handwörterbuch der Physiologie, [illegible] Elsässer's Essay, Ueber die Magenerweichung der Säuglinge, 8vo., Stuttgart, [illegible] They are the authorities for the statements in the text.

condition of the stomach, and the absence of a healthy secretion of gastric juice.

The nature of the food is the first point that requires attention in the management of these cases of infantile dyspepsia. If the child had been fed on cow's milk, the symptoms may have been produced by the gastric juice being unable to redissolve the hard curd formed by the coagulation of its casein. In this case the infant may sometimes be restored to health without the employment of any medicine, by diluting the milk, by substituting asses' milk for it, or even by giving whey for a day or two, until the stomach recovers its powers of digesting casein. The addition of a small quantity of some alkali—as the carbonate of potash, or prepared chalk, or lime-water—to the milk, is another precaution which should not be omitted, since, while it does not at all interfere with digestion, it tends to prevent the matters taken into the stomach so readily undergoing the acetous fermentation. The indiscriminate employment of alkalies as medicines is, however, not to be recommended;—they are of service combined with minute doses of laudanum, when the irritability of the stomach is extreme, as in those cases which were referred to at the commencement of this lecture;—they are also useful in cases of a more chronic kind, where the sour smell of the evacuations, and the frequent occurrence of acid eructations, indicate the presence of an excess of acid in the *primæ viæ*. I do not give them by themselves, but in combination with some tonic, as the infusion of calumba, to which the extract of dandelion and the tincture of rhubarb may be added, if, as sometimes happens,[1] the functions of the liver appear to be but ill performed.

Vomiting of the milk in a coagulated state is no proof of the presence of an excess of acid in the stomach. It may indicate a condition in which the secretion of the gastric juice is either disordered or insufficient, and in which the acetous fermentation is set up in the contents of the stomach, because the organ is inadequate to the proper discharge of those vital functions which would prevent its occurrence. Such cases—and they are many, and among them may be classed all those in which the breath is offensive and the infant is distressed by nauseous eructations—are benefited by the mineral acids in combination with some bitter infusion; as, the infusion of cascarilla with hydrochloric acid,[2] and recently I have employed Morson's pepsin wine, in ten or fifteen minim doses three or four times a day, with considerable advan-

---

[1] (No. 26.)

℞. Sodæ Sesquicarb., gr. xxiv.
Extr. Taraxaci, ℈ij.
Tinct. Rhei, ʒj.
Inf. Calumbæ, ℥xj.
Aquæ Carui, ℥iv. M.
Two teaspoonfuls twice a day.

[2] (No. 27.)

℞. Acid. Hydrochlor. dil., ♏xvj.
Syr. Aurantii, ʒj.
Tinct. Aurantii, ʒj.
Inf. Cascarillæ, ℥x. M.
[...]ul three times a day.

tage. I have often observed the action of the bowels become [illegible] and the appearance of the evacuations healthy, during the [illegible] tion of these remedies. The use of mercurials, indeed, [illegible] resorted to in order to correct some real or fancied disorder [illegible] has become too indiscriminate a practice. The diarrhœa with [illegible] pale light yellow evacuations, that comes on in some of these [illegible] often arrested by a spare diet and by the administration of [illegible] doses of sulphate of magnesia and tincture of rhubarb; such [illegible] grains of the former and ten minims of the latter three times a [illegible] a child a year old.[1] In cases where diarrhœa has been long continued, or where the evacuations are very white, and resemble putty, mercurials are generally needed; as they are also, in those cases where the horribly offensive odor of the evacuations proves that the contents of the intestines have been undergoing a process akin to putrefaction. The mercury and chalk powder, in small doses night and morning, is the mildest preparation that can be given. Sometimes, however, it causes nausea or vomiting, and very small doses of calomel must then be substituted for it; while, if the mercurial should excite the bowels to overaction, this tendency may generally be checked by combining it with Dover's powder.

The same rules must guide us in the management of children in whom, though they are still at the breast, the symptoms of dyspepsia make their appearance. Disorder of the digestive function is, however, much less common before weaning than afterwards. It may depend on the mother's milk being from some cause or other ill adapted to the support of the child; and hence the condition of the parent's health must in all these cases engage our attention.

With these general rules I must dismiss the subject of indigestion, content to have pointed out the principles that should guide you; it must be left to your own experience in future years to supply the details. I have touched on the subject, too, only with reference to the infant, for as the child grows older and its food becomes the same as that of the adult, the symptoms of disorder of its digestive organs become the same too, and require a similar treatment.

In most works on the diseases of childhood we used to meet with an enumeration of rather obscure symptoms which were stated to indicate the existence of gastritis or gastro-enteritis, and to be followed by more or less considerable *softening of the stomach or intestines*, or of both. A similar condition of the stomach was observed by John Hunter in the adult, and was conceived by him to be the result of the action of the gastric juice upon the tissues after death. The carefully conducted experiments of Dr. Carswell have completely confirmed the opinion of Mr. Hunter with reference to the agent by which this softening is effected; while they have further shown that it is independent of the

---

[1] (No. 28.)

℞. Magnesiæ Sulphatis, ʒj.
Tinct. Rhei, ʒij.
Syr. Zingiberis, ʒj.
Aquæ Carui, ʒix. M.

A teaspoonful three times a day. For children a year [illegible]

person's previous health. Some writers, among whom may be mentioned those eminent authorities M. Cruveilhier and Professor Rokitansky, have however dissented in a measure from these views, and have endeavored to distinguish between two kinds of softening, one of which they regard as a post-mortem occurrence; the other, which is that chiefly observed in infancy, they consider to be the result of disease. This distinction, however, is now generally, and I believe correctly, regarded as untenable, and softening of the stomach in both its forms may be considered as equally due to change in the tissues after death.[1]

This conclusion, however, has not been definitively arrived at sufficiently long to warrant me in passing over the condition without some notice, or without reference to the grounds which have led to the opinion which I have just expressed so unhesitatingly.

The state is met with varying in degree from a slight diminution in the consistence of the mucous membrane, to a state of complete diffluence of all the tissues of the organ, in which it breaks down under the finger on the slightest touch, or even gives way of its own accord, and allows of the escape of its contents into the abdomen. When the change is not far advanced, the exterior of the stomach presents a perfectly natural appearance, but on laying it open, a colorless or slightly brownish, tenacious mucus, like the mucilage of quince-seeds, is found closely adhering to its interior, over a more or less considerable space at the great end of the organ, and extending along the edges of its rugæ. This mucus is easily washed away, and the muscular coat of the stomach in those parts to which it had adhered is then left almost or altogether bare, and denuded of its mucous membrane. When the change has gone further, the stomach at its great end presents a semi-transparent appearance, though not uniformly so, but in streaks running in the direction of the rugæ; the destruction of the tissues having in those situations reached deeper than elsewhere, and involved a portion of the muscular as well as the mucous coat of the organ. If roughly handled, the stomach in many cases gives way, an irregular rent taking place at its great end, where the coats of the organ are found to be soft and pulpy, and to break down easily under the finger. In the next degree, the coats of the stomach are found to have been already dissolved in some parts, so that the contents of the organ have escaped into the abdominal cavity. The whole of the great end of the stomach, and a considerable extent of the posterior wall, are now reduced to a gelatinous condition, in which no distinction of tissues is apparent; and the parts thus altered are either transparent and colorless, or else of a pale rose-red hue. The interior of the organ sometimes presents a similar tinge, even beyond the limits to which the softening of its tissue has extended. This, however, is by no means constantly observed, while in no case is there any injection of the vessels of the stomach, or any evidence of its having been the seat of real inflammatory action. The opaque and brownish appearance of the

[1] No better summary of the reasons for this opinion is given anywhere than by Vogel, in his Lehrbuch der Kinderkrankheiten, 4th ed., Erlangen, 1869, p. 121.

tissues—characteristic of pulpy softening—is but seldom met with in infancy.

Softening of the intestines, though much less frequent than softening of the stomach, is observed in similar circumstances, and presents the same characters. The exterior of the intestines is generally anæmic, and the softened parts show no traces of increased vascularity; they are either colorless or of a pale rose hue. The mucous membrane of their interior is neither ulcerated nor abraded, but is found in some parts to be much softened, or even altogether absent in small patches. The muscular coat too is sometimes destroyed, though no abrupt edge marks the limits of its destruction, but there is a gradual attenuation of the tissue down to the spot where the peritoneum is laid completely bare. Several of these softened patches are generally met with in the same subject, and at some of them the bowel is often found to have given way, or it breaks down in the attempt to lay open its cavity.[1]

The allegation, that softening of the stomach in the adult occurs with greater frequency in persons who have died from some diseases than in those who have died from others, has led to the hypothesis that in the former case a diseased and superabundant secretion of gastric juice during the life of the individual had caused the softening of his stomach after death. The same hypothesis has been applied to account for its peculiar frequency in infancy, since at no period of life is gastric disorder so common as then. Some writers have advanced still further, and have endeavored to connect the existence of a softened state of the stomach after death with certain well-marked symptoms of disorder of its functions: for my own part, however, I have not been able to discover any peculiarity in the character of such symptoms, nor even any constancy in their occurrence.

The much greater frequency of softening of the stomach and intestines in infancy and early childhood than in adult age, and the greater amount and wider extent of the alterations, have received considerable elucidation from the researches of Dr. Elsässer.[2] He found that a much more rapid action upon animal tissues than that exerted by the gastric juice, was put forth by any substance capable of undergoing the acetous fermentation, combined with pepsin. Such substances are furnished by the milk as well as by the various farinaceous and saccharine matters on which infants almost exclusively subsist. The tendency of these substances to undergo the acetous fermentation is checked by the presence of healthy gastric juice, while, as we know by experience, it takes place very readily in infants who are dyspeptic, and to a very

[1] The very elaborate work of MM. Herrich and Popp, Der plötzliche Tod aus inneren Ursachen, 8vo., Regensburg, 1848, contains, at p. 380, a table of [illegible] in which softening of the stomach was found after death from different causes [illegible] at various ages. In no instance were symptoms observed that would have [illegible] any one to pronounce beforehand that softening of the stomach would be [illegible] after death. In by far the greater number of the cases the stomach was [illegible] showing that the occurrence very often did not depend on digestion going on [illegible] time of death; while the period of childhood, the rapid course of the fatal [illegible] and death from cerebral affections, were the only circumstances which appeared [illegible] have any clearly appreciable influence in favoring its production.

[2] Die Magenerweichung der Säuglinge, 8vo. Stuttgart, 1846.

remarkable degree in many cases of infantile diarrhœa. Facts bear out to a very great extent the opinion of M. Elsässer. Out of 104 cases of softening of the stomach that came under the notice of two very eminent German physicians, MM. Herrich and Popp, 72 were met with in the period of infancy or early childhood. My own notes on this point, though too few to be of any weight, yet point to a similar conclusion; for of 14 cases of softening of the stomach or intestines, or of both, observed out of a total of 61 cases in which the condition of those viscera was carefully recorded, 11 were met with in children under two years of age; while out of a total of 389 examinations of infants under the age of three months in the Foundling Hospital at Vienna, M. Bednar[1] met with 100 instances of softening of the stomach or intestines; in 61 of which death had taken place from diarrhœa. I need scarcely add that this theory of M. Elsässer's is only supplementary to Mr. Hunter's, and is perfectly reconcilable with the correctness of his observations, and of those of Dr. Carswell.

Among those rare diseases, too seldom met with for any person to have what can be called real experience about them, may be mentioned the *vomiting and purging of blood* occasionally observed in infants and young children. In the greater number of cases the occurrence has taken place within a few days[2] after birth, sometimes within a few hours, and in some instances has followed a tedious or difficult labor, in which the head of the child has been much compressed, or its abdomen has been pressed on, or otherwise injured during attempts at its extraction; while in other cases the difficult establishment of respiration has seemed to be the predisposing cause of the hemorrhage. Very often, however, no reason can be assigned for it; and the vomiting of blood, sometimes associated with its discharge per anum, has been unattended with other indications of disorder of the abdominal viscera. In most cases the hæmatemesis has not recurred above two or three times in any quantity; and the children, though at first very much exhausted by the loss of blood, have, in about half the cases, eventually recovered. In a few instances, however, recovery has been partial, and the children have sunk into a cachectic condition, in which they died. When death has taken place from the immediate effects of the hemorrhage, the liver and the abdominal veins have sometimes been found gorged with blood, and blood has been found within the intestines, or extravasated within their coats, constituting what has been termed abdominal apoplexy—appearances which have been supposed to indicate that some impediment to the establishment of the new course of the circulation which the blood should follow after birth, had given rise to the accident.

I have nothing to say about the treatment of an accident which in general occurs too causelessly to furnish indications for its prevention,

---

[1] Die Krankheiten der Neugebornen, &c., 8vo, p. 76. Wien, 1850.

[2] Within 6 days in 17, and within 36 hours in 9 out of 20 cases collected by M. Rilliet, in his Essai sur les Hémorrhagies Intestinales chez les Nouveaux-nés, published in Gaz. Méd de Paris, No. 53, 1848; and reproduced in vol. ii of the second edition of his and M. Barthez's Traité des Maladies des Enfans, pp. 295–310.

and too suddenly to allow of the employment of measures [illegible] but I will give you the result of my scanty experience [illegible] which amounts to three cases. In one of these cases the [illegible] occurred without apparent cause soon after birth, and [illegible] ously; while in the other two it took place at a later period [illegible] proached in its characters more nearly to similar occurrence [illegible] age.

The subject of the first observation was a male child, who [illegible] of a healthy mother, after a short and easy labor, at 11 A.M. on [illegible] tember 23, 1845. The infant was well grown, and apparently [illegible] and healthy, and continued so till 2½ A.M. on the 24th, when, [illegible] any previous sickness, or other indication of illness, he vomited [illegible] half a teacupful of blood. This vomiting was not attended [illegible] pain, nor was any large quantity of blood rejected afterwards, [illegible] child continued at intervals of not more than an hour to throw up [illegible] quantities of dark greenish matter, resembling meconium, and [illegible] with mucus; and on the morning of the 25th he vomited a small [illegible] tion of coagulated blood, as big as the top of the little finger. [illegible] the time of the child's birth and the morning of the 25th, the [illegible] acted seven times; the motions were rather scanty, and consisted [illegible] tirely of meconium. The child sucked well, did not appear in [illegible] its surface was warm, and its abdomen neither full nor tender. [illegible] matters vomited did not decompose, although they were kept for [illegible] days; and when examined under the microscope, they were seen to [illegible] made up of a great number of granular globules, with which [illegible] termixed some scales of tessellated epithelium.

The 27th of September was the last day on which the dark [illegible] matter like meconium was vomited; but the child continued to [illegible] occasionally until October 7, although the attacks of sickness [illegible] seem to be excited by sucking, but occurred in general when the [illegible] was empty, and ended with the rejection of a small quantity of [illegible] occasionally of a greenish color. The bowels were rather [illegible] and the evacuations for the first week after the child's birth [illegible] very dark-colored; they afterwards assumed a more natural color, [illegible] the bowels remained very constipated during the whole of the [illegible] life. The child never throve; it lost flesh, occasionally vomited [illegible] milk, had a frequent and troublesome cough; its strength decayed, [illegible] it died exhausted on April 28, 1846, at the age of seven months. [illegible] examining the body, nothing was found to explain the child's ill[illegible] there was no tubercle in any organ; the viscera were anæmic; no [illegible] of inflammatory action was visible anywhere. A few lobules in [illegible] lungs were in a collapsed condition; the small intestines [illegible] several recent intussusceptions; and the stomach was remarkably [illegible] and undeveloped in form as well as in size; but no other [illegible] pearances existed in any part of the body.

In the second case, the child, likewise a boy, had perfect [illegible] health till he was two months old, when he began to appear [illegible] his chest, and had frequent though not severe cough. At [illegible] ten weeks, he brought up a small quantity of dark blood [illegible] ing, and afterwards had frequent attacks of retching and [illegible] dependent of cough. During these attacks he brought up a dark-red fluid, like blood, sometimes in as large a quantity as two-thirds of a teacupful. On February 17, 1844, after these symptoms had continued for four days, I saw the child, whose face was slightly flushed, and the expression of his countenance dull. His abdomen was full and rather tender, especially in the right hypochondriac region; his urine was very high-colored, and his evacuations were quite white. From February 17 to April 13, the child remained under my care, and during this time the above-mentioned symptoms continued, although with a gradual amelioration in the child's condition. Within a week after I first saw him, he had a severe conslusive seizure, and attacks of a similar kind occurred a great many times afterwards, independent of any obvious cause. The bowels were always constipated; the evacuations usually very white, though occasionally almost black, sometimes accompanied with a slight discharge of blood; and blood was now and then voided unmixed with fecal matter. The stomach became very irritable, and the child suffered from frequent vomiting; the matters rejected being untinged with blood for days together, and then, without any apparent reason, blood was abundantly mingled with them. Sometimes the infant cried much, and appeared in very great pain; and these attacks often terminated in the rejection of a considerable quantity of nearly pure blood.

The face soon lost its flush, and became pale; but the puffiness continued, and was evidently due to a slight degree of anasarca. From the tender age of the child, I was unable to obtain any of his urine, in order to ascertain whether or not it contained albumen. The treatment followed was directed to diminish the abdominal tenderness, by the application of a couple of leeches over the right hypochondrium, and to overcome the constipated state of the bowels, and induce the healthy action of the liver, by the employment of small doses of mercurials, and of the sulphate of magnesia, to which it became sometimes necessary to add the administration of an active purgative. In May, 1844, the child was sent to Margate, where the convulsive attacks and other symptoms altogether ceased. On his return to London, after a stay of six months at the seaside, his health failed—partly, as it seemed, in consequence of his mother's poverty preventing her from supplying him with proper food. In November, 1846, when much out of health, and suffering from diarrhœa, he came again under my care, but died suddenly of hemorrhage into the arachnoid.[1] There was no appearance in the abdominal viscera after death which threw any light on the cause of the hæmatemesis and melæna, from which the child had suffered for so many months during his early infancy.

The subject of the third observation was a little boy, the child of a healthy father but strumous mother, who had thriven well at the breast till he was four months old, when he cut some of his incisor teeth; and his health had seemed less good since that period. There was, however, no marked ailment until he was weaned at nine and a half months; but after that he drooped, became much less cheerful, and his evacua-

---

[1] The particulars of his last illness are given in Lecture V, p. 66.

tions were seen to be white and unhealthy. He was in this [illegible] when ten months and a week old; his abdomen, though large, was generally soft; but pressure in the left hypochondrium seemed to give pain; and careful examination detected a tumor there of the size of a small apple. On the evening of the same day on which he was first seen, the bowels having acted spontaneously in the morning, the child suddenly, and without any effort or straining, voided between three and four ounces of pure blood, partly fluid, partly coagulated. The discharge of blood occasioned faintness, and left the child very pallid, but apparently not suffering. He slept tolerably well during the night, but the ensuing morning at 7 A.M. voided nearly the same quantity of blood as on the previous evening, unmixed with fæces, but apparently somewhat diluted with intestinal mucus. Some warm water thrown up the bowel returned, stained with blood, but unmixed with fecal matter, as did a second enema administered six hours afterwards. In the course of the same day he had two scanty evacuations, both composed almost entirely of bloody mucus, and with such slight admixture of adhesive, white, fecal matter, almost like putty in appearance, that I did not feel my anxiety lest the case should turn out to be one of intussusception of the intestines entirely removed until nearly twenty-four hours afterwards, when, after a dose of castor oil, two tolerably healthy evacuations were passed. The tenderness of the abdomen had now completely subsided, the swelling in the left hypochondrium (possibly the enlarged and congested spleen) had entirely disappeared; and the child, in spite of the quantity of blood it had lost, appeared much better than before the hemorrhage occurred.

This amendment, however, was not of long duration; no hemorrhage, indeed, returned, but the child had an attack of very severe diarrhœa, attended with great emaciation and much abdominal pain, which lasted for nearly six weeks. After the diarrhœa ceased, the child still continued weak and thin, and suffering, and died convulsed in the middle of June, after vague head symptoms of two days' duration.

In this last case no post-mortem examination could be made, so that we are uncertain what connection, if any, subsisted between the hemorrhages at the outset of the child's illness, and the obstinate diarrhœa which came on soon after, and had so large a share in occasioning its death. One thing, at any rate, these cases illustrate, and one worth bearing in mind, viz., that formidable as the occurrence is, and large as the quantity of blood which is lost may be, still the immediate danger to life is far less than, but for this evidence to the contrary, we should most naturally apprehend.[1]

It will not be necessary to do more than allude to cases of wh[illegible] been called *spurious hæmatemesis*, in which an infant vomit[illegible] drawn from some crack or ulceration of its mother's nipple, [illegible] has been furnished by some little vessel cut in dividing the [illegible] linguæ, or in performing some other operation on its [illegible]

[1] The affection is, however, much more serious in infancy than [illegible] of twenty-three cases referred to by M. Rilliet (loc. cit., p. 807), [illegible] termination.

would at once suspect the source of the blood vomited after the operation on the infant's mouth, and an examination of the mother's nipple in a case of hæmatemesis will guard you against the other possible source of error.

LECTURE XXXV.

ICTERUS OF NEW-BORN CHILDREN.—Generally a trivial affection—Not usually dependent on intestinal disorder, but on imperfect performance of functions of skin and respiratory organs—Sometimes results from absence or closure of hepatic or cystic ducts—Is then associated with great tendency to hemorrhage, and proves speedily fatal. It occasionally occurs in children in the same circumstances as in the adult.

CONSTIPATION sometimes results from mechanical obstruction of intestines.—Which may be congenital—As from imperforate anus or impervious rectum—Varieties of these malformations—Their general symptoms—Special signs of each—Their comparative danger and appropriate treatment.

Obstruction of intestines from causes not congenital—Strangulated hernia very rare in infancy—Intussusception of intestines—Its symptoms—Usually more characteristic than in the adult—Its generally fatal result—But occasional spontaneous cure—Suggestions for its treatment.

IT is curious to watch the changes which take place in the color of the infant during the first few days after its birth, and to notice how the vivid red fades by degrees into the pale rose-tint of the skin of a healthy baby. But there is often a transition state between the two when the skin, neither red nor pale, has a dull yellow tinge, which comes on about the third day after birth, and, deepening for a day or two, subsides but very gradually: the child, however, all the time seeming quite well, the bowels acting properly, and the urine not being high-colored. Though to this condition the name of *jaundice* has been applied, it yet is no real jaundice; but is merely the result of the changes which the blood, in the overcongested skin, is undergoing: "the redness fading as bruises fade, through shades of *yellow*, into the genuine flesh color."

This icteroid tinge of the skin is unassociated with the altered hue of the conjunctiva, which is seldom absent when the functions of the liver are disordered; and it has, therefore, been proposed[1] to distinguish the physiological change in the color of the skin, which takes place after birth, by the name of *local icterus*, and to apply the term of *general icterus* to cases in which the yellow hue of the surface is an indication of hepatic disorder.

Even the general icterus, however, is not often of serious moment, though the assumption that it is a perfectly natural state in which the

---

[1] ... op. cit., p. 280.

skin, and other secreting organs, are called on for a few days [illegible] in disposing of the bile, until the demand for it to minister [illegible] gestive functions becomes equal to its abundant supply, is shown [illegible] erroneous, by the circumstance that jaundice does not affect [illegible] healthy children, who have been born at the full time, have been [illegible] ished exclusively at the mother's breast, and been sheltered [illegible] without being overburdened with clothing or confined in a [illegible] atmosphere. In the Dublin Lying-in Hospital, where the children are defended by the most watchful care from the evils either of cold [illegible] of a vitiated atmosphere, the occurrence of infantile jaundice is [illegible] while in the Foundling Hospital at Paris, jaundice is so common that comparatively few infants escape it. Almost all the children at the Foundling Hospital have been exposed to the action of cold while being brought to the institution, and suffer from the combined influence of cold and bad air while inmates of it—causes which interfere very seriously with the due performance of the functions of the skin and of the respiratory organs.

The children in whom jaundice is most frequent and most [illegible] are the immature and the feeble; while in none is it so often met with, or in such an intense degree, as in infants affected with induration of the cellular tissue, in whom the yellow color is often so deep as to be manifest in the serum infiltrated into their cellular tissue, or [illegible] out into the cavities of their chest or abdomen. Interruption of the function of the skin, and great impairment of that of the lungs, are, as you know, the grand characteristics of that affection; while in many instances of it the fœtal passages are still pervious, and the blood circulates in part through channels which ought to have been closed from the time of birth. These facts seem to substantiate the opinions entertained by many writers of high authority, that the jaundice of young children is not due to any cause *primarily* seated in the liver, but rather to the defective respiration, and the impaired performance of the functions of the skin, of which the hepatic disorder and consequent jaundice are but the effects.

As the respiratory function, and that of the skin, increase in activity —which they will do if the cause of their imperfect performance is but slight or temporary—the jaundice disappears of its own accord. [illegible] attention must be paid during its continuance to avoid exposure of the child to cold, while no other food than the mother's milk should be given. If the bowels are at all constipated, a grain of Hyd. c. [illegible] may be given, followed by a small dose of castor oil, and the [illegible] will often seem to hasten the disappearance of the jaundice; but [illegible] large number of cases even this amount of medical interference is [illegible] needed.

Besides these cases, however, in which the jaundice is at most [illegible] very trivial ailment, instances are sometimes met with where [illegible] symptom of very serious import. Thus, for instance, it has been [illegible] served to attend upon the peritonitis of new-born infants, and [illegible] enteritis which, like the affection of the peritoneum, is one [illegible] demic diseases of foundling hospitals. It sometimes depends [illegible] mation of the liver, occasionally on phlebitis of the umbilical [illegible] diseases, all of them, to which in private practice we are strangers. Lastly, it is occasionally due to congenital absence of the hepatic or cystic biliary ducts, or to the obstruction of those ducts by inspissated bile.

When dependent on the former of these causes, death takes place sooner or later; and though now and then life is prolonged for several weeks or months, during which time, as might be expected, the evacuations are destitute of bile, yet in the majority of instances the fatal issue takes place within a fortnight after birth; and this in consequence of hemorrhage from the umbilicus immediately after the separation of the funis. It is characteristic of the bleeding which occurs in these circumstances that it is not furnished exclusively—sometimes, indeed, not at all—from the umbilical vessels, but is rather a constant oozing of blood from the granulating surface of the navel. The blood, too, is almost completely destitute of the power of coagulation, so that it is neither restrained by styptics nor controlled by tying the umbilical vessels. The only means indeed, on which we can rely for checking the bleeding is the ligature *en masse*, as it has been termed; or, in other words, the transfixing the integuments at the root of the navel with a couple of hare-lip pins, and twisting around them several coils of strong silken ligature. In the only case of this form of hemorrhage which has come under my observation, the bleeding was suppressed by these means, though the child died apparently exhausted in the course of the ensuing twenty-four hours, or about thirty-six hours after the separation of the navel and the commencement of the bleeding. Of course, when bleeding is dependent on a congenital malformation of the hepatic ducts, all interference is useless as far as the preservation of the child's life is concerned; but, at the same time, the death of an infant from hemorrhage will leave a more painful impression on the parents' minds than its sinking somewhat later from the remote though inevitable consequences of the condition. Now and then, too, in spite of the coexistence of hemorrhage and jaundice, the former has been checked, and the latter had disappeared; the child completely recovering; and, in other instances which terminated fatally, though the umbilical vessels have been found open, and no clots within their canals, and the fœtal passages for the blood still pervious, yet the bile-ducts have sometimes been found quite pervious and arranged in a perfectly natural manner.

In some rare instances, as has been mentioned, life is prolonged; and when that is the case, a condition of general atrophy comes on, attended with enlargement of the abdomen in both hypochondriac regions; and some intercurrent attack of diarrhœa generally exhausts the feeble powers when only a few months have passed. Some years ago, through the courtesy of Mr. Jones of Tenby, I saw a remarkable case of this kind, where life was prolonged for six and a half months, in spite of absence of the gall-bladder; but in almost all instances death takes place within the first two months. In the case which I have just referred to, no hemorrhage took place at any time; but on the third day after birth, the surface began to be yellow, and, at the end of three weeks, the yellow tinge was very deep. At the same time a swelling of the size of an egg was first noticed in the right hypo[illegible] while the evacuations from the second day after birth [illegible] cream, and the urine was habitually high-colored.

The child was thirteen weeks old when I first saw [illegible] small, ill-thriven, sallow, icteroid, but not intensely [illegible] abdomen measured twelve inches and three-quarters at [illegible] and fourteen and one-third two inches lower down. [illegible] was due to a tumor which dipped down on the right side [illegible] the pelvis, sloping off on the left side, so as to project [illegible] though its hard edge was still distinctly traceable.

In three months more the child died, much emaciated, [illegible] abdomen was distended by a pint and a half of fluid in the [illegible] cavity. The spleen was much larger than natural, forming a [illegible] tumor in the left iliac and lumbar regions. Its color was [illegible] its tissue firmer than natural. On examination of the liver, [illegible] much enlarged, and weighed eleven ounces and a half, it was [illegible] that the gall-bladder was absent, and in its place were two small [illegible] without any outlet, one of them of the size of a pea, the other [illegible] large, containing a tenacious matter of a greenish color, and [illegible] inspissated bile; while the hepatic ducts were impervious and [illegible] dilated.

The interest of such cases is chiefly that which they offer [illegible] morbid anatomist; but one sad and somewhat strange peculiarity [illegible] reference to them is, that they are apt to be met with in several [illegible] sive children of the same parents. I knew one lady who lost [illegible] cession three out of five children, soon after their birth, with [illegible] intense jaundice, which in one instance was ascertained to be [illegible] with malformation of the biliary ducts; in the second, no examination was made after death; and in the third, malformation was said, [illegible] scarcely on adequate authority, not to have existed. Another [illegible] of whose children I saw die of infantile jaundice from impervious biliary ducts, had already lost three infants from the same cause; [illegible] her sister's only infant had also died in similar circumstances. [illegible] hereditary tendency to this condition receives a fresh illustration [illegible] the circumstance, that, in twenty-six out of seventy-nine cases of [illegible] bilical hemorrhage in the new-born infant, collected by Dr. [illegible] Smith,[1] of New York, other children of the same parent had died [illegible] the same untoward accident; while the more elaborate statistics [illegible] Dr. Grandidier, of Cassel,[2] give a total of forty-one infants of [illegible] mothers in whom umbilical hemorrhage occurred.

---

[1] In New York Journal of Medicine, July, 1855, vol. xv, p. 73. [illegible] occurred in two children of the same parents, twice in three, and [illegible] Further information on the subject of umbilical hemorrhage with jaundice [illegible] found in a paper by Dr. A. B. Campbell, in the Northern Journal, [illegible] in the valuable paper of Mr. Ray, in Med. Gazette for March, 1849; [illegible] Manley, in the same journal for May, 1850; in the dissertation of M. [illegible] which an abstract is given in the Arch. Gén. de Médecine for October, [illegible] essay by Dr. Bowditch in the American Journal of Medical Science, [illegible] and in a lecture by M. Roger, of Paris, republished in the Journal für [illegible] heiten, July, 1853.

[2] Journal für Kinderkrankheiten, May, 1859, vol. xxxii, p. [illegible]

Jaundice may also occur in older children in the same circumstances as in adults, and associated with similar symptoms; the evacuations being white, the urine high-colored, and more or less pain and tenderness being experienced in the hypochondriac region. Such cases are most frequently met with during the summer or autumn, especially at times when diarrhœa is prevalent, the skin sometimes assuming a generally yellow tinge as the purging subsides; while in other instances the jaundice occurs as an idiopathic affection, though apparently due to the same causes as have produced diarrhœa in other children.

In the instances that have come under my notice, the skin has not assumed a very deep yellow tinge, and the constitutional symptoms have seldom been severe. Now and then, however, considerable febrile disturbance precedes the appearance of the jaundice for two or three days; the skin is dry, though not very hot; vomiting occurs; and the child complains much of headache and dizziness, and rests ill at night, or awakes in a state of alarm. The resemblance between these symptoms, and some of those which occur in cases of real cerebral disease, is almost sure to excite much apprehension in the mind of the parents, and may even render it a difficult task for you to form a correct diagnosis. The following circumstances will, however, usually suffice to preserve you from error: the attack has not, in most instances, been preceded by those indications of generally failing health which so often exist during many days before the symptoms of tubercular meningitis manifest themselves, and it is not attended either by the anxious expression of countenance, the heat of head, or the intolerance of light, by which cerebral disease is accompanied. Though the sleep may be disturbed, it is usually less so than in tubercular meningitis; the pulse is less frequent; and though the child vomits occasionally, it does not suffer from constant nausea. When to these symptoms tenderness on pressure in the hypochondriac region is superadded, with the appearance in a day or two of high-colored urine and of white evacuations, and lastly, of the yellow tinge of the skin, no further possibility of error remains.

The *treatment* of jaundice in the child calls for but very simple remedies. The employment of small doses of the sulphate of magnesia, in combination with the tincture of rhubarb, every four or every six hours, with three grains of the Hyd. c. Cretâ for a child of five years old, at bed-time, will generally suffice to restore the patient to health in the course of four or five days. Should the appetite continue bad, and the child fretful and languid, after the subsidence of the jaundice and the return of the evacuations to a more healthy character, the compound infusion of roses, either alone or in combination with small doses of sulphate of magnesia, will be found of much service. In some cases, however, removal to the country, or to the seaside, appears to be absolutely necessary to the child's complete recovery.

Far more frequent than cases of actual jaundice, are instances of what is popularly termed sluggish liver in children, in which the bowels are usually constipated, and the evacuations almost always pale and deficient in bile. Without being positively ill, children thus affected are usually sallow and look out of health; their appetite is variable, and their tongue never quite clean, but slightly coated with yellowish fur. In such cases it not infrequently happens that mercurials become almost a domestic remedy, and that calomel is the aperient constantly resorted to as often as the costive bowels require the employment of medicine. Other cases, too, of a somewhat different kind are not unusual, in which calomel is again considered a panacea. They are the cases of children, for the most part somewhat older than those who constitute the former class, whose general health is good and their bowels are usually regular, but who, every few weeks or months, are attacked by a severe headache accompanied by bilious vomiting which lasts for several hours, and then subsides, leaving the patients in a state of extreme exhaustion, from which they do not recover for many days.

Cases of this latter class are far less serious than the others. They are for the most part instances of congestion of the liver, brought on either by some error in diet, or, as is far more commonly the case, by a system of habitual overfeeding. It is by no means necessary for the production of these symptoms that the food should be improper, or that its quantity should be very excessive, but it quite suffices that it should be a little in excess of the actual necessities of the system, and of the power of the digestive organs to assimilate. In these cases there can be no sort of objection to the administration of a dose of calomel to arrest the sickness, and by its purgative action to assist in relieving the liver; but it is the careful regulation and due restriction of the diet which will alone prevent the frequent recurrence of the attack.

Cases of the other kind are by no means so simple. They are met with in delicate children: often in those in whose family there exists some taint of scrofulous or tubercular disease; and in them not infrequently the symptoms of habitual intestinal disorder, and deficiency of the biliary secretion, become at last merged in the signs of general tuberculosis or of tabes mesenterica. I do not know what is the actual state of the liver in these cases, but I am sure that the empirical recourse to mercurials, which do but remove for a short time some of the symptoms of a deepseated constitutional disorder, is not a judicious proceeding. In a large proportion of instances, indeed, with increased health and strength, there comes almost spontaneously an improved state of digestion and a more efficient performance of the functions of the liver. And to this amendment of the general health our first endeavors must in these circumstances be directed,—air, situations, climate; all those points to which in cases of threatening tubercular disease our attention is always turned, are here, too, of far more importance than mere medicine, though that of course cannot be dispensed with. I often find the nitro-muriatic acid[1] specially serviceable, both as a tonic, and also as a remedy which acts upon the liver and increases the secretion of bile; while, if an aperient is needed, the powdered aloes, or powdered extract of rhubarb, will either enable us to dispense with mercurials altogether, or at least will allow us to give

[1] See Formula No. 22, p. 426.

them in smaller doses than otherwise we should be compelled to employ. Sometimes, however, this treatment seems of no avail, and we are compelled to put the patient on a regular course of mercurials. This has seemed to be best done by the employment of small doses of the perchloride of mercury; not alone, but in combination with the infusion of bark, or the Liquor Cinchonæ, and Liquor Taraxaci;[1] and from the steady continuance of this treatment I have seen recovery take place, even where little appeared to promise a favorable issue. The danger of tuberculosis is the one great risk which in these cases must be borne in mind; low diet, violent purgatives, must be avoided, and the constitutional symptoms rather than the mere amount of disorder of the functions of the liver must govern our prognosis and regulate our conduct.

I have nothing to add to what has already been said on the subject of *constipation*—which is to be regarded as a symptom of various diseases rather than as a special idiopathic affection. To this rule, however, an exception must be made in those cases in which the due action of the bowels is prevented by some mechanical impediment. Such an impediment is, in some rare instances, presented by *congenital malformation of the intestines,* whose calibre has been found greatly diminished, or their canal completely obstructed, or even their continuity altogether interrupted. These occurrences, although of great interest and importance, from their relation to the laws that regulate fœtal development, yet for the most part afford no scope for the interference of medical or surgical skill. But while we pass over, as foreign to our purpose, the general study of these malformations, we must take some notice of one variety of them, in which the obstacle to the escape of the fæces is situated low down in the large intestine, since their diagnosis is often easy, and their cure not always beyond the resources of our art.

The cause of the obstruction in these cases is not always of the same kind, nor is the patient in every instance exposed to the same amount of danger. But *three different classes of the malformation* may be recognized, in each of which our prognosis must somewhat differ, although in almost all it must be doubtful, and in many extremely unfavorable.

To the *first* class may be referred all those cases in which the rectum is perfect, but the canal is closed either by a false membrane obstructing its orifice, or situated higher up in the intestine, or by the cohesion of the opposite sides of the gut.

The *second* class includes cases in which, although the natural aper-

---

[1] (No. 29.)

℞. Liq. Hydr. Perchlor., ʒj.
Liq. Taraxaci, ʒij.
Liq. Cinchonæ, ʒj.
Tinct Aurantii, ʒj.
Syrupi, ʒiij.
Aquæ destil., ℥iij M.

A tablespoonful twice a day for a child three years.

ture is absent, yet the intestine terminates by opening into the urethra, bladder, or vagina.

To the *third* class belong those instances in which the intestinal canal is not merely occluded, but also malformed, or altogether absent, for a more or less considerable extent.

The affection in any form is so rare as to render a correct estimate of the comparative frequency of its varieties by no means easy. Dr. Collins observed only one instance of it out of 16,654 children born in the Dublin Lying-in Hospital during his mastership;[1] and Dr. [illegible], of Vienna,[2] mentions that he met with it only twice out of 50,000 new-born children. A comparison of seventy-five cases derived from different sources yields seventeen belonging to the first class, twenty-nine to the second, and twenty-nine to the third; but it is probable that many instances of simple closure of the anus have passed unrecorded, while all the instances of more serious malformation have been described.

Whatever be the seat of the obstruction, its existence is betrayed by much the same train of *symptoms* in all cases. Attention is first excited by the infant not having voided any meconium, although from twelve to twenty-four hours may have elapsed since its birth. A dose of castor-oil or of some other aperient, given with the view of exciting the bowels to action, fails of producing this effect, while it is either returned by vomiting, or, if not actually rejected, it causes nausea and retching. Before long, the child shows indications of uneasiness, and has attacks of pain, in which it cries, and seems to suffer much. In some cases it remains quiet in the interval between these attacks, and seems drowsy, but in other cases it appears to be in a state of constant discomfort, which it betrays by a whimpering cry. The attempt to suck is almost always followed by retching, frequently by actual vomiting; and attacks both of retching and vomiting often come on when the stomach is quite empty. In some cases nothing more is thrown up than a little mucus, which is sometimes of a greenish color; while in other instances vomiting of meconium takes place: but this occurrence is by no means constant. The abdomen becomes distended and tympanitic, and grows larger and more tense the longer that life continues, while at the same time the child's discomfort is much aggravated by any pressure upon it. The restlessness increases, and the attacks of pain grow more severe, the child often making violent straining efforts during their continuance; but as the powers of life decline, these efforts become more feeble, though the retching and vomiting often continue to the last. The period at which death takes place varies much, for though, in the majority of instances, the child dies within a week from its birth, yet cases are on record in which it has survived for several weeks; and an instance has been mentioned to me by Mr. Arnott, in which he saw a child live for seven weeks and three days, although the colon terminated in a blind pouch, and the rectum was entirely absent. Death usually occurs under a gradual

---

[1] System of Midwifery, p. 509

[2] Oesterr. med. Wochenschr. and Canstatt's Jahresber. für 1842, Bd. i, S. [illegible].

aggravation of the previous symptoms; but now and then it is ushered in by the sudden supervention of a state of collapse, owing to the over-distended intestine having given way. This is, however, a rare occurrence, for I find mention of it having happened only in three out of the seventy-five cases to which I have referred.

Coupled with the general signs of intestinal obstruction, there are in each case some special indications of the peculiar form of malformation to which the obstruction is due. If the anus is merely closed by a membrane or by the cohesion of its edges, the collection of the meconium above may give rise to the formation of a distinct tumor between the buttocks; while sometimes the dark color of the meconium shows through the thin integument by which its escape is prevented. In other cases the anus itself is well formed, but the introduction of the finger or of a bougie into the rectum detects the existence of some obstruction within the gut. Again, in other instances, there is no trace of an anus, or a small depression is all that marks the situation which it should occupy; the rectum either ending in a blind pouch, or communicating with the vagina, urethra, or bladder.

Although the diagnosis in all cases is sufficiently easy, yet the carrying out the very obvious indication of relieving the patient, by providing for the escape of the contents of the intestines, is often very difficult; and even, when accomplished, its result is in many instances extremely uncertain. If the obstruction is situated at the orifice of the anus, a crucial incision through the membrane which closes it or the introduction of a trocar, will afford immediate relief. Our prognosis also may, in these circumstances, be very favorable; for of fifteen cases of this kind, all but one had a favorable issue. After the opening has been established, however, some attention must be paid to prevent its becoming closed, or much contracted. For this purpose it has been recommended that a tent should be kept in the anus for some days, though to this it has been objected that a constant straining effort is thereby produced, and the frequent introduction of the finger or of a bougie into the passage is therefore recommended, as preferable to leaving any body constantly within it.[1]

If the obstacle is occasioned by a membrane seated higher up in the rectum, we may still hope to succeed, though our prognosis must be more guarded, since two out of four cases of this description had a fatal result. In one of the fatal cases it appeared that rupture of the intestine had already taken place before any operation was performed; in the other, the death of the child was accounted for by the discovery

[1] I may just mention having seen great pain and difficulty in defecation produced in an infant aged seven months by congenital smallness of the anal opening. For the first three months of life the child had not suffered from this condition, but afterwards, when the motions began to be slightly more consistent, constipation became very troublesome, defecation difficult, painful, and attended by great tenesmus, while the evacuations were not infrequently streaked with blood. The opening admitted the finger with difficulty, and its edges tightly constringed it, while the rectum above was much dilated, and permanently distended with fæces. The daily employment of a bougie relieved the inconvenience, which I refer to here only on account of its rarity.

of a second septum higher up in the rectum than that which [illegible] divided.

The existence of an anus, and a small extent of gut above it, although a decidedly favorable feature in a case, does not warrant quite so hopeful a prognosis as we might in the first instance feel disposed to adopt. The probabilities, indeed, are that the distance is not great between the end of the rectum and the cul-de-sac in which the anus terminates, yet a considerable space may intervene between the two, or, as in a case which Mr. Arnott was so good as to communicate to me, the rectum may be found altogether absent, the colon terminating in a blind extremity, and floating loose in the abdominal cavity. In the majority of instances, the two blind pouches are connected together by the intervention of an eighth or a quarter of an inch of dense cellular tissue, which sometimes presents an almost ligamentous character; and in these cases the end of the large intestine is situated anterior to the extremity of the cul-de-sac that leads from the anus. Owing to this latter circumstance, the operation for the relief of this condition has sometimes failed, the instrument, although introduced deep enough, yet passing behind the distended bowel. Out of nine cases of this kind, eight had a fatal termination; the bowel on four occasions not having been reached at all, while once the opening made in it was too small to allow of the free escape of the meconium. It may be added, that in three of the fatal cases there existed such contraction of the calibre of different parts of the large intestine as would of itself have opposed a serious obstacle to the child's recovery.

In twelve cases the anus was absent, and in some of these instances no trace of it existed, while the rectum terminated in a cul-de-sac at from one to two inches from the surface. In five of these cases the attempt to open the intestine was successful, and the child eventually did well; while in two other cases, although temporary relief followed the operation, yet symptoms of inflammation of the bowels came on, which terminated fatally in the course of a few days. In three instances it was not found possible to reach the bowel; and in two others, although an opening was made, yet its size was insufficient to afford a free vent to the accumulated meconium; and the fatal issue, though deferred, was not prevented. Failure to reach the intestine seems to have depended either on the trocar not having been introduced sufficiently deep, or on its having been directed too far backwards. The danger of hemorrhage, or of wounding the bladder, of which some operators seem to have been apprehensive, is not much to be feared; for I find but one instance on record in which the bladder was accidentally wounded, and not one of fatal or even of serious hemorrhage. Better success also appears to have been obtained in those cases in which a sufficiently deep and free incision was made with a bistoury in the direction of the rectum, than in those in which a trocar was at once introduced. The suggestion of M. Amussat, that in these cases the blind sac of the intestine should be drawn down, and its cut edges attached by sutures to the margin of the external skin, in order to prevent the infiltration of fecal matter between the end of the rectum and the wound in the integuments, is one

diminish the danger of the aperture closing, is worth bearing in mind. It was adopted with apparent advantage by Mr. Waters in a case of this kind recorded by him in the Dublin Journal for May, 1842, on which he operated with success; and I was a witness to its advantages in a little boy on whom Mr. Shaw operated successfully some years since at the Middlesex Hospital.

Several years ago I was present at the post-mortem examination of a child, aged fourteen months, whose history illustrated very forcibly the importance of the precaution to which I have just referred. The rectum was imperforate at birth, though an anus existed. Relief was readily afforded by puncture with a trocar, but no attempt was made to bring down the intestine to the edges of the opening. The child soon passed from under observation, and when seen again, it was asserted that no evacuation had taken place for a month, and that for a long time constipation had been growing more and more obstinate. The child died speedily: its abdomen being enormously distended both with fæces and flatus. The circular fibres of the large intestine had undergone the most extraordinary hypertrophy; doubtless to enable them to overcome the resistance offered to the expulsion of their contents; a task to which at last they had proved unequal. This resistance was seen to be due to the contraction of the original opening just above the anus, while the intestine was quite permeable beyond; a misadventure which might have been obviated by care in the performance of the operation, and by watchfulness afterwards.

Beside these cases in which the malformation was confined to the rectum, I find mention of three others in which the rectum was entirely absent, and the intestine terminated in a cul-de-sac as high up as the colon. In two other cases in which the attempt to discover the rectum failed, the life of the child was preserved by the establishment of an artificial anus. M. Amussat has of late recommended that, in all cases in which fluctuation cannot be detected through the skin, an artificial anus should at once be formed in the left lumbar region, as being a safer proceeding than the attempt to open the bowel from the perineum. When we consider, however, the loathsome nature of the infirmity to which a person is condemned in whom an artificial anus exists, we shall probably be disposed still to regard the operation for its formation as a last resource, to be employed only in the event of our failing to discover the rectum by an operation instituted on the perineum.

In some cases, although the anus is absent, yet the intestine is not imperforate, but opens either into the vagina in the female, or into the bladder or urethra in the male subject. In either case the malformation is due to a similar cause—namely, an arrest of development, whereby the separation between the bowel and the sinus uro-genitalis has never been completed. The malformation in the female subject is not attended with immediate danger to life, and fortunately it admits of cure in the great majority of instances. I find, indeed, that in seven out of ten cases of this description, an operation was attempted, and that in every instance it proved successful. In some cases the mere establishment of the natural opening of the anus, with the introduction of a tube into the rectum, was sufficient to effect a cure; [illegible] complex operation was in general necessary, the principle of [illegible] sisted in dividing all the parts from the vagina into the rectum; [illegible] the details of the proceeding, and the means whereby a [illegible] two canals was prevented, varied in different cases.

The result is very much more unfavorable when a communication subsists between the intestine and the bladder or urethra in the [illegible], for eight out of eleven cases of the former kind, and the same [illegible] out of nine of the latter kind, ended in the death of the infant. The connection with the bladder is generally established by means of a very slender canal which enters that viscus at or near its neck; but in one instance in which the rectum was wanting, the colon terminated by opening with a wide aperture into the upper part of the bladder. A slender duct is likewise the usual channel of communication between the rectum and the urethra, and this duct generally enters the membranous portion of the urethra, just in front of the prostate. Cruveilhier, however, met with an instance in which the rectum opened under the glans penis; and a somewhat similar case, in which there was a small aperture through which meconium passed in front of the scrotum, came under the notice of Mr. South, and is mentioned by him in his edition of Chelius's Surgery.

The existence of a communication between the rectum and the urethra or bladder is generally indicated by the urine voided being tinged with meconium; but it seldom happens that the contents of the intestines are discharged by the urethra with freedom sufficient to preserve the child from the suffering and danger that attend upon an imperforate state of the rectum. Even when life has been prolonged for some time, yet the infant's death is in general merely deferred, for the symptoms of obstruction appear, and at length prove fatal, after the fæces have acquired a firmer consistence than they possessed during the first few months of existence. These cases, too, do not appear to be favorable for an operation, since the rectum usually terminates high up, and in five out of ten cases in which it is stated that the attempt was made to puncture the intestine, this attempt was unsuccessful. In Mr. South's case the rectum was punctured by a trocar introduced an inch deep, and though much difficulty was experienced in keeping the passage free, yet the child survived and grew up to manhood. Of the other two successful cases, one of which is recorded by Mr. Miller,[1] and the other by Sir W. Fergusson,[2] both were cured only with much trouble and difficulty. For a full account of the difficulties these gentlemen had to contend with, and the means by which they overcame them, I must refer you to the history of the cases in the Edinburgh Medical Journal. A third successful case has since been recorded by the late Professor Wutzer, of Bonn,[3] in which there was no [illegible] anus, and the incision was carried an inch and three-quarters [illegible] the intestine was reached. I saw the child in this case [illegible]

[1] Edinburgh Medical and Surgical Journal, No. 96, p. 63.

[2] Ibid., vol. xxxvi, p. 868.

[3] Rheinische Monatschrift für praktische Aerzte, June, [illegible]

months old; he was a healthy infant, and passed his evacuations generally per rectum, though a small quantity of fæces was still frequently intermixed with his urine.[1]

An insuperable obstacle to the action of the bowels may occur in children, just as it sometimes does in older persons, either from the *strangulation of an external hernia*, or from the *invagination of a portion of intestine.* Although hernia is by no means an uncommon affection in early life, yet it is, I believe, a very rare occurrence for the intestine to become strangulated. Such an accident, however, may take place, even in very young infants, of which a case related by Sir W. Fergusson, where he operated for strangulated inguinal hernia on an infant only seventeen days old, may be mentioned as a striking illustration. Bearing in mind its possibility, therefore, you would examine any infant or child, in whom abdominal pain, vomiting, and obstinate constipation came on, just as carefully as you would an adult in similar circumstances, lest it should be found out, when too late, that the symptoms had been due to some unsuspected external hernia.

The strangulation of an external rupture is probably a rarer accident in early infancy than the occurrence of *intussusception* of one or more portions of the intestines. This condition, indeed, is frequently met with in the bodies of children who have died of various diseases, and wholly independent of any symptoms of disorder of the bowels during the patient's lifetime. Sometimes a single intussusception exists, but oftener there are several; ten, twelve, and even more, have occasionally been observed in the same subject. They are almost invariably confined to the small intestine, are most numerous in the ileum, and though seldom involving more than three or four inches, have been found to include more than double that extent of bowel. Their great frequency, the absence of any symptom of them during life, and of any indication of inflammation about the intestines after death, all confirm the general opinion that they take place during the act of dying.

But while this form of intussusception, limited to the small intestine, and producing no symptoms during life, is extremely common in early childhood, few accidents are rarer than the invagination of the large intestine, so that MM. Rilliet and Barthez state that they have not met with it even once in 500 post-mortem examinations of children between the ages of two and fifteen years. In early childhood, the various causes which in the adult may produce insuperable obstruction of the bowels seem not to exist; and our diagnosis is made easier, I think that I may even say our prognosis less absolutely hopeless, from a knowledge of the fact that the symptoms of intestinal obstruction in the infant point almost invariably to invagination of the large intestine.

Children in whom intussusception takes place are generally infants

[1] I cannot do better than refer, for a detail of all the important surgical questions involved in cases of imperforate anus, to Mr. Curling's able treatise on Diseases of the Rectum, 2d ed., London, 1868, pp 192–282; as also to Holmes, Surgical Treatment of Diseases of Infancy and Childhood, 2d ed. London, 1869, pp 152–180: Guersant. Notices sur la Chirurgie des Enfans, 8vo., Paris, 1867, pp. 196–201; and Giraldes Maladies Chirurgicales des Enfans, 8vo., Paris, 1868, pp. 118–139.

under a year, often under six months old.[1] Their previous history does not in general display any liability either to constipation or to diarrhœa; nor, in the greater number of instances, has the manifestation of the symptoms followed the administration of any aperient medicine. Sudden and violent vomiting, followed by loud cries and other indications of uneasiness, which, ceasing for a time, return at uncertain intervals, and are accompanied by violent straining, and efforts to empty the bowels, are the earliest symptoms of the accident. At first some fæces are voided during these efforts, but afterwards the matters dis-

---

[1] Nine cases of intussusception have come under my own notice, of which 4 recovered, 5 died.

The 4 recoveries were:

1 Male,	aged	6 months.
1 Female,	"	6 "
1 Male,	"	14 "
1 Female,	"	10 years.

The 5 deaths were:

1 Male,	aged	4 months,	who died in	36 hours.
1 Female,	"	6 "	"	"	48 "
1 Female,	"	8 years	"	"	18 days.
1 Female,	"	12 "	"	"	9 "
1 Male,	"	8 "	"	"	3 months.

The two male children recovered under a soothing treatment, with a careful avoidance of aperients; the elder of the female children recovered under the use of inflation of the intestine by the rectum; while in the younger the invagination yielded to the copious injection of warm water after inflation had been tried without success. The two youngest of the fatal cases were moribund when they came under my notice. In the child twelve years old the intussusception affected three inches of the small intestine about a foot above the ileo-cæcal valve; and in the one aged 8 years, 7 inches of the small intestine were invaginated through the valve. The case of the boy was very singular, for the whole of the large intestine was invaginated, so that during the expulsive efforts which the child made, the inverted cæcum with the opening of the appendix vermiformis was protruded beyond the anus, while the finger could be passed by the rectum through the ileo-cæcal valve, and the large intestine was for all practical purposes abolished. Death took place at last from peritonitis. The case was under my observation for only three days before the patient's death.

The most complete statistics of this condition are furnished by Rilliet, in his valuable essay published originally in the Gazette des Hôpitaux, 1852, but reprinted at p. 806 of the 2d ed., of the 1st vol., of his work on Diseases of Children; by M. Duchaussoy, in vol xxiv, of the Mémoires de l'Académie de Médecine, 1860; and lastly in the very able paper of Dr. Smith, of New York, published in the American Journal, January, 1862 and reproduced in his work on Children's Diseases, of which the 2d edition, published in 1872, is now before me. Deducting those cases which are common to his table and M. Rilliet's, and also 3 in which no age is given, and adding my 9 cases, we have a total of 71 cases in children under 15, of which 40 occurred during the first year of life, 31 in the succeeding 14 years.

3	were under		3	months old.	
11	"	"	4	"	"
3	"	"	5	"	"
9	"	"	6	"	"
4	"	"	7	"	"
2	"	"	8	"	"
4	"	"	9	"	"
2	"	"	10	"	"
1	"	"	11	"	"
1	"	"	12	"	"
40					

2	were between		1 and	2	years old.	
11	"	"	2	5	"	"
18	"	"	5	15	"	"
31						

charged from the bowels are either mucus tinged with blood,[1] or else pure blood, and that sometimes in considerable quantities. If an enema is given, the fluid thrown up immediately returns, it appearing not properly to enter the intestine; while on a few occasions the existence of an obstruction has been discovered on introducing the finger into the rectum. The vomiting is almost immediately renewed whenever either food or medicine is given, but fecal matters are seldom if ever discharged by the mouth. The child has intervals of quiet, from which it is roused by the returns of pain; it is often thirsty, and though the sickness continues unabated, yet it seems eager for the breast, and sucks frequently. The condition of the addomen is variable; and though a distinct tumor may be detected in some cases, at a spot which is found afterwards to correspond to the situation of the intussusception, yet it happens, in at least as large a number of instances, that the most careful examination fails to detect anything unnatural in its state, and that it continues uniformly soft up to the time of the patient's death. The continuance of the intussusception leads to the exhaustion of the infant's strength; its pulse grows more and more feeble, its face becomes anxious and sunken, and it falls in the intervals between its attacks of pain into a quiet, half-comatose condition. In the majority of cases convulsions come on a few hours before death, which always takes place within a week, oftener in from forty-eight to seventy-two hours. Now and then, however, instead of going on from bad to worse, the symptoms abate, the pain ceases, the vomiting subsides, the bowels act spontaneously, and were the indications of invagination less characteristic, we might, on seeing the speedy and complete recovery of the patient, almost doubt whether our first diagnosis had not been erroneous. Such a case was that of a little boy fourteen months old, well-nourished and previously healthy, who was suddenly attacked, at 5 A.M., on June 12, 1855, by pain and sickness. He at that time passed one fecal motion, but the pain continued, and at 8.30 A.M., he voided a second, which consisted of pure blood. At 10 A.M. I saw him; he looked very ill, his face was extremely anxious, he shivered sometimes, the pain returned at intervals, and he was still frequently sick. The abdomen was neither full nor tender except in the cæcal region, where there was a firm oblong tumor, about the size of a hen's egg, very tender to the. touch. A linseed poultice was applied over the abdomen, hydrocyanic acid was given to allay the sickness, and the child was allowed only a very small quantity of drink at a time to allay the thirst, which was very urgent. In eight hours the child was better, the bowels had acted twice spontaneously, and but very little blood was contained in the evacuations. On the next morning all traces of the tumor had disappeared, and the abdomen was equably soft and tolerant of pressure; and no symptom recurred from this time to excite any apprehension.

Another somewhat similar case came under my notice in a child

[1] The credit of drawing attention to the value of the intestinal hemorrhage in these cases as a sign of intussusception, belongs to Mr Gorham, whose essay on this affection, in No. 7 of the Guy's Hospital Reports, may be consulted with profit.

aged six months, in whom symptoms equally characteristic [illegible] exception of the abdominal tumor, which was not present, [illegible] ceased spontaneously. Such a result is nevertheless not to be [illegible] looked for, and M. Rilliet states the results of fifteen cases [illegible] in children between four months and four and a half years [illegible] yield ten deaths to five recoveries.

The *treatment* of intussusception in the child must be conducted [illegible] the same principle as would govern our conduct if the patient [illegible] adult, though, as the symptoms enable us to arrive at a tolerably certain knowledge of the nature of the case earlier in the infant than in the grown person, we should be absolutely without excuse if we were to persevere in the use of active purgatives in order to overcome the constipation. It was during the suspension of the active remedies which had been previously employed, that the second of the two cases which I have referred to took a favorable turn; and the studious avoidance of any other than soothing measures was succeeded by the spontaneous disappearance of the symptoms and removal of the abdominal tumor in the other. I should regard the supervention of the symptoms of intussusception as calling for the immediate discontinuance of all aperient medicines administered by the mouth; and for the steady adoption of a soothing plan of treatment. Warm poultices to the abdomen, hydrocyanic acid, for the sake not merely of its power in allaying sickness, but also of its generally sedative properties, and the administration of opium in small doses to control the pain and allay the spasm, would be the remedies to which I should trust, while I should insist on all food being given in extremely small quantities. If at the end of twelve or at most of twenty-four hours, the symptoms had not disappeared, I should without further delay resort to the inflation of the intestine with air, as a means of mechanically unfolding the invagination likely to be more effectual than the employment of large enemata, which yet in some instances, one of which came under my own observation, has proved successful. In three of the cases which have come under my own observation, inflation was resorted to; in one (that to which Sir T. Watson has referred in his Lectures[1]) it was followed by the disentanglement of the involution, and [illegible] child's recovery; in a second, after its failure, the abundant injection of warm water was successful; while, in a third, where the small intestine was concerned, the experiment, as might be expected, [illegible] successful, and the child died. In infancy, however, by far the [illegible] proportion of cases of intussusception affect the large intestine, and it is especially in infants under the age of one year that the [illegible] ment of inflation has proved successful. But even in older [illegible] as the case just mentioned shows, life has sometimes been [illegible] employment; and it is by an oversight, which I notice [illegible] of its rarity, that Mr. Holmes, in his valuable work [illegible] Diseases of Children,"[2] refers to it as an "idea," and [illegible] results as "imaginary."

With reference to the question of surgical interference [illegible]

[1] 5th ed., vol. ii, p. 553.

[2] [illegible]

observations on the child that tend specially to elucidate it. One point, however, deserves consideration; namely, that as in infancy the seat of the obstruction is almost invariably in the large intestine, the uncertainty as to the possibility of liberating it which, in the adult, often causes hesitation, does not beset us here. I am not acquainted with any data from which to determine the comparative risks of gastrotomy at different periods of life; but it is not without moment to know that the detachment of the invaginated portion of bowel, and subsequent recovery of the patient, which now and then happen in the adult and in the child, appear never to occur in the infant, who sinks before such processes have time to take place.

LECTURE XXXVI.

DIARRHŒA.—Its two forms, the simple and the inflammatory—Causes of the affection—Influence of age—Of process of dentition—Of temperature, and season of the year.

Symptoms of simple diarrhœa—Not usually a dangerous affection—Occasional hazard from great exhaustion that it produces—Cessation of purging sometimes independent of real amendment—Danger of secondary diarrhœa.

Inflammatory diarrhœa.—Occasional want of correspondence between the symptoms and morbid appearances—Latter observed chiefly in large intestine—Very similar to those discovered in dysentery of the adult.

Symptoms of inflammatory diarrhœa.—Occasional disturbance of nervous system at the outset—Progress of the disease—Its tendency to a chronic course. Life sometimes cut short by intercurrent bronchitis—By head symptoms—By relapse after temporary amendment.

In a systematic course of lectures like the present, subjects of very various interest and importance come successively before us. We were engaged yesterday in the study of some affections which fortunately are of very rare occurrence; but to-day we pass to the examination of one of the most common, and at the same time one of the most serious disorders of infancy and childhood. The importance of *diarrhœa* in early life indeed, is not to be estimated merely by the number of deaths which our tables of mortality represent it to have occasioned; for the figures that they display would warrant our dismissing it with a comparatively short notice.[1] But we shall come to a very different conclusion, if we consider the frequency of the affection, and the slight causes which often suffice to induce it; the dangers to

[1] According to the [illegible] Report of the Registrar-General, the deaths in London [illegible] as compared with the total deaths from all [illegible] year old, in the proportion of 8 9 per [illegible] to five, 6 per cent.; from five

health which result from its long continuance; and the greatly increased hazard to which its supervention in the course of some other disease exposes the patient.

Under the common name of diarrhœa, many of the older writers on the diseases of children have included all cases, without distinction, in which there is an unnatural increase in the alvine discharges. On the other hand, some among the moderns, rejecting the word diarrhœa from their medical nomenclature, have treated only of certain inflammatory affections of the intestines of which they believe the flux to be symptomatic. Neither of these arrangements, however, is free from objection, for while the former draws no adequate distinction between cases in which the disorder of the functions of the bowels is the result of some accidental and temporary cause, and others in which it is the consequence of organic disease, the latter involves an attempt to distinguish, on purely anatomical grounds, between affections which present the same symptoms and require the same treatment.

In the present state of our knowledge, it will perhaps be the safer way to attempt no further subdivision than into the two grand classes of *simple diarrhœa*, or *catarrhal diarrhœa* as it has been termed by some writers, and *inflammatory diarrhœa*, or *dysentery*. Even in this arrangement it must be confessed that there is something arbitrary, for the two affections are closely allied to each other. In the child, as in the adult, they often prevail at the same time—they are to a considerable degree dependent on the same causes, and are in a measure amenable to the same remedies; while the milder complaint not infrequently passes into the more severe. Before we proceed, therefore, to the study of the special characters of either affection, it may be well to examine into some of those conditions which are alike favorable to the production of both.

The following table, deduced from 2129 cases of diarrhœa or dysentery that came under my notice at the Children's Infirmary, shows that the *age* of the child has much to do with the occurrence of the affection:

Cases of diarrhœa in children at the following ages.	Were to all cases of diarrhœa in children under 15 in the proportion of	Were to all diseases at the same age in the proportion of
Under 6 months	9.7 per cent.	16.1 per cent.
Between 6 " and 12 months	15.7 "	20 0 "
" 12 " " 18 "	20.9 "	26.8 "
" 18 " " 2 years	13 9 "	25.4 "
" 2 years " 3 "	12.1 "	15.0 "
" 3 " " 5 "	11 2 "	9.3 "
" 5 " " 10 "	11 5 "	7 9 "
" 10 " " 15 "	4.7 "	7.7 "

You will observe that the period of the greatest prevalence of diarrhœa coincides exactly with that time during which the *process of dentition* is going on most actively, and that exactly half of all cases of diarrhœa occurred in children between the ages of six months and two years. So close, indeed, is the connection between teething and diarrhœa, that a French physician, M. Bouchut,[1] found that only twenty-six out of 138 children entirely escaped its attack during the period of their first dentition, while forty-six suffered from it severely. The older writers on medicine, whose notice this fact did not escape, attributed the disturbance of the bowels to a sort of sympathy between the intestinal canal and the gums, swollen and irritated by the approach of the teeth to their surface. The frequent observation of cases in which an attack of diarrhœa attends the eruption of each fresh tooth, and ceases when it has cut through the gum, shows that such an hypothesis is not altogether without foundation. But besides the influence of nervous irritation in quickening for a time the peristaltic action of the bowels, and thus inducing diarrhœa, it must be borne in mind that there exists during the period of teething a more abiding cause, which strongly predisposes to its occurrence. All parts of the digestive canal, and of its dependencies, are now undergoing an active evolution to fit them for the proper assimilation of the varied food on which the young being will soon have to subsist. Just as the salivary glands now begin to secrete and pour out saliva in abundance, so the whole glandular system of the intestines assumes a rapidity of growth, and an activity of function, which under the influence of comparatively slight exciting causes, may pass the just limits of health. In too many instances, causes fully adequate to excite diarrhœa are abundantly supplied in the excessive quantity or unsuitable quality of the food with which the infant is furnished; for it is forgotten that its condition is one of transition, in which something more than ordinary care is needed; while, in accordance with that mistaken humoral pathology so popular among the vulgar, the profuse secretion from the irritated glands is regarded as the result of a kind of safety-valve arrangement whereby nature seeks to moderate the constitutional excitement attendant upon teething.

But, besides these conditions seated within the organism which predispose to diarrhœa, and those occasions furnished from without by the food with which the child is supplied, *atmospheric influences* constitute a third, and a very important class of causes, which at one time render diarrhœa very frequent, and at another greatly check its prevalence.

On a comparison of the result of eight years' observation at the Children's Infirmary, I find that

In the 3 mos.	Nov., Dec., Jan ,	diarrhœa formed	7.9	per cent.	of all cases of disease.
"	Feb., March, April,	"	9.5	"	"
"	May, June, July,	"	15.8	"	"
"	Aug., Sept., Oct.,	"	23.0	"	"

The above-mentioned causes dispose alike to diarrhœa and dysentery; but among the dwellings of the poor in this metropolis, as in every large city, conditions abound which often stamp on the disease the characters of the more serious malady. Before investigating them, however, we may first study the *symptoms of the milder affection*, which,

[1] Manuel Pratique des Maladies des Nouveaux-Nés, 2d ed., 8vo., p. 580. Paris, 1852.

though much the more frequent, yet, if uncomplicated, is almost never fatal.

When the attack comes on in perfectly healthy children, it usually sets in quite suddenly, with vomiting of the contents of the stomach, and afterwards of mucus, which sometimes has a yellow or greenish color. The sickness does not in general continue, though exceptions are met with in some of the more severe cases, in which the stomach remains very irritable during the whole period that the affection lasts. In either case the vomiting is almost immediately succeeded by increased action of the bowels, the matters discharged being at first the healthy fæces; but they soon assume a bright yellow color, like that of the yolk of egg, and are often intermixed with slime, or in other cases they present a frothy appearance. The bright yellow color of the evacuations often, though by no means always, changes to green under exposure to the air; while, if the diarrhœa should continue, the fæces present in many instances a green color when voided, similar to that which is frequently produced by the administration of mercury. In other cases the green and yellow colors appear intermixed in the evacuations, while the presence in them of numerous white specks, the casein of the undigested milk, shows that the function of the stomach is interfered with by the same cause as produces the overaction of the bowels. The source of the green color of the evacuations has not yet been quite satisfactorily determined. In some cases it probably depends on the action of the acids of the alimentary canal upon the coloring matter of the bile; but the late Dr. Golding Bird's investigations have proved it not to be always due to this cause, and have rendered it probable that, in many instances, it results from the presence of altered blood in the evacuations. As the child returns to health, the fæces become less watery, and then resume their yellow color; or stools of a natural character alternate with others of a green color and unhealthy aspect, or in which a very large quantity of mucus is present. The action of the bowels, too, becomes less frequent, and the child often regains its usual health in four or five days, though sometimes a disposition to diarrhœa is left behind, and the disorder is liable to be re-excited by very slight causes.

In the majority of cases this overaction of the bowels is not attended by much fever or constitutional disturbance, though, if it should come on during teething, the general feverishness of the child is often somewhat aggravated. The appetite is usually much impaired, while the thirst is often considerably increased, and the child seems very desirous of cold water. The tongue is moist, in general thinly covered with mucus, through which the papillæ appear of a brighter red than natural; but the tongue is neither very red, nor much coated. The abdomen is soft, seldom either full or painful; and the pain which attends the diarrhœa is very variable; sometimes it is completely absent, the stools being expelled without either effort or suffering; while in other cases pain comes on severely at intervals, and then ceases as soon as the bowels have acted. Although there is seldom much tenesmus, yet a slight degree of it attends upon simple diarrhœa in the child much more frequently than in the adult. There is, as might

pated, a loss of the natural look of health—the face grows pale, the eyes appear sunken, and the child becomes fretful and languid—while, if the attack sets in severely, a day or two sometimes suffices to reduce the child to a state of extreme weakness and exhaustion; and in young infants, all the symptoms of spurious hydrocephalus sometimes make their appearance.

The diarrhœa that occurs in connection with the irritation occasioned by teething is in general more gradual in its onset, and slower in its progress, than that which depends on some more transient cause. It is likewise often associated with catarrhal symptoms; and both the catarrh and diarrhœa frequently continue until the tooth having pierced the gum the irritation of the mucous membrane subsides; but to be renewed when a fresh tooth approaches the surface.

Although the dangers attendant on simple diarrhœa, especially when it occurs in healthy children, are not considerable, yet the affection is one which it is never wise to make light of. On more than one occasion I have seen an infant reduced by it to a state of such extreme exhaustion as seriously to endanger life. Diarrhœa, indeed, is the exciting cause of the greater number of cases of that spurious hydrocephalus,[1] in which cerebral disturbance from debility simulates real inflammatory disease of the brain. In such circumstances, too, the diarrhœa has not infrequently ceased for some time before the other more alarming symptoms made their appearance. The cessation of diarrhœa may be due, not so much to the quieting of irritation, as to the exhaustion of the nervous energy which is essential to the performance of their secretory function by the glands of the intestines, or to the due maintenance of the peristaltic movements of the bowels. In infants prematurely weaned or improperly fed after being taken from the breast, we often see this fact exemplified in the cessation, some twelve or twenty-four hours before death, of the diarrhœa from which they have been suffering for weeks together. Nor must we ever make too sure that because purging has ceased, therefore danger is over; or venture to relax our watchful care, until the continuance of amendment for twenty-four hours or more, shows that there is indeed no longer anything to fear.

This, however, is not the only danger to which previously healthy children are exposed by an attack of simple diarrhœa; for if not quickly checked, it sometimes assumes the more serious characters of dysentery, and occasions severe and long-continued suffering. When diarrhœa supervenes in children who are recovering from some disease, such as measles, in which a tendency to relaxation of the bowels often marks the period of convalescence, or who have been suffering from a protracted ailment, such as hooping-cough, it sometimes occasions the patient's death, although it may leave behind in the intestinal canal no traces of serious mischief. Still more frequently is this the case with infants who have been brought up by hand, or who have thriven badly at the breast. A troublesome purging, continuing for weeks together, exhausts the strength of such infants, and at length occasions

---

[1] See Lecture XI, p. 181.

their death; but yet the intestinal canal in many instances presents no trace of more serious mischief than an unusual degree of distinctness of the follicles of the small intestines, and of the solitary glands of the colon and rectum.

In proposing at the commencement of this lecture, to distinguish between simple and *inflammatory diarrhœa*, I yet was forced to acknowledge that the distinction was one rather of degree than of kind; or perhaps it would be more correct to say, that our observation has not hitherto been minute enough to enable us to draw the line of demarcation strictly between the two affections. Even MM. Rilliet and Barthez,[1] whose opportunities have been so extensive, and whose industry was so untiring, confess their inability to refer the symptoms that attend upon the different varieties of diarrhœa to any distinct and invariable anatomical lesions. They remark that not merely are exceedingly different appearances discovered after death in cases where the same symptoms have been observed during life, but that likewise there is often no proportion between the intensity of the two; and that sometimes no morbid appearances are found, even where well-marked symptoms had existed. Usually, indeed, in cases where the morbid appearances are slight, the symptoms during life have not been severe. Occasionally, however, the reverse has occurred; and the diarrhœa has been intense, the pain considerable, and the abdomen tense and tympanitic. MM. Rilliet and Barthez state, that out of 127 children who had died of different diseases, 84 had presented the symptoms of inflammatory diarrhœa, or entero-colitis, and the characteristic appearances of that affection were manifest on an examination of their intestines after death; in 24, though no symptoms had existed during life, similar changes were discovered; while in 19, the signs of disease were present during life, but its morbid appearances were absent. It is true that these observations refer to children above two years of age, and to cases in which diarrhœa had occurred as a secondary affection; but my own observations would lead me to believe that a similar statement might be made with reference to younger children, and to cases of idiopathic diarrhœa.

These circumstances prevent our deducing from the *results of anatomical investigation* those practical conclusions which we should otherwise be inclined to draw from them; but they do not warrant us in altogether omitting to inquire what changes we shall be most likely to meet with in cases of fatal diarrhœa.

These changes will be found chiefly, though not exclusively, in the large intestine; and though usually much less serious than those which are observed in cases of fatal dysentery in the adult, they yet present very similar characters. In those cases in which the structural alterations have been least considerable, the attention is arrested less by any great increase of vascularity in the intestine, than by the remarkable distinctness of the orifices of the solitary glands, which appear like almost innumerable dark spots upon the surface of the mucous membrane. In many cases, and especially in those in which the diarrhœa

[1] Op. cit., vol. i, pp. 509–12; and 2d ed., vol. i, p. 747.

was profuse at the time of the patient's death, not merely are the openings of these follicles distinct, but the glands themselves are enlarged, and project like small millet-seeds, or small pins' heads, beyond the level of the surrounding tissue. This enlargement of the solitary glands is usually associated with increased vascularity of the mucous membrane; which does not, however, assume the characters of a general erythematous redness, but is confined to that part of the membrane which covers each gland, or which surrounds its base. If the disease advances further, ulceration succeeds to this inflammation of the glands. A small circular or slightly oval spot appears upon their summit, and increases in size and depth, until it has destroyed the glandular structure and the mucous membrane, and has produced a deep cup-like depression or ulceration, the base of which is formed by the muscular coat of the intestine. On one occasion I observed, in the midst of enlarged and ulcerated glands, some others equally large, but on which the excavated ulcer had not yet formed; their summits presenting a small round or oval spot, of a yellowish color—most probably a minute slough not yet detached from the surface. Besides that loss of substance which results from the ulceration or sloughing of the glands themselves, a process of thinning and destruction likewise affects other parts of the mucous membrane, especially in those situations which correspond to the edges of the intestinal rugæ. In some parts the membrane appears to be merely attenuated, while in others it seems to have entirely disappeared, though the limits of its destruction are not marked by the same well-defined edges as circumscribe the ulcers of the glands, nor is the loss of substance so deep. On the inner surface of an intestine thus affected may be seen a number of narrow, white lines, inclosing between them islets of mucous membrane, and often having such an arrangement as to give to those portions of membrane the form of irregular parallelograms. This superficial destruction of the mucous coat of the intestine is often much more complete in the rectum and in the sigmoid flexure of the colon, than elsewhere; and when this is the case, the surface of the bowel presents a uniformly rough appearance. It is also in the lower part of the large intestine that the ulcerative process is most frequent and most extensive; and if care is not taken to examine the last few inches of the rectum, we may come to the mistaken conclusion that ulceration is altogether absent, in cases where more careful investigation would have easily convinced us of its existence. On one occasion, I found the disease in the lower part of the large intestine to be so far advanced that the interior of the sigmoid flexure of the colon and of the rectum presented an irregular tuberculated surface, of an ash-gray color, which appeared eaten into holes by a number of small circular pits or ulcers, with sharply cut edges. Besides these changes in the interior of the large intestine, a thickening of its submucous coat is almost always observable, whenever the diarrhœa has continued for any considerable length of time. It is in the rectum and sigmoid flexure of the colon that this thickening is most perceptible; and in this situation a gelatinous-looking matter is sometimes deposited in such abundance beneath the mucous membrane, as to prevent the intestine from becoming collapsed when it is divided.

But it is not merely in the morbid appearances presented by the large intestines, but also in the subsidiary changes observed in other parts of the intestinal canal, that the close relation is manifested between the diarrhœa of the infant and dysentery in the adult. The changes in the small intestine are almost always confined to the lower part of the ileum, and become more striking the nearer we approach to the ileo-cæcal valve. They consist in a more or less intense redness of the mucous membrane, which sometimes appears thickened, and presents something of a velvety appearance, studded over with numerous dark spots,—the orifices of the solitary glands. In other instances, the surface of the reddened mucous membrane appears slightly roughened, as if sprinkled over with fine sand; while near to the cæcum this roughening is often greater, the membrane appearing elevated into rough orange-colored prominences, separated by narrow lines of a dead white color, which mark the situations where, by the destruction of the mucous membrane, the subjacent tissue is exposed. Besides this affection of the mucous membrane of the ileum, Peyer's glands are not infrequently very well marked in the lower part of the small intestine, and their surface presents a punctated appearance, due to the unusual distinctness of the orifices of the sacculi which compose each gland. Occasionally a few of them are congested and swollen, and once or twice I have observed one or two spots of ulceration on that cluster of Peyer's glands which is situated close to the ileo-cæcal valve; but in every instance the affection of the small intestine has appeared to be secondary and quite subsidiary to the disease in the colon. Lastly, I may observe that the mesenteric glands, even in the vicinity of the diseased large intestine, deviate but little from a state of health, being at most a little larger, and of a somewhat redder color, than usual,—a condition which contrasts remarkably with their serious affection in cases of typhoid fever in childhood, where yet the intestinal lesion is often much less considerable.

The *symptoms of inflammatory diarrhœa* sometimes become developed very gradually out of what had seemed at first to be nothing more than a simple looseness of the bowels; but, in the majority of cases, they present, almost from the outset, a graver character than those of simple diarrhœa, and are associated with more serious constitutional disturbance. When the attack comes on suddenly, it often commences with vomiting; and though in many instances the sickness does not recur frequently, yet sometimes the irritability of the stomach continues for twenty-four or forty-eight hours to be so extreme, that every drop of fluid taken is immediately rejected, and that frequent efforts at vomiting are made even when the stomach is empty. Violent relaxation of the bowels occurs almost simultaneously with the vomiting; and the child sometimes has as many as twenty or thirty evacuations, or even more, in the course of twenty-four hours. The motions are at first fecal; but they soon lose their natural character, and become intermixed with slime, often streaked with blood. At first they are abundant, and are often expelled with violence; but before long they become scanty, though sometimes they still gush out without much effort on the part of the child. The character of the evacuations again changes; in the severest cases they not only lose their fecal appearance, but become like dirty-green water, with which neither blood nor intestinal mucus is intermingled. Usually, however, when the first violence of the purging has a little abated, although some serous stools may still be voided, yet the evacuations consist chiefly of intestinal mucus intermixed with a little fæces, and more or less streaked with blood. The scanty mucous stools are generally expelled with much straining and difficulty; a few drops of blood sometimes follow them; and once or twice at an early period of the attack, I have known an infant void as much as a tablespoonful of pure blood.

The constitutional symptoms which accompany an attack of this description are usually very severe; the skin becomes dry and very hot, though unequally; the pulse is quickened, often very much so; the head is heavy; the child fretful and irritable if disturbed, though otherwise it lies drowsily in its nurse's lap, with its eyes half open, and scarcely closing the lids even when they are touched with the finger. Now and then, too, the disturbance of the nervous system at the commencement of one of these attacks of diarrhœa is so considerable, that a state of excitement alternates with one of stupor, that convulsions seem impending, and that there are distinct carpopedal contractions, or startings of the tendons of the wrist or forearm. Now and then, too, I have known convulsions actually occur, and be succeeded by a comatose condition, from which the child never recovered to more than a sort of semi-consciousness; exhaustion speedily following the first violent disturbance of the nervous system. The abdomen is usually full, and rather tympanitic, but seldom very tender; nor does the child seem to suffer much pain, though sometimes a degree of tormina appears to precede each action of the bowels. The tongue at first is moist, coated slightly with mucous fur; its papillæ are often of a bright red, as are also its tip and edges; while, if the disease continues, the redness becomes more general, and the tongue grows dry, though it is not often much coated. The thirst is generally intense, the child craving for cold water, and crying out for more the moment that the cup is taken from its lips; and the thirst is quite as urgent even in those cases where the stomach is so irritable that it immediately rejects whatever is swallowed. There is scarcely any affection in which the loss of health and of flesh is so rapid as in the severer forms of diarrhœa; and a period of twenty-four hours will in some cases suffice to reduce a previously healthy infant to a condition in which its eyes are sunken, its features sharp, its limbs shrunken, and its strength so impaired that, though I have never seen an instance of it myself, I can yet well understand that death may sometimes take place in the course of a few hours from the commencement of the attack. This rapidly fatal termination is far from unusual in some of the Southern States of America, where diarrhœa, under the various names of Cholera Infantum, the Summer Complaint, or Gastrofollicular Enteritis, annually destroys many thousands of children.[1]

[1] The essential identity of this disease with the infantile diarrhœa of our own and other temperate climes is conclusively established by Dr. Parker, of New York, in a paper published in the American Monthly Journal for May, 1857.

A rapidly fatal termination, however, is not that which is generally observed in this country; but, how urgent soever the symptoms may have been, there is in most instances a spontaneous subsidence of them in the course of forty-eight hours at furthest; or a measure of abatement of their severity follows the use of remedies. The sickness entirely ceases; the bowels act much less frequently, probably not above ten or twelve times in the twenty-four hours; but they act irregularly, five or six evacuations being passed within an hour or two, and then no action of the bowels occurring for four or five hours together. The appearance of the motions likewise varies, and apparently without cause, being mucous, green, watery, intermingled with blood, all in the course of a single day, and with no accompanying modification in the infant's symptoms. The tenesmus in general continues; and in weakly children, or in those who have previously suffered from diarrhœa, prolapsus ani not infrequently occurs; though this accident happens less commonly in infants than in children of two or three years old.

There is much uncertainty in the further course of the affection, and in the way in which it tends in one instance towards recovery, and in another to a fatal issue. Many fluctuations generally interrupt the progress of those cases which terminate favorably; while, when it eventually proves fatal, the affection often assumes a chronic character, and does not end in death until after the lapse of several weeks.

In such *chronic cases* the patient's condition, though progressively tending from bad to worse, presents but little difference from day to day. The loss of flesh goes on until the child is reduced to a degree of emaciation as great as is ever witnessed even in the most advanced stage of mesenteric disease or pulmonary consumption, though its extreme attenuation is sometimes concealed by the anasarcous swelling of its face and hands. The appetite fails completely, or becomes very capricious; and the child refuses to-day the food which yesterday it took with eagerness. In course of time, the desire for drink is lost too; for though there may be no return of vomiting, yet nausea is excited by everything which the child takes. The tongue grows red and dry, coated with brown or yellow fur towards its root, or aphthæ appear upon its tip and edges, or the whole inside of the mouth becomes coated with thrush. The diarrhœa continues much as it was before, except that the action of the bowels is now almost immediately excited by either food or drink. The evacuations are usually of a green color, often particolored, and though generally watery, yet they vary both in their consistence and in their other characters, without apparent cause. Slime, blood, and pus are sometimes present in the stools, at other times absent; and it does not often happen that purulent matter is present in large quantity in the evacuations, or for many days together, though I have observed this in some cases that recovered, as well as in others which had a fatal termination. The body is no longer able to maintain its proper temperature, but the extremities are almost invariably cold; small indolent abscesses occasionally form about the buttocks; and on one occasion I saw an eruption of large vesicles, like those of pemphigus, make their appearance on the hands, arms, and neck of an infant eight months old, about ten days before her death. In the condition of weak-

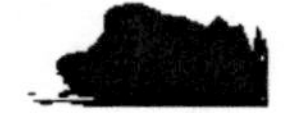

ness to which the child is now reduced, a slight aggravation of the diarrhœa, or a return of vomiting, suffices to put out its feeble life; or, even should no such accident occur, death takes place from pure exhaustion.

But various causes may abridge this protracted course of the affection; and hence it results that death not infrequently takes place before the mischief in the intestines has become so serious as it is usually found to be in cases of fatal dysentery in the adult. Bronchitis is one of the most frequent of these intercurrent maladies, while the symptoms that attend it are often so slight, that danger to the patient from this source is very frequently overlooked. It happens, indeed, in many cases, that almost from the outset of an attack of diarrhœa, the mucous membrane of the respiratory organs sympathizes with the irritation of the intestinal canal, and from the very commencement of its illness the child has slight cough, the continuance or even the aggravation of which attracts but little notice. Unless, therefore, auscultation is carefully practiced, and often repeated, there is little in such cases to call attention to the state of the respiratory organs until the accumulated secretions in the bronchi have already seriously interfered with the entrance of air into the pulmonary vesicles, and have occasioned the collapse of a considerable extent of the substance of the lungs.

Life is sometimes cut short by other causes in the course of infantile diarrhœa. The disturbance of the nervous system that attends the attack issues now and then in convulsions, and these convulsions end in a state of stupor which terminates in death—an occurrence fortunately rare, but of which instances may be observed during those hot seasons of the year when bowel complaints are usually epidemic. Less rare than a fatal termination of this kind is the infant's death under symptoms of a gradually deepening coma, which may have supervened on the suppression of the diarrhœa, or on its great mitigation. Many of the symptoms by which this condition is accompanied are such as to indicate the exhaustion of the infant's powers; but it happens in many instances that there is an occasional flush of the face, or a temporary heat of skin, or some other passing sign of an attempt at reaction, just sufficient to mislead the practitioner, and to betray him into a vacillating line of practice that proves fatal to his patient.

Lastly, there are cases, and those by no means few, in which the onset of a severe attack of diarrhœa has been promptly met and judiciously treated, in which the symptoms have yielded, and the child has appeared convalescent. Some slight error in diet, however, a variation in the temperature, or the too early withdrawal of medicine, is followed by a return of the vomiting and purging; or the *relapse* may take place without our being able to assign for it any adequate cause. The active symptoms which attended the original seizure are absent now; the evacuations, though very watery, generally contain neither blood nor slime; but medicine is often wholly unable to check them. The vital powers fail speedily, and death often takes place in three or four days from this exacerbation of the symptoms; while an examination of the body after death shows no evidence of recent mischief in the intestines, but only the traces left by the first attack, and these manifestly in process of disappearance.

We must postpone until the next lecture the very important subject of the treatment appropriate to all the varieties of diarrhœa and its different complications.

LECTURE XXXVII.

DIARRHŒA, continued.—Close resemblance between inflammatory diarrhœa and the dysentery of the adult—Local conditions favoring its occurrence, as want of drainage, &c.

Treatment of simple diarrhœa.—Of diarrhœa in connection with teething—Use of astringents.

Treatment of inflammatory diarrhœa.—In its acute stage—Treatment of certain symptoms—As the irritability of the stomach, the cerebral symptoms—Indications for the use of stimulants—Of astringents—Management of the chronic stage—Use of enemata—Diet in this stage.

Management of intertrigo excited by diarrhœa.—And of prolapsus ani.

THOSE of you who were present at yesterday's lecture could hardly fail to be struck by the close resemblance which exists between the severer forms of infantile diarrhœa and the true dysentery of the adult. In both cases similar morbid appearances are discovered, occupying the same parts of the intestinal canal; in both the symptoms during life are almost identical, their resemblance being disturbed mainly by the greater excitability of the nervous system in early life; whence it arises that convulsions and other signs of serious cerebral disorder are often observed in the infant affected with diarrhœa, while they are but seldom noticed in the adult suffering even from severe dysentery. But this difference is one of degree rather than of kind, since the morbid poison, whatever be its nature, to which dysentery is due in the adult, produces in favorable circumstances disorders of the nervous system analogous to those which we may have frequent opportunities of observing in the infant. If dysentery, for instance, break out epidemically in a large prison, the inmates of which have had the excitability of their nervous system increased by the debilitating influence of long confinement, tremors, cramps, spasms, convulsions, or stupor may attend upon the affection, and death may take place under symptoms that betoken disturbance of the brain or spinal cord. You will find ample proof of this in Dr. Latham's account of the Disease at the Penitentiary in the year 1823; and in Dr. Baly's Gulstonian Lectures on Dysentery, which are based on observations at the same establishment. Among the striking examples of this complication given by those writers, some are recorded in which, though death [illegible] neither the brain nor the spinal cord presented any sign of disease. Just of the same kind, and equally independent of any appreciable change of structure, are the nervous symptoms that often come on in the course of infantile diarrhœa. I shall have presently to refer to the important practical bearings of this fact, when we come to consider the treatment of diarrhœa and its complications.

Before we pass to that subject, however, we must inquire whether there are any *special conditions that tend to engender* the severer forms of bowel complaint in childhood, over and above those general causes of diarrhœa to which your attention was directed in the last lecture. I believe that such special conditions do exist—that they abound in the locality where most of my observations have been made—and that they are precisely the same as prevailed far more extensively in this metropolis at the time that the bloody flux annually carried off large numbers of its inhabitants.

In almost every country and climate, and in circumstances in many respects very different, dysentery has been known to occur, but in each instance it has been possible to connect the prevalence of the disease with some source or other of malaria. Although while I was a physician to the Finsbury Dispensary, a large amount of disease among children came under my notice, yet my acquaintance with those severer forms of infantile diarrhœa which approach to the characters of dysentery, and which give rise to similar lesions, has been derived almost exclusively from observations made in Lambeth and the adjoining parishes.[1] The children in both districts are alike subjected to the evils of improper and insufficient food, and of close and ill-ventilated dwellings; but in the latter there are superadded certain very important influences of a local character. A considerable portion of the district on the Surrey side of the Thames lies below high-water mark; and the kitchens and cellars of some of the houses near the river become flooded at unusually high tides. The sewage throughout is very defective: in many parts it is effected entirely by open drains, while in some places there are mere cesspools, which have no communication with any drain whatever. Cases of infantile dysentery do not occur with the same frequency in all parts of this district, but they are most numerous and most severe wherever these noxious influences are most abundant. Proof, too, of the intimate connection that subsists between these conditions and the occurrence of infantile dysentery is afforded by cases such as the following:

With the return of every spring, a poor woman brought to me her younger children suffering from diarrhœa, which they seemed to outgrow when about three years old. This diarrhœa was always obstinate, very apt to assume a dysenteric character, and was almost sure to return if medicines were discontinued before the return of the cold season. On one occasion, her infant, aged about fifteen months, who

[1] To this statement I may now add, that since the opening of the Hospital for Sick Children, the patients of which come from much the same district as that inhabited by my former patients at the Finsbury Dispensary, the severer forms of infantile dysentery have again come less frequently under my notice.

had had diarrhœa severely in the previous autumn, [illegible] of it with the returning warmth of spring. The [illegible] were very alarming, and the child had frequent convulsions; [illegible] account I visited her at home. I then found that the [illegible] whole of the day in a back room on the ground floor which [illegible] upon a little yard, at the bottom of which there was a large [illegible] whence there came a most offensive smell during the whole [illegible] warm weather. I urged the mother to remove her infant from [illegible] room, and to occupy instead a front room on the first floor in the [illegible] house, which looked upon the street. When this had been done, [illegible] convulsions ceased almost at once, and the diarrhœa was not [illegible] before it disappeared. I attended this woman's children for [illegible] affections on several occasions during the ensuing eighteen months, [illegible] after their removal to the more wholesome room I heard nothing [illegible] their suffering from diarrhœa. I may just add, that in similar [illegible] stances I have met with a few instances of the sudden and apparently causeless occurrence of convulsions, in two or three children of the same family. Some years since, a little girl, five years old, was [illegible] with convulsions, which recurred frequently for between two and three days, leaving her in a state of stupor. By degrees the symptoms of very severe typhoid fever developed themselves out of this disturbance of the nervous system; the disease during the whole of its course [illegible] sented an adynamic character, and required the free employment of wine and stimulants. While she was convalescent, the health of [illegible] elder sister, who was eight years old, began to fail, and before long [illegible] experienced convulsive attacks of an anomalous character not [illegible] fits of hysteria, which returned at intervals of two or three days, [illegible] several weeks together, three or four fits sometimes recurring in the course of a single day. These seizures were accompanied by much debility, and they disappeared by degrees under the use of preparations of iron, and a generally tonic plan of treatment.

In studying the *treatment* of diarrhœa and dysentery in early life we will pass successively in review the different forms of the disease, beginning with the simplest and least dangerous, and passing to the more formidable varieties of the affection, and to those complications which add so greatly to its hazard.

In a large proportion of cases of *simple infantile diarrhœa*, the [illegible] ment tends to subside in a day or two, and finally to cease of its [illegible] accord. While, therefore, in consideration of the tender years of [illegible] patient, no such case can be regarded as altogether trivial, yet in [illegible] instances, but little medical interference is needed. Great care, [illegible] ever, is required in this, as well as in the more serious forms of [illegible] rhœa, to prevent the affection being aggravated by any error of [illegible] even by the infant being allowed to partake too freely of food [illegible] wise suitable for it. If, therefore, the sickness with which the [illegible] sets in has not altogether subsided, the child should be taken [illegible] pletely from the breast for a few hours, and should have [illegible] more than a few spoonfuls of water or barley-water, till the [illegible] of the stomach has abated. If the disposition to vomit has [illegible] ceased, it will yet be right to put the infant less frequently [illegible] breast; while it is supplied, if thirsty, with water, or barley-water, in small quantities at a time. In children already weaned, a similar plan must be carried out; solid food being for a time withdrawn, and thin arrowroot, or barley-water and milk, in equal parts, being substituted for it, or whey, if, as happens not very rarely, the child should be unable to digest the curd, which then irritates the bowels and passes through them unchanged. If the attack is clearly traceable to some improper article of food, a dose of castor-oil will sometimes get rid of the irritant cause and of the diarrhœa together. Unless this is the case, however, it is better not to give the aperient, since its action in these circumstances is somewhat uncertain; and instead of relieving, it may aggravate the diarrhœa. Provided there is neither much pain nor much tenesmus, and the evacuations, though watery, are fecal, and contain little mucus and no blood, very small doses of the sulphate of magnesia and tincture of rhubarb have seemed to me more useful than any other remedy;[1] and I seldom fail to observe from their use a speedy diminution in the frequency of the action of the bowels, and a return of the natural character of the evacuations. In these cases also I have tried the sulphuric acid, which has of late been so much vaunted as almost a specific in catarrhal diarrhœa. I have given it in doses of four minims every four hours, to infants a year old, sweetened, and mixed with caraway-water. Though successful in some instances, it has in my hands failed to control the diarrhœa more frequently than the sulphate of magnesia and rhubarb mixture; and the only cases where it seemed to possess a decided superiority over that remedy were those which were attended with frequent vomiting and great irritability of the stomach.

In the *diarrhœa that comes on in connection with teething*, it has seemed to be better to pursue a somewhat different plan. It is usually attended by a greater amount of constitutional disturbance than is observed in the diarrhœa of younger infants, and by some degree of febrile excitement. There is, likewise, in many instances, a considerable disposition to catarrhal affection of the respiratory mucous membrane, which needs to be carefully watched, lest by its increase it should become a source of serious danger to the child. The diarrhœa in the majority of these cases comes on gradually, and its subsidence takes place gradually too. Now and then the gum may appear at one spot so tense and swollen as to induce us to scarify it; and if the tooth is very near the surface, this proceeding may sometimes greatly diminish the diarrhœa, by relieving the irritation which excited it. Any such marked benefit, however, is quite an exceptional occurrence; and unless the state of the gums is such as of itself to indicate the propriety of scarifying them, it would be a cruel and useless piece of empiricism to subject the child to the distress of the operation. Instead of the saline and rhubarb mixture which I have just mentioned, I usually employ in these cases small doses of ipecacuanha in combination with an alkali; and think that I have found great benefit from this plan. Three or four drops of liquor potassæ, and the same quantity of vinum ipecacuanhæ, mixed with mucilage,[2]

---

[1] See Formula No. 28, p. 494.

[2] See Formula No. 23, p. 466.

and given in a little milk about every four hours, is a suitable dose for an infant a twelvemonth old. At the same time the child should be placed in a tepid bath every night; and a powder of one grain of Dover's powder, and one of mercury with chalk, given to it afterwards, will often be found to procure for the little patient, previously restless and fretful, some hours of quiet repose. If the child should appear much exhausted, a slight stimulant, such as four or five drops of the spirit of nitrous ether, may be advantageously combined with each dose of the mixture; and in all cases of simple diarrhœa it behooves us to watch most carefully against the powers becoming too much depressed, either by the profuseness of the purging or by its continuance.

Supposing in any case that a considerable degree of looseness of the bowels should continue after a lapse of two or three days astringents must be resorted to; and I know of none better than the extract of logwood, in combination with tincture of catechu.[1] The logwood, moreover, is something besides a mere astringent; it is a very valuable tonic in all cases where gastro-intestinal disorder has existed; and it is one which children take readily. It is, however, not very popular in the nursery, because it imparts to the evacuations a deep pink color, which leaves an indelible stain upon the napkins—a fact which it is as well to mention when you prescribe the medicine. The mercury and chalk and Dover's powder may be still continued at bedtime if the evacuations, though less frequent, are still slimy and unhealthy. If either the evacuations or the infant's breath have a sour smell, three grains of the sesquicarbonate of soda may be added to each dose of the mixture; or if the child is not wholly fed at the breast, a drachm of prepared chalk may be stirred up with each pint of milk given to it; and after the powder has been allowed to settle, enough will still remain suspended in the fluid to counteract any slight acidity in the alimentary canal. If, after the bowels have become quite regular, some tonic should still be required, the extract of bark, with small doses of the tincture,[2] will be one of the best that can be given. You will observe that all the remedies mentioned occupy but a very small compass,—a point the importance of which is never to be forgotten in prescribing for children.

But there are cases which wear a much more serious aspect than those the treatment of which we have hitherto considered. Even in true *inflammatory diarrhœa*, however, depletion is but seldom needed; for either the abdominal tenderness is inconsiderable, or if the attack set in with great severity, it will be generally found to have occasioned so much depression as to contraindicate the abstraction of blood. Still, in cases of recent date, if the abdominal tenderness is considerable, and if it is associated with much heat of skin and febrile disturbance, a few leeches may be applied in either iliac region. The child should be care-

---

[1] (No. 30.)

℞. Extr. Hæmatoxyli. ℥j.
Tinct. Catechu. ℥ij.
Syrupi. ℥j.
Aquæ Carui. ℥ix. M.

A teaspoonful three times a day. For a child a year old.

[2] See Formula, No. 4, p. 57.

fully watched for some hours afterwards, in order to prevent any excessive loss of blood; since considerable hemorrhage not infrequently follows the application of leeches to the abdomen, and it is not always very easily arrested. On this account, I think you may find it the better plan to apply the leeches to the margin of the anus, in which situation they will relieve the bowels at least as much, while the bleeding from them will be completely under your control. In the majority of instances the pain and tenderness of the abdomen are much eased by the application of a large hot bran poultice; the frequent renewal of which often affords great comfort to the child.

If the irritability of the stomach is not so great as to prevent its administration, no medicine is of such general application, or of such essential service, in these cases, as a mixture containing a small quantity of castor oil diffused in mucilage, with the addition of a few drops of tincture of opium, which I was led to use in the inflammatory diarrhœa of children from observing the great benefit which followed its employment by my friend the late Dr. Baly, in the treatment of dysentery among the prisoners in Millbank Penitentiary.[1]

Although this medicine may relieve all the symptoms considerably, and although the general state of the child may be much improved, yet it sometimes happens that a considerable degree both of tenesmus and of purging continues. These symptoms will now be more effectually soothed by an opiate enema than by any other means. Three minims of laudanum will form an enema of sufficient strength for an infant a year old; and this should be given suspended in half an ounce of mucilage, since a more bulky injection is almost sure to be immediately expelled. Supposing the symptoms not to yield to these means, or that the case presented from the first a great degree of severity, small doses of Hyd. c. Cretâ and Dover's powder may be given every four hours, in addition to the castor-oil mixture; which, however, should now be given without the laudanum.

In some cases the *irritability of the stomach* is so great that almost everything taken is speedily rejected; and when this condition is present, none of the medicines already mentioned can be borne. In these circumstances a small mustard poultice should at once be applied to the epigastrium, the child should be taken from the breast, a teaspoonful of cold water or cold barley-water should be given at intervals, and a powder of a third of a grain of calomel, and a twelfth of a grain of opium, should be laid upon its tongue every three hours for three or four times. The sickness will generally subside in four or five hours, though the stomach often remains too irritable to bear any change in the remedies, and the greatest caution will be needed in restoring the infant

---

[1] (No. 31.)

℞. Ol. Ricini, ℥j.
Pulv. Acaciæ, ♏xx.
Sacchari albi, ℨss.
Tinct Opii, ♏iv.
Spt. Myristicæ, ♏xx.
Aquæ Flor. Aurant., ℨxi. M.

A teaspoonful every four hours. For a child a year old.

to the breast. It may be necessary indeed, to confine the [illegible] twenty-four or thirty-six hours to cold barley-water, cold water [illegible] ened with isinglass, the white decoction of Sydenham, or equal [illegible] cold milk and water; and when the child has been seen early [illegible] disease, I have never observed any evil to follow the perseverance [illegible] this short period in a rigorous diet.

The tepid bath employed twice a day, or even more frequently, [illegible] be found of great service in soothing that general *irritability of the nervous system* which often continues through the whole course of the affection, and which sometimes issues in convulsive seizures, or in other symptoms that are occasionally mistaken for the indications of [illegible] cerebral disease. It cannot be necessary to reiterate here the often-repeated caution against regarding the symptoms of disturbance of the nervous system as being always the signs of active cerebral disease, calling for depletion to relieve the congestion of the vessels of the brain, and for antiphlogistic measures to moderate the excited state of the circulation. At the very commencement of this course of lectures I endeavored to set before you the various circumstances in which convulsions come on in early life; and some days ago[2] I tried to delineate the characteristic features of spurious hydrocephalus. On that occasion I related the history of two children, both of whom had been [illegible] by severe diarrhœa. In one case, the child passed every few minutes from a state of listless drowsiness to a condition of extreme restlessness and alarm; the tendons of the forearm were in a state of subsultus, and general convulsions seemed impending. In the other case, the irritability of the nervous system was rapidly subsiding under the general exhaustion of the vital powers, and probably in a few hours more the infant would have sunk into a profound coma, from which no means would have been adequate to rouse it. The tepid bath and an opiate enema in the first-mentioned case, and the free employment of stimulants in combination with small doses of Dover's powder in the second, speedily averted dangers that had seemed so threatening. I need not, however, tread again over all the ground we have already passed, but will content myself with repeating the remark I then made—that if in cases of this kind, you fall into the error of regarding the cerebral symptoms as the signs of active disease, and withhold the Dover's powder or the opiate enema, that might have checked the diarrhœa and soothed the irritability, while you apply cold lotions to the head, and give the child nothing more nutritious than barley-water in small quantities, because the irritability of the stomach, which results from weakness, seems to you to be the indication of disease of the brain, the restlessness will before long alternate with coma, and the child will die either comatose or in convulsions.

As to the time when *stimulants* are to be given, or the quantity in which they are to be employed, no definite rule can be laid down. Each case must be treated for itself; and to be treated successfully must be watched most closely. The necessity for stimulants [illegible] suddenly, or the need of their administration may be but [illegible]

---

[1] Lecture III, p. 43. [2] Lecture [illegible]

while the infant's state in the morning affords, in cases of severe diarrhœa, no sure criterion by which to judge what its condition will be at night. In general, it is not until the active symptoms have begun to decline that stimulants are needed, nor even then are they required in a large number of instances. I have, however, met with some instances in which they were absolutely necessary as early as the second or third day of the disease. This has occurred in cases in which there was great irritability of the stomach, as well as violent action of the bowels; in which no medicine could be borne except the calomel and opium powders, nor any drinks except such as were given cold. In such circumstances a state of extreme debility is sometimes very rapidly induced, and the vomiting, which at first was a sign of the gastric disorder, continues when it is nothing else than an effect of the general exhaustion. About half a drachm of brandy given every two or three hours to a child of a year old, in a quantity of a few drops at a time, mixed with the cold milk and water, or the thin arrowroot with which it is fed, will often have the effect of arresting the sickness, as well as of rallying the sunken energies of the system. No stimulant has appeared to answer the required ends better than brandy; and, when sufficiently diluted, children take it very readily. Occasionally, however, when it has been necessary to continue it for some time, it has seemed to produce pain in the stomach, and even to nauseate the child; and in this case the compound tincture of bark, or the aromatic spirits of ammonia, or the two together, may be substituted for it; and there is seldom much difficulty in administering them, if they are mixed with milk and sufficiently sweetened.

The proper time for the employment of *aromatics* and *astringents* is not during the acute stage of the affection; but when the disease has already begun to decline, these remedies will be found of most essential service in checking that looseness of the bowels which otherwise is very apt to degenerate into a state of chronic diarrhœa. In these circumstances the logwood and catechu mixture, mentioned at an early part of this lecture, is a very valuable medicine, or the watery extract of Bael, and the syrup of the Australian Red Gum.[1] If, notwithstanding its employment, the bowels still continue to act with excessive frequency, small doses of the compound powder of chalk and opium may be given twice a day,[2] or the use of the opiate enema may be continued if there be much tenesmus. By these means, coupled with the most

---

[1] (No. 32.)

℞. Extr. Belæ liquidi, ʒiij.
Syr. Gummi rubri, ʒiss.
Tinct. Camph co., ʒij.
Tinct. Aurantii, ʒij.
Glycerina purificati, ʒiij.
Aquæ Anisi, ʒvj.
Aquæ puræ, ad ℥iij. M. ft. Mist.
Two teaspoonfuls every six hours. For a child a year old.

[2] (No. 33.)

℞. Pulv. Cretæ co. c. Opio, ℈j.
Inf. Catechu Co., ℥iss. M.
[illegible] times a day. For a child a year old.

sedulous attention to the child's diet, and the greatest [illegible] either animal broths or meat or other solid food, a complete [illegible] usually be brought about in the course of two, or at the [illegible] weeks.

There are some cases in which, after the disease has passed [illegible] stage, it still retains much of its dysenteric character; the bowels [illegible] merely acting with undue frequency, but the evacuations [illegible] mucus, pus, or blood, and their expulsion being attended with [illegible] considerable tenesmus. The strength in such *chronic* cases [illegible] greatly reduced, and emaciation goes on to a greater degree [illegible] almost any other affection with the exception of phthisis and [illegible]teric disease; while the bowels are excited to almost immediate [illegible] by even the simplest food. The treatment of these cases is [illegible] with considerable difficulty; recovery, when it does take place ([illegible] is consolatory to know that it often does, even from a condition [illegible]ently desperate), is brought about very slowly, and each [illegible] employed seems speedily to become ineffectual. Throughout [illegible] course two objects are to be borne in mind,—one being to check [illegible] diarrhœa; the other to support the child's strength during [illegible] required for nature to effect the cicatrization of the ulcerated [illegible] membrane, and to restore it to a state of health. The utility of [illegible]curial preparations has appeared to me to be almost exclusively [illegible] to the early stage of dysentery, and to cease when the disease has [illegible] into the chronic form. On the other hand, astringents may [illegible] employed with the most marked benefit, and when one fails, [illegible] may be substituted for it. In cases where the stomach has been [illegible] irritable, so that almost everything has been speedily rejected, I [illegible] sometimes employed the gallic acid in combination with [illegible] and have seen much benefit from its use. At other times I have [illegible] the acetate of lead with opium,[2]—a combination which retains its [illegible]cacy when given in the form of mixture, notwithstanding the decom[illegible] position that takes place. The sulphate of iron combined with [illegible]

[1] (No. 34.)

℞. Acidi Gallici, gr. viij.
Tinct. Cinnamomi co., ʒj.
Tinct. Opii, ♏viij.
Syrupi. ℥ij.
Aquæ Cinnamomi. ℥v.
Aquæ puræ, ℥iv. M.

Two teaspoonfuls every six hours.

[2] (No. 35.)

℞. Plumbi Acetat., gr. vj.
Aceti destillati, ♏xx.
Tinct. Opii, ♏viij.
Muc. Acaciæ, ℥ij.
Syrupi Zingib., ʒj.
Aquæ puræ, ℥xiij. M.

Two teaspoonfuls every six hours.

The above are all suited for children one year old.

[3] (No. 36.)

℞. Ferri Sulphatis, gr. iv.
Tinct. Opii, ♏vj.
Syrupi Aurantii, ℥j.
Aquæ Carui, ℥x. M.

Two teaspoonfuls every six hours. For a child [illegible]

is another highly useful remedy in these cases, and appears to have the advantage over the sulphate of zinc, which has likewise been used in similar cases, of not exciting the irritability of the stomach.

Our remedies are not to be confined to those administered by the mouth; for much may be done towards relieving the symptoms and curing the disease by suitable enemata. In some cases of unmanageable diarrhœa, M. Trousseau employed an enema of nitrate of silver in the proportion of a grain to an ounce of distilled water, which I have sometimes tried in combination with a few drops of laudanum, with very good effect. I have employed the gallic acid in enema in a similar manner; and throughout any case of chronic diarrhœa, occasion will often arise for altering our remedies in various ways, not so much to meet any changes in the character of the symptoms, as because all medicines, even the most appropriate, after having been employed for a time, seem to lose their power. In the majority of instances I have begun with the administration of clysters of laudanum diffused in mucilage, or in a small quantity of starch, while occasionally, in protracted cases, where the tenesmus was very distressing, I have used the black wash as a vehicle for the laudanum; and on one occasion, in which a copious discharge of pus continued for several days in a little boy two years old, this symptom was greatly relieved by the administration, twice a day, of an enema containing two grains of sulphate of zinc.

The support of the child's strength is a matter of no less importance in chronic dysentery than the suppression of the diarrhœa. The great weakness of the patient, and the manifest distaste for nourishment of all kinds, often render it necessary to continue the use of brandy for several days, or even for several weeks. For an infant not weaned, there can be no better food than that which is furnished by the breast of a healthy nurse. In the majority of cases, however, the child has been either in great measure or altogether weaned before the affection came on, and consequently it is a less easy matter to supply it with suitable food. Farinaceous articles, such as arrowroot, sago, &c., are less easily assimilated in early life than in adult age, and in cases of this kind they not infrequently pass through the alimentary canal unchanged. Milk, too, does not always agree, and is sometimes rejected almost at once, unless it be given in a state of extreme dilution; and in many of these cases whey may be advantageously substituted for it. In these circumstances we must not hesitate to give strong beef or veal tea in small quantities, but at short intervals, to the patient; for though it is true that the bowels are often excited to increased action in cases of chronic diarrhœa or dysentery by animal broths, yet this is a smaller hazard than that of the child dying for want of sufficient nutriment. I may add that, when prepared with care, and quite free from salt or any seasoning, and when given cold, I have seldom observed any serious increase of the diarrhœa to follow their use in these circumstances. In some instances, too, beef tea prepared cold by means of hydrochloric acid is retained by the stomach, which rejects almost everyhing else. In some of these cases, however, we encounter an addi- to the child's distaste for almost every kind of food, which it either positively rejects, or having taken a [illegible] to be nauseated by it, and refuses any more; and this, even though [illegible] eager manner and its plaintive cry plainly announce its hunger. [illegible] these circumstances there is still one article of food—raw meat—which is often eagerly taken, and almost always perfectly digested.[1] Dr. Weisse, of St. Petersburg,[2] first recommended its employment in children suffering from diarrhœa after weaning, and it has since then been very frequently given by other physicians in Germany in cases of long-standing diarrhœa. The lean, either of beef or mutton, very finely shred, pounded to a pulp in a mortar, and if the stomach be very irritable, rubbed through a fine sieve, may be given in quantities at first of not more than an ounce in the course of the day, and in small quantities at a time to children of a year old; and afterwards, if they crave for more, an ounce and a half even may be allowed. I have seldom found any difficulty in getting children to take it—often, indeed, they are clamorous for it; it does not nauseate if given in small quantities, neither does it ever aggravate the diarrhœa, while in some instances it has appeared to have been the only means by which the life of the child has been preserved. With returning convalescence the desire for this food subsides, and the child can without difficulty be placed again on its ordinary diet.

Two accidents are occasionally met with in connection with protracted diarrhœa in infants and young children, concerning each of which a few words must be said. It is not unusual to observe a general erythematous redness of the buttocks and nates in infants suffering from severe diarrhœa, and sometimes the irritation of the acrid discharges produces an *attack of intertrigo*, and a serous fluid exudes abundantly from the inflamed skin. This condition, which is the occasion of very considerable suffering to the child, almost always depends upon neglect of that most scrupulous cleanliness which is of such essential importance in early life. In order to prevent its occurrence, the nates and buttocks must be sponged with warm water immediately after each evacuation; the surface may afterwards be smeared with a little zinc ointment, while any part at which the skin seems disposed to crack should be dusted over with the oxide of zinc in powder. These simple precautions will usually suffice to prevent a condition which, in some of the hospitals of Paris, where such sedulous care is almost impossible,

---

[1] The greater digestibility of raw meat than of that which has been cooked, constitutes doubtless its great advantage in these cases. The fact, though contrary to the opinions formerly entertained on the subject, appears to be substantiated, not merely by carefully conducted experiments on artificial digestion, but also by observations on the subject, for which opportunity was afforded by a case resembling that of the Canadian, who was for so long a time under the notice of Dr. Beaumont. See a dissertation, Succi Gastrici Humani Vis Digestiva ope Fistulæ [illegible] Indagata. Auctore Ernesto de Schrœder. Dorpat, 1853. The author arrives at the conclusion, "carnem crudam in ventriculo hominis facilius quam carnem [illegible] solutam esse." M. Trousseau, at p. 128 of vol iii, of the 2d edition of his [illegible] Médicale, bears the strongest testimony to the utility of raw meat in [illegible] rhœa, and more especially of that form which succeeds to weaning.

[2] Journal f. Kinderkrankheiten, vol. iv, 1846, p. 99.

degenerates into a state of unhealthy ulceration that exhausts the infant's powers, and sometimes contributes to its destruction quite as much as the diarrhœa in the course of which it came on.

Prolapsus of the anus is another troublesome accident which sometimes takes place in the course of protracted diarrhœa. It abates, however, almost always, as the diarrhœa diminishes, and generally ceases altogether as the child regains its strength. When there is a disposition to it during the acute stage of the affection, this may often be controlled if the nurse be instructed to support the margin of the anus during each evacuation, and thus to prevent the descent of the bowel, while the opiate enema which relieves the tenesmus is of most essential service, by thus removing the cause of the prolapse. The child's attendant should also be taught how to return the bowel if it should come down; and this is best effected by means of gentle pressure with a napkin wrung out of cold water. If, as the diarrhœa abates, the prolapse should still continue, the nurse must still support the edge of the bowel during each effort at defecation, if the child cannot be induced to pass its evacuations lying down. If, however, the gut should come down independent of efforts at defecation, it may be necessary to confine the child to bed for some little time, while the buttocks may be kept close together by a couple of broad strips of plaster passed round from one hip to the other. I have seen many cases which, as out-patients, were most rebellious to all treatment, completely cured by a few weeks' stay in bed. When the child begins to go about again it may be wise to let it wear a pad and bandage for a short time, while some advantage may be gained by the daily employment for a week or two of a small enema of cold water or of the decoction of tormentilla, or of some other astringent.[1]

---

[1] It does not come within my province to discuss the surgical treatment of long-standing prolapsus ani. Cold enemata, however, or any proceedings not addressed to the paralyzed state of the sphincter itself, are in such cases entirely useless; and the removal of some of the folds of skin at the margin of the anus, or the application of the actual cautery at four opposite points in that situation, are the only measures likely to be of service. With reference to the latter proceeding, which has the advantage of being the less severe, and in the young child is said to be generally effectual, see a paper by M. Duchaussez, in the Archives de Médecine, September, 1853. See also Holmes, op. cit., p. 577.

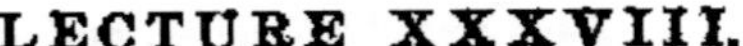

LECTURE XXXVIII.

PERITONITIS.—Sometimes occurs during fœtal existence, or in very [illegible]—Is then possibly dependent on syphilitic taint—When epidemic in [illegible] tutions, is often connected with infantile erysipelas.

Peritonitis in after childhood—A rare occurrence—Generally [illegible] febrile attack—Case illustrative of its symptoms, which are much [illegible] in the adult—Occasional escape of the fluids effused, through the [illegible] walls, and recovery of the patient—Inflammation sometimes [illegible] especially in connection with disease about the appendix [illegible] cases—Treatment of peritonitis.

Chronic peritonitis—Almost always a tubercular disease—Morbid [illegible] Symptoms—Their vagueness—Pauses in the advance of the [illegible] and often obscure forms which it assumes—Close analogy between its [illegible] and those referred to tubercular disease of the mesenteric glands.

TABES MESENTERICA.—Rarity of extensive disease of the glands—[illegible] symptoms when uncomplicated—Treatment of it, and of tubercular [illegible]

FROM the study of the affections of the mucous lining of the [illegible] tinal canal, we pass by a natural transition to that of the disease [illegible] serous investment. *Peritonitis*, however, which is not very [illegible] as an idiopathic affection at any period of life, is still more rare [illegible] the greater number of the years of childhood; while its [illegible] not deviate in any important respect from those which [illegible] in the adult. It would be idle to spend our time in speculating on [illegible] reasons for the rarity of inflammation of the peritoneum in early [illegible] Some connection may perhaps be thought to subsist between the [illegible] irritability of the intestinal mucous membrane, and its [illegible] disease during the greater part of childhood on the one hand, [illegible] immunity from disease which the peritoneum exhibits during the [illegible] period. At any rate, it is certain that in the new-born infant, in [illegible] the former peculiarity has not yet become developed, inflammation [illegible] the peritoneum is of more common occurrence than in subsequent [illegible] hood.

Inflammation of the peritoneum, giving rise to adhesions between [illegible] intestines, and to the effusion of lymph and serum into the cavity of the abdomen, occurs sometimes even *during intra-uterine life*, and [illegible] sions the death of the fœtus. It is not possible to say with [illegible] to what cause the disease should be attributed at a time when the [illegible] is sheltered from all those influences from without which may [illegible] inflammation after birth; but it is worthy of notice that in many [illegible] stances of peritonitis in the fœtus, traces of syphilitic disease are [illegible] upon it; or there is clear evidence of the existence of venereal [illegible] the mother. In such cases, the inflammation of the serous [illegible] the abdomen is probably due to the altered state of the [illegible] a cause to which, in after life, inflammation of the serous [illegible] is frequently owing.

My own experience of non-congenital peritonitis in early infancy is extremely small, and consists of only two cases; in one, which recovered, it was obviously connected with syphilitic taint, but in the other, which proved fatal, and which ran an acute course, it was impossible to assign any cause whatever for its occurrence. In this instance, the infant, seven months old, who had been brought up by hand since the age of four months, was put to bed perfectly well, but awoke in the night screaming with pain. The child became very sick, its abdomen was tense and tender, and the urinary secretion exceedingly scanty. In six days the child died under a continuance of these symptoms, and after death there was found a large quantity of sero-purulent fluid in the abdomen; the intestines and the abdominal peritoneum were coated with a thin layer of lymph, and their vessels were congested. There was no tubercle in any organ, no obstruction of any kind; and, indeed, the bowels had acted from mild aperients; no disease was to be found except the simple acute peritonitis.

The other case was that of a little boy, five weeks old (whose mother had twice before been confined prematurely with stillborn children), who began to have snuffles at the age of three weeks. In the course of the next week a few copper-colored spots appeared about his face; his scrotum next grew sore, then his voice became hoarse and his lips cracked; and at the end of the fourth week he grew sick and his abdomen enlarged and became tender. When brought to me, the child was extremely small; he was greatly emaciated; the skin of his face wrinkled; his appearance distressed; his chin covered with copper-colored blotches; the angles of his mouth were ulcerated; his lips cracked; and small sores beset his scrotum. His abdomen likewise was very large; it was remarkably prominent about the umbilicus, and its superficial veins were much enlarged. It was extremely tense, somewhat tympanitic, and though dull in places, it yet did not yield the impression of distinct fluctuation anywhere. The abdomen was exceedingly tender to the touch, but the child seemed in pain also even when quite quiet; he had been very sick for nearly a week, and vomited almost immediately after sucking, besides which he threw up a yellow fluid at other times. His bowels were purged several times a day. His mother, who did not suffer at that time from any syphilitic symptom, was put upon a mild mercurial course, with iodide of potassium and sarsaparilla; and the mercury with chalk was likewise administered to the child. By degrees, as the syphilitic spots faded, the abdomen grew less tender, and less swollen—it became soft; and in the course of time the infant regained perfect health.

The symptoms in this case ran a chronic course; but peritonitis of an acute character, and tending to a rapidly fatal termination, is sometimes observed to occur among very young infants when collected together in large numbers, and under conditions unfavorable to health. A French physician, M. Thore,[1] during a year's observation at the Hospice des Enfans Trouvés at Paris, found that acute peritonitis

[1] De la Péritonite chez les Nouveau-nés, in the Archives Gén. de Méd. for August and September, 1846.

existed in about six per cent. of the infants who died at that institution. The disease, such as he observed it, seems to be ... affection of early infancy, since, though the hospice contains ... of all ages, yet no child above the age of ten weeks was attacked by it, while thirty-five out of fifty-nine were less than a fortnight old. The previous health of the children had in some instances been good, but in many cases the peritonitis appeared as a consequence or complication of some other affection. A sudden tympanitic swelling of the abdomen was often the first symptom of the disease, and was ... associated with vomiting of a greenish matter; which phenomenon, however, was seldom of long continuance. The bowels were generally constipated throughout, the respiration and pulse soon became accelerated, and the heat of the skin increased, while the child evidently suffered pain in the abdomen. With the advance of the disease the countenance altered, the skin grew cold, and the pulse feeble; ... the majority of cases the child died within twenty-four hours, ... life was not in any instance prolonged beyond the third day.

The appearances found after death were much the same as those which characterize peritonitis in the fœtus. In none of the sixty ... cases which were examined was there any puriform matter in the abdominal cavity, but only a dirty serous fluid, in which flocculi of lymph were often floating; while the intestines were more or less coated with false membrane, which was especially abundant about the spleen and liver. Pleurisy was found associated with the peritonitis in a third of the cases; and the frequency of this complication is another point of resemblance between the disease as it occurs during fœtal life and in early infancy. Its causes, too, appear to be ... act through the medium of the circulating fluid; for in seventeen ... of sixty-three cases the peritonitis followed upon erysipelas, and in ... upon phlebitis of the umbilical vein—affections which, it is known, are immediately dependent on epidemic causes, and are excited by the same atmospheric conditions as induce puerperal fever in lying-in women. The influence of such agencies is still further shown by the fact that forty-two per cent. of the cases of peritonitis recorded by M. Thore occurred during the months of April and May, while the others were somewhat unequally distributed over the remainder of the year.

When the child grows older it is no longer so susceptible of noxious influences as before; and when they come into play, the mucous membrane of the bowels suffers, rather than their serous investment. Hence acute idiopathic *peritonitis* becomes a very rare disease in children, and peritoneal inflammation usually occurs as a sequela of some affection which has been attended with considerable alteration in the circulating fluid. It sometimes succeeds to an attack of scarlatina, ... the possibility of its occurrence should lead us to look with ... suspicion upon any complaint of pain in the abdomen made by ... during their convalescence from that disease; while, though the ... of its supervention after other febrile affections is less considerable, ... risk is by no means to be forgotten.

The *symptoms* and course of the disease appear to be ...

whether it occurs as a primary or as a secondary affection; but there is a great difference between the severity of the symptoms and the amount of danger to which the patient is exposed, in different cases.

I do not recollect ever to have witnessed more intense suffering than was endured by a little boy, nine years old, who, after recovering from fever, yet seemed to regain his health by but slow degrees, and had almost habitual constipation. He came under my notice on May 25, and was much benefited by alterative and slightly aperient medicines; when he was suddenly, and without any known cause, seized on the 3d of June with profuse diarrhœa, and severe pain in the abdomen. On the following day, when I saw him, his face was haggard and anxious, and his abdomen excessively tender; while the diarrhœa continued even more profusely than before. Some leeches were applied to the abdomen and calomel and Dover's powder were given every four hours; but the leeches drew but little blood, and though the purging ceased, the pain in the abdomen increased in severity. On the 5th of June I found the boy lying on his back, with his legs stretched straight out; while the slightest movement, or any attempt to sit up, produced excruciating pain. The abdomen was tympanitic, very tender to the touch, and especially so just below the umbilicus. The pulse was frequent and sharp; the tongue moist, and uniformly coated with yellow fur. Leeches were again applied, in greater numbers than before; and the mercurial was given every three instead of every four hours. Towards evening he was rather better, but the pain, which was referred especially to the neighborhood of the umbilicus, came on severely during the night, and was aggravated in paroxysms. He had passed no urine for many hours, but only half a pint was drawn off by the catheter, and this was dark-colored, and had a very strong smell. The bowels had acted only once, and then scantily. The same remedies were continued, but the child's condition continued to grow worse; and during the night he was in such pain that he frequently shrieked aloud, so as to alarm the neighborhood. On the morning of the 7th he had turned round upon his right side, and lay with his knees drawn up towards his abdomen, his head supported in his mother's lap; his face expressed the most intense suffering, and he shrieked frequently with pain. The abdomen was much distended, and so tender that it could not endure the slightest touch. The pulse had become frequent and thready. He had made water twice of his own accord. The abdomen was now covered with a large blister; beef tea and brandy were given to support the vital powers; and while the mercurial was continued, an endeavor was made by a full dose of opium, to procure a temporary abatement of the child's sufferings. When seen at 6 P.M. he had vomited frequently a dark green fluid, and had passed three natural liquid evacuations. He was lying in the same attitude as before, dozing with half-closed eyes, his forehead wrinkled, the corners of his mouth drawn down, terror and pain stamped on his countenance,—seeming as if dying, till roused by a return of pain, when he called with loud and piteous cries on his mother for help. His pulse was now smaller and more thready. During the night his sufferings were unceasing; towards morning he became quieter, and died quietly at 9 A.M. on June the 8th.

On opening the abdomen, thin pus, unmixed with [illegible] forth in great abundance. It quite concealed the intes[illegible] and must have amounted to at least a quart. The perit[illegible] the abdominal walls was highly vascular, especially in the [illegible] region; that covering the intestines had lost its natural [illegible] was softer, and seemed thicker, but was not much injected. [illegible] no lymph effused on any part of the parietal peritoneum, [illegible] there any adhesions between the intestines; but the spleen [illegible] the latter especially on its convex surface, were coated [illegible] The whole tract of the intestines was examined with great [illegible] was found to be quite healthy; the mucous membrane being [illegible] pale. There was some crude tuberculous matter in the [illegible] glands. The right side of the chest contained a pint of pus, [illegible] that in the abdomen; the right pleura was intensely vascular, [illegible] condition was especially remarkable in that part of it which [illegible] diaphragm; a patch of lymph, of small extent, formed a [illegible] between the two surfaces of the lung, while the right lung [illegible] had a rather thick coating of false membrane. Some tubercle [illegible] bronchial glands, and a compressed state of the substance of the [illegible] lung, formed the rest of the morbid appearances.

There can be no doubt but that, in the early stages of this [illegible] more active plan of treatment ought to have been adopted. [illegible] lated, however, not as an illustration of the therapeutical princi[illegible] which you should be guided, but as affording a remarkably good [illegible] men of the symptoms of acute peritonitis. The inflammation [illegible] pleura was doubtless secondary to that of the peritoneum, [illegible] effusion into the cavity of the chest probably coincided with the [illegible] when the child assumed the position on his right side. We learn [illegible] this case, that pain, coming on suddenly, referred particularly [illegible] part of the abdomen, but extending over the whole, greatly aggra[illegible] on pressure, or on the slightest movement, so as to compel the pa[illegible] to remain in the recumbent posture, with the legs extended and [illegible] tionless, characterizes the disease. The abdomen before long [illegible] tympanitic, and this tympanitis, if considerable, greatly aggravates [illegible] patient's sufferings. The state of the bowels varies: frequently [illegible] are relaxed at the outset of the illness; sometimes they continue [illegible] throughout, while they are but rarely constipated. Vomiting is [illegible] constant symptom; and when it does occur, the irritability of [illegible] stomach varies, both in its degree as well as in the time at which [illegible] appears. The symptoms sometimes continue to increase in [illegible] until death takes place; at other times they undergo a sudden [illegible] inution, or even cease altogether; though this seeming amend[illegible] attended, or rapidly followed, by sinking of the vital po[illegible] soon afterwards by the patient's death.

Acute general peritonitis is fortunately very rare in chil[illegible] only four other instances of it as an idiopathic affection [illegible] under my notice; and still rarer is its termination by the [illegible] pus into the cavity of the abdomen. Even in these appa[illegible] less circumstances, however, nature does sometimes [illegible] at cure. The active symptoms diminish in intensity; [illegible] parietes grow thin at some spot, where a passage at length is formed through which the pus is discharged, and recovery sometimes slowly follows,—the result of a process precisely analogous to that which nature has recourse to in pleurisy, when she brings about the evacuation of the fluid through an opening spontaneously formed in the parietes of the thorax. An instance of this mode of cure of peritonitis, in a child seven years old, was related by Dr. Aldis, at a meeting of the Medico-Chirurgical Society, in November, 1846.[1] A few similar cases may be found in medical journals;[2] and three have come under my own observation,—one in the person of a little child, whose history I formerly related[3] as affording an illustration of that rare affection, thrombosis of the sinuses of the dura mater; a second in a little girl aged six and a half years, in whom puncture of the prominent umbilicus on the 27th day from the attack of acute peritonitis was followed by the discharge of forty-eight ounces of pus; a renewal of the puncture on the 33d day was again succeeded by the escape of twenty-four ounces, and some discharge continued from this time until the death of the patient, from exhaustion, fifty-three days after the onset of her illness. In the third case, that of a girl aged eight years, the peritonitis was chronic in its character, and associated with tubercular disease.

The peritoneal inflammation which comes on during scarlatinal dropsy is not in general of a very active character, and seldom produces any morbid appearance of greater gravity than numerous slight adhesions between the intestines. It generally succeeds to ascites; and the abdominal affection seldom exists alone, but is usually associated with pleurisy, and abundant serous effusion into the chest; and the symptoms of disease of the respiratory organs very often mask those of abdominal inflammation, which latter indeed seem in many instances to have but a very subsidiary share in bringing about the patient's death. But to this there are occasional exceptions; and I have seen a few instances of peritonitis of a most acute character coming on in the course of scarlatina independent of dropsy, but as one of the secondary results of the disease, due in short to blood-poisoning, and belonging to the same category with cervical bubo, and the inflammation of the joints. This form of peritonitis is not in general attended with severe pain; but is accompanied by great depression, and is characterized after death, which takes place in the course of two or three days, by abundant effusion of sero-purulent fluid just like that which one meets with in cases of fatal puerperal fever. Like many of the sequelæ of scarlet fever, the frequency of the condition varies much in different epidemics; not occurring, perhaps, for several years, and then being met with on several occasions, within a few weeks. I have never seen it, however, except during the time of epidemic prevalence of scarlet fever.

Besides those cases in which the peritonitis is general, there are

---

[1] Reported in the London Medical Gazette, November, 1846.

[2] For instance, Bernhardi, in Preuss. Med. Zeitung, 1842, No. 10; and Beyer, Casper's Wochenschr., 1842, No. 5.

[3] See Lecture VIII, p. 108.

others in which the *inflammation is circumscribed to a* [illegible] times to a small part of the *peritoneum*. Now and [illegible] affecting only a very small extent of surface prove [illegible] (though no such instance has come under my own notice) [illegible] there is correspondence between the severity of the sym[illegible] extent of the disease. I imagine the inflammation to have [illegible] scribed in some cases in which the principal pain was [illegible] part of the abdomen, while the tenderness was almost [illegible] situation, in which, moreover, the abdomen did not become [illegible] tense or tympanitic, and all the symptoms yielded with [illegible] ness to the employment of remedies, though the disposition [illegible] tenderness in one spot was some time before it wholly disapp[illegible]

Lastly, some notice must be taken of a highly dangerous [illegible] *peritonitis*, circumscribed in some cases, but general in [illegible] *succeeds to inflammation of the cæcum, or of its vermiform* [illegible] This affection, however, of comparatively rare occurrence [illegible] presents no such peculiarities in early life as to require [illegible] lengthened description. It has come under my observation [illegible] times; the patients in every instance were male children, of the [illegible] tive ages of seven, eight and a half, six and a half, nine, and [illegible] and a half years; and the remaining three were all ten years [illegible] the first three cases it terminated fatally; in the fourth it [illegible] protracted suffering, in the formation of an abscess in the [illegible] region, which was opened a little above the centre of Poupart's [illegible] ment, the child eventually recovering; while I am ignorant [illegible] issue of the fifth case. In the first fatal case, no foreign body, [illegible] intestinal concretion was discovered; but in the second, a small [illegible] cretion, which weighed two grains, was found impacted in the [illegible] ity of the vermiform appendix, which was ulcerated around [illegible] though no escape of the intestinal contents had taken place. In [illegible] third fatal case, permission was not obtained to make a post-[illegible] examination.

The main symptoms are the same in all cases. First, there [illegible] order of the bowels, which sometimes are constipated, less [illegible] laxed; but in either case there is pain in the abdomen, which [illegible] first for that of ordinary stomach-ache, though a little inquiry [illegible] ascertain that it is more abiding, and that besides it is chiefly [illegible] to the right side, and is still experienced there, even when [illegible] where else it has ceased for a season. Next, there comes, it may [illegible] one day, or it may be not until after four or five, an increase [illegible] severity of the pain, attended with tenderness on pressure [illegible] abdomen, and this tenderness is more marked on the right [illegible] elsewhere. Treatment perhaps mitigates it; but as it does [illegible] at the same time to bring out more clearly the characteristic [illegible] of the ailment. The right side of the abdomen now becomes [illegible] and swollen, and hard, and dull on percussion, which, though [illegible] elsewhere, causes much pain in this situation. The prominence [illegible] right side sometimes assumes the form of a distinct, somewhat [illegible] gated tumor, reaching down to the ramus of the pubes, upwards [illegible] into the right hypochondrium, and backwards towards, [illegible] general into, the lumbar region, while the integument above it presents a peculiar unyielding, brawny hardness. In addition to the swelling in this situation, it will now be observed, that while the child is able to extend the left leg without pain, so much suffering is induced by any attempt to stretch out the right, as to compel him at once to desist, and the posture which he adopts is accordingly peculiar,—one leg usually extended, the other drawn up towards the abdomen, and all the abdominal muscles kept as rigidly immovable as those of a marble statue.

While these peculiarities stamp, almost beyond the possibility of error, the nature of the ailment, it may yet run its further course in different ways, and to various issues. The extension of the inflammation to the general peritoneum may speedily prove fatal; having betrayed its existence, not by intense pain, but by a state of general collapse, in which, while the skin is cold and the pulse scarcely perceptible, the intellect is clear and the temper unruffled. It was thus I saw a little boy die, who was eight and a half years old, and who, though liable to constipation, was as well as usual till August 11th. He then had stomach-ache, which was not relieved by an aperient, and on the next day was more severe, though chiefly referred to the right side of the abdomen. On the 13th some leeches mitigated the pain, but their application produced extreme faintness. On recovering from this faintness there was no longer any tenderness of the abdomen, but the two most remarkable symptoms were a peculiar tension of the abdominal muscles, and inability to move the right leg without pain. Swelling, too, was now apparent in the right pubo-iliac region, and on the 14th this was still more marked, while, though there was no increase of pain, the pulse had risen in frequency to 130. In the afternoon of that day, after scanty relief from the bowels, consequent on the administration of an enema, the child, without pain, sank into a state of collapse, in which his pulse became almost imperceptible, and his surface was bathed with cold sweat. In four hours he rallied somewhat, and his face, though pale and anxious, by no means suggested that dissolution was impending, for his manner was quite calm, and his gentle consideration for others, which had formed part of his very lovely character, was quite remarkable. His pulse, however, was like a thread, and his surface cold like that of a cholera patient. He said that he had scarcely any pain, and that his great distress was from thirst, which no fluids quenched, though he took water abundantly, and very seldom vomited. He grew colder and colder, his pulse became more and more feeble: now and then he wandered for a moment, but was self-possessed the moment he was spoken to, and the last words that he spoke just before his death, which took place eight hours after the state of collapse came on, were, "Thank you, sir," to one who gave him a draught of water. The death which came so gently though so quickly, seemed due in this case not to the intensity of the inflammation, but to its extension over the whole of the peritoneum. This, however, does not appear to be the most common issue of the affecti[illegible] ly the mischief remains circumscribed to the [illegible] originated. It did so in another fatal case [illegible] though the irritation extended to the chest, and pleurisy [illegible] side, which issued in abundant sero-purulent effusion, [illegible] largely to bring about the death of the child. Sometimes [illegible] mation subsides, the tenderness abates, the swelling disappears [illegible] convalescence gradually takes place. I believe, however, that [illegible] the mischief is slight, resolution is a rare occurrence, and that [illegible] tion of the cellular tissue about the cæcum, and the formation [illegible] abscess, which points either in the lumbar or the iliac region [illegible] mode in which recovery is usually effected; a mode tedious indeed [illegible] painful, but one that, judging from one's experience of iliac [illegible] in the female sex, one would count on as almost always certain, [illegible] slow.[1]

The indications for *treatment* in cases of acute peritonitis, are so [illegible] that it would be superfluous to occupy much time in laying down [illegible] for your guidance. You have to deal with the active inflammation [illegible] parts in which acute disease cannot go on long without destroying [illegible] Depletion, both general and local, and the employment of [illegible] combined with opium or Dover's powder, in order to mitigate the [illegible] fering which attends on the disease, are the remedies to which [illegible] must have recourse, and which you must employ with an [illegible] hand. When the abdominal tenderness has been mitigated by [illegible] a warm poultice, frequently renewed, will often afford [illegible] comfort; and in some cases of local peritonitis I have seen [illegible] hip-bath give much relief. The error into which you are likely [illegible] in the management of these cases is not that of pursuing a wrong [illegible] but of following the right one with too little vigor.

In the peritonitis that follows scarlatina, the symptoms are [illegible] urgent than in other circumstances; but you will bear in mind [illegible] when the function of the kidneys is disturbed, and urea is [illegible] in the blood, the serous membranes are very apt to become [illegible] and you will, therefore, keep on the lookout for any indication [illegible] suffering. I shall hereafter have to point out to you, that in [illegible] well as in so many other cases, prevention is not only better, [illegible] than cure; and that if, on the first appearance of the dropsy [illegible] on scarlet fever, you have recourse to active antiphlogistic [illegible] you will, in the large majority of cases, escape the risk of these [illegible] dary inflammations. Concerning the treatment of the peritoneal [illegible] flammation which I have referred to as an occasional [illegible] rather than sequela of scarlet fever, I have little indeed to say. [illegible] secondary inflammations which attend on blood-poisoning run [illegible] course to a fatal issue, as we know but too well, unchecked [illegible] treatment which we can devise.

The circumscribed inflammation of the peritoneum which [illegible] ated with mischief in the cæcum or its appendix, calls for very [illegible] treatment. The tendency of the ailment even when it terminates [illegible] favorably, is to run a slow course, and unless you could [illegible]

[1] The papers of Dr. Burne, in vols. xx and xxii of the Medico-Chirurgical [illegible] actions, still contain the most valuable information of which we are [illegible] this subject.

local irritation in which it originated, it would be idle to expect that you could cut it short by heroic measures. The application of a few leeches over the cæcum, and their repetition once or twice at intervals of two or three days, the sedulous employment of a warm poultice and the administration of small doses of calomel with opium or Dover's powder, while the bowels are kept regular by castor oil, and the diet consists entirely of milk and farinaceous substances, constitute all that we can venture on during the active stage of the inflammation. When that has passed, and the abiding swelling, hard and tense and tender, remains behind, indicating that the inflammation has ended in the formation of matter, the support of the patient's strength, the employment of bark, the use of wine and animal broths (though still we must be most careful in allowing solid food), are no less indicated; while, even at the best, we must not look for the speedy approach of the matter to the surface, or expect other than a very tedious convalescence.

Acute peritonitis indeed, in all its forms, like the acute inflammation of any other tissue, may subside, but not altogether cease; it may pass into a chronic state, and the patient may still suffer from the consequences of the disease long after the disease in its original form has disappeared. But it is not to an affection of this kind that I wish to call your notice in speaking of *chronic peritonitis;* but to a disease, the progress of which is slow from its commencement, which is weeks or months in running its course, but which yet demands your closest attention, since in a very large number of cases that course is to a fatal issue.

It is not, however, its tardy progress which alone distinguishes the chronic from the acute inflammation of the peritoneum, but the former is almost invariably associated with the tuberculous cachexia, and, indeed, generally succeeds to the deposit of tubercle upon the serous membrane of the abdomen. The occasional recovery of a child in whom the symptoms of chronic peritonitis have existed, by no means disproves that connection between it and the phthisical disease, of which dissection in fatal cases affords such convincing proof.

The *bodies of children who have died of this affection* are usually found to be exceedingly emaciated; and their face retains after death the suffering expression which it had worn during their protracted illness. The lungs and bronchial glands contain tubercle in greater or less abundance, and the pulmonary disease is sometimes so far advanced as to have obviously had no small share in bringing about the fatal event. On dividing the abdominal parietes, long, slender, cellular adhesions are often found connecting the peritoneum and the subjacent viscera; while in other instances the peritoneum and intestines are agglutinated together, so as to render it difficult thoroughly to expose the abdominal cavity. The intestines, too, are closely connected by adhesions, some of which are very easily broken down, while others are so firm that the coats of the bowels give way in the attempt to separate them. This difference does not depend on the age of the adhesions (although in this respect they vary greatly, some being apparently of very recent date, others of long standing) so much as on their nature. Those connections which are formed by the mere effusion of lymph, even when they have acquired considerable firmness, can generally be broken without much difficulty; and at any rate the attempt will not [illegible] rupture of the intestines. When, however, different portions of the bowel are matted together so inseparably that it is easier to [illegible] than to detach them from each other, it will be found that something more than the mere effusion of lymph has produced this union; it will be seen to have been effected by means of a yellow granular matter, like that which connects the opposite surfaces of the arachnoid in a case of tubercular meningitis, and made up like it in part of lymph, in part of tubercular deposits. Adhesions are thus formed between the opposite surfaces of the peritoneum, at first of small extent, but fresh deposits of tubercle soon take place in the vicinity, and the attendant inflammatory process unites together a still greater extent of intestine. Nor is this all; but in time, the tubercle thus deposited undergoes a process of softening, in the course of which the muscular tissue of the intestines becomes destroyed, and their mucous membrane may then eventually be perforated, so that distant parts of the intestinal canal, which at first were merely adherent together, are sometimes brought by this means into direct communication with each other. The abdomen generally contains a small quantity of transparent serum; but if, as sometimes happens, life should have been cut short by the supervention of acute peritonitis upon the old disease, the effusion may be of a puriform or sero-purulent character; though this is seldom abundant.

In addition to the evidences of inflammatory action presented by the peritoneum, that membrane and the various abdominal viscera are the seat of a more or less generally diffused tubercular deposit. In some instances the peritoneum lining the abdominal walls is greatly thickened, and abundantly beset with small gray semitransparent granulations, or even with yellow tubercle, usually in the miliary form, though sometimes small distinct patches of tubercle are interspersed. In the majority of cases, however, the affection of the parietal peritoneum is less considerable, and almost invariably the deposit on it is greatly exceeded by that on other parts of the membrane. That part of the peritoneum which lines the diaphragm or the abdominal walls in the immediate vicinity of the spleen, is one of the favorite seats of tubercular deposit. In some instances the omentum is the seat of the chief tubercular deposit; and though it usually assumes the miliary form, yet now and then masses of crude tubercle of considerable size are met with in this situation. The peritoneum covering the liver and spleen seldom fails to show an abundant deposit of tubercle; and tubercles usually abound in the substance of the latter organ. The mesenteric glands likewise are tuberculous, though the degree of their degeneration, and the size which they have in consequence attained, vary much in different cases. The same remark holds good with reference to the amount of tubercular disease in the interior of the intestines, which, though in some cases very considerable, yet is not so in by any means the majority of instances, while it bears no invariable relation with the degree of the affection of the peritoneum, or to that of the mesenteric glands. Perforation of the intestines, too, is produced in these cases from without inwards, not by destruction of the coats of the bowel by tubercular ulceration on its interior.

In cases of this affection, those vague indications of decaying health which characterize the early stages of the tuberculous cachexia often precede any *symptom* of special disorder of the abdominal viscera. But this is not always the case; for in some instances the child begins, without any previous indisposition, to complain of occasional pains in the abdomen, which last but for a moment, and which cause the less anxiety from the appetite being good, the bowels regular, and the general cheerfulness undisturbed. In the course of a short time, however, the appetite fails, or becomes capricious; the bowels begin to act irregularly, being alternately constipated and relaxed; while the motions, always abundant, are usually unnatural in character,—dark, loose, and slimy. The child now grows restless and feverish at night, its thirst is considerable, and the abdominal pain becomes both more severe and more frequent in its recurrence. Sometimes the stomach grows very irritable, and food taken is occasionally vomited; but this symptom is often absent; while the tongue, throughout the early stages of the affection, continues for the most part clean and moist, and deviates but little from its appearance in health. The symptoms just enumerated seldom continue long without being accompanied by a marked change in the size of the abdomen; and sometimes the alteration in the abdomen takes place rather suddenly, and is one of the earliest signs of the affection from which the child is suffering. The abdomen becomes large, tense, and tympanitic, while its parietes often seem glued to the subjacent viscera; and that manipulation which causes no discomfort, even when practiced somewhat roughly on the big abdomen of a rickety child, is sure to occasion uneasiness, often even considerable pain, when tried with ever so much gentleness in the child suffering from chronic peritonitis.

In this, as in other forms of tubercular disease, the progress from bad to worse seldom goes on uninterruptedly. Pauses take place in its course, though each time they become shorter; and signs of amendment now and then appear—but they too promise less and less with each return. The child loses flesh; the face grows pale, and sallow, and anxious; the skin becomes habitually dry, and hotter than natural, and the pulse is permanently accelerated. The abdomen does not grow progressively larger; often, indeed, it shrinks in the more advanced stages of the disease, and at the same time it becomes more and more tense, although this tension varies without any evident cause, and sometimes disappears for a day or two, to return again as causelessly as it disappeared. When the tension is diminished, the abdomen yields a solid and doughy sensation, and the union between the contents of the abdomen and the abdominal walls becomes very perceptible. In many cases, too, a vague sense of fluctuation may be detected in the hypogastric region, which seems more distinct at one time than at another, is never as marked as is the fluctuation in cases of ascites, and is doubtless due, as suggested by MM. Rilliet and Barthez,[1] in some [illegible] transmission of the shock by the agglutinated mass of [illegible] one side of the abdomen to the other. The superficial [illegible] now become enlarged in many instances, and the skin [illegible] desquamates, and looks as if it were dirty. The pain in the [illegible] tains the same colicky character as before, but it returns [illegible] and is sometimes exceedingly severe, while the child is [illegible] a sense of uneasiness. The tenderness of the abdomen [illegible] seldom increases in proportion to the increase of pain. [illegible] in general habitually relaxed, though the degree of [illegible] well as the severity of the abdominal pain, vary much in [illegible] As the disease advances, the child becomes confined to [illegible] length reduced to a state of extreme weakness and emaciation [illegible] is often hastened by the concomitant affection of the lungs [illegible] rarely by the occurrence of tubercular meningitis; but should [illegible] be the case, the patient may continue for many weeks in this [illegible] dition, till life is destroyed, after a day or two of increased [illegible] some renewed attack of peritoneal inflammation, or till, in [illegible] stances, the child sinks, almost painlessly, from sheer exhaustion.

Such, now, is the ordinary course of tubercular peritonitis [illegible] as it would not be possible to draw a picture of pulmonary [illegible] which would represent with perfect accuracy every case of the [illegible] so it is with our attempt to delineate the features of this malady [illegible] main diversities, of which the differences in the appearances [illegible] death are far from affording a satisfactory explanation, [illegible] the various degrees in which pain is experienced, in the [illegible] the course of the affection, and in the alternation of constipation [illegible] diarrhœa, or sometimes in the complete substitution of the [illegible] tion for the other. One form of tubercular peritonitis, in [illegible] early stages are very likely to be unnoticed, is that which [illegible] when it supervenes upon one of the eruptive fevers—usually [illegible] measles; the diarrhœa, the feverishness, the loss of flesh, are [illegible] merely as attendants upon a tardy convalescence; the abdominal [illegible] probably by no means severe, is supposed to be of little moment [illegible] the abiding tenderness is altogether overlooked. The chief [illegible] against this error is found in our being fully alive to the [illegible] the danger, and in the most sedulous watching of every child [illegible] convalescence is tedious. Another class of symptoms which [illegible] cite our suspicion are those which are sometimes presented by [illegible] who, having suffered from dyspepsia, become liable to occasional [illegible] of colic and constipation, the severity of the pain being not [illegible] tion to the duration of the previous constipation, the effect of [illegible] in inducing action of the bowels being uncertain, and the [illegible] follows their operation neither immediate nor complete. [illegible] disease is sometimes observed attended by scarcely any pain [illegible] grows pale and thin, and has occasional diarrhœa but [illegible] plaint of pain, or at most of nothing beyond a sense of [illegible] ness of the belly; but emaciation goes on, perhaps rapidly [illegible]

[1] Op. cit., tome iii, p. 784.

becomes habitual, and medicine loses much of its control over it; the strength fails, and the little one dies, worn out and weary, but quietly, and without pain. It would be easy, but I do not think it necessary, to relate a history illustrative of each of these varieties of the disease; they would each point to the same moral,—that, under all modifications of symptoms, when a child loses flesh, and has in conjunction with that emaciation, abiding even though but slight tenderness of the abdomen on pressure, you are to suspect the existence of *tubercular peritonitis*.

Some of you have probably been struck by the many points of resemblance between the symptoms that have just been described and those which are often enumerated as characteristic of mesenteric disease. Nor is it at all surprising that a very close analogy should subsist between chronic peritonitis and *tabes mesenterica*, since not only are both affections the results of the tubercular cachexia, but in both the abdominal viscera are chiefly involved in the disease, and both are in consequence characterized by a remarkable impairment of the functions of nutrition. It was natural, too, that in former times, when morbid anatomy was less carefully cultivated than at present, the attention of the observer should have been chiefly drawn to the increased size and altered structure of the mesenteric glands—appearances which must have been often discovered on an examination of the bodies of children who had died after a slow wasting of their flesh, attended with more or less enlargement of the abdomen and disturbance of the bowels. The physiology of those days, too, knew of no means whereby the absorption of the chyle could be effected except through the medium of the mesenteric glands; and the coarse appliances which then subserved the purposes of anatomical investigation did not suffice to show that, even when these glands outwardly present a considerable degree of tuberculization, their lymphatics in many instances are still pervious.

We know that the nutrition of children is often much impaired from other causes besides tubercular disease; and that, when the digestive organs perform their functions ill, nothing is more common than for the abdomen greatly to exceed its natural size. Our predecessors had observed similar facts; but, owing to the imperfection of their physiological knowledge, they drew from them erroneous conclusions. Disease of the mesenteric glands was in their eyes the almost exclusive cause of the atrophy of children, and a preternatural enlargement of the belly was looked upon by them as an almost infallible sign that such disease had already begun. Tabes mesenterica was consequently regarded as a very common affection; and though its frequency is now well known to have been much overrated, yet the appearance of those symptoms that were once supposed to be characteristic of it, still excites much needless alarm among non-professional persons.

The mere presence of tubercle in the mesentery is, it must be owned, of very common occurrence, since MM. Rilliet and Barthez met with it in nearly half of all children in whom that morbid deposit existed in some one or other of the viscera. But though the existence of tubercle in the glands is thus frequent, its presence in any considerable quantity is extremely rare, since, according to the same authorities, it was found in abundance in only one out of every sixteen children [illegible] organs contained tubercle.

The general character of tuberculous mesenteric [illegible] same with that of tuberculous bronchial glands, [illegible] usually surrounded by a more delicate cyst; and [illegible] seldom exceeds that of a chestnut, yet they [illegible] degree of development which far exceeds that of [illegible] glands, and three or four of them coalescing together, [illegible] a mass as big as the fist, or even bigger.

The effects produced even by an advanced degree of [illegible] of the mesenteric glands are smaller than might be [illegible] much smaller than those which result from a considerably [illegible] of disease of the bronchial glands. Nor will this at all [illegible] we bear in mind the difference between their [illegible] The bronchial glands are not merely situated in a cavity [illegible] bounded by comparatively unyielding parietes, but the [illegible] which they are in contact are solid and resisting, and they [illegible] adherent to the trachea and the larger air-tubes, so that any [illegible] their size is sure to produce compression of parts whose [illegible] vital importance. The mesenteric glands, on the contrary, [illegible] tained in a cavity whose yielding walls allow them to [illegible] in size, while the loose attachments of the mesentery still [illegible] mit them to attain even to considerable dimensions, without [illegible] upon any viscus; so that it is an exceedingly unusual [illegible] them to cause the perforation of any part of the intestines, [illegible] them to contract adhesions to their exterior.

To these causes it must be attributed that there is no [illegible] thognomonic of tubercle of the mesenteric glands, except [illegible] perceptible through the abdominal parietes. This, however, [illegible] never are during the early stage of the affection; and though [illegible] occasions I have felt a tumor in the abdomen, which, [illegible] associated with the evidence of tuberculous disease in other [illegible] have been led to attribute to the enlarged mesenteric glands, [illegible] have only once had the opportunity of confirming the [illegible] examination after death. There can, however, be no doubt [illegible] they do sometimes become perceptible through the abdominal [illegible] though at a season when, their cure being hopeless, little [illegible] can be made of the certainty of our diagnosis. In its earliest [illegible] no symptoms at all are present, or only the indications of that [illegible] tuberculous disease of which the affection of the mesentery is [illegible] but a subordinate part. At a later period, when the disorder [illegible] digestive organs attracts attention, the symptoms are generally [illegible] the same with those of chronic peritonitis, save that, if the [illegible] be free from disease, the abdomen is in most cases both less [illegible] less tender.

I the less regret that so little time remains for the [illegible] the *treatment of chronic peritonitis and of tabes mesenterica,* [illegible] subject may be dismissed in a few words. In each of these [illegible] two periods may be distinguished. During the first, while [illegible] sis is still uncertain, general principles guide our conduct, [illegible] to subject the child to the same dietetic and hygienic management as we should adopt if we feared the approach of any other form of phthisis. In the second, the advancing mischief has removed all doubt from our minds, but at the same time has chased almost all hope from our spirits; and we now minister to symptoms as they arise, and try to mitigate sufferings which we can seldom cure.

The dyspeptic symptoms, the unhealthy appearance of the evacuations, and the frequency with which diarrhœa occurs, enforce the necessity for the diet being as mild and unstimulating as possible. The abdominal pain which is experienced in tubercular peritonitis is almost always relieved by the application of a few leeches; but even local depletion must not be practiced without absolute necessity; and in many instances a large poultice to the abdomen, frequently renewed, will remove pain the severity of which at first seemed to call for the abstraction of blood. Now and then, however, symptoms of acute peritonitis come on in children who have previously manifested unmistakable signs of tubercular disease, and nevertheless yield to free local depletion, and the administration of mercury. I would therefore advise you not to allow any notion, how well founded soever, of the probable connection of the symptoms with tubercular disease, to betray you during their presence in an acute form into an inert course of treatment; nor, I may add, into the too positive expression of a gloomy prognosis. Still these are exceptional cases; and our treatment in the majority of instances is confined to relieving the more urgent symptoms. Next in importance to the pain, or sometimes even more important, is the diarrhœa, which we must try by all means to keep in check; and for this purpose few astringents are better than the logwood and catechu mixture mentioned in the last lecture. Sulphate of iron and opium, in the form either of pills or of mixture, may be given if the diarrhœa is very obstinate, though we may be compelled to abandon their use, from finding that they add to the fever, and thus aggravate the patient's illness; but I have not observed the mere suppression of the diarrhœa by astringents to be followed by any exacerbation of the other abdominal symptoms. Astringents, however, are far from being the only remedies to be employed; but mercurials in a mild form, and continued for a long period, have often seemed to be of much service. When the tenderness of the abdomen has been sufficiently relieved to admit of it, I generally direct the use of a liniment twice a day, consisting of the Linimentum Hydrargyri, soap liniment, and olive oil, in equal parts, which has seemed useful as a counter-irritant even independent of the mercury which enters into its composition. It is generally better to apply the liniment by soaking a piece of lint in it twice a day and spreading it over the abdomen; covering it with oiled silk; or, if the pain is considerable, an ointment of two drachms of the extract of belladonna and six drachms of mercurial ointment may be applied in the same manner, and often with much benefit. Besides this I usually give equal parts of the Hydr. c. Cretâ and Dover's powder once or twice a day. The Dover's powder prevents the mercurial from irritating the bowels, and also allays the restlessness and feverishness at night—an end to which the use of the tepid bath every evening likewise conduces, often in an eminent degree. The comfort of the child is frequently much promoted by wearing a well-adapted flannel bandage over the abdomen both by night as well as by day; and the support this affords may be increased with advantage by a piece of thin whalebone at either side.

If diarrhœa is absent, or if, though it is present in a slight degree, the skin is very hot and dry, and the child very thirsty and feverish, the tepid bath, the mercurial with Dover's powder, and small doses of liquor potassæ and ipecacuanha, are the remedies on which I chiefly rely; and to these the extract of dandelion may often be added with advantage. If it seems likely that a mild tonic will be borne, a mixture containing the extract of dandelion, extract of sarsaparilla, and sesquicarbonate of soda,[1] may be given; or the liquor cinchonæ, or the infusion of calumba may be employed for the same purpose; or the combination of the bichloride of mercury with bark, which I recommended a short time ago.[2] It is only with much caution that we can administer chalybeates in these cases, and after having found that the milder vegetable tonics are well borne. The ferrocitrate of quinine, or the citrate of iron, are the preparations which it will generally be desirable to employ in the first instance; and even their effect should be watched attentively. When well borne the cod-liver oil is, I think, more useful in this than in any other form of the tuberculous cachexia in early life. The cases in which it causes nausea or diarrhœa are comparatively few, and its effects in fattening children who were greatly emaciated are sometimes very remarkable. In conclusion, I need hardly mention the importance of change of air, and the benefits likely to arise from a sojourn on the seacoast; for you know how much more powerful nature's remedies are in diseases of this kind than the remedies of man's devising.

---

[1] (No. 37.)

℞. Extracti Taraxaci, ʒij.
Sodæ Sesquicarbonatis, ʒj.
Extr. Sarzæ, ʒiv.
Syr. Aurantii, ʒiv.
Decoct Sarzæ Co., ℥v. M.

A tablespoonful three times a day in a little milk. For a child four years old.

[2] See Formula 29, p. 507.

LECTURE XXXIX.

INTESTINAL WORMS.—Their varieties, symptoms, and treatment.

DISEASES OF THE URINARY ORGANS.—Inflammation of the kidneys—Albuminous nephritis—Generally follows one of the eruptive fevers, oftenest scarlatina—Its symptoms—Modes in which it proves fatal—Condition of the urine—Appearances after death—Essential nature of the changes in the kidneys—Treatment.

Calculous disorders.—Frequent in early life—Deposits in the urine in childhood almost always consist of the lithates—Other causes of dysuria besides gravel and calculus—Congenital phimosis as a cause of dysuria—Treatment of dysuria in early life—Lithic acid deposits connected with chronic rheumatism in children—Symptoms of ill health associated with them—Importance of not overlooking them.

Diabetes.—True saccharine diabetes very rare in early life—Simple diuresis less uncommon—Symptoms of disordered health that attend both affections.—Treatment.

Incontinence of urine.—Circumstances in which it occurs—Treatment.

OUR study of the diseases of the digestive organs would be incomplete if we took no notice of those parasitic animals which frequently inhabit the alimentary canal in children. It will not, indeed, be necessary to say much respecting them; for we know that the older medical writers greatly overrated their frequency and importance, when they saw the proofs of their existence in almost every variety of gastric and intestinal disorder, and even commonly attributed to their presence many forms of serious disturbance of the nervous system. Still, they are in many instances the occasion of considerable discomfort; they often aggravate, or even give rise to, disorder of the digestive organs, while the irritation excited by their presence, being propagated to the spinal cord, sometimes produces convulsions or other formidable nervous symptoms.

Although *intestinal worms* are much more common in early life than in adult age, yet no species of them is peculiar to the child, but they belong to one or other of the five sorts ordinarily met with in the grown person.[1]

The *ascaris vermicularis*, or small threadworm, which lives principally in the rectum, is by far the most common of all these entozoa, and is very troublesome, from the local irritation which it excites. The long threadworm, the *tricocephalus dispar*, appears much less frequently in the evacuations; it inhabits the upper end of the large intestines, and in some cases coexists with the presence of ascarides in the rectum. When it is present alone, I am not aware that it gives rise to any unpleasant symptoms. The *ascaris lumbricoides*, or round-

[1] The work of Dr. Küchenmeister, Die Parasiten, &c., 8vo., Leipsig, 1855, contains the fullest details concerning the anatomy and physiology of intestinal worms, and particularly all those ingenious observations by which the development of the tænia from the cysticercus cellulosæ has been established. Its translation by the Sydenham Society has rendered the book accessible to all readers.

worm, is of much less common occurrence than the small [illegible], though observed more frequently than the tricocephalus; [illegible] the small intestines, and sometimes, entering the stomach, [illegible] by vomiting. Occasionally only one of these worms is present; [illegible] though there are oftener several, yet it is but seldom that they [illegible] in the child in very considerable numbers. The tapeworm, of which there are two kinds, the *tænia solium* and *tænia lata*, is much the [illegible] of these entozoa in early life, and is seldom met with in children under seven years of age, though once or twice I have known it to [illegible] infants who were still in part nourished at the breast; and I appre-hend it is altogether more frequent in early life in this country than in France,[1] or at least than in Paris.

Various *symptoms* have been said to indicate the presence of worms in the intestines, but most of them are of small value; and nothing short of actually seeing the worms can be regarded as affording con-clusive evidence of their existence. No one who is at all familiar with the disorders of early life will be disposed to attach much weight to symptoms such as the altered hue of the face, the appearance of a livid circle around the eyes, the loss of appetite, or its becoming irregular or capricious. Many causes besides the presence of worms give rise to a tumid state of the abdomen, to colicky pains, and to occasional sick-ness and vomiting; and itching of the nose or anus, though often pres-ent when the intestinal canal is infested with worms, yet is sometimes the occasion of much annoyance independently of their existence. An irregular or intermittent pulse, widely dilated pupils, occasional drowsi-ness, with uneasy rest at night, and starting during sleep, are evidences of disturbance of the nervous system, but do not specially indicate the presence of worms as the cause of such irritation.

The small threadworms, which are of all the most frequent, pro-duce a most distressing itching and irritation about the anus, which always become more troublesome at night than they are in the day-time, and frequently prevent the child for hours from getting to sleep. Sometimes, too, they give rise to a troublesome diarrhœa, attended with considerable tenesmus; while in female children they occasion-ally creep up the vulva, and not merely cause much irritation there, but excite a leucorrhœal discharge, which ceases on their expulsion.

The roundworms often give no evidence at all of their presence, so long as they are but few in number, and as the child affected by them is otherwise healthy; the discharge of a lumbricus by stool, or its expulsion by vomiting, being often the first indication of their exist-ence. The common opinion, indeed, which associates inordinate appe-tite with the presence of lumbrici, is probably not devoid of truth; since these creatures appear to live on the contents of the intestines; not, as the tapeworm does, on the juices of the living structures them-

[1] MM. Rilliet and Barthez, op. cit., 2d ed., vol. iii, p. 862, pass over tapeworm without notice, on account of its extreme rarity in early life. At Geneva, how-ever, M. Rilliet states that he has seen it several times, even in an infant of fifteen months; while, though I have kept no exact account of the instances of it which have come under my notice, the occurrence of tapeworm in children from five to ten years old is far from having been extremely uncommon.

selves. The more marked symptoms of gastro-intestinal disorder are dependent either on the presence of a great number of these parasites (an occurrence which seems to be far rarer in this country than in many parts of the Continent, especially in Italy), or on some circumstance exciting in them an unusual restlessness, and causing them to wander from one part of the intestines to another. According to the excitability of the patient, and according also to the course taken by the worm, the symptoms thus produced will be more or less formidable. The diarrhœa that sometimes attends the expulsion of lumbrici is of all the accidents the least serious, or rather it is by the supervention of diarrhœa, or its artificial induction, that these intruders are most frequently got rid of. Much discomfort often precedes their expulsion by vomiting, though sometimes I have known a worm to be rejected almost without warning, and with very little difficulty or annoyance. Strange instances, indeed, are on record of these worms getting into the œsophagus, and thence passing out of the nostrils; and of death being produced by their entering the larynx; but such are wholly exceptional accidents, from which no inference can be deduced as to the ordinary consequences of their presence. Violent convulsions, and other cerebral symptoms, are alleged to be more frequently produced by the presence of lumbrici than of any other varieties of these entozoa. It chances, however, that the most formidable convulsions which I ever observed to be excited by worms, were due to the presence of an immense number of small threadworms, and ceased immediately on their expulsion. M. Legendre,[1] too, has called attention to the great frequency of symptoms of disorder of the nervous system in connection with the presence of tapeworm; "such symptoms having been present in twenty out of thirty-three cases. They consisted, in twelve instances, of more or less frequently repeated convulsive seizures, which eight times assumed the character of epilepsy, four times of hysteria; while on eight occasions the convulsive movements were partial, and affected either the face or one of the limbs."

It would seem, then, that the presence of worms of any kind, just like any other source of irritation, may excite convulsions, or may disturb in other ways the functions of the nervous system. In the symptoms themselves, there does not seem to be anything which could enable us at once to distinguish between convulsions produced by the presence of worms and those dependent on some other cause. In most instances, however, it will be found that the child has passed worms frequently before the cerebral symptoms made their appearance, while the absence of any other adequate cause for their occurrence should at once direct our attention to the possibility of their arising from this source; and an examination of the evacuations will seldom fail to discover evidence to justify our suspicions.

The symptoms of tænia are not pathognomonic of that peculiar form

[1] Sur les Symptomes Nerveux que détermine le Tænia: tiré des Archives de Médecine, 1850, and a second paper in the Archives for December, 1854. In this latter paper he gives the particulars of several cases of convulsions in children from the presence of tænia, and has collected statistics to show that the rarity of this worm in early life has been somewhat exaggerated.

of entozoon, but are common to it and to the lumbrici, [illegible] tion, perhaps, that tapeworm is apt to produce a more [illegible] ment of the general health, and that from the difficulty [illegible] its complete expulsion its symptoms are usually more [illegible] once, however, our suspicions are excited, we are seldom [illegible] receiving complete confirmation of them in the [illegible] the worm intermingled with the evacuations, since, when [illegible] has attained to maturity, the spontaneous detachment of [illegible] from time to time is a purely physiological occurrence.

The different varieties of worms are not to be got rid of [illegible] treatment; nor is the cure of all equally easily effected. [illegible] remedies are of comparatively little use against the small [illegible] though their destruction is by no means difficult if they [illegible] by enemata in the lower bowel, which they chiefly inhabit. [illegible] of lime-water usually answer for this purpose extremely well; [illegible] ascarides are very numerous, or have been frequently [illegible] remedy may be made more efficacious by the addition to [illegible] lime-water of two drachms of the solution of perchloride [illegible] Küchenmeister, to whose elaborate treatise on helminthology [illegible] already referred, speaks of having employed santonin in an [illegible] the proportion of from four to eight grains; but I have no [illegible] of its employment in this manner. He further gives a hint [illegible] expediency in cases which are at all obstinate of introducing [illegible] elastic tube, in order that the fluids injected may reach [illegible] creatures as have travelled high up beyond the sigmoid flexure [illegible] colon. Though I have never employed santonin in an enema, [illegible] satisfied with the results obtained by lavements of lime-water [illegible] I very generally employ it as a vermifuge, giving three or four [illegible] twice a week, at bedtime, to children of five years of age, and [illegible] it by any simple aperient in the morning. It is always well [illegible] the parents of the peculiar change in the color of the urine [illegible] tonin sometimes produces, imparting to it a greenish-yellow, or [illegible] instances a scarlet hue, such as might be supposed due to the [illegible] of blood in the urine. During the continuance of the [illegible] well as afterwards, when the threadworms have been got rid of, [illegible] arations of iron are also of much service. I believe the remedy [illegible] these cases, not merely as a tonic, but also, by its admixture [illegible] secretions, it renders the intestinal mucous membrane [illegible] serve as a nidus for the reproduction of the worms.

A vast number of remedies have been employed for the cure of [illegible] roundworm and tapeworm, some of which are mere drastic [illegible] and act by dislodging the worms, while others exercise a [illegible] sonous influence on them, and destroy as well as expel them. [illegible] treatment of tænia, remedies of the latter class are absolutely [illegible] since, unless the head of the creature be detached from its [illegible] intestinal mucous membrane, no permanent cure is effected, [illegible] detached joints are speedily reproduced. Mere mechanical, [illegible] such as tin filings, appear, according to Dr. Küchenmeister's [illegible] to be absolutely useless as far as the destruction of worms is [illegible] though by no means without a mischievous influence on [illegible] the intestines. For the roundworm, a very efficacious proceeding, and one which has the advantage of not distressing the child, consists in giving a small dose of santonin, as two or three grains for a patient six years old, over night, and a full dose of castor oil the next morning, and repeating this two or three times in succession; and I have never myself seen from the use of santonin any of the unpleasant symptoms which some persons have experienced from its employment.

I have not satisfied myself that santonin exercises any very decided influence upon tapeworm; for the cure of which, as well as of lumbrici, when the persistence of the symptoms leads to the suspicion that they have not all been got rid of, the kousso, the oil of male fern, or the kamella, is far more effectual. For the success of any of these remedies against tapeworm it is, however, very necessary that the intestines should be previously well emptied of their contents. This is best accomplished by giving a dose of castor oil some three hours after an early dinner, and afterwards allowing the child only a small cupful of milk during the remainder of the day, the vermifuge being given on the following morning fasting. The great bulk of the kousso almost excludes it from use when our patients are children, and it may be added that Küchenmeister's investigations seem to show that it is actually inferior in efficacy to several other anthelmintics. The same drawback, too, attends the use of the seeds of the pumpkin, which in their fresh state have much, and apparently well-merited, reputation as an anthelmintic in America and in parts of Southern Europe. For a child of ten years old three ounces made into a paste with honey or sugar is the dose. I imagine it acts simply by its irritant properties. I have tried the dried seeds bruised and mixed with sugar, but without result; though I have seen the use of the fresh seeds followed by the expulsion of a worm which every other remedy had failed to dislodge. I believe turpentine to be a very efficacious remedy, but the violent effects which it sometimes produces, as well as the temporary intoxication which follows its administration in a large dose, have withheld me from giving it to children. Still it is to be borne in mind as a most energetic vermifuge; while the unpleasant symptoms that follow it are not dangerous, and soon pass away, especially if the turpentine be given with an equal quantity of castor oil. The oil of male fern has proved itself more efficacious in my hands than any other medicine in cases of tænia; and the sickness which it sometimes causes seems to me to be the chief drawback from its employment.[1] I have almost completely abandoned the use of the pomegranate bark, in spite of the strong evi-

---

[1] I subjoin a formula, according to which the remedy is tolerable.

(No. 38.)

℞. Olei Filicis Maris, ʒj.
Pulv. Acaciæ, gr. xl.
Spt. Myristicæ, ♏v.
Syr. Tolutan, ʒiv.
Aq. Cinnamomi, ad ℥j. M.

To be taken mixed with an equal quantity of hot milk. For a child of eight or ten years old.

dence borne to its utility,[1] in consequence of the bulk of the [illegible] which I have found it impossible to induce children to take in [illegible] cient quantity and sufficiently often repeated to be of much [illegible]. Küchenmeister, however, speaks of a watery extract which is [illegible] in India, and which possesses great efficacy; but of this I have [illegible] experience.

Closely connected with the disorders of the digestive organs [illegible] *affections to which the urinary apparatus is liable.* [illegible] special difficulties attend their investigation in early life, and [illegible] information which it is in my power to give you with reference to [illegible] diseases is less complete than I could have desired.

In childhood, as in adult age, congestion and inflammation [illegible] exciting cause of by far the greater number of affections of the [illegible] and the proof of their existence is furnished by an albuminous [illegible] the urine. Hence the designation of *albuminous nephritis*, [illegible] seems to me convenient to retain in speaking of the disorder as [illegible] monly occurs in childhood; sometimes as dependent primarily on [illegible] altered state of the blood, as in diphtheria, pyæmia, and the [illegible] of scarlatina; sometimes as produced by the direct influence of [illegible] when checking of the action of the skin is followed by [illegible] the kidney; or in other instances, and those the most frequent [illegible] early life, where the urinary tubules become choked by the [illegible] tion of their epithelium during the desquamative stage of [illegible]

It is after scarlatina that we meet with three-fourths of the [illegible] albuminuria that occur in early life; and the peculiar condition [illegible] I have referred to as then producing it has led to the adoption of [illegible] term *desquamative nephritis* by Dr. G. Johnson to distinguish [illegible] other forms of the disease dependent on a different cause. It [illegible] first be expected that this condition would be found to occur after [illegible] latina with a tolerably uniform regularity, or at any rate that [illegible] be easy to determine the peculiarities of the disease which [illegible] But neither the one nor the other is the fact. Its varying frequency [illegible] shown by a statement of Dr. Vogel, that, "while in some epidemics [illegible] scarlet fever almost every patient becomes dropsical, in others [illegible] number is so small as not to amount even to 1 per cent.

[1] See paper by Mr. Breton, in Med.-Chir. Trans., vol. xi, p. 301; and Küchen-meister, op. cit., p. 122.

[2] Of 120 cases of albuminuria of which I chance to have preserved a record ([illegible] in which it complicated diphtheria not included, since examination of the [illegible] sometimes omitted),

85	succeeded to	Scarlatina.
1	"	Measles.
3	"	Typhoid fever.
1	"	Ague.
1	"	Acute rheumatism.
2	"	Empyema.
1	"	Pyæmia.
2	"	Pneumonia.
1	"	application of a blister.
In 14	the disease was	acute and idiopathic.
" 9	" "	chronic "
120		

In an epidemic described by	Haidenheim,	albuminuria occurred in	80	per cent.
"	"	James Miller,	"	"	27	"
"	"	Wood, in Edinburgh,	"	"	12½	"
"	"	Rösch,	"	"	10	"
"	"	Frerichs,	"	"	4	"

Scarlet fever has now for many years been endemic in Munich, but only slightly contagious. I have treated at least 50 or 60 cases, but have only twice met with albuminuria out of this number, and in both of them it was very temporary."[1]

The common opinion that albuminuria is rare after severe scarlet fever, and frequent after cases of the disease in a mild form, is, I believe, correct; but my impression is, that in other respects there is no constant relation between the characters of the disease and liability to dropsy or immunity from its occurrence. It is an accident, not only, as I have already shown, rare in some epidemics of scarlet fever, frequent in others;[2] but its fatality is liable to at least as great variations as its frequency; for it appears that while in the first quarter of 1848 only 7 per cent. of the mortality of scarlatina was owing to the consecutive dropsy, 20 per cent. of the deaths from scarlet fever in the last quarter of the same year were due to that cause.[3]

That cold and interruption of the cutaneous function favor the occurrence of dropsy after scarlatina, is a fact supported by universal testimony; and that the maintenance of the functions of the skin, and the securing an unvarying temperature about the patient during convalescence from the fever, will go far to prevent it, is also abundantly proved. The early adoption of a stimulating plan of diet or treatment during convalescence from scarlet fever is also reputed to have a marked influence in inducing dropsy after it. It must be remembered, however, that injudicious management in this respect seldom goes alone, but is usually associated with carelessness in other points; so that the influence of this cause cannot be exactly estimated. I am, however, quite sure that the employment of stimulants in such cases of severe scarlatina as appear to indicate their administration, and even the freest use of wine in such circumstances, in no respect increases the risk of dropsical effusion occurring subsequently.

The date of appearance of the dropsy is liable to very considerable variation, occurring sometimes within the first week, at other times as late as the end of the third week, or even later. In the great majority of instances, however, its symptoms appear after the end of the first, but before the completion of the second week; while it but seldom happens, if its appearance is delayed till far into the third week, that its symptoms are formidable, or that its course is acute. It sometimes

---

[1] Vogel, lib. cit., p. 370.

[2] M. Jaccoud's able article, Albuminurie, in the Nouveau Dictionnaire de Médecine et de Chirurgie, 8vo., Paris, 1864, abundantly confirms, by a reference to numerous authorities, the above statement as to the varying prevalence of albuminuria in different epidemics of scarlatina.

[3] As deduced from data in the Registrar-General's office, by Dr. Tripe, whose papers on Scarlatinal Dropsy, in the British and Foreign Medico-Chirurgical Review, for January and July, 1854, are models for inquiries of this kind in laborious research, lucid arrangement, and cautious in[illegible]ed premises.

sets in with considerable febrile disturbance, but even then has a great tendency to assume a chronic character; while in by far the majority of cases its attack is gradual, and its advance is slow. In these circumstances, the child who has passed through the fever perhaps with less than the average amount of suffering, and who for a day or two had seemed rapidly advancing to convalescence, begins to droop, grows languid, feverish, and restless. The skin becomes dry and hot; the process of desquamation is arrested while still incomplete; the appetite is lost, though the thirst is often considerable; the bowels become constipated and the urine diminished in quantity, although the desire for voiding it is very frequent. After these signs of interrupted convalescence have continued for two or three days, or even longer, the face becomes slightly swollen, a puffiness appearing about the eyelids in the morning, which probably disappears later in the day; so that in many instances the attention of the parents is not particularly directed to the child's condition until œdema has extended to the hands and feet. The degree of anasarca varies much in different cases, and likewise fluctuates at different periods in the same patient. Usually, though by no means invariably, there is a distinct relation between the degree of swelling and the severity of the general symptoms; and in most cases which terminate fatally there is considerable serous effusion into the different cavities of the body. In very mild cases the febrile disturbance is inconsiderable, the anasarca slight, and confined to the face; and after a few days of poorliness the kidneys resume their proper functions, the anasarca disappears, and the child's health returns. In severe cases the symptoms exist for a longer time; the swelling extends to the cellular tissue of most parts of the body, the secretion of urine is extremely scanty, and sometimes, though certainly in the smallest number of instances, there are complaints of pain in the back, or more frequently of tenderness on pressure in the lumbar region. The danger of the affection, however, depends almost entirely on its complications; for if they do not destroy the patient, amendment generally becomes apparent in the course of a week or ten days, the urine gradually increasing in quantity and becoming less albuminous, the anasarca also diminishing, and the patient regaining health; though in cases where the attack has been severe, traces of albumen often remain in the urine long after all signs of ailment, with the exception of those of simple debility, have disappeared; and I have occasionally found the urine to be still albuminous even one or two years after an attack of scarlatina.

I have spoken of the dropsy, which is only one of the symptoms, and of the albuminuria, almost as if they were convertible terms; and in the earlier years of my practice, when my patients were seen only at their own homes, I thought them so to be. This, however, has been abundantly proved not to be the case; serous effusion is sometimes entirely absent; in other instances it is but slight and temporary; and in the great majority of cases the presence of albumen in the urine precedes by a day or two not merely the occurrence of the dropsy, but even any indication of increased constitutional disturbance, except perhaps some elevation of temperature, though observations are not at present sufficiently numerous to determine whether this takes place invariably.

It must further be added, that while the rule unquestionably is for the amount of dropsy and the degree of danger to bear some relation to each other, the rule is subject to numerous exceptions; for of 35 fatal cases of scarlatinal albuminuria, dropsy was present in 26, absent in 9.

In the 26 cases associated with dropsy,

Death took place from effusion into the serous cavities in	11 cases.
" " the same cause associated with pleurisy or pneumonia, or both, in	6
" " pleurisy or pneumonia independent of considerable effusion, in .	4
" " convulsions or other uræmic symptoms, in	5
	26

In the cases which were unassociated with dropsy,

Death took place from the direct effect of the fever in .	2 cases.
" " pleurisy or pneumonia, or both, in .	4
" " intercurrent diphtheria, in . .	2
" " uræmic convulsions, in . . .	1
	9

When death takes place from effusion into the chest, the anasarca has usually been considerable from the outset, and in the course of a few days, after having undergone apparently causeless variations, it becomes extreme as well as universal: the features are disfigured by the dropsy, the legs greatly swollen, and the abdominal parietes much infiltrated, while fluctuation often becomes perceptible in the abdomen. The quantity of water voided is very scanty; it is high-colored, very albuminous, and generally contains blood, while it is now and then suppressed for several hours together, and in one instance none whatever was secreted for thirty-six hours before the patient's death. Pain in the back is sometimes complained of, but the chief suffering is referred to the chest; the respiration is labored and accelerated, the child is distressed by a frequent, short, hacking cough, and becomes unable to assume the recumbent posture. In these circumstances life is sometimes prolonged for several days, though in a state of great suffering, remedies proving unable either to relieve the dropsy or to increase the action of the kidneys; death at length taking place under a sudden but usually short aggravation of the disorder of the respiratory organs—an abundant effusion of serum into the pleura generally associated with œdema of the pulmonary tissue being the most important appearances discovered on a post-mortem examination. This effusion sometimes takes place with so little previous warning as to occasion the sudden death of children whose symptoms had not presented any special urgency, and had not seemed to warrant serious anxiety. It was so in the case of a little boy eight years old, in whom slight anasarca appeared on the nineteenth day after a moderately severe attack of scarlet fever. On the third day from the appearance of the dropsy the child walked to and from the Infirmary for Children—a distance of two miles; and though he appeared oppressed and exhausted, he yet manifested no symptom of particular urgency. He had a somewhat restless night, but seemed better rather than worse in the morning, when he [illegible] relieve his bowels, which acted scantily. Soon after being [illegible] bed he began to struggle faintly, and in less than five minutes was dead. The presence of half a pint of fluid in the cavity of each pleura, and the consequent compression and condensation of the lower part of each lung, were the only appearances which could account for the child's sudden death. Other instances of almost equally sudden death in cases of dropsy after scarlet fever have come under my observation. The possibility of such an occurrence should lead us always to watch a patient with great care, in whom the want of due resonance, or the absence of clear respiration in either infra-scapular region, informs us that fluid is present in the chest; since the scanty effusion may increase with extreme rapidity, and symptoms which had seemed of little moment may, in a few hours, jeopardize life, or even destroy it.

A slight degree of inflammation of the pleura giving rise to increase of its vascularity, or to a scanty deposit of lymph on its surface, is very often observed in connection with the abundant effusion of fluid into the cavity of the chest. Acute pleurisy terminating in the formation of pus, or pneumonia running rapidly into the third stage of the disease, is a less frequent but by no means a less formidable complication of albuminous nephritis. The occurrence of either of these affections is often independent of the existence of anasarca, though it is, I believe, always associated with an albuminous state of the urine, and preceded by those general febrile symptoms which almost invariably accompany that affection when it succeeds to scarlatina. Both diseases run in these circumstances an exceedingly rapid course; and I have known death take place, and nearly the whole of one lung pass into the second and third stages of pneumonia, within thirty-six hours from the appearance of the first symptom of disorder of the respiratory organs—a fact which gives a peculiar gravity to all affections of the chest succeeding to scarlet fever.

Lastly, death is sometimes due to convulsions, similar to those which take place occasionally in the adult in the course of granular degeneration of the kidneys. In the child, however, this accident is very unusual; while, even when it does take place, it does not in general lead to a fatal result: inasmuch as, of twelve cases which came under my own observation, seven recovered; and of thirteen, particulars of which are collected by M. Rilliet,[1] ten issued in the recovery, only three in the death, of the patient. These convulsions are sudden in their occurrence, coming on without any premonitory symptoms, except the almost invariable great diminution of the urinary secretion for at least twenty-four hours. They are sometimes immediately preceded by [illegible] headache; and are followed by a more or less complete unconsciousness, and a repetition of the attack takes place almost always in the [illegible] of from one to three hours. The violence of the fits varies, [illegible] is not, in general, so severe as those which succeed to it, and [illegible]

[1] Op. cit., 2d ed., vol. iii, p. 165.

to which consciousness returns in the intervals between the fits is uncertain; though, whenever recovery takes place, the complete restoration of all the powers, both of mind and body, proves that no abiding injury has been inflicted on the brain. When recovery takes place, the restoration of the cerebral functions is not only complete, but rapid; and if the child survive twenty-four hours from the first convulsive seizure, we may, I think, look upon the danger from that source as at an end, though it must not be forgotten that the same state of blood as predisposes to the convulsive attack is a very influential cause of inflammation of the serous membranes, and that, as happened in one case which came under my own observation, the patient may outlive danger from the one source only to sink under that arising from the other.

Supposing the patient to escape the dangers arising from these various causes, convalescence eventually takes place, the dropsy seldom persisting, at the longest, above a fortnight or three weeks; though the child often remains long afterwards languid and feeble, with a weak pulse and an anæmic aspect, while any serious complication may obviously enough retard recovery almost indefinitely. Accidental exposure to cold, too, may suffice, even months after apparent convalescence, to disorder once more the functions of the kidneys, to reproduce an albuminous condition of the urine, attended as before with anasarca, though the dropsical symptoms are not in general considerable.

The symptoms of constitutional disturbance already described, and which in the main are those of inflammatory dropsy, are associated with changes in the *composition of the urine*, as well as, in most instances, with a diminution in the quantity of the secretion. In very slight cases, in which the dropsical symptoms are scarcely indicated, or in which there is simply a little poorliness retarding the rapid advance of convalescence, the urine may be a little less transparent than natural, and present very slight traces of albumen on examination. It has, indeed, been doubted whether the presence of slight traces of albumen for a very short time, possibly not more than twenty-four hours, is not invariable during some period or other of the convalescence from scarlet fever; and the tendency of recent researches is to lend increased probability to the supposition. Be this as it may, however, the changes in the urine are from the first much more considerable, or very speedily become so, in all instances in which any marked constitutional disorder is present. Though transparent when passed, it is of a deeper color than natural, and speedily becomes turbid on cooling, when it deposits a more or less abundant precipitate. It has a strong acid reaction; somewhat exceeds the usual specific gravity of healthy urine; is at first rendered clear by the application of heat, but again becomes cloudy, as the albumen which it contains is coagulated, and falls down in a flocculent precipitate. If the attack is more severe, the urine, which is very scanty, is of a brown or smoke color, deep red, or coffee-colored, and throws down a deposit chiefly of a reddish-brown color; which, however, does not entirely disappear when heated, while albumen is present in it in extreme abundance. It is to the presence of the coloring matter of the blood that this d 'ine of the urine is partly to be attributed; but in many instances blood [illegible] in great abundance, and for a season the case is strictly [illegible] turia; though the symptom in this extreme degree is usually [illegible] not continuing for above thirty-six or forty-eight hours [illegible] recurring sometimes causelessly more than once during the [illegible] illness. Usually, though not invariably, the presence [illegible] large quantity of blood in the urine indicates a very serious [illegible] of the functions of the kidney, and forebodes a slow and [illegible] convalescence. On the other hand, an extreme degree of [illegible] hæmaturia are by no means generally associated; nor does the [illegible] disappearance of blood from the urine constantly imply a [illegible] improvement in the patient's general condition. Of all [illegible] furnished by the urine none is of such constantly evil [illegible] marked diminution in the quantity of that secretion, especially [illegible] such diminution takes place suddenly; and in whatever other [illegible] the state of a patient may differ, complete suppression of urine [illegible] period much exceeding twelve hours almost invariably [illegible] speedy approach of death.

Microscopic examination of the urine in cases of this disease [illegible] crystals of lithate of ammonia, mucus corpuscles, scales of [illegible] casts of the urinary tubules, and in many instances blood-[illegible] very little altered. These matters, however, disappear by [illegible] the patient's symptoms abate, as the quantity of the urine [illegible] and its natural appearance returns: though long after it looks [illegible] and has ceased to throw down any deposit, it may be shown by [illegible] cal reagents not to be entirely free from albumen; and I have [illegible] traces of its presence more than two years and a half after an [illegible] scarlatinal dropsy.

The degree of *alteration presented by the kidneys* in fatal cases [illegible] to depend partly on the duration of the disease, partly on the [illegible] ate cause of the patient's death, being more considerable when [illegible] resulted from the dropsy itself than when it has been produced [illegible] some intercurrent inflammation. When least affected, the kidneys [illegible] swollen, dark, heavy, and gorged with venous blood; but not [illegible] altered. In a more advanced stage of disease their surface [illegible] pale color and mottled appearance, and is sometimes distinctly [illegible] ular, while spots of vascularity, remarkable for the stellated [illegible] ment of the small vessels of which they are composed, are [illegible] over it. On a section being made, a marked contrast is [illegible] between the pale, fawn-colored, cortical structure of the [illegible] their deeply injected tubular parts; whilst the lining of [illegible] and infundibula generally displays a greatly increased [illegible] The granular appearance characteristic of the second [illegible] disease is also still more obvious on a section of the [illegible] on the examination of their surface, while the change [illegible] further shown by the facility with which it tears or [illegible] the finger. The time required for the production of [illegible] the kidneys varies much. I have seen them present [illegible] degree in the case of a little boy aged five and a [illegible] of serous effusion into his chest on the twenty-second day from the appearance of the rash of scarlet fever, and the thirteenth from the commencement of the dropsy; but this is the only occasion, in my experience, on which such extensive alterations have been wrought within so short a period. No instance has offered itself to my notice in which the changes characteristic of the third stage of Bright's disease have been found after death; for though children may continue feeble and much out of health long after the acute stage of the disease has passed away, and may even die of its remoter consequences, yet I believe that the fatal issue, in such circumstances, is usually brought about by the development of tuberculosis, not by the progressive advance of disorganization of the kidney.

The use of the microscope has of late enabled us to advance a step farther than we otherwise could have done towards understanding the pathology of this disease. It has shown us that the morbid process begins in the cortical part of the inflamed kidney, the urinary tubules of which are stimulated to an increased production of their epithelial lining, or even to a pouring out of solid fibrinous matter into their cavities. The urine carries away with it some of these matters, and thus frees the tubules for a time: but as their contents are reproduced in quantities too large to be thus eliminated, some of the tubules become plugged and impervious, sometimes even so overdistended that they give way, and are completely destroyed. Nor is this all, but the capillaries of the organ necessarily bear a part in the mischief. At first, from overcongestion, they become dilated and varicose, and afterwards (in part, probably, from the formation of fibrinous clots within them, in part as the result of a process of adhesive inflammation) they become obstructed or even obliterated. Supposing this morbid process to have gone on to any considerable extent, the kidney must be left by it prematurely injured; while even its slighter degrees must for a time seriously disturb the functions of the organ. In the earlier stages of the disease, the presence of albumen in the urine is in part due to the actual escape of blood from the overloaded capillaries of the kidney, in part to the temporary suspension of its functions. If at a later period, when the urine has lost its preternaturally deep color, and has regained much of its healthy appearance, albumen should still exist in any quantity, there will be reason for apprehending that some serious injury has been inflicted on the organ. At the same time, the reparative power characteristic of early life tends, I believe, to the ultimate removal of the mischief, and warrants a more hopeful prognosis as to the ultimate complete recovery of a child from the effects of scarlatinal dropsy, than would be justifiable in a case of albuminuria in the adult.

The *treatment* of this affection is, on the whole, that of inflammatory dropsy, from what cause soever it may arise. If it has set in with severity, the urine being [illegible], extremely scanty, and loaded with [illegible] of blood is most [illegible] or the applica- [illegible] for [illegible] re-excitement of the cutaneous function; and in proportion as we succeed in this shall we avert danger and expedite convalescence. For this purpose the hot-air bath is one of the most efficacious means with which I am acquainted; it not only stimulates the skin much more powerfully than the warm-water bath, but has the further advantage that it can be employed without removing the patient from bed, and consequently without the risk of catching cold. It may be used once or twice in the twenty-four hours, and seldom fails, even when its action is most transitory, in inducing, for the time at least, a copious perspiration. Among internal remedies, the tartar emetic deserves to hold the highest rank; and I know of no medicine to the utility of which, in the acute stage of scarlatinal dropsy, there are so few exceptions. It should be given in nauseating doses every four hours, and at bedtime; if headache or a constipated state of the bowels does not contraindicate its use, a small dose of Dover's powder may be advantageously combined with it. When, by the employment of these means, the skin has been excited to action, the anasarca has ceased to increase, and the albumen in the urine has much diminished, some of the milder diuretics may be combined with the mixture—as the acetate of potash, the extract of taraxacum, the spirits of nitrous ether, or the benzoic acid, of which latter remedy I have recently made much use, while at the same time the dose of the tartar emetic may be reduced; but any change of the urine to a darker color, or the increase of albumen in it should be regarded as indicating the propriety of discontinuing them, and of returning to the previous treatment.

The obvious desirability of increasing the quantity of urine without irritating the kidney, led Dr. Dickinson[1] to suggest the administration of a large quantity of water, on the principle on which Dr. Wade has advocated a similar proceeding in diphtheria. There is not in scarlatinal albuminuria the difficulty in its employment which is presented by the sore throat in diphtheria; and there is no doubt but that in some instances the plan is very serviceable, producing an increase in the quantity of the urine, a diminution in its specific gravity, and almost absolute lessening of the albumen. The limit of this latter result, however, seems to be speedily arrived at; and, those mild cases excepted in which the ailment tends spontaneously to pass away, nothing whatever that was observed during its use among my patients at the Children's Hospital seemed to justify one's regarding the drinking of two or three pints of cold water in the twenty-four hours as more [illegible] useful adjunct to the treatment.

My experience does not lead me to form a favorable opinion of the utility of cathartics in the treatment of this affection. They are uncertain in their action, their operation is often attended by much distress to the child, and by unavoidable risk of catching cold, while the occurrence of diarrhœa is a very troublesome and very unmanageable complication. On this account, therefore, I think it preferable [illegible]

[1] In a paper read before the Medico-Chirurgical Society in March, [illegible] reported in abstract at p. 355 of vol. iv of its Proceedings.

aperients only when a constipated condition of the bowels absolutely requires their employment.

In very mild cases of dropsy it suffices to give the antimony in small doses, so as to produce merely its diaphoretic effects; while in cases of long standing the feebleness of the patient's pulse and the occasional irritability of his stomach often completely contraindicate its use. In those instances too in which the quantity of blood in the urine is considerable, the restraining its discharge from the kidneys becomes the first indication. For this purpose the gallic acid, in doses of five grains every four hours for a child of five years old, is the best remedy that we can employ; while a small dose of antimony may still be given in the evening, at the time when the hot-air bath is used, with the view of helping to keep up the proper action of the skin. In the chronic stage of the disease, even though no blood be present in the urine, yet if the quantity of albumen is large, the gallic acid will again be indicated in preference to any other remedy.

With reference to the complications of the disease, I do not know that their association with scarlatinal dropsy furnishes any special indications for their treatment, though it certainly destroys much of the hopefulness which we might otherwise feel with reference to the success of our remedies. This remark applies with especial force to the inflammatory affections that sometimes supervene in its course, and more particularly to the pneumonia, which though not a very frequent, is a most dangerous accident, and one in which, if depletion and tartar emetic fail, I know not to what remedy to have recourse. In four of the cases of convulsions which recovered, large depletion was resorted to; but of late years, since I have been conversant with the employment of chloroform in puerperal convulsions, I have also used it in those which succeed to scarlatina, and have done so with manifest advantage, arresting in some instances convulsions which had previously been going on for hours. As in puerperal convulsions too, so here, the chloroform has seemed to enable me to dispense with the very copious abstraction of blood, which, how useful soever in some cases, yet at the best weakened the child, and rendered its subsequent convalescence tedious. I now, therefore, always try chloroform first as a means of controlling the attack, and limit the depletion to such an amount as the state of the child subsequently may seem to require, being guided by the persistence of the coma, and the character of the pulse.

The convalescence from scarlatinal dropsy requires much care in restoring the child to its usual diet, and long-continued precaution against cold and damp, together with great attention to maintain the active performance of the cutaneous functions; on which account it is always desirable that flannel be worn next the skin. In mild cases the observance of these precautions is all that is needed; but in many instances the child is left weak and bloodless, and with its digestive powers much enfeebled. In these circumstances tonic remedies are always indicated, and either the extract of bark or the tincture of the perchloride of iron will generally be found most appropriate, while wine is not infrequently needed to restore the [illegible] any instances seems completely lost. [illegible] tinute detail:

the great principles which should govern your [illegible] be sufficiently obvious.

I have dwelt thus at length on albuminuria as it [illegible] tina because that is by far the most frequent, and by [illegible] portant form of the disease. We meet with it, however, [illegible] we do in the adult, in consequence of exposure to cold; [illegible] rheumatism, pneumonia, or pleurisy are produced by [illegible] childhood with far greater frequency than acute dropsy. [illegible] dropsy from cold generally recover more quickly, and, [illegible] more completely than in the adult; I suppose because [illegible] in general more healthy, and the powers of repair greater [illegible]

Chronic albuminuria is very rare, and, I believe, dates [illegible] great majority of instances, to some attack of scarlatina, [illegible] haps as scarcely to have been noticed, and of which the [illegible] so slight as to have been altogether forgotten. Now and [illegible] nuria occurs in the course of the so-called albuminoid [illegible] liver; and is then an evidence of the kidney having become [illegible] the same kind of interstitial deposit as that to which the [illegible] of the liver was due. Chronic albuminuria is also [illegible] with in connection with a state of general tuberculosis; but [illegible] disorder plays, in these cases, a subordinate part in the [illegible] the symptoms which seem to be due to disturbance of function [illegible] than to alteration of structure. The same applies, too, to [illegible] minuria coming on in the course of disease of the heart in [illegible] In the few instances of uncomplicated idiopathic chronic [illegible] in childhood which I have met with, anasarca has been almost [illegible] bly present; calling attention at once to the kidney and its [illegible] and with scarcely an exception, this anasarca has been the [illegible] tom to arouse the attention of the friends to the health of the [illegible] is in accordance with this, that the large white kidney is the [illegible] degeneration of the organ, which I believe is almost always [illegible] in fatal cases of chronic idiopathic albuminuria in early life.

Although most diseases of the urinary organs are less [illegible] children than in grown persons, yet *calculous disorders* are [illegible] frequent in early life than in adult age. It appears, indeed, [illegible] statistical data furnished by Dr. Prout, that out of 1256 [illegible] ceived into the Bristol, Leeds, and Norwich Hospitals, for the [illegible] of being operated on for stone, 500, or nearly 40 per cent., [illegible] ten years of age. If we bear in mind the intimate connection [illegible] sists between the assimilative and the excretory functions, it [illegible] surprise us that in early life, when the former, though so active, [illegible] readily disturbed, the latter should be often thrown into [illegible]

Very slight and very temporary causes often suffice to [illegible] posits in the urine of children; and these deposits almost [illegible] sist either of the amorphous lithate of ammonia, or of the [illegible] dish-brown crystals of lithic acid. These deposits, indeed, [illegible] much moment, and one might perhaps say that the younger [illegible] the less is their importance, since the presence of lithic [illegible] erable quantity in the kidneys of new-born children seems [illegible] a physiological condition. Its frequency was first noticed, [illegible] ago, by Professor Schlossberger; and his original statements have been confirmed both by his own subsequent researches, as well as by those of Professor Martin, of Jena.[1] Dr. Schlossberger, on an examination of 199 children who died within thirty days from birth, found lithic acid gravel in the tubuli uriniferi of 32 per cent. of the number, in many but not all of whom some degree of icterus had existed. The frequency of this condition is probably connected with the peculiar changes in the processes of assimilation which take place after birth; and any interruption to their performance, or any disturbance of the cutaneous function, increases, as in the case of infantile icterus, the probability of its occurrence. The same causes exert a similar influence both in infancy, and also to a considerable degree even in subsequent childhood. A trifling cold, slight gastric disorder, or the feverishness and general irritation which sometimes attend upon dentition, not infrequently produce these deposits, while they disappear as soon as the brief constitutional disturbance subsides. While it lasts, however, the condition of the child is often one of very considerable suffering, each attempt to make water being attended by much pain, the patient crying and drawing up its legs towards its abdomen; while frequently a few drops only of urine are voided at each time. Now and then, the suppression of urine is complete for twelve, eighteen, or twenty-four hours; but this seldom happens, except in children previously much out of health, and in whom, in these circumstances, the febrile symptoms and the constitutional disturbance are very severe, the bowels usually constipated, and the evacuations very unnatural in appearance. But besides cases of this acute kind, which occur almost exclusively in infants in whom the process of dentition is not yet complete, similar symptoms are often observed in older children; and though at first of a much less urgent character, they are yet of more serious import, since they frequently indicate the existence of a calculus in the bladder, instead of betokening a merely temporary excess of lithic acid deposits in the urine.

In many instances the formation of lithic acid in the kidneys goes on without giving rise to any very obvious symptoms; and I have but rarely seen a child suffer from pain of that severe character which in the adult not infrequently accompanies the descent of a calculus from the kidney to the bladder. Sometimes, however, after frequent attacks resembling seizures of ordinary colic, a child begins to manifest the symptoms of stone in the bladder; and in these circumstances it is probable that the previous attacks of abdominal pain were due to the disordered function of the kidneys, rather than to any primary affection of the intestinal canal. The occurrence of colic in children of three or four years old indeed, should always direct our most sedulous attention to the state of the urine, which will very often be found to deviate widely from a healthy condition,—frequently to abound in lithic acid gravel.

The *symptoms* of stone in the bladder are much the same at all ages;

[1] Archiv f. physiol. Heilkunde, vol. ix; also Schmidt's Jahrbücher, Dec. 1850, p. 333.

the pain in voiding urine, and immediately afterwards, the frequent desire to pass water, the occasional abrupt stoppage of the stream of urine, and the irritation about the penis, owing to which the child keeps its hand almost constantly on its genitals, can hardly fail to awaken suspicion as to the nature of the case.

In the child, however, we sometimes find the symptoms produced by difficulty in making water owing to the length of the prepuce and the extreme narrowness of its orifice, which may even be scarcely large enough to admit the head of a pin. This congenital phimosis is, I may add, not an infrequent occasion of incontinence of urine in children, and also an exciting cause of the habit of masturbation owing to the discomfort and irritation which it constantly keeps up. In every case, therefore, where any difficulty attends the passing or the retention of the urine, or where the practice of masturbation is suspected, the penis ought to be examined, and circumcision performed if the preputial opening is too small. This little operation, too, ought never to be delayed, since, if put off, adhesions are very likely to form between the glans and the foreskin, which render the necessary surgical proceeding less easy and more severe. Another occasional cause of irritation of the bladder, and of difficult, painful, or even frequent micturition is furnished by the presence of ascarides in the rectum, and against this possible source of error it behooves us to be likewise on the watch.

The *treatment* of dysuria in early life, connected, as the affection almost always is, with an excess of lithic acid in the urine, is sufficiently simple. Those acute attacks which come on during infancy, and for the most part during the period of teething, and which are attended with much fever, with a constipated or otherwise disordered condition of the bowels, and with severe suffering, obviously call for antiphlogistic and soothing measures. The warm bath is often very serviceable in these cases in relieving the febrile symptoms; besides which, the occasional immersion of the child in hot water, as high as the hips, soothes the pain which is so apt to attend upon every attempt to empty the bladder. The bowels should be acted on freely by castor oil; and, afterwards, no medicine has appeared to me to afford so much relief to pain, or so effectually to excite the kidneys to action, as the castor oil mixture which I have already mentioned to you, in combination with small doses of liquor potassæ, laudanum, and nitrous ether. Barley-water, milk and water, and thin arrowroot, should constitute the child's nourishment during the severity of its attack; and, even when the symptoms are on the decline, much prudence must still be exercised in keeping to a very mild and unstimulating diet. It is generally wise to continue the use of alkalies for some time after the active symptoms have subsided; and small doses of liquor potassæ, either alone or in combination with the vinum ipecacuanhæ, may be given three or four times a day in a little milk. Once or twice I have seen a sudden suppression of urine, attended with great aggravation of the child's sufferings, follow after the existence of severe dysuria for two or three days; and have found this occurrence to be due to the mechanical obstruction of the urethra by a small calculus which had become fixed pacted in its canal. The dysuria which is produced by the excessive length and extreme narrowness of the orifice of the prepuce can be relieved only by the removal of a portion of the superfluous foreskin; while, when it is excited by ascarides, an enema of liquor calcis, with a dose or two of castor oil, will often produce an immediate cure of symptoms which had been very troublesome.

The treatment of calculus in the bladder hardly requires special notice here; but you will bear in mind that the calculi which form in childhood are just of that kind on which medicinal agents are best calculated to act; and that we have but little reason for dreading those changes in the precipitate thrown down from the urine which take place in later life. The deposits that occur and the calculi that form in childhood consist almost invariably of the lithates, and hence we may employ the alkaline carbonates without apprehension; and under their continued use I have seen very copious sediments completely and permanently disappear from the urine. Their action, however, is far too slow to be relied on in any case where unequivocal signs are present of the existence of a stone of considerable dimensions; while, fortunately, the anæsthetic agents which we now possess, by depriving the operation of lithotomy of the pain that once attended it, have robbed it of many of its terrors.

The importance of lithic acid deposits in the urine is, however, by no means dependent on the temporary suffering associated with its elimination in some instances, or the dangers of the formation of vesical calculus in others. Deposits of lithic acid are observed in the urine of children, as the consequence and the indication of a state of general constitutional disorder, which manifests itself by dyspeptic symptoms and imperfect nutrition, and is often associated with chronic cutaneous affections. Not infrequently the deposits in the urine and the state of general ailment succeed to some attack of rheumatism. I have already told you that rheumatism in the child runs its course frequently with a much smaller amount of local pain, and with less swelling of the joints than generally attend it in the adult. Its remote effects also very seldom show themselves in those abiding pains which characterize chronic rheumatism in the grown person, but in a state of general ill-health such as that to which I have just referred. A child is brought to you with a vague history of failing health; or loss of flesh, of variable appetite, sluggish bowels, and occasional night perspirations. On further inquiry you learn that he is nervous and excitable in the highest degree; sometimes depressed and sullen, at other times so high-spirited as to be almost uncontrollable: each of these fluctuations in his condition, whether for better or for worse, is found to be more marked at some seasons of the year than at others; and often also modified by change of residence, his health being manifestly worse in cold weather, and in exposed situations, than in a sheltered spot, and during the summer season. Anxiety lest consumptive disease should be impending is often needlessly entertained in these cases; but if you examine the urine you will at once discover the clue that will help you to their thorough understanding. The urine will be found acid, of a very high specific gravity, 1025° or upwards, depositing on cooling abundant red crystals of lithic acid, and on the addition of nitric acid giving [illegible] speedy crystallization that takes place, of the presence of [illegible] urea. On close inquiry you will probably learn that some [illegible] viously the child had had an attack of rheumatism, not [illegible] very severe, and that since then his health had never been so [illegible] before; or, if not, you will almost certainly find that [illegible] disease from which, in some one or other of its numerous [illegible] bers of his parents' family have suffered. It is to cases [illegible] that the term of the lithic acid diathesis[1] is applicable.

The treatment of this condition does not require much [illegible] residence in a sheltered and warm situation, and the habitual [illegible] of flannel next the skin, are two points of much importance. [illegible] of at least equal moment, is the careful regulation of the [illegible] should be simple, unstimulating, and moderate in quantity. [illegible] erence to medicine, the alkalies and alkaline carbonates may be [illegible] with a vegetable bitter if some decided tonic appears [illegible] you must bear in mind, and clearly explain to your patient's [illegible] that the condition is not one to be overcome in a short [illegible] potent remedies, but one which will require watching and [illegible] well-considered system of diet and regimen, to be carried on [illegible] and years, and from which it is scarcely safe to depart [illegible] of puberty has been passed in safety. I referred to it, not [illegible] had any special cautions to give you about its treatment, but [illegible] attention to a set of symptoms, the real signification of which [illegible] readily overlooked.

An unnaturally profuse flow of urine occurs at all ages as a [illegible] symptom in the course of many disorders. Its permanent [illegible] when associated with certain changes in the composition of [illegible] and the presence of saccharine matters among its elements, [illegible] *diabetes*. This disease, although not common at any period [illegible] occurs in the adult sufficiently often for us to become [illegible] characters, and to dread it as one of the most formidable [illegible] order of the assimilative processes. In the child, however, [illegible] exceedingly rare affection, for Dr. Prout, out of his immense [illegible] in diseases of the urinary organs, states that he has seen but [illegible] of it in a child of five years old, and only twelve in [illegible] between the ages of eight and twenty years, out of a total [illegible] of diabetes.[2] Five cases only of it have come under [illegible] whether in hospital or in private practice; one in a [illegible] three years and a half, whose brother had died at the [illegible] and her sister at two years and a half, with precisely [illegible] toms as she presented, and from the first appearance of [illegible] [illegible] in both cases only six weeks elapsed. [illegible] [illegible] been drooping for about two months [illegible] [illegible] had not then begun to experience [illegible] [illegible] She was pale, thin, and rather [illegible]

[illegible] the reader of Dr. Todd's [illegible]
[illegible] Gout, Rheumatism, &c.
[illegible] 8vo., p. 34, note.

tongue was slightly coated, but not at all characteristic of her disease. Her urine, of which she passed about four pints in the twenty-four hours, had a specific gravity of 1045, became of a dark color when boiled with liquor potassæ, and yielded with Trommer's test indications of sugar in abundance. The parents, who had lost all heart, in consequence of the death of their other children, could not be persuaded to restrict her diet, or to put her on any plan of treatment, and I never saw the child but on one occasion. The second case I saw but twice. It was that of a girl ten years old in whose family a phthisical taint existed; and in whom the first symptom of diabetes had appeared on convalescence from measles eighteen months before. She had at one time voided as much as ninety ounces of urine of a specific gravity of 1035; and it had ranged as high as 1040 to 1050. Judicious treatment, however, had reduced the quantity to fifty ounces, and the specific gravity to 1036; while the urgent thirst had ceased; and a gain of several pounds in weight justified the hope that the child might survive, though the urine was still laden with sugar. Of the three other cases: one, a girl, aged ten, died suddenly four months after the commencement of her illness, and apparently as the immediate result of mental shock; the second, aged seven years and nine months, sank from general tuberculosis at the end of six months; while the third, a boy seven years of age, has now been kept in moderate health for fifteen months since the nature of his illness was discovered; but only by the most unremitting attention to his health, by the use of iron and cod-liver oil: while the slightest relaxation of rules with reference to his diet is followed by the reappearance of sugar in his urine, and the return of all the signs of diabetes. *Simple diuresis*, or diabetes insipidus indeed, is less rare than true saccharine diabetes; and though where it exists in a marked degree, it is most rebellious to all treatment, yet it has no such decided or rapid tendency to a bad issue as the saccharine form of the disease. Cases, too, are sometimes met with in which there is a great increase of the quantity of urine voided, though not so extreme as to constitute diabetes and not accompanied with the intense thirst of the diabetic patient, but associated with considerable disorder of the digestive organs. In these cases the gastro-intestinal disorder usually precedes for some time the excessive flow of urine; and Dr. Prout states that in the earlier stages of infantile diuresis the urine is loaded with lithates and diminished in quantity, though as the disease advances the quantity of urine becomes considerably increased; and it sometimes contains albumen, or more rarely yields signs of sugar. So far as my observation goes, indeed, the disturbance of the functions of the kidney is in these cases purely secondary, and subsidiary to the gastric and intestinal disorder. The quantity of urine has either been speedily diminished under a due attention to diet and the regulation of the digestive organs, or the symptoms have become merged by degrees in those of phthisis, which has gradually developed itself. My experience concerning these affections amounts, in short, to this,—that whenever the processes of digestion and assimilation are seriously disturbed for any considerable time in early life, the functions of the kidney are very apt to become excessive in degree as well as disordered in kind. Further, such disorder is especially likely to occur just at that period when the simple but highly animalized food of the suckling is exchanged for the more varied diet of the infant after weaning. And, lastly, its existence may be suspected, whenever, coupled with more or less evident indications of gastro-intestinal disorder, there is a rapidly increasing emaciation, for which no adequate cause appears. It will, however, often happen, even when the amount of urine greatly exceeds the healthy average, that the parents of an infant take no notice of the circumstance, imagining it to be either an accidental and unimportant occurrence, or accounting for it as the natural result of the thirst, which induces the child to drink very abundantly. Hence, unless you make special inquiries with reference to this point, you may remain in ignorance of a very important symptom.

When once you have become aware of the existence of this affection, its *treatment* is attended by no particular difficulty, and, if undertaken sufficiently early, will often prove successful. The state of the bowels requires most careful attention: mild alteratives are frequently serviceable, but drastic purgatives are very unsuitable. The Hydr. c. Cret., in combination with Dover's powder, is often very useful in promoting a healthy condition of the evacuations; while the Dover's powder alone is also beneficial in calming the child's excessive irritability, as well as in diminishing the amount of urine secreted. Dr. Prout adds a caution, however, with reference to the use of opiates in these cases, as well as to the sudden withdrawal of fluids, since a suppression of urine may follow the incautious adoption of these measures, and that condition is almost sure to end in coma and death. Change of air to a dry and temperate situation, especially on the seacoast, is of much importance, and the tepid or warm sea-water bath is often beneficial; while tonics of various kinds are generally of service. The different preparations of iron appear to have advantages over other medicines; and Dr. Venables, who was the first to call the attention of the profession to this affection, bestows high commendation on the phosphate of iron. Dr. Prout insists, moreover, on the importance of a suitable diet, into which albuminous matters should enter freely, in preference to, though not to the entire exclusion of, those which contain gelatin. Milk should form a chief element in the diet; while of farinaceous matters, those are to be preferred which have undergone the fermentative process. These precautions too must be observed, not for a short period only, but until the child has for some time regained its health, since a slight error is very likely to be followed by a serious relapse. I need not add that these remarks of mine apply to cases of simple diuresis, not to established diabetes, whether in the form of diabetes insipidus, or the saccharine diabetes. In them, however, the principles of treatment are the same, although the prospects of a successful issue are very slender.

Incontinence of urine is a very distressing infirmity from which children sometimes suffer, and which, in many instances, it is found very difficult to cure. In most cases this inability to command the flow of urine exists only in the night-time, but sometimes it is present also by day; and both forms of the affection are met with in children of both sexes and of all ages, even up to the period of puberty. The nocturnal incontinence of urine is often associated with the presence of an excess of lithic acid in the secretion; and in such cases the first step towards remedying the infirmity consists in correcting the morbid state of the fluid. Now and then it appears to be dependent upon the irritation produced by ascarides in the rectum, while in the majority of cases, so long as the affection is recent, a connection may be clearly traced between it and gastro-intestinal disorder. If not remedied, however, all the functions of the body may return to a healthy state, while yet the incontinence is perpetuated by a kind of habit which it is found very difficult to break through.

The involuntary discharge of urine by daytime as well as at night is a still more troublesome affection, except when it depends, as is by no means seldom the case, on the child's indolence and indifference, when one or two judicious whippings cure an apparently deep-rooted evil. We must, however, in every instance examine a case with the greatest care before we come to the conclusion that the apparent infirmity is within the power of the child to prevent. Sometimes there is an absolute want of control over the bladder, so that the urine is almost constantly dribbling away; while in other cases the desire to pass water is distinctly felt at certain short intervals, but the patient is unable to resist this desire even for a minute. This affection, too, is sometimes associated with a morbid condition of the urine: in other instances it seems to depend on a state of general weakness; while in some cases there is no apparent cause, either general or local, to which it is possible to ascribe it. Cases of this last kind are of all the most troublesome; they are sometimes met with in several members of the same family, especially in girls, though, according to my experience, the other more curable forms of incontinence are much more common in male children.

In the cure of nocturnal incontinence of urine much may often be gained by attention to certain precautionary measures; such as limiting the quantity of drink taken at the last meal, preventing the child from lying on his back when in bed (a position which seems greatly to favor the occurrence of the accident) and rousing him from bed to empty his bladder two or three times in the night. To gain any good, however, from this the child must each time be awoke completely so as to put forth a conscious effort of the will. The mere mechanical emptying of the bladder, which the child soon gets a habit of doing, while still fast asleep, is absolutely useless. If the urine is loaded with lithates, the diet must be most carefully regulated, and medicines must be given to restore the urine to a healthy state, and to insure the due performance of the functions of the digestive organs. Tonics are often extremely useful afterwards; and there is none from which I have seen so much benefit as from the tincture of the perchloride of iron. At the same time cold sponging to the back and loins is often decidedly serviceable, and, if the case resists these milder measures, the frequent application of a blister to the sacrum seldom fails to do great good. But there are two remedies which seem to have a special influence over this infirmity, and one which they seldom fail to exert, though in very different ways. The one of them is strychnine, or nux vomica, the latter of which I generally prefer on account of the greater safety of its administration in children; the other is belladonna. The nux vomica has appeared to me to be most suitable in those cases where there is manifest general debility, and I commonly give it in combination with iron about every six hours; and this combination often succeeds in cases where iron alone had previously been given without result. Belladonna has proved most useful in those cases where the incontinence of urine was quite a chronic evil, and was unassociated with any manifest constitutional disorder. It must of course be given carefully and in doses gradually increased, four times in the twenty-four hours, and very large doses are sometimes taken before the specific influence of the drug is exerted, and this without the production of any of its poisonous effects. It must be borne in mind, that whatever be the remedies used or the precautions taken to overcome the ailment, it is quite essential for the permanence of the cure that they should be continued for some weeks after the child's apparent recovery.

Lastly I must just mention an ingenious suggestion of Sir Dominic Corrigan,[1] which I regret that I have never had a fair opportunity of putting to the test. Regarding the inability to retain the urine at night as dependent usually on relaxation of the sphincter vesicæ or on a lax condition of the urethra, he advises that the child should lie with the feet raised higher than the pelvis, so that the urine may collect towards the fundus, not towards the neck of the bladder, and next that the edges of the prepuce, or still better the lips of the urethra should be stuck together with collodion which can easily be removed in the morning. How far a radical cure may be thus effected I cannot say, but I should fear the evil would be left unmitigated; though even then, something is gained by preventing the bed from being wetted. At any rate the plan deserves a trial.

LECTURE XL.

ABDOMINAL TUMORS.—Large abdomen natural in childhood—Causes of [illegible] enlargement various, as rickets, disorders of digestive organs, [illegible] from flatus, from fluid.

DISTINCT TUMORS.—From enlarged liver—From simple hypertrophy—[illegible] posit—Albuminoid deposit—Hydatid cysts—Malignant disease—From [illegible] spleen—Its connection with leucæmia, and disposition to hemorrhage—[illegible] kidney, which is almost always due to malignant disease—[illegible] mesenteric glands—From disease of intestines, or from [illegible] in abdominal walls.

[illegible] this lecture to a brief notice of some [illegible] [illegible] and in their importance, which have [illegible]

---

[1] [illegible] vol. xcvii, p. 118, referred to in Canstatt [illegible]

in common, that they produce enlargement of the abdomen; and this abdominal enlargement is usually the first thing which excites the anxiety of the friends, and which leads to the patient being brought under your notice.

But before speaking of *abdominal tumors* in children, I must say something concerning tumors which are no tumors; apparent, not real ones.

If you go into a gallery of the old masters, and look at any of the pictures of angels, which are generally to be seen there in such abundance, you will probably be struck in the case of all the child angels, by what will seem to you to be the undue size of their abdomen. You will notice this even in the works of painters, who, like Raphael, most idealize their subjects, while in those of others, who, like Rubens, interpret nature more literally, the apparent disproportion becomes grotesque; or in the coarser hands of Jordaens, even repulsive.

But these painters are after all true interpreters of nature. In infancy and early childhood, the abdomen is much larger comparatively, than in the adult. Two causes chiefly conduce to this; the one, the much smaller size of the pelvis, the other the greater size of the liver, which Frerichs[1] estimates as being in proportion to the weight of the whole body

as 1 : 17 in the 7 months' fœtus.
1 : 20 at birth, and in early infancy.
1 : 40 in adult age.

Now this excess in the size of the abdomen may be much exaggerated if the child is small, weakly, or premature; if the lungs have been but imperfectly inflated at birth, and the chest is consequently ill-developed, and if, in addition, the general muscular power is feeble, so that the intestinal gases are subjected to a smaller amount of compression from the coats of the bowels than would be exercised upon them if the child were robust.

In cases where the child is not merely weakly but is also affected by rickets, other causes come into play which greatly increase the abdominal enlargement.

1st. The chest is not merely small and unexpanded, but it is actually deformed; and this chest deformity is associated with displacement downwards of the abdominal organs.

2d. Rickets arrest the development of the pelvis and of the lower limbs to a very considerable degree, and thus tend to produce an enlargement of the abdomen which not infrequently remains very marked even in adult age.

3d. The disease is associated not only with great feebleness of the muscular powers, but also with very imperfect digestion. The intestines then become distended, not merely from the contained gases being subjected to but little compression, but also from the generation of flatus which is the symptom and consequence of dyspepsia.

4th. In many cases the abdomen in rickets is also enlarged by a dis-

[1] Klinik der Leberkrankheiten, 1858, vol. i, table at p. 20.

tinct tumor or tumors, produced by the amyloid or albuminoid hypertrophy of liver and spleen. This cause of abdominal enlargement, however, unlike the other three, is not invariable, and the cases are decidedly exceptional in which it is the chief cause of the enlargement.

In subsequent childhood the abdomen is found much enlarged wholly independent of any disposition to rickets, but as a symptom and a result of indigestion.

You will often be asked whether you do not think a child is suffering from worms, and just as often whether you do not think it is suffering from mesenteric disease, when the only reason assigned, or indeed assignable for either suspicion, is the unusual size of the abdomen.

Now with reference to both of these points it is well to bear in mind,

1st. That there is no special condition of the abdomen in itself characteristic of the presence of intestinal worms.

2d. That even when much larger than natural, so long as the abdomen is not tense, you need entertain no apprehension of the existence of organic disease; and

3d. That sometimes, especially in infancy, you may meet with extreme tension of the abdomen, and even with enlargement of the superficial veins of the abdominal walls, such as is usually associated with mesenteric disease, due in reality to mere flatulent distension of the intestines.

In such doubtful cases, however, you will be preserved from error by observing two points:

1st. That there is no general glandular enlargement to be discovered, and especially that there is no enlargement of the inguinal glands, for they never fail to participate in any considerable increase in size that may affect the glands of the mesentery.

2d. That the resonance on percussion of the abdomen is equal and universal. In cases of tubercular peritonitis, or of at all advanced mesenteric disease, this is not the case, but about or below the umbilicus there is either absolute or relative dulness on percussion, and, in addition, in the case of tubercular peritonitis, a doughy feeling of the abdomen in that situation owing to the adhesion of the coils of small intestine to each other and to the peritoneum.

On a few occasions, almost always in young children between the ages of two and three, I have found the abdomen extremely distended, hard, tense, even slightly tender to the touch, and with marked enlargement of the superficial veins, but yet everywhere resonant on percussion. The enlargement has been so considerable as to force upon me the conviction that some deepseated disease must underlie it, and yet it has entirely disappeared, just as the phantom tumor of a hysterical woman does, when the child was put under chloroform. A somewhat similar state, too, has occasionally come under my notice in older children who were subject to colic, and in whom the distinct outline of a tumor seemed sometimes perceptible; due to the spasmodic contraction of the abdominal muscles, and recognizable both by its outline never being complete, but undistinguishable at one side, though clearly perceptible at the other, by its not being invariably to be felt, and also by its disappearance under the use of chloroform. Such cases are rare, but it is well to be aware of them.

A word or two ought, perhaps, to be added with reference to the enlargement of the abdomen from fluid in childhood. Though often suspected by the friends of our patients, abdominal enlargement from the collection of fluid is a comparatively rare occurrence. It is, of course, met with sometimes, in cases of albuminuria, whether acute or chronic; the ascites bearing some proportion to the degree of general œdema; and it also occurs, though not so frequently as in the grown person, in cases of disorganization of the heart from long-standing valvular disease; and in such circumstances no diagnostic difficulty presents itself. Every now and then, too, the same exposure to cold as, more commonly, gives rise to acute anasarca, occasions the outpouring of fluid into the abdominal cavity, an accident by no means always associated with albuminous urine; but the fluid in such cases is in general speedily absorbed if the patient is kept in bed, the abdomen gently swathed in flannel, the action of the skin promoted by the vapor or hot-air bath, and that of the kidneys by mild diuretics. Now and then ascites occurs in early life, in connection with a general state of cachexia; the fluid, however, in these cases is seldom considerable in quantity; and disappears simultaneously with the general improvement of the health which tonics and chalybeates bring out.

But besides these cases, we sometimes meet with a large collection of fluid in the abdomen, which has formed gradually in connection with an apparently causeless failure of the general health, and which may be due to cirrhosis of the liver. It is true that cirrhosis is rare in childhood; but still not so rare that the possibility of its existence should be absent from our minds. But over and above these cases I have on a few occasions observed ascites with failure of the general health, an ill-defined state of fever and considerable emaciation with a dry and harsh skin; and symptoms of general illness, suggestive of grave organic disease; but in reality due to the influence of malaria; the health improving, the fever ceasing, and the fluid becoming absorbed under the steady employment of quinine. It is very difficult, I own, to discriminate these cases; but a careful inquiry into the possible exposure of the child to the influence of malaria, and the fact that irregular febrile attacks of a remittent if not of an actually intermittent character have preceded for some weeks the effusion into the abdomen, will do much to put us on our guard, and to prevent us from at once attributing to hopeless organic disease symptoms that may really be due to a perfectly removable cause.

In some cases of mesenteric disease fluid is effused into the abdominal cavity; rarely indeed in large quantity, or so as to contribute much to the enlargement of the abdomen. Still when present it is a condition of much moment, since I fear in any case of disorder of the digestive organs of long continuance, associated with loss of flesh, tumefaction of the abdomen, and enlargement of the inguinal glands, the presence of fluctuation even though indistinct greatly adds to the gravity of our prognosis.

In some few cases of tubercular peritonitis, small collections of pus form between the coils of intestines, and as already mentioned a few days ago point and discharge at the umbilicus. Here, however, the gravity of the other symptoms is such as rarely to leave doubt as to the nature of the case, or as to the cause of the abdominal enlargement.

We have now I think disposed of all the more important conditions to which enlargement of the abdomen in childhood may be due, with the exception of those in which there exists some actual definite growth or tumor, or some distinct collection of matter.

Such tumors may be due:

1st. To the liver.
2d. " spleen.
3d. " kidneys.
4th. " mesenteric glands.
5th. " disease of the intestines themselves; an occurrence, however, of extreme rarity, or to ovarian disease.
6th. To abscesses in the abdominal parietes.

We will examine these in the order in which I have enumerated them; and

1st. Of abdominal tumors due to *enlargement of the liver.*

1st. Sometimes we meet with very perceptible enlargement of the liver in cases of heart disease, when of course we attach to it no special importance, but regard it only as one of the consequences of the obstructed circulation. In these circumstances, too, the enlargement is rarely so considerable as to constitute a distinct abdominal tumor, while the other symptoms with which it is associated are such as to prevent all risk of error.

A similar enlargement of the liver, though likewise seldom to a remarkable degree is also sometimes met with in children of two or three or four years old. It is accompanied by dyspeptic symptoms, with white evacuations, and considerable deposits of lithates in the urine; but neither with jaundice nor with distinct tenderness in the region of the liver. Some loss of flesh attends it, and general flatulent distension of the abdomen, but it is not associated with evidence of tubercular disease, and the symptoms disappear, the abdomen grows smaller, and the liver resumes its natural size, under the employment of mercurials, sometimes in purgative, but oftener in alterative doses.

I refer to this condition, not so much on account of the mere enlargement of the liver, as on account of the general symptoms, which are not infrequently regarded as those of mesenteric disease. The abdomen, however, is softer, it is less tender, or not tender at all; percussion does not elicit the diminished resonance around and below the umbilicus, generally perceptible in cases of tubercular disease, the tongue is not morbidly clean, nor are any distinct symptoms of glandular enlargement or of phthisical disease present.

2d. At a still earlier age; in infancy, and early childhood, up to the age of two years, we meet sometimes with an enlarged liver owing to fatty deposit. In its less marked degrees, it is merely an exaggeration of the fatty liver of infancy. It sometimes, however, is very considerable, is accompanied with complete non-performance of the functions of the liver, and with extreme emaciation, and yet by no means of necessity with the deposit of tubercle.

This condition of the liver, too, is sometimes found to exist in cases of laryngismus stridulus, and appears to be at the root of that malassimilation which is often the exciting cause of the convulsive affections of early life.

The subject calls for and will repay further investigation than it has yet received. It is, however, well to bear in mind the possible connection of convulsions with a state of fatty liver, and the possible existence of extreme and even fatal atrophy in infancy independent of tubercular deposit. The existence of this state explains, perhaps, to some degree the cases in which young children have failed to be nourished by the milk and farinaceous diet which commonly suits their tender age, but have improved on animal broths and on the raw meat which in some instances we find so extremely valuable.

I have, however, referred to these two classes of cases rather to suggest an explanation of the conditions with which you may find hepatic enlargement associated, than because the increased size of the liver is such as at once to attract your notice. You discover it in the course of that examination of the abdomen, which in the case of infants and children you should never omit. I have merely tried to give you a clue to its meaning.

3d. The albuminoid, amyloid, or waxy liver is the most common form of those enlargements of the organ in which it attains such a size as to force itself on the notice even of the unobservant.

It is one of the common attendants upon rickets, and is then usually associated with a similar enlargement of the spleen. The latter organ, indeed, is commonly the first to be affected, and its enlargement is in general proportionately greater than that of the liver.

A boy three years old, but unable to walk, was admitted into the Children's Hospital. His thighs and legs were much bent by rickets, and his head was large and had the characteristic square form which one commonly meets with in rickety children. He was emaciated, was reported to have been always delicate, to have suffered at different times from diarrhœa, and for the previous four months to have lost much flesh, to have suffered from occasional sickness, and from general dyspeptic symptoms.

On examining his big abdomen, the sharp, firm edge of the liver was felt two inches below the margin of the ribs on the right side, and in the middle three inches below the ensiform cartilage; and three-fourths of an inch below the tenth rib on the left side. The enlarged spleen, presenting the same characters of hardness with a distinct sharp edge, reached down to within half an inch of the anterior superior spine of the ilium, and across the abdomen to within two and a half inches of the mesial line.

My business now is not to pursue the history of this case further. The boy, indeed, left the hospital after a short stay somewhat better in health, but with the liver and spleen as large as ever. That which it behooves you to remember is that in almost all cases where the cachexia of rickets is well marked, and the dyspeptic symptoms are severe, you will meet with enlargement of the liver and spleen; that this enlargement is usually associated with considerable emaciation, but that it has no necessary relation to tubercular disease; nor in the case of the rickety child to any scrofulous taint in the system.

I do not know what changes take place in the albuminoid liver during convalescence from rickets, nor am I prepared to say whether a great degree of enlargement of the liver produces or implies such an intensity of the rickety cachexia as to preclude the child's recovery. Both these points require elucidation.

This state of the liver is associated with various cachexiæ. It has been ascertained by Dr. Gubler of Paris[1] to exist in congenital syphilis whenever the constitutional symptoms are well marked, though it does not occasion the same degree of enlargement of the organ as one constantly observes in cases of rickets.

It is a not infrequent attendant on scrofulous disease of the bones, and Dr. Budd,[2] who was the first to call special attention to it, believes this affection of the liver to be always or almost always found in this connection. This, however, is by no means invariably the case, for I have met with it not only in cases of rickets, or of syphilis, but also in instances where no special constitutional taint could be alleged as producing it.

Some years ago the child of healthy parents came under my notice at the age of fourteen months. She was healthy when born, and was suckled by a healthy wet nurse up to the age of eight months. At that time the wet nurse fell ill with fever at Nice, where the family had been residing for half a year, and some unavoidable difficulty and delay occurred in obtaining another. During this time the child drooped, and a distinct enlargement of the abdomen was now noticed. In spite of being restored to a healthy wet nurse emaciation went on, and was not arrested either by a return to England at the age of nine months, or by an attempt at artificial feeding at the age of twelve months. The artificial feeding not having succeeded, and an attack of convulsions having occurred, a third wet nurse was obtained, and about a fortnight after I saw the child.

She was very thin, and her general aspect was like that of a child with tubercular disease, except that her face was less distressed and she seemed even somewhat cheerful. The tongue was clean and moist, and the mouth quite free from aphthæ.

The limbs were very much emaciated, but the abdomen was very large. It measured twenty-one inches at the umbilicus, where six weeks before its girth was but nineteen. The superficial abdominal veins were much enlarged, the surface of the abdomen was smooth, not tender.

The enlargement of the abdomen was due to two firm tumors. One on the left side extended from below the floating ribs down into the

[1] Mémoires de la Société de Biologie, Paris, 1853, 8vo., p. 25.

[2] In his Treatise on Diseases of the Liver, at p. 304; where, and in Henoch's Klinik der Unterleibs-Krankheiten, vol. i, Berlin, 1852, p. 130, and in Frerichs's Klinik der Leberkrankheiten, vol. ii, Braunschweig, 1861, p. 165, is to be found the best account of this affection.

pelvis. It had a sharp straight edge which reached very nearly to the mesial line. The other tumor, which occupied chiefly the right half of the abdomen, did pass over somewhat to the left, a deep notch in the mesial line marking out its two halves. The edge of the right half descended considerably below the umbilicus; the notch was about on a level with it, while the left half sloped by degrees upwards and passed out of reach below the ribs.

Six weeks afterwards the child died exhausted by diarrhœa, but never having presented that peculiar pallor of the surface characteristic of leucæmia, and with which splenic enlargement is frequently associated.

It is not in infancy only that this condition comes on; it may be met with at any time and unassociated with any complication, though I believe for the most part, if not invariably, with a distinct history of a scrofulous diathesis in the parents or in other members of the family.

A boy, eight years old, several members of whose family had died of strumous ailments, began to fail in health about a year before he came under my notice. At that time there was perhaps a slight fulness of the abdomen, but no distinct tumor was discovered till three months before I saw him, though since that time it had increased rapidly. The abdominal enlargement had not been attended by any pain, but with failing appetite, an irregular state of the bowels in which constipation alternated with diarrhœa, pyrosis and occasional vomiting.

The boy was tall, thin, his complexion sallow, but his appearance not particularly unhealthy, and his tongue clean.

His abdomen measured 22½ inches at the umbilicus. Its enlargement was due to a tumor which came from beneath the ribs on the right side, and reached down exactly to the umbilicus, about which it was particularly prominent. It thence sloped up gradually to the left side, and passed out of reach then under the ribs. There was no enlargement of the spleen.

The boy's health fluctuated; the tumor at first enlarged so that the abdomen was an inch and a half bigger at the end of three months than when I first saw him. It afterwards remained stationary, but then again enlarged. It grew most where it encountered least resistance, as all tumors do, so that at the end of a year, when I saw him for the last time, although the abdomen was not increased in circumference, the tumor extended down below the iliac crest.

These tumors are generally easily recognized by their smoothness, hardness, by their sharp edge, their painlessness, and the history obtained of their slow growth. They are unattended by any pathognomonic symptoms as far as the disturbance of the general health is concerned, although they are almost always associated with more or less serious dyspeptic disorder.

In young children, death, when it occurs, seems to be due to the general advance of the rickety cachexia; or if rickets are not present, and the liver is very large, the spleen also is almost invariably enlarged too, and the symptoms under which death takes place are very much those of leucæmia.

In children after the period of dentition, life does not seem to be jeopardized so long as the affection is confined to the liver; though of course some intercurrent scrofulous or tubercular disease may prove fatal. Sometimes, however, while the liver disease seems to remain stationary or slowly increases, the peculiar deposit invades the kidney also. The urine then becomes scanty in quantity and highly albuminous, evidencing the existence of a peculiarly intractable form of granular degeneration of the kidneys which on one or two occasions I have met with and have seen prove fatal.

4th. The liver may be enlarged by the development of cysts in its substance.

These cysts, when they attain to any such size as to form a distinct tumor perceptible during life, are almost if not quite invariably produced by the development of hydatids.

Of all causes of hepatic tumor, hydatid cysts are, according to my experience, by far the rarest. I have met with them but twice; once in a patient who died, and a second time in a girl in whom the puncture of the cyst would seem to have been followed by the cure of the [illegible] tion, for six years have now passed without any sign of its reappear- ance.

In the fatal case the tumor, which no doubt must have existed [illegible] time previously, was first discovered at the age of eleven years [illegible] formed in the right side, and its growth was unattended by general [illegible] disposition, though as it increased in size occasional attacks of [illegible] severe pain came on. These attacks were, I believe, due [illegible] measure to the pressure of the enlarging cyst outwards against the [illegible] walls as well as upwards agains the diaphragm. With these [illegible] the general health was not disturbed until six weeks before the [illegible] death at the age of seventeen. Gastric disorder, occasional [illegible] and severe abdominal pains then came on, fluid was poured [illegible] the abdominal cavity, and death took place six weeks after the com- mencement of these symptoms.

I am not pursuing the subject of the pathology of these tumors [illegible] considering the question of their treatment, though I cannot [illegible] observing to you that the question of the puncture of the cyst [illegible] its earlier stages to have been considered.

When death occurred the tumor had attained to such [illegible] that while on the left side it descended somewhat below the [illegible] false ribs, and not quite so low on the right, it had pushed [illegible] diaphragm a little above the level of the upper margin of the [illegible] on the right side, and the second on the left.

It did not in short obey that law of growing downwards in the [illegible] tion where it encounters the least resistance to which I called [illegible] [illegible] the development of the slowly growing [illegible]

[illegible] was first discovered in the [illegible] [illegible] told, during an attack [illegible] [illegible] panied with [illegible] [illegible] to a higher [illegible]

[illegible]

raised the ribs and merged gradually into the liver. It resembled a segment of a large orange, projected at its most prominent part about two inches; was smooth, elastic, vibrating, almost fluctuating on percussion; and on inspiration the liver and it descended together.

The cyst was punctured, 27 ounces of fluid were withdrawn; at the end of three months the cyst appeared to be refilling, but it shrank again in the course of a few months, and I hear that the child continues perfectly well six years since the puncture, though I have not seen her for the past five years, when a distinct firm lump was perceptible in the situation of the hydatid; but not yielding any sense as of fluid within it.

The diagnosis of these tumors is not attended by much difficulty. Their growth is unattended by any pathognomonic symptom, nor at all constantly either by dyspepsia, disorder of the functions of the liver, or by pain; while whenever pain does occur it is due almost or quite invariably to mechanical pressure.

The hydatid tumor is smooth, globular, yielding fluctuation, or at least a sense of tremor on percussing it. You will remember that small, tense cysts often yield no distinct fluctuation, but at most a sort of sense of elasticity. Your experience of the occasional diagnostic difficulties in the case of small ovarian cysts situated within the pelvic cavity will impress this on your minds.

It is almost needless to observe that these tumors are attended by no general enlargement of the liver, but are developed in its substance and to a certain degree at its expense. There is nowhere the sharp edge to be felt so characteristic of the albuminoid enlargement of the liver, nor the general nodosity of its surface characteristic of malignant disease. There is no history of acute illness at its commencement, nor any sign of cachexia from its continuance.

5th. The liver may be enlarged by malignant disease.

One of the inconveniences attendant upon the practice of medicine in a large city is that many fragments of cases come under one's notice, but few cases in their entirety; that one sees the beginning of one, the middle of a second, the termination of a third. It is thus that while I have had several cases of what I believe to have been malignant disease of the liver under my notice, I have never followed but one from its commencement to its end.

In that case the affection was attended by vague indications of abdominal disease, in which there was nothing that pointed especially to any one viscus; while the morbid growth having originated from the under surface of the right lobe of the liver was supposed to be due to enlargement of the mesenteric glands. The patient was a little boy, who was 8 months old when the first indications of disordered health appeared in diarrhœa, fretfulness, and loss of flesh and appetite; and at the age of nine months his mother noticed some solid masses in his abdomen, which from the commencement of his illness had been hard and rather tender. The child lived to the age of one year; and for the last six weeks of his life, during which I had the opportunity of watching him, he suffered from diarrhœa, which was occasionally very profuse. He became extremely emaciated, and his skin assumed an exceedingly sallow color; but the evacuations, though relaxed, were otherwise natural. No hemorrhage took place from the intestines, and the urine was found to be perfectly natural whenever it was passed. During the last month of life he had a slight cough, and wheezing respiration; but death seemed due to the constant diarrhœa and the severe pain which the child suffered, his exhaustion being doubtless in great measure the consequence of the blood, which should have nourished his body, being diverted to supply the enormous mass of [illegible] disease of the liver.

During the six weeks that the child was under my observation, his abdomen increased from 21 to 25 inches in circumference; and the tumor, the surface of which was uneven, was always much larger on the left than on the right side. It turned out, however, on examination after death, that the left lobe of the liver was almost completely healthy, but that it had been driven up under the ribs by the enlarged right lobe; while part of the organ was converted into a soft white brain-like matter, intermingled with which were portions of a firmer, highly vascular, fibro-cellular substance. A few deposits of medullary cancer existed also in the right lung, but the other viscera were healthy.

I saw once a little girl three years and four months old whose health had been failing for the previous three months. She had been noticed to lose flesh rather rapidly, to become indisposed to exertion, and to walk with some apparent difficulty, while her skin had assumed a general icteroid tinge. Her appetite had become bad, her bowels irregular, and her abdomen enlarged, though attention had been somewhat turned away from that by a gradually increasing prominence of the right eye, and next by the occurrence of ecchymosis of both eyelids which gave the child a most singular appearance. The globe of the right eye projected when I saw the child fully half out of its orbit; and there were two specks of extravasated blood in the conjunctiva.

The abdomen was enlarged by a tumor, firm, non-fluctuating; its surface uneven, its edge rounded, and the superficial veins of the abdomen were generally much enlarged. The tumors occupied the situation of the liver, passing down from the right hypochondrium to below the iliac crest, then sloping up to the left side, where it passed out of reach under the floating ribs, but not occupying at all the splenic region, clear percussion being elicited for three inches to the left of the outer edge of the swelling.

In this case the protrusion of the right eyeball and the general history of the patient seemed at once to direct the attention to the probable existence of malignant disease.

Independently of that, however, the general features of the case were sufficiently characteristic. The causeless failure of health, the well-marked cachexia, the rapid development of the disease, the irregular surface of the tumor, the rounded edge unlike the sharp well-defined edge of albuminoid enlargement of the liver, and the absence of the slightest enlargement of the spleen, stamped upon the case these peculiarities which when well-marked will I think always justify you in pronouncing on the existence of malignant disease of the liver.

2d. Tumor of the abdomen may be produced by *enlargement of the spleen.*

That enlargement of the organ consequent on frequent attacks of ague is extremely rare in the neighborhood of London, and the only instance of it which I have met with in childhood where a distinct abdominal enlargement was due solely to the hypertrophied spleen was in the case of a little girl aged six and a half years who had had frequent attacks of fever on the west coast of Africa. The enlargement of her spleen first attracted attention at the age of five years, and when I saw her, her abdomen measured 21½ inches in circumference, and the spleen reached from under the ribs quite down into the pelvis, and forward as far as the mesial line of the abdomen.

In the great majority of instances which we meet with in this country, the enlargement of the spleen is associated with enlargement of the liver, and the causes which produce the one are the same as those which give rise to the other. Hence we meet with it in rickets, in congenital syphilis, and in the same scrofulous constitution as favors the albuminoid enlargement of the liver. In most of these instances, however, the enlargement of the spleen is rather a condition found by those who seek for it, than one so marked as to force itself on the unobservant.

But besides these cases we sometimes meet with great enlargement of the spleen in infancy in connection with that general condition known as Leucæmia from its supposed dependence on imperfect blood-formation, and on the predominance of white corpuscles in the blood. My friend and colleague Dr. Gee informs me, indeed, that the connection between the general symptoms and the microscopic state of the circulating fluid has not seemed to him to be so close as has been alleged.

Be this as it may the general symptoms are sufficiently marked to be easily recognizable, and are just those which were observed in an infant 8½ months old; the third child of tolerably healthy parents though the father had been supposed at one time to have presented some of the early symptoms of phthisis. The child had been nursed by its mother for six weeks, and afterwards by a healthy wet-nurse up to the age of six months. It was alleged to have been always healthy though remarkable for its pallor. Dentition had not commenced, but save that the bowels were always costive there was nothing which excited the parents' anxiety until the discovery, not much above a week before, of a tumor on the left side of the abdomen.

The child looked well-nourished; but of extreme pallor—"the faded hue of sapless boxen leaves," as Dydren has it in his version of the Knight's Tale; true to nature as the true poet always is.

The abdomen was remarkably full; it was tympanitic on the right side; but on the left there was a solid tumor which reached up under the floating ribs, down below the crest of the ilium, and extended an inch across the mesial line, but did not reach quite back into the lumbar region. The superficial abdominal veins were somewhat enlarged over it; it was hard, smooth, painless and presented a distinct sharp edge, which ran almost straight downwards; while, apart from the difference in history, these characters clearly distinguished it from any tumor due to enlargement of the kidney, with which [illegible] have been confounded.

The constitutional symptoms in these cases are, indeed, [illegible] to be overlooked. They would run but little risk of being [illegible] preted, if the simple precaution were always taken of undressing [illegible] fant or young child who suffers from some apparently causeless [illegible] and examining it carefully before forming a diagnosis. I believe [illegible] this state of spleen, as well as the constitutional condition with [illegible] it is associated, often date back to early infancy. I have, indeed, [illegible] with them in a child only three months old, and though in the [illegible] of cases which I have observed, the age of the patients varied from [illegible] to fifteen months, yet the size that the spleen then presented, clearly showed that its enlargement must have begun long before that time. The early age at which this condition has been noticed, [illegible] tives its supposed dependence on protracted lactation;[1] while its [illegible] rence among the children of the wealthier classes, as well as [illegible] those of the poor, shows that it depends on constitutional [illegible] merely on bad air, or other unfavorable hygienic influences. [illegible] minor degree, the enlargement of the spleen is not infrequently over looked, owing to neglect of the precaution I have just insisted on; [illegible] I have discovered it in cases where it had not been at all suspected, but where the pallor of the child, the peculiar waxen hue of [illegible] face, its failing strength, and loss of flesh, yet unassociated with the evidences of tuberculosis, betrayed to those who were familiar with [illegible] features the real nature of the ailment. In such cases the enlarged spleen sometimes returns to its proper size in proportion as the health of the child improves; as it often does under a tonic treatment [illegible] bined with the employment of preparations of iron and quinine. When the depravation of the blood, however, is very considerable, no [illegible] ment follows treatment; while not only does the enlargement of the spleen become more and more considerable, but in very many instances the liver also participates in the change; and two distinct tumors may then be perceived in the abdomen; the one of an elongated form, [illegible] on the left side, and often dipping down into the pelvis; the other of a more rounded shape, principally occupying the right side, and [illegible] descending so low. When the enlargement is very considerable, the circulation through the abdominal vessels is interfered with, and the superficial veins in consequence become enlarged; but it is decidedly unusual for ascites to be produced. The smoothness of surface of these tumors, and their equable firmness, serve to distinguish them from growths of a malignant kind; all of which, by the by, are of far greater rarity than those of which I am now speaking.

It now and then happens in connection with this affection that a great disposition to hemorrhage manifests itself; and this not only in the appearance of petechiæ on the surface, but also in the occurrence

[1] An idea suggested by Dr. Battersby, to whose article on Enlargement of the Liver and Spleen in Children, in Dublin Med. Journal, May, 1846, p. [illegible], [illegible] indebted for calling the attention of the profession to cases of this description.

of formidable or even fatal epistaxis, or hæmatemesis.[1] I believe, however, that this accident is to be looked for in children of five years old and upwards rather than in infants. They indeed generally fade away with no very definite symptoms, but grow feebler and feebler, just as women with large ovarian tumors may often be observed to do, when the blood which should nourish the body is diverted to the supply of the morbid growth. The appetite usually keeps up, and not infrequently the bowels continue regular, though diarrhœa occasionally takes place; and the loss of strength, the increasing pallor, and the more and more waxen hue of the surface, are in general more remarkable than even the loss of flesh, though towards the end of life that too is often very considerable. Slight irregular febrile disturbance is seldom absent as the disease advances, and seems, just as in cases of general tuberculosis, to contribute not a little to exhaust the patient. I do not know indeed how more shortly or more correctly to sum up the symptoms of this affection, than by saying that they are those of general tuberculosis, but with greater pallor of the surface, less apparent suffering or distress, less disturbance of any one set of functions, less rapid loss of flesh; and with an enlargement of the spleen, which gives a clue to the understanding of the whole train of phenomena.

3d. *Enlargement of the kidney*, producing abdominal tumor, is usually, though not quite invariably, due to malignant disease; and of this I have the record of seven instances, of which four occurred in male, three in female children. Their respective ages at death, or when so ill that life could obviously be prolonged only for a few weeks, were in two, between one and two years; in one, between two and three; in two, between three and four; in one, between six and seven; and in one, between seven and eight years.

The cases all presented very remarkable similarity to each other; and in all, though there may have been some slight failure of the general health, the discovery of a tumor in the lumbar region was the first thing that excited real solicitude about the patient. The characters of the tumor were in every instance sufficiently well marked; though

---

[1] I have seen five cases of that tendency to hemorrhage which, while sometimes associated with splenic enlargement, is not so by any means invariably, and which the Germans have described as a distinct and independent form of disease.

My patients, of whom the youngest was a boy aged six weeks, the other four, girls aged seven, eight, ten and eleven years respectively, died of hemorrhage, which took place from the bowels, the stomach, and, in the four elder children, from the nose also. In three of the girls the hemorrhage was accompanied by a general purpurous eruption, and ecchymoses appeared on the infant. In one girl the attack succeeded to measles, but there was no assignable cause for it in the others.

I do not dwell further on these cases here, because their occurrence is not limited to early life, and because, be their cause what it may, it is by no means identical with that which constitutes leucæmia.

With reference to leucæmia, the reader may consult with advantage a paper by Löschner, at p. 265 of his Aus dem Franz Joseph Kinder-Spitale, 8vo., Prag., 1860. Concerning the hemorrhagic diathesis, the best account is still that given by Lange, in Oppenheim's Zeitschrift, Oct. 1850. See also Virchow's Specielle Pathologie, vol. i, p. 263; two papers by Leudet, in the Mémoires de la Société de Biologie for 1858 and 1859; and two others by Veit, in Virchow's Archiv for 1858.

when it is situated on the left side, a doubt may be entertained as to whether it is formed by the kidney or by the enlarged spleen. I believe, however, that error may be avoided, if it is borne in mind that the spleen presents a sharp edge towards the mesial line, while the contour of the kidney is rounded; and further, that while the spleen reaches higher up under the floating ribs, it does not extend into the lumbar region so completely as the kidney, but always leaves an interspace close to the spinal column, where percussion yields a clear sound.

The history of the cases, too, is widely different. Generally, probably always, if one had the opportunity of continually watching the cases, the urine at some period or other would be found tinged with blood. My own experience would lead me to believe that this is oftener an early symptom, than one of the disease in an advanced stage; while most certainly it is never constantly present; nor, indeed, does disorder of the urinary function play the important part which might be expected in such circumstances. General causeless failure of health is sometimes associated with the development of the disease; but even when the growth has attained a large size, the peculiar waxen hue of the surface already referred to, as attendant on splenic hypertrophy, is absent; and cachectic symptoms are less marked, and less speedily developed than in those cases in which the liver is the seat of malignant disease.

The bulk of the tumor, the diversion to its nutrition of the blood which should supply the body generally, the consequent wasting of the tissues, and general loss of vital power, and all the discomfort produced by mechanical pressure on the other abdominal viscera, have seemed to me to be the causes which destroyed the patients' health and eventually occasioned their death. Severe pain is not frequent, and when experienced has seemed to be due to mechanical pressure rather than to suffering seated in the tumor itself.

To sum up, I think I may say, that an abdominal tumor developing rapidly in one or other side of the abdomen, neither preceded nor accompanied by any grave constitutional disturbance, though sometimes associated with intermittent hæmaturia, ovoid in shape, apt to descend into the pelvis rather than to rise under the ribs; solid to the touch, but smooth on its surface; rounded at its edge, and projecting back completely into the lumbar region, may be assumed with almost absolute certainty to be a tumor, and that malignant in its character, of one or other kidney.

Such tumors belong to the class of fungoid cancer, into which the whole substance of the enormously enlarged kidney becomes converted; and, in obedience to the law which seems to govern fungoid cancer in general, they are very rapid in their growth, and usually bring a fatal issue within six months, while I have not known any instance of the prolongation of life beyond a year.

It would appear that cystic disease of the organ runs a somewhat slower course, for I once saw a male child in which a tumor, recognized as the enlarged left kidney, was first discovered at the end of 3 months, but did not prove fatal until 17 months.

The post-mortem examination alone made manifest the difference between it and malignant disease of the kidney, but, I believe that, at no period in the history of the case had hæmaturia been noticed. With this exception, however, there was nothing to distinguish the case during life from one of malignant disease.

The disease which occupied the left kidney weighed 14 pounds. It was non-adherent to any of the surrounding structures, and on examination, the kidney, flattened out but unaltered in texture, was found on its posterior surface.

On dividing its substance, it presented an alveolar texture, in the meshes of which there was a clear fluid.

Some parts were much more solid than others, and projected, when cut, so as to look like medullary cancer.

In connection with this subject, I must warn you of the possibility of mistaking the *swelling formed by a psoas abscess* for that produced by enlargement of the kidney. When psoas abscess occurs in young children, its early stages may readily be overlooked, partly because the patient is unable to describe those vague sensations of uneasiness in the loins by which it is attended,—partly because impairment or loss of the power of walking is so common a result of indisposition of any kind in early life that it seems scarcely necessary to seek for any special cause to explain its occurrence. The gradual failure of the health, the loss of flesh, and the occasional disturbance of the bowels, are symptoms that attend upon various disorders of the abdominal viscera, and that present nothing pathognomonic of any. The tumor, like that formed by enlargement of the kidney, occupies the lumbar region, projecting forwards into the abdomen; while fluctuation in the abscess is often so obscure as to be scarcely, if at all, perceptible. The tumor of psoas abscess, however, reaches less high up in the abdomen than that formed by enlargement of the kidney; its contour is usually more circular, less oval, and the tenderness over it is in general greater, than in cases of malignant disease of the kidney. As the affection advances, and the matter gravitates into the thigh, or points in the lumbar region, its nature becomes clearly manifest; but though, as far as the final issue of the case is concerned, an error of diagnosis is but of little import, it is yet very desirable for your own reputation that you should not at any period have fallen into a mistake as to its nature. A somewhat similar error, too, I have sometimes seen committed in cases where inflammation going on to the formation of matter has attacked the cellular tissue beneath some part or other of the abdominal viscera just as one often sees it do in women after delivery. In these circumstances there is a hard, imperfectly circumscribed swelling, slow in its progress, and attended by but little suffering. Its real nature is indeed obvious enough if the swelling is carefully examined, but if the possibility of the accident is not borne in mind, its nature is likely to be misinterpreted.

Every case of enlargement of the kidney is not due to malignant disease: for once I saw a large abscess, which had distended the kidney by slow degrees, point at last in the lumbar region, death taking place from exhaustion a few days after a puncture had been made and the pus evacuated. For some months, too, I watched a case of hydronephrosis in the Children's Hospital, under the care of [illegible]lier; but it is needless to dwell on cases whose chief interest [illegible] their great rarity.

4th. The abdomen may become enlarged in consequence of disease *of the mesenteric glands.* I must, however, repeat what I have already said, that in no instance have I found tumors of the abdomen due wholly or even in any considerable degree to enlargement of the glands. You may meet, indeed, with a big abdomen in cases of mesenteric disease, and may be able by firm pressure to distinguish the irregular lumps of enlarged glands, though this even is exceptional; but the bulk of the enlargement is due either to the presence of flatus in the intestines, or to the tubercular peritonitis with which mesenteric disease is commonly associated. The enlarged abdomen from tubercular peritonitis is due either to matting of the intestines together about and below the umbilicus, or to the effusion of seropurulent fluid between their coils, or to both of these causes combined. The shape of the abdomen in such cases is sufficiently characteristic. The enlargement is most marked in the hypogastrium, and the greatest prominence is about and around the umbilicus, which not seldom projects a little. A dull sound is elicited everywhere on percussion, the abdominal walls are found agglutinated to the intestines, and pressure is painful, often extremely so. All these conditions may, and frequently do, coexist with tubercle of the mesenteric glands, but are not due to it alone.

5th. Rare cases are now and then met with in which a distinct tumor *is produced by disease of the intestines* themselves, *or* in the female child long before puberty *by ovarian disease.* Thus I once saw a boy ten years old in whom an irregular nodulated tumor in the left iliac fossa, and extending across the mesial line, was due to cancerous disease of the descending colon, and cancerous outgrowth from its walls. The tumor in this case was very rapid in its growth, accompanied with great failure of general health, but with no interferance with the action of the bowels. Death took place under an attack of peritonitis within a month after the first discovery of the tumor, the real seat and nature of which were discovered only on a post-mortem examination. It can scarcely be necessary for me to remind you of the deceptive characters sometimes presented by fecal accumulation in the child as in the adult, or of the necessity to clear out the intestines both by aperients and by enemata, before attempting to settle the nature of any obscure abdominal enlargement.

Two years since, a little girl, seven years of age, died after a year's illness of medullary cancer of the right ovary, which burst into the abdominal cavity. The tumor had been observed for four months before the child came under my notice, and she continued in the hospital for a month, when she died apparently from exhaustion.

The nature of the case was diagnosed during life, and, indeed, no special difficulty attended the discrimination of its nature. The physical signs were the same as one would meet with in ovarian disease in the adult; the mass manifestly sprang from within the pelvis, although it reached up to the under surface of the liver. The mass weighed 5[illegible] pounds, and it was limited entirely to the right ovary. There were some secondary deposits in the omentum but none elsewhere.

Two or three similar cases have been in the Children's Hospital within the past twenty-two years. I have mentioned them, and the case of cancer of the intestines, in order that in a doubtful case you may have the various possibilities present to your minds.

6th, and lastly. *Abscesses in the abdominal walls* may give rise to distinct circumscribed enlargements which it may not always be easy to distinguish from tumors seated within the cavity of the abdomen. I have indeed seen much uncertainty in the minds of very experienced practitioners with reference to the nature of swellings of this kind, and the rather since they come on in many instances without any definite exciting cause, and are also extremely chronic in their course, and often almost or altogether painless. They may be seated almost anywhere. I have seen one follow a subacute attack of rheumatism in a boy seven years old, occupying the crest of the left ilium. I have seen another on the right side just over the region of the liver, and concerning which the question arose whether it was not a swelling formed by a hydatid, since there was no history of injury, and the swelling had remained stationary for many weeks.

I once observed a swelling which had formed beneath the rectus abdominis on the left side, and had not altered at all for many months; concerning the nature of which most conflicting opinions had been hazarded. I expressed my belief that it was a chronic abscess, and heard some long time afterwards that I had been right. It is, however, in one or other iliac region, or on the right side of the abdomen in the neighborhood of the cæcum, that these collections of matter are most frequent, and at the same time that their diagnosis is the least difficult, for they will generally be found to have succeeded to some inflammatory symptoms not in general either acute or formidable, but referred to the abdomen, and accompanied with constipation, painful defecation, and other evidences of peritoneal or of intestinal mischief.

Now and then, if the nature of such abscess has been altogether misapprehended until the matter has approached near the surface, I have known the abdominal swelling covered by the tense and shining skin, through which large veins were seen meandering, raise the suspicion that the case was one of some malignant tumor.

I do not think, however, that with due care there is much difficulty in the diagnosis of these cases. Something, indeed, of the probability of your coming to a correct conclusion depends, as on so many other occasions, on the habit of your own minds. If you are restless hunters after curiosities, or vain and self-conscious, anxious in every case at all obscure to signalize yourselves by the display of your wonderful ingenuity, you will be very likely to make mistakes. Let me advise you, if you would escape from error, always to credit the practitioner in whose care the patient has previously been, and with whom you may be called to consult, with the possession of common sense and common powers of observation. Do not listen to his statements as if you were the opposing counsel, and as if it were your business to find every argument that can be adduced against his opinion. Remember, too, that as a mere question of chances, the more frequent [illegible] the more likely is it that on any occasion you will meet [illegible] you are bound therefore first to disprove the common, before you are justified in looking out for the rare. Forgive my saying [illegible] but using one of the privileges of age. Every day I am [illegible] and more, with the degree to which simplicity of mind helps in arriving at a correct diagnosis, as well as in leading to the adoption of right treatment, and I have, therefore, ventured to warn you [illegible] which is especially that of the young, the ingenious, and the accomplished.

But to return. These abscesses are characterized by the [illegible] of their surface and the regularity of their contour; by their situation rarely tallying exactly with that which would be occupied by any internal growth; by the deficient mobility of the abdominal integuments over them, and by their margin not being anywhere as defined as in some part at least of its outline the edge of an internal tumor would be sure to be. The absence of the general constitutional symptoms and of the cachexia which attend upon internal tumors, would further help you, while though if matter were formed in large quantity the general health might be much impaired, still you ought not to allow yourself to be misled by a mere superficial resemblance to some malignant disease, against which in such conditions the obvious fluctuation in the swelling would guard you. Lastly, in doubtful cases, when, as often happens if the abscess is small and somewhat deepseated, there is no distinct evidence of fluid, and merely a certain vague sense of elasticity, the aspirator will enable you with perfect safety to apply a crucial test, and to settle all doubt by the very means which serve at the same time in many instances to get rid of the disease.

LECTURE XLI.

THE CACHEXIÆ OF EARLY LIFE.—Syphilis, Scrofula, and Rickets.

Infantile Syphilis.—Its symptoms—Character of the syphilitic cachexia—Morbid appearances supposed to be due to it—Tendency of the symptoms to return after apparent cure—Treatment.

Scrofula.—Not identical with tuberculosis—Its characteristics—notice of a few of its symptoms—Scrofulous abscesses—Swelling of glands, otorrhœa, and [illegible] Leucorrhœal discharges.

Rickets.—Due almost entirely to injurious hygienic influences—Alleged occasional occurrence as a congenital condition—Its general characteristics seen in the skeleton—age at which it commences—General symptoms—Influence on the skull, chest, and skeleton generally—Mode of production of deformities investigated—Diseases complicating rickets—Albuminoid disease of different organs—Spasm of glottis—Hydrocephalus—Bronchitis—Principles of treatment of rickets.

WE pass next by no inapt transition from the study of a set of affections connected for the most part, more or less, with some radical defect in the circulating fluid, to the consideration of what may be regarded as the special *cachectic diseases* of early life.

These are three in number: Syphilis, Scrofula, and Rickets; and each of these would well justify a far longer notice than we have leisure to bestow.

Syphilis, as it occurs in the infant, presents many important differences from the characters which it assumes in the adult; nor is there in this anything to excite our surprise, if we bear in mind the very different circumstances in which in the two cases the poison affects the organism. In the adult, the symptoms are almost always the result of the direct inoculation of the system with the venereal virus. In the child, infection by that mode seldom occurs; and the communication of the disease from the mother to the child during its birth, which was once supposed to be the ordinary mode of origin of infantile syphilis, is now justly regarded as of great rarity. The infection of a child by sucking the milk of a syphilitic nurse is, to say the least, a very unusual occurrence; and the weight of evidence is decidedly against it ever taking place. Cases, indeed, are by no means rare, in which the nipple of a previously healthy nurse having been excoriated by the mouth of a syphilitic nursling, the disease is communicated to her own child, who shares the breast with its foster-brother; but between this accident and the direct transmission of syphilis by the milk, there is obviously no analogy. In by far the greater number of cases, the infant has, without doubt, contracted the disease in the womb, although its indications comparatively seldom show themselves until at least fourteen days after birth. In many of these cases the mother has, during her pregnancy, been the subject of primary syphilis, or if not, has presented well-marked secondary symptoms; and under either of these conditions we can understand that her infected blood may deteriorate that of her infant, and give rise to consequences more or less analogous to those from which she has recently suffered herself. Cases, however, are now and then met with, in which the venereal taint appears to have been derived entirely from the father; the mother, as far as can be ascertained, not having suffered at any time either from primary or secondary symptoms; although she has given birth to an infant affected with all the characteristic marks of syphilitic disease.[1]

Through whatever medium the infant becomes infected with syphilis, *symptoms* of the same kind appear, though there is no invariable order in which they show themselves; and coryza is its earliest indication in one case, a cutaneous eruption in a second, ulceration about the corners of the mouth in a third. When we consider the frequency with which abortion or premature labor appears to be due to the influence of the syphilitic poison, it might naturally be expected that cases would be by no means unusual in which infants at the moment of their birth have presented evidences of the venereal taint. This, however, is very seldom the case—so seldom, indeed, that I do not remember to have met with an instance of it, and M. Trousseau, of Paris,[2] whose appoint-

---

[1] Ample evidence of this is collected by M. Diday, at p. 22 of his Traité de la Syphilis des Enfans Nouveau-Nés, 8vo., Paris, 1854.

[2] See Trousseau's valuable memoir on "Infantile Syphilis," in the Archives Gén.

ment at the Hôpital Necker in that city gave him most [illegible] tunities for observing the diseases of early infancy, [illegible] to its extreme rarity. Children, although infected with [illegible] in whom the signs of the disease speedily show themsel[illegible] generally well nourished, and apparently in good health, at [illegible] birth. This, too, is observed to be the case even when the [illegible] suffered severely from secondary symptoms, has already [illegible] quently, or has given birth prematurely to dead children [illegible] was peeling off—a condition generally regarded, though far [illegible] satisfactorily proved, to be an effect of the venereal poison. [illegible] at length produces a living child, there is nothing for the first [illegible] three weeks after its birth to distinguish it from the offspring of the most healthy parents. After the lapse of that time the first symptom of disease shows itself; and most commonly this is nothing [illegible] the occurrence of a degree of snuffling with the child's breathing, and slight difficulty in sucking—the signs in short of ordinary coryza. Now and then, as I have already stated,[2] no other indication of syphilis appears; but nevertheless the coryza does not yield until after the child has been brought under the influence of mercurial remedies—a fact which would seem to show that, although unaccompanied with other signs of venereal taint, the snuffles of young infants are sometimes produced by that cause. In the majority of instances, however, the coryza does not continue long without characteristic signs of disease appearing about the nostrils themselves, and without syphilitic eruptions breaking out upon the surface of the body. The mucous membrane of the nostrils secretes a yellow ichorous matter, sometimes slightly streaked with blood, which, drying, obstructs the opening of the nostrils, and renders breathing and sucking very distressing to the child. The voice, too, before long becomes affected and assumes a peculiar hoarse tone, which has been not inaptly compared to the sound of a child's penny trumpet, and which, when you once have heard, you will at once recognize as almost pathognomonic of syphilis. This change of voice depends no doubt on the affection of the throat, which you will often see, in common with the interior of the mouth, to be red and shining, and to present many superficial ulcerations. The skin of the upper lip, over which the discharge from the nostrils runs, often becomes excoriated, or if not, it assumes a peculiar yellowish-brown color, like the hue of a faded leaf. Should the disease be unchecked, large patches of the skin upon the face and forehead put on this appearance, which

de Médecine for October, 1847; and his lecture on the subject at p. 291 of vol. iii. of his Clinique de l'Hôtel Dieu, 2d ed., Paris, 1865. Two important contributions to our knowledge of this subject must further be noticed: first, M. Roger's papers in the Union Médicale, Jan. 1865, No. 10–17, and J. f. Kinderkr., vol xliv, p. [illegible]; and Mr. Hutchinson's researches on vaccino-syphilis in Medico-Chirurgical Transactions, vol. liv, p 317, and Proceedings of Medico-Chirurgical Society, vol. vii, No. 3, of which more hereafter.

[1] Diday has collected the particulars of 158 cases, in which the date of the appearance of the first symptom of syphilis was accurately noted. It showed itself in [illegible] within the first month, and in 110 within six weeks, while there were but twelve instances in which it was deferred beyond the third month. Op. cit., p. 164.

[2] In Lecture XIX, p. 261.

seems due to a kind of staining of the part, and is unaccompanied with any alteration of its texture. Both lips before long become affected; a number of minute perpendicular fissures take place in them, which bleed whenever the infant sucks; and small ulcerations appear at either angle of the mouth. It generally happens, however, before these effects of the disease have become very obvious about the mouth, that the skin in various parts presents appearances equally characteristic. Though not limited to any situation, the eruption of syphilis usually makes its appearance about the buttocks and nates, in the form of small circular spots of a coppery red color, having a slightly shining surface and disposed to become somewhat rough at their centre from the desquamation of the epidermis in that situation. The spots in the neighborhood of the anus often degenerate into small, soft, spongy ulcerations, with a slightly elevated base; the margins of the anus become fissured; and the skin about the scrotum and along the inside of the thighs grows red, sore, cracked, shining, and denuded of its epidermis. The eyes become weak, the margins of the eyelids sore, and a scanty, adhesive, puriform secretion is poured out from the Meibomian glands, attended with but little redness of the conjunctiva. Sometimes, too, the hair of the head drops off, as small, red, sometimes slightly elevated spots, extend over the scalp.

The child is generally by this time reduced to the last stage of weakness and attenuation; but, even when the disease proves fatal, it does not, as in the adult, affect the bones. I have chanced, indeed, to see one instance of destruction of the bony palate from this cause in an infant of a few months old; but so rare is the occurrence, that the late Mr. Colles, of Dublin,[1] notwithstanding his immense experience, states that he had never observed it. Should life be prolonged after the disease has reached an advanced stage, its further manifestations consist in the formation of small pustules about the mouth, especially upon the lower lip and chin, which destroy the cutis, and leave the surface after they have healed much scarred by their cicatrices. The epidermis, too, in some bad cases peels off the hands and feet; it generally becomes thickened to a kind of crust, like that which forms on the hands in psoriasis palmaria, and then cracking, falls off in patches, leaving the skin fissured, and sometimes deeply ulcerated at the bend of the wrist, or at the flexures of the fingers and toes. The new and delicate epidermis in its turn undergoes a similar thickening, and becomes detached in the same manner, or else it continues white and thin, but shrivelled, and looking like the sodden and wrinkled skin of a washerwoman's hand, and peeling off in little fragments, leaves the cutis, especially at the tips of the fingers and toes, red, and bleeding slightly, even on the gentlest touch.

Although such are the effects that may flow from infantile syphilis when it runs its course unchecked, it yet happens but rarely that we meet in any case with all the symptoms that have just been described. Most serious constitutional disturbance is associated with the local mischief, and the child often falls a victim to the former, when the out-

[1] Practical Observations on the Venereal Disease, 8vo., p. 271. London, 1837.

ward signs of syphilitic disease are yet comparatively slight, it [illegible] rapidly, it suffers from sickness, or its bowels become much purged; it is constantly fretful and uneasy; the advance of ossification is retarded, the head feels soft, and the anterior fontanelle is large, conditions which sometimes lead to the suspicion that chronic hydrocephalus has come on, though, if the poison of syphilis should be eradicated from the system, the completeness of the patient's recovery shows that no serious cerebral disease had existed. In children affected by this syphilitic cachexia, not only are the loss of flesh, and that withered aspect which gives to infancy the appearance of old age, very remarkable, but also the bloodless state of the conjunctiva, and the yellow, waxen tint of the skin, like that of a person who has been reduced to the most extreme degree of anæmia. Even in children who have survived their earliest infancy, and in whom the disease though not completely eradicated has yet been kept in check, this color of the skin continues, and seems indeed to be an almost pathognomonic sign of the affection from which they are suffering.

When imperfectly cured, other indications of the disease remain besides the impairment of the general health, the loss of flesh, and the peculiar color of the skin; or at least, if not constantly present, they show themselves from time to time, reappearing at uncertain intervals, without there being any fresh cause for their manifestation. Such symptoms are the return of the small copper-colored spots, which, however, seldom reappear in considerable numbers; the general loss of hair; the existence of a slight degree of coryza; the appearance of one or two soft tubercular elevations, with ulcerated summits, about the organs of generation, or the outbreak of a very severe and unmanageable intertrigo. In other instances, there are few local signs of the disease beyond the occurrence of small ulcerations at each angle of the mouth, or the development of large soft condylomata at the verge of the anus, or in a few instances the formation of exceedingly troublesome ulcerations, having a slightly elevated base, between the fingers and toes, which last appearances seem to belong to the tertiary rather than to the secondary consequences of syphilitic disease.

The duration of the disease, and the mode in which it proves fatal, vary in different cases; for while death sometimes takes place speedily under the first outbreak of its symptoms, life is in other instances prolonged for several months. In cases of this kind the more marked signs of the disease recede for a time, either spontaneously or under medical treatment, but the evidences of the syphilitic cachexia continue; the child never regains its health, glandular enlargement takes place, and it either dies phthisical, or else drags out a miserable existence until some intercurrent disease, as pneumonia or diarrhœa, supervenes and destroys it.

Within the last few years anatomical research has discovered certain organic affections of the viscera connected with the syphilitic cachexia, to which the fatal termination of the disease is, at any rate, in some measure, to be attributed. Suppuration of the thymus gland, the formation of small indurated nodules throughout the lungs passing rapidly into a state of suppuration, and the occurrence of that albuminoid degeneration and enlargement of the liver of which I spoke the commencement of this lecture, are the more important changes with which the researches of MM. Dubois,[1] Depaul,[2] and Gubler[3] have made us acquainted. With reference to the alterations in the lungs, their relation to genuine lobular pneumonia seems to be uncertain, and it also appears to be somewhat doubtful whether their connection with infantile syphilis is anything more than the result of mere accidental complication; but the evidence of the dependence of the affection of the thymus and of the liver on the syphilitic poison must be regarded as conclusive.

Though the consequences of infantile syphilis are so serious, if it is either let alone or inefficiently treated, a fatal result seldom takes place if remedies are employed before the syphilitic cachexia has become fully established, and if *treatment*, when once begun, is perseveringly continued for some time after the complete disappearance of every symptom. This, indeed, sometimes implies the continuance of treatment for two or even three months; for so long as any symptom remains, be it only a slight spot of eruption, or a small condyloma about the anus, the suspension of remedies will be certainly followed by the reappearance of the whole train of symptoms. Even after the apparent cure of the affection, it is not wise hastily to omit all medicines, since, just as in the adult, the symptoms have a great tendency to recur.

Mercury in some form or other appears to be indispensable to the cure of this affection. It has been recommended by some writers not to administer it directly to the child, but to content ourselves with bringing the mother's system gently under the mercurial influence, and to cure the infant through her medium. In some slight cases this may suffice, and in almost all, the cure of the infant is materially expedited by the administration of the remedy to its mother; but I think that, as a general rule, it is expedient to give mercury likewise to the child. For internal administration I prefer the Hydrargyrum cum Cretâ to any other form of the remedy, and give it in doses of a grain twice a day to a child of six weeks old, combining it with two or three grains of chalk if the bowels are disturbed at the time of commencing the treatment, or if they become so during its continuance. I have never found it seriously disagree, though sometimes it causes sickness, in which case small doses of calomel, or of the solution of corrosive sublimate, may be substituted for it. In some cases, whatever be the form of mercurial employed, its protracted use occasions such great irritability of the stomach, that we are compelled to discontinue the remedy. Usually, the child becomes able to take it again, after a pause of two or three days; but if this should not be the case, we must leave it off, and content ourselves with ordering a scruple of mercurial ointment to be rubbed into the thighs or the axillæ twice a day; or with letting the child wear the mercurial belt. This simple contrivance, which consists in nothing else than swathing a piece of flannel, the inner surface of which is smeared daily with the Unguentum Hydrargyri, around the abdomen of

[1] Gaz. Méd. de Paris, 1850, p. 392.

[2] Ibid., 1851, p. 288.

[3] Mémoires de la Société de Biologie, 1853, p. 25. Se- these subjects, the recent work of M. Diday, already referr-

the infant, is spoken of by those who have employed it [illegible] an exceedingly efficacious method of bringing the system under the influence of mercury, and as free from all the risks of [illegible] child's health which attend upon the internal administration of [illegible] remedy. In hospital practice I confess that I have scarcely [illegible] merits; for I found that while I could give powders without [illegible] the mercurial ointment was known; and inconvenience arose from [illegible] remedy betraying the nature of the disease. This objection might probably have been got rid of by coloring the ointment with [illegible]; but my experience of the gray powder was on the whole so satisfactory that I felt the less anxious to try a new plan of treatment.

As a local application to the sores, the black wash usually agrees better than anything else; but the large soft condylomata, which form about the anus, often require to be touched with the solid nitrate of silver. It very often happens that as the syphilitic symptoms disappear, the health of the child becomes perfectly restored under the use of no other remedy than mercury. If this is not the case, however, some tonic medicine or other must be given. If the bowels are disordered, the liquor cinchonæ, or the extract of sarsaparilla, will be found very useful. If there is no gastric or intestinal irritation, minute doses of iodide of potassium may be given in combination with the extract of sarsaparilla; but if the syphilitic cachexia is well marked, and the child has suffered long from the disease, or has had frequent returns of its symptoms, no remedy has appeared to be so serviceable as the iodide of iron, which may be given in the form of syrup, and is in most cases taken by the child very readily, while it is seldom found to disagree.

Concerning *Scrofula* I have but little to say, for its more important manifestations are of a kind which custom and convenience have assigned to the care of the surgeon rather than to that of the physician. Closely allied in its essential nature to tuberculosis; like it, hereditary, like it induced by scanty food, defective ventilation, and an unhealthy dwelling, and proving fatal in many cases by becoming associated with phthisis, or with tubercular meningitis, there yet are differences between tuberculosis and scrofula at least as marked as those which separate diphtheria from scarlatina, and the tendency of pathological research appears to be to render these differences more and more obvious. Scrofula is much more limited than tuberculosis to early life; it affects the bony structures, the skin and the mucous membranes continuous with it, and the absorbent glands, in preference to the lungs, the brain, or the serous membranes. Fatty degeneration of the liver accompanies tuberculosis; the albuminoid or amyloid affection of that organ is a not infrequent attendant on scrofula.

Scrofula and tuberculosis do not mutually pass into each other. It is true that the manifestations of the latter often supervene in the course of the former, but the converse of this does not hold good, and we do not usually find children suffering from tuberculosis in whom the signs of scrofula become superadded, while not infrequently whole families display one or the other diathesis in its most aggravated forms perfectly uncomplicated.

Having thus expressed my opinion with reference to the relation

which subsists between scrofula and tuberculosis, it remains for me to say a few words concerning some of those most frequent manifestations of the scrofulous cachexia with which I have become practically acquainted.

Apart from the impetiginous and eczematous eruptions on the face and scalp which not infrequently make their appearance in strumous children even before dentition has commenced, one of the earliest signs of the scrofulous habit consists in the occurrence of small abscesses in the subcutaneous cellular tissue. These abscesses form usually on the extremities, though not in general in the neighborhood of the joints. They are extremely indolent in their character—at first they are felt beneath the skin as small round indurations of the size of a bean or of a small marble, and slightly movable. They are not at all tender to the touch; they increase in size very slowly; sometimes indeed they disappear spontaneously, but in the majority of instances they approach by slow degrees to the surface, and then project above it. After they have done so, however, the skin sometimes continues unchanged for a week or two; and even after it has become red, and the abscesses have seemed about to burst, they may still remain so for many days, before a small opening forms through which their contents escape. They then collapse, and finally disappear; a slight depression of the skin, and a degree of lividity of the surface, marking for a considerable time the situation which they had occupied. Occasionally such collections of matter form under the scalp, and this even independently of any previous cutaneous affection; but their usual seat is that which I have indicated. Sometimes they may be observed near the elbow-joint, and then they raise the apprehension, which is often groundless, of their being related to some grave mischief going on in the immediate vicinity of the joint. Their import is much more serious when they occupy a seat about the palm of the hand, or on one of the phalanges of the fingers, since in those situations they are almost always associated with thickening of the periosteum, and their tendency unquestionably is in the majority of cases ultimately to involve the bone itself.

I believe that in whatever situation these abscesses are met with, they ought to be let alone, and all treatment should be essentially constitutional. When they form in the hand, or on the phalanges of the fingers, the affected parts should be kept as quiet as possible by means of a splint of gutta-percha; but while mere periosteal thickening sometimes disappears more quickly if the surface is painted from time to time with tincture of iodine, I have not found any benefit from its application in the vicinity of the abscesses, wherever they may have been seated.

Swelling of the superficial absorbent glands, especially of those situated near the angle of the jaw and down the side of the neck, is another very characteristic sign of the scrofulous habit. The irritation attendant on the latter stages of the first dentition often seems to give the first occasion to some slight enlargement of these glands, though it is not in general before the fifth or sixth year, often not till a considerably later period, that the increase becomes so remarkable as to attract notice. In consequence, however, of some accidental exposure to cold, after an attack of measles, or of some debilitating disorder, or sometimes altogether independently of any obvious exciting cause, [illegible] these glands will somewhat rapidly increase in size. It may [illegible] tinue enlarged but not otherwise altered, but usually it [illegible] ful, tender to the touch, adherent to the skin which before [illegible] over it; and then, inflammation going on both in it and the [illegible] cellular tissue, an abscess forms which eventually discharges [illegible] by an irregular opening, that leaves on healing a depressed [illegible] ered scar. The inflammation is often slowly propagated [illegible] glands, and several abscesses may then form in succession [illegible] which leaves a similar scar and thus increases the deformity [illegible] this all: but the abscesses often continue to discharge for [illegible] and sinuses not infrequently lead from one to another; while the [illegible] healthy state of the edges of the wound interferes with its healing [illegible] thus increases the size of the scar, and tends to produce those [illegible] cicatrices which seam the neck of many scrofulous patients.

There are besides some instances of much rarer occurrence in which the glands increase to the size of a hen's egg or even to larger dimen[illegible] sions, but show no disposition to suppurate, although they may [illegible] both sides of the neck and produce a deformity similar to that which is occasioned by goitre. The glands, I believe, in these cases [illegible] undergone the albuminoid or amyloid transformation, rather than [illegible] infiltration with scrofulous or tuberculous material which is their [illegible] common change.

I have no faith, in cases of scrofulous enlargement of the [illegible] glands, in the influence of applications of iodine or of any other supposed discutient as a means of producing their absorption. [illegible] some cases indeed I admit that, in combination with tonic [illegible] and a protracted stay at the seaside, these local means have appeared to conduce, perhaps have really contributed, to this end; but on the other hand I have seen not a few instances in which inflammation [illegible] appeared to be excited by them, and in which the occurrence of sup[illegible] puration has seemed to me entirely due to local applications [illegible] to promote the absorption of the swellings. I confine myself [illegible] to the mere application of dry cotton-wool covered with oiled [illegible] which I direct to be worn constantly even for months together, [illegible] to preserve the uniformity of temperature around the part. If, in [illegible] of this precaution, and of all means calculated to promote the [illegible] health, suppuration should take place, the abscess must not be [illegible] to burst spontaneously, but when thinning of the skin has [illegible] begun to be apparent, a very small puncture must be made [illegible] narrow-bladed lancet, and the opening allowed to close as [illegible] possible; no other application being made than simple water [illegible] for the first few hours, and afterwards a piece of dry lint [illegible] oiled silk.

Obstinate otorrhœa is another of the most troublesome [illegible] of the strumous constitution; but at the same time I believe [illegible] independent of disease of the internal ear, its persistence [illegible] extent due to want of perseverance in the employment [illegible] means. The daily syringing of the ear with tepid [illegible] solution of sulphate of zinc, in the proportion of [illegible] of water, and the employment of mild counter-irritation by painting the tincture of iodine behind the ear, almost invariably arrests the discharge. It is apt indeed to return again and again, but the same means almost always relieve it, and if resorted to immediately on each occasion of its reappearance, the discharge finally ceases as the general health becomes more robust. Now and then indeed chronic discharges from the ears assume a graver character, and may even, as I have already said,[1] become the point of departure, whence disease of the bones and eventually of the brain itself may originate.

Strumous ozæna is another peculiarly distressing ailment, and all the more so perhaps because it occurs with greater frequency in girls than in boys, and sometimes befalls those whose appearance of health and good looks may render them otherwise objects of general attraction. Though often associated with a rather abundant thin seropurulent defluxion from the nostrils, this is by no means of constant occurrence. Neither, I may add, does it, as a rule, depend on disease of the turbinated bones, though unquestionably that is present in some instances. Either with or without discharge from the nares the offensive odor will sometimes continue even for years together, rendering the patient's bedroom almost intolerable after the night has been passed there, and any near approach to the person, even by day, extremely repulsive.

Much may be done, however, by the employment of a weak solution of the permanganate of potass in the proportion of a drachm of Condy's fluid to a pint of water, some of which should be sniffed up the nostrils two or three times a day, to diminish the offensive odor. When this ceases to produce any effect, the chloride of soda or chloride of zinc, in very weak solutions, may be substituted for it with advantage, while the internal use of the chlorate of potass in rather large doses, as a drachm in the course of the day for a child ten years old, has seemed in some cases to have something of an almost specific influence over the condition. I need not say that during the whole time, fresh air, sea-breezes, good food, and tonics have the same kind of influence as they exert in the whole class of strumous affections.[2]

The only other scrofulous ailment which I would wish to bring before your notice is the occurrence of purulent or mucopurulent discharges from the vagina or vulva in young girls. Such discharges were once erroneously supposed to be due to some impure cause; an opinion which, though now justly abandoned by the profession, still retains its hold among the vulgar. They take place occasionally in female children of all ages, from the time when dentition commences down to the period of puberty, but are most frequent between the ages of two and seven years. They are almost always essentially chronic in their character, being associated in general with very little swelling of the sexual organs, and with little or no pain; but proving extremely annoying from their disposition to continue for a long time, from their obstinate resistance to remedies, and their great tendency to recur

[1] See Lecture VIII, p. 104.

[2] There is scarcely a subject noticed in these lectures which does not suggest a [illegible] Trousseau. See his remarks on Ozæna at p. 509 of [illegible]

under very slight exciting causes. Even when the discha[illegible] profuse, there is no great redness of the parts from which [illegible] out; while it will be seen to be furnished almost entirely b[illegible] surface of the labia, by the nymphæ and the vulva [illegible] come scarcely at all from the canal of the vagina. The [illegible] of swelling of the parts; the source of the discharge almo[illegible] from the parts anterior to the hymen; and the absence [illegible] the very slight degree in which it has attended the onset [illegible] tion, coupled with the integrity of the hymen, and the a[illegible] appearances of injury, are sufficient to distinguish this [illegible] gonorrhœa. Sometimes, indeed, when this discharge [illegible] during teething, it has been preceded by considerable [illegible] older children rarely suffer more than a degree of itching [illegible] of the parts, which is troublesome from its persistence rather [illegible] its severity. When it occurs during dentition, the discharg[illegible] general abundant, and ceases so soon as the tooth has cut [illegible] gum, though probably returning with a renewal of the [illegible] Sometimes it occurs in children who are much troubled by [illegible] when it is kept up in many instances not merely by the [illegible] excited by their presence in the rectum, but in a measure also [illegible] creeping about the vulva. In some instances it takes place [illegible] of the eruptive fevers, especially of scarlatina; and though [illegible] never met with it in these circumstances, except as a chronic [illegible] accompanied by great general debility, cases have been [illegible] which it came on with acute symptoms on the decline of the [illegible] Generally, however, it neither succeeds to any previous fever [illegible] dependent on any local cause, but occurs in strumous children [illegible] nection with general impairment of health, or following [illegible] erable fatigue. Where no special cause can be assigned for [illegible] rence, its appearance is yet, in general, preceded for a day [illegible] some slight increase of indisposition; such as an attack of [illegible] ness, or catarrh, or diarrhœa.

Be the cause what it may, our great difficulty in almost [illegible] stance is to effect a permanent cure, so that the suspension of [illegible] may not be followed by a return of the discharge. When it [illegible] nected with teething, or with the presence of worms, the indi[illegible] are plain enough, and cure is in general comparatively easy. [illegible] but abundant ablution with tepid water, repeated every hour or [illegible] the first appearance of the discharge, will, in conjunction with [illegible] priate general treatment, not infrequently suffice for its comple[illegible] If the discharge, however, continues for more than one or [illegible] astringents must be had recourse to, such as the Liquor Plumbi, [illegible] or lotions of sulphate of zinc, or of alum, each of which [illegible] ployed for a few days, and then changed for another. At [illegible] time frequent cold sponging of the nates and vulva should be [illegible] and it must be impressed on the child's attendants that [illegible] ever can supply the place of frequent ablution. Now [illegible] at the onset of the discharge there has been more [illegible]

[1] By Dr. Cormack, in the London Journal of Medi[illegible]

mon, I have given small doses of copaiba and liquor potassæ; and have obtained from their administration just the same kind of relief as those remedies afford in acute vaginitis in the adult. Such cases, however, are quite exceptional; and usually tonics and especially preparations of iron are the only internal remedies which are required, while it is in general necessary to begin their administration early. These medicines, especially if associated with change to the seaside, and sea-bathing, usually suffice, even in the most obstinate cases, to effect a cure. It is however in general a wise precaution to continue the employment of frequent ablution, and in addition to sponge the parts twice a day with alum lotion, even for weeks after the discharge has completely ceased; while once I found the employment of a lotion of a scruple of nitrate of silver to an ounce of water necessary to arrest a discharge which had bid defiance to all other remedies.

Between the various manifestations of scrofula and *rickets* there seems to be no other relation than that which subsists between two conditions, each of which is dependent in great measure on unfavorable hygienic conditions. Between those conditions too which beget scrofula and those which promote the occurrence of rickets there are many differences; insufficient food appears to be the great occasion of the former, insufficient air of the latter; while the absence in the case of rickets of any marked tendency to the perpetuation of the disease from parent to child forms a distinct peculiarity which separates it from syphilis, tubercle, and, though possibly in a less marked degree, also from scrofula.

Rickets, though known on the Continent, and especially in Germany, by the name of the English Disease, is by no means limited to this country, but is, I believe, quite as prevalent in many parts of Germany[1] as in England, though by no means so frequent in its occurrence nor met with commonly in such serious forms, in France. The rooms overheated in winter by the close stove, the complete want of ventilation, and the absence of attention to personal cleanliness, are conditions favorable to the occurrence of rickets, which exist throughout the whole of Northern and Central Germany, and to which a greater analogy is found in the habits of the English than of the French poor. The comparative rarity of rickets in the purely agricultural population of England furnishes a further proof of the paramount influence of bad air and insufficient ventilation in the production of the disease.

At the same time, however, this disease occurs sometimes in cases where no injurious influences have been previously at work, and cases have even been published of the child presenting at birth all the deformities of the skeleton which are characteristic of rickets.[2] Of such

---

[1] A recent writer on this subject, Ritter von Rittershain, estimates the number of rickety children at 81 per cent. of the total number who came under his notice as outpatients at Prague, and Professor Henoch of Berlin, at p. 518 of his translation of my Lectures, confirms this estimate from his own experience in that city.

[2] See various references in Graetzer, Krankheiten des Fötus, 8vo., Breslau, 1837, p. 170. Of the more recent cases, one of the most remarkable is described and de- [illegible] Symbolæ ad Ossium recens natorum Morbos, [illegible]

cases I can offer no explanation, though their [illegible] unquestionable, and I am also unable to say whether [illegible] tion that was made there was any such careful [illegible] state of the internal organs as would have been [illegible] whether, and in what degree, they presented the changes [illegible] in those who after birth have suffered severely from [illegible]

The general characters of a rickety child retained [illegible] those who have suffered severely from it in their early [illegible] iar to us all. The stunted stature, the large head, [illegible] shapen chest, twisted long bones, and enlarged wrists and [illegible] a physiognomy so peculiar that the effects of rickets [illegible] founded for a moment with those produced by any other [illegible] servers looking at these changes in the skeleton have [illegible] of rickets as though it were a disease exclusively of [illegible] that the absence from them of the due amount of earthy [illegible] its sole and essential characteristic.

But this is by no means the case. The deformity of the [illegible] but one, although the most remarkable, of the effects of [illegible] there are minor degrees of the affection well worth attention [illegible] which, though ossification may be tardy, and the develop[illegible] skeleton somewhat arrested, no actual deformity is produced.

Rickets is essentially a disease of childhood, and of early [illegible] commonly attracting attention towards the end of the first [illegible] though often, I believe, beginning anterior even to the com[illegible] of that process; while, though I have known its symptoms [illegible] and more grave up to the end of the fifth year, I have [illegible] begin later than the age of three.

I have never seen an infant, while efficiently suckled by [illegible] nurse or mother, present any of the symptoms of rickets, [illegible] the hygienic influences by which it was surrounded were [illegible] respects unfavorable. It is commonly at the period of [illegible] when, with the diminution of the supply of the mother's milk, [illegible] food is first had recourse to, that the premonitory symptoms [illegible] appear. The ordinary coincidence of that change in diet [illegible] demand on the constitution made at the time of the commence[illegible] teething, often renders the advance of the disease very rapid, [illegible] efforts that a child commonly makes to stand or walk be[illegible] ages of nine and fifteen months occasion that bowing of the [illegible] more than anything else attracts the attention of the friends. [illegible] frequently, however, and this especially in children who [illegible] up wholly or in part by hand, the symptoms of rickets [illegible] selves at a far earlier period. Dr. Stiebel of Frankfort [illegible] has observed them as early as the fourth or fifth week.

The infant loses, or never attains, that brightness which [illegible] istic of the healthy babe. It is dull, dislikes being distur[illegible] peevishly at the gentlest handling, or at any change of pos[illegible] were sore and actually pained by touching; but though [illegible]

[1] In the article "Rachitis," in vol. i of Virchow's Specielle [illegible] Therapie.

body as quiet as possible, it rolls the head fretfully from side to side, so as to wear the hair completely off the occiput. It has irregular feverish attacks, not limited to any particular time of day or night, nor of any fixed duration, attended with increased fretfulness and restlessness passing off in sleep, during which there is a great disposition to sweat about the head and upper part of the trunk; and with the advance of the disease these sweats become more and more abundant, standing in large drops upon the forehead, and running down so as completely to soak the pillow. The skin at the same time loses its transparency, and becomes dull and dirty-looking; digestion is ill performed, but the disposition is rather to constipation than to diarrhœa; while, though the infant loses flesh, there is very rarely either the extreme emaciation of the tuberculous child or the glandular enlargement attendant on scrofula.

With these symptoms of general disturbance there will be found associated the three never-failing evidences of rickety disease—retarded ossification of the skull, enlargement of the wrists, and thickening of the ends of the ribs, coupled with the commencement of the pigeon-breast deformity of the chest.

I have already noticed the peculiarities of the rickety cranium when speaking of some of the convulsive affections of early infancy,[1] and have told you how we are indebted to Dr. Elsässer for calling our attention to this condition, which from its most striking characteristics he termed "craniotabes," and the "soft occiput." The fontanelles and sutures not only remain unossified long beyond the usual time, but bone-matter already deposited is removed, so that the occipital and parietal bones become yielding just like tinsel. Coupled with this change in the bones themselves, there is almost always an undue development of the head; due not to the occurrence of serous effusion into the ventricles, as in chronic hydrocephalus, but to the overgrowth of the brain itself. The forehead becomes projecting, but this projection is not accompanied with that downward direction of the eyes which occurs in chronic hydrocephalus, and which is due to the pressure of the fluid on the roof of the orbits. The head becomes elongated, and square in form, and though the occiput projects, we do not find the occipital bone depressed from its proper position at the hind head, quite to the base of the skull, as in cases of chronic water on the brain. The undue size of the head is further exaggerated in appearance by the same arrested development of the bones of the face as takes place in chronic hydrocephalus, while it must not be forgotten that the two conditions are not infrequently associated, and that chronic water on the brain is a by no means rare complication of rickets.[2] The interrupted bone formation is displayed in an equally characteristic manner in the retarded dentition. The teeth appear late and irregularly, while the undeveloped jaws do not allow them adequate space, and they are crowded together, some behind the others, and some growing edgewise from want

[1] See Lecture XIII, p. 165.

[2] See, for a contrast between the [illegible] head, plates 6 and 7 in Beylard's essay. Du [illegible]

of space to admit of their being ranged properly. In ... too, the bony sockets which should surround the ... formed, so that the teeth are held in their places by the ...

It is in the skull that rickets first shows itself in a ... of cases. The earlier the age at which the disease comm... marked will be the affection of the cranium, while in ... in which the disease does not appear till the age of ... months, the bones of the head often escape it altogether.

At how early an age soever rickets begins, the affection ... of the skull is invariably associated with some enlargem... of the long bones. This enlargement, which is most ... wrists, is not, as has been suggested, a merely apparent ... brought out by contrast with the generally attenuated limb... to a real heaping up of bone-matter in excess; in other ... W. Jenner says in his valuable "Lectures on Rickets," ... cessive preparation for the process of ossification, and arrest ... pletion of the process."

It is to the same excessive preparation for bone formation ... the thickening of the end of each rib, which gives to the ... chest that peculiar beaded appearance on either side famili... on the Continent as the rickety rosary. This peculiar ... is often brought into striking prominence by being associ... extreme degree of the pigeon-breast deformity of the thorax. ... of the chest are flattened, the sternum is carried forwards, ... ribs are bent inwards at an acute angle at the point where ... and cartilage unite, rendering all beyond this spot a sort ... appendage to the chest, while its boundary is defined by the ... pendicular groove marked out by the beading of the ribs. ... nipple the chest widens out again, owing to the resistance of ... stomach, and spleen, which prevents its walls from collapsing ... do higher up under the pressure of the external air. The ... walls of the chest, the feeble inspiratory power, and the pressure ... external air contract the chest, give to it its great depth and ... capacity from side to side, and produce the perpendicular groove ... follows the situation of the ends of the ribs. The presence of ... dominal viscera, the stomach, liver, and spleen, prevents this ... from extending through the whole depth of the chest; and the ... constriction which divides the chest into an upper and a ... represents, as Sir W. Jenner was the first to point out, the upp... of these viscera, and not the points of insertion of the diaph...

Associated with this contracted chest we find a prominent ... Many causes contribute to produce it. First, the abdomin... are carried below their natural situation by the contracted ... chest, and the small amount of lateral expansion of which it ... tible in inspiration. In the next place, some degree of en... both of the liver and spleen from albuminoid infiltration ... substance, is a frequent attendant on rickets. Thirdly, ... pelvis which characterizes infancy often continues still ... in its development, and hence presents a greater contrast ... to the size of the abdomen; and, lastly, the general want of ...

power affects the involuntary as well as the voluntary muscles, so that the intestines are constantly more distended with air than in the healthy child.

The most striking characteristic of rickets, however, is found in that softening and bending of the long bones which become most marked when the child has begun to walk about, and this deformity increasing daily in proportion as the weight of the child increases, has led to the statement, now abundantly disproved, that the disease begins at the lower extremities, and thence travels upwards.

It would not be easy, and I do not know that it would answer any important end, to describe the exact form in which each limb is peculiarly contorted. Even while the child still lies in bed the deformities are very striking. The softened clavicles become greatly curved, and this gives to the upper part of the chest the appearance of a greater degree of contraction than really exists, since the head of the humerus is thereby thrown forwards to the front of the chest, instead of retaining its natural position at the side. This bending, too, is not infrequently increased by actual fracture of the bones (usually the so-called green-stick fracture which takes place in early childhood); and this fracture is rendered all the more noticeable by the heaping up of bone-material just at the point where it has taken place. The arm and forearm become much curved, and this curving is usually most remarkable in the latter, where the bend sometimes almost amounts to a fracture. All the joints are loose, owing to the yielding of the ligaments, and this is especially observable in the joints of the wrists. Muscular action has been invoked to explain the deformities of the upper part of the trunk; but I think with Sir W. Jenner, and to a great degree also with Professor Trousseau,[1] that simple pressure on the softened bones will explain them all. The child who cannot walk endeavors to raise and support itself by its arms, which bend under the weight of the body, while the same pressure communicated by the head of the humerus to the clavicle produces its exaggerated curve, and even occasions its fracture. It is remarkable too to how great an extent this deformity of the upper limbs rectifies itself in after life, while the legs, which now bear the weight of the body, not only become more and more deformed, but retain this deformity permanently.[2] I need not observe that, were muscular action the cause of the deformity, the legs indeed might grow worse, but the upper extremities would show no tendency to grow better.

It is in the legs that the greatest rickety deformities present themselves. At first there is some curving outwards and forwards of the thighs, owing, as Sir W. Jenner has observed, to the mere weight of the legs and feet, which even as the child lies in bed is not without its influence in bending the bones, though this becomes much more marked so soon as the child is able to sit up in a chair or in its mother's lap. From this early period, too, dates that bowing out-

[1] Clinique, &c , vol. iii, p. 465.

[2] In illustration, see in plate iii of Beylard's essay the contrast between the upper and lower limbs of a man the subject of an extreme degree of rickets.

wards of the spine in the dorsal region which sometimes excites the apprehension of friends lest it should imply the existence of actual disease of the bones. It takes place just at that part of the spine which, when the infant is carried in its mother's arms, is left unsupported; it is due to no disease of the bones, but to the yielding of the ligaments, and disappears at once if the child is held up by the arms, or even if it is turned over on its abdomen. Later in life the spine becomes deformed from other causes. It yields to the superincumbent weight of the head, and bends inwards somewhat in the cervical and upper dorsal region; the weakened ligaments give way, and lateral curvature takes place just as it does in many cases of mere general debility of the system. The weight of the body is borne by the sacrum, but the weakened pelvic ligaments do not hold it—the keystone as it were of the arch—firmly in its position. Its promontory is driven downwards and forwards, contracting the pelvis, as obstetricians know, and at the same time producing the sinking in of the loins which gives to the adult who in early life has suffered from rickets that peculiar gait so characteristic of the affection.

The pelvic deformity, as you know, is not limited to the altered position of the sacrum, but the counter pressure of the thighs drives the anterior pelvic wall much above its natural level. At the same time too the pubic arch becomes widened and flattened, and the acetabula assume a position in front of the pelvis instead of at its sides; a condition which still further increases the waddling gait of the rickety patient, and compels the very upright attitude by which alone the tendency to fall forwards in walking is counteracted. Extreme rickety softening of the bones, and its persistence to a later period than usual, sometimes obliterates these characteristics, and gives to the pelvis the triangular form which is usually seen in mollities ossium. With these exceptional cases, however, we have nothing to do.

With the erect posture of the child, and its gradually increasing weight, there come too the striking deformities in the legs which stamp on the rickety frame its most indelible marks. The curvature of the thighs increases greatly, the tibiæ and fibulæ bend forward to an arch, and the convexity of their anterior surface looks inwards instead of forwards, and sometimes, in addition to the bowing at their centre, there is a second deep notch in the bones, or second abrupt curve with its convexity turned backwards a few inches above the malleoli, as if the bones were there doubled on themselves. The ligaments are weakened as at the wrist, so that the child walks in many cases almost on the inner ankle, while if the relaxation is less, and the child still walks on the soles of the feet, the arch of the foot is entirely destroyed, and the child becomes completely flat-footed.

If to this be added the general influence of rickets in arresting growth, so that the patient is dwarfed not by deformity only, but by the actual shortness of the different long bones, we have, I think, a plete summary of the different modes in which rickets in the skeleton.

With improved health many of the minor conse pear; much of the superfluous bone-material larged wrists and ankles diminish in size, and the bones of the upper extremities on which there is no permanent pressure regain much of their straightness, though the dwarfed growth is never altogether made up for. In cases where the disease has been severe, however, and almost always to a considerable degree in the lower extremities, the evidences of bygone rickets are more abiding. The bones do not straighten, nor is the superfluous bone-matter which was deposited along their concavity and at their ends absorbed. It undergoes a process of hardening, concerning the nature of which opinion has differed, some persons regarding it as identical with ordinary ossification, while the majority see in it a process of calcification similar to that which occurs in enchondromata—a pathological, not a physiological occurrence.[1] The tissue thus changed presents an ivory-like density and hardness, so as to become susceptible of a high polish. It is in the long bones, and especially in the seat of an old fracture, or at the concavity of the arch into which they have bent when softened, that the petrifaction of the bone-matter is most remarkable; though it is by no means confined to those situations, but is observable, though in a less degree, in the flat bones, and is sometimes strikingly marked in those of the skull.

I have already described the evidences of general ill health and of imperfect nutrition which are characteristic of rickets, and it sometimes happens that the child dies with no definite disease, but apparently as the result of the aggravation of all these symptoms. In such cases there is usually a considerable degree of albuminoid infiltration of the liver, spleen, and lymphatic glands, and the degree to which the latter are sometimes distinctly enlarged gave rise to the opinion which once prevailed as to the essential identity of scrofula and rickets. The condition of the glands in the two cases is, however, entirely different; and instead of there being any real connection, there is rather a condition of antagonism between tubercle and scrofula on the one hand, and rickets on the other.

In the majority of instances, death is not due to the mere intensity of the rickety cachexia, but to the supervention of some intercurrent disease. I have already alluded to the connection between spasm of the glottis and that imperfect ossification of the skull which is one of the early indications of rickets; and rickety children are not seldom carried off either by distinct laryngeal spasm, or by some other form of those convulsions, which, where teething is tardily and ill accomplished, often attend upon it. When the disease comes on in very early infancy, too, it is by no means unusual to find it associated with a slow form of chronic hydrocephalus, which develops itself during the general febrile disturbance of the system. The effusion of fluid in these cases is never very considerable, but the head assumes the regular hydrocephalic form, while the general deformity of the skeleton is often so trivial that, unless the patient's history is carefully inquired into, the relation of the

---

[1] Professor Kölliker took the former view, while Trousseau, op. cit., vol. iii, p. 472, and Sir W. Jenner more authoritatively, because based on independent microscopical examination, take the latter; see Jenner's Lecture in Med. Times, March 17, 1860, p. 261.

hydrocephalus to rickets may be altogether over[illegible] learned, however, that the symptoms had no acute onset, [illegible] very gradually, that they did not come on until the fifth [illegible] at the earliest, and that the enlargement of the skull was [illegible] fuse sweats about the head. Children in whom this [illegible] appear to suffer much; their emaciation is usually very great, [illegible] digestive functions are very ill performed. For the most [illegible] under some attack of intercurrent diarrhœa, or are carried [illegible] convulsions at an early stage of the process of dentition. [illegible] ever, is the great enemy of the rickety child. The malformed [illegible] as you know, the evidence, and the cause as well as the [illegible] the imperfect performance of respiration, while an emphysem[illegible] of the lungs due to the same cause is habitual in every instance [illegible] siderable thoracic deformity. It suffices for a comparatively [illegible] tack of bronchitis to interfere with the entrance of air into the [illegible] for large portions of lung at once to become collapsed, and for death [illegible] follow suddenly and unexpectedly on what in any other child [illegible] have been a comparatively slight attack of catarrh or influenza.

The *treatment* of rickets need not detain us long, for, notwithstand[illegible] ing the importance of the disease, the principles to be borne in mind alike for its prevention and its cure are abundantly simple. Bad [illegible] and defective ventilation are its two great causes; and causes which among the poor it is often difficult, sometimes impossible, to remove. Even among the comparatively wealthy these causes of rickets are not infrequently met with. The nurseries are overcrowded; the infant is laid in a deep cot, wrapped up overwarmly in blankets, and left to breathe for hours the atmosphere which is inclosed within the curtains or the sides of the cot; and which, moreover, is not seldom rendered still more impure by a want of the most sedulous attention to cleanli[illegible] ness on the part of the nurse. If to this be added the attempt to bring up the child entirely, or in great measure, on artificial food, we have at once the two conditions combined which are most certain to generate rickets.

Remove them; nourish the infant at the breast of a healthy [illegible] place it in a large room, and in a cot which admits the air to [illegible] freely over the child; let there be most careful attention to clean[illegible] and improvement will become almost immediately apparent. If the disease is advanced, combine with all these precautions country [illegible] better, sea air, and even where marked deformity has already [illegible] place, amendment will be sure to follow.

As the child grows older, and other food than the mother's [illegible] milk becomes necessary, let too exclusively farinaceous food [illegible] Beef tea at the age of eight or nine months, and a little under[illegible] at fifteen or twenty months, are always desirable, while [illegible] always form an important part of the diet.

There is no specific for rickets—nothing which furnish[illegible] hand, in a way in which it can be appropriated, the [illegible] which the bones are deficient, and the notion that [illegible] supplied in large quantities to the child would [illegible] cure is but an unphysiological fallacy. Iron and [illegible] two great remedies on which, in this as well as in other cachectic diseases, we mainly rely. Their continuous employment, however, requires that attention be specially paid to the state of the digestive organs; but the simpler aperients, as rhubarb and magnesia, or castor oil, or syrup of senna, are to be preferred to the mercurial preparations which are so often employed without due occasion.

It would be needlessly to occupy your time were I to speak of the management of all those complications to which, as I have already said, the main danger of rickets is due. The diarrhœa, the laryngismus, and the bronchitis are to be treated in accordance with the principles which I have already laid down. One point, however, is always to be borne in mind, that whereas rickets is a disease of debility, a cachexia, all its complications must be treated with a full recognition of this fact. Depletion and antiphlogistics are out of place; a tonic plan of treatment should in all cases be adopted.

LECTURE XLII.

FEVERS.—Chiefly belong to the class of Exanthemata—Mistakes with reference to simple fever in childhood—Its identity with fever in the adult.

INFANTILE REMITTENT FEVER, identical with TYPHOID FEVER, which is a fitter name, occurs in two degrees.—Symptoms of its milder form—Of its severer form—Signs of convalescence—Modes of death—Diagnosis—Treatment.

INTERMITTENT FEVER OR AGUE.—Peculiarities characterizing it in childhood.

WE come now to the last part of this course of lectures; namely, to the study of *the febrile diseases incidental to infancy and childhood.* They belong, for the most part, to the class of the Exanthemata—diseases characterized, as you know, by very well-marked symptoms, by a very definite course, and by usually occurring only once in a person's life. These peculiarities have always obtained for them the notice of practitioners of medicine, and few of the affections of early life have been watched so closely, or described with so much accuracy, as small-pox, measles, and scarlatina. Hence it will be unnecessary to occupy so much of your time with their investigation as we have devoted to the study of other diseases, which, though not so important, have yet been less carefully or less completely described.

While the well-marked and unvarying features of the eruptive fevers, however, have forced those diseases on the attention of all observers, the more fluctuating characters of continued fever have been so masked [illegible] [illegible]ences between youth and age, that the affection as it occurs [illegible] [illegible]ntirely overlooked, and its nature was, in many respects, still longer misapprehended. [illegible] of the older writers on medicine, have spoken of [illegible] among children at all ages; but under this [illegible] together several diseases in which febrile disturbance [illegible] effect of the constitution sympathising with some local [illegible] mistake was committed with especial frequency in the [illegible] affections of the abdominal viscera; many of which are [illegible] considerable degree of sympathetic fever, while their [illegible] respects, are often so obscure that the imperfect [illegible] days failed to discover their exact nature. As medical [illegible] creased, many of these disorders were referred to their [illegible] but, nevertheless, the descriptions given of the so-called [illegible] worm fever, and hectic fever of children, present little [illegible] character, and are evidently the result of a blending [illegible] symptoms of various affections. The disease described [illegible] different names was supposed to be a symptomatic fever, [illegible] gastric or intestinal disorder, and limited in the period of its [illegible] to early life; while the absence of the well-marked shivering [illegible] usually attends the onset of fever in the adult, the rarity of [illegible] escence on the surface of the body, and the comparatively low [illegible] mortality which it occasions, led persons altogether to overlook [illegible] close connection between it and the continued fever of the adult.

It was not to be wondered at that the identity of continued [illegible] different periods of life should escape observation, so long as the [illegible] types of the disease in the adult, though separated by essential [illegible] ences, were yet confounded together. The recognition of the [illegible] character of typhus and typhoid fevers, which we owe to Sir W. [illegible] was a necessary step towards this object; and this once [illegible] alogy between the latter affection in the adult, and remittent [illegible] the child, could not long remain unnoticed. To M. Rilliet [illegible] indebted for a most elaborate inquiry into this subject, which [illegible] so close a resemblance to subsist between the two diseases, as [illegible] removed all doubt with reference to their identity. They are both [illegible] duced by the same unfavorable hygienic influences, they both [illegible] similar definite course, and have the same duration, while both, [illegible] generally affecting isolated individuals, have also their seasons [illegible] demic prevalence. Though varying in severity, so that in [illegible] confinement to bed for a few days is scarcely necessary, while [illegible] cases the patient hardly escapes with his life, yet medicine has [illegible] able to cut short the course even of their mildest forms. [illegible] though the local affections associated with both vary much [illegible] cases, yet in every instance we meet with that assemblage of [illegible] which makes up our idea of fever. Or if, from the examination [illegible] symptoms during life, we pass to the inquiry into the traces [illegible] disease on the bodies of those to whom it proves fatal, we [illegible] further evidence of the close relation that subsists between [illegible] the child and that of the adult. Enlargement, tumefaction [illegible]

[1] De la Fièvre Typhoïde chez les Enfans: Thèse de la [illegible] des Maladies des Enfans, vol. ii, p. 663.

ation of Peyer's glands, constitute one of the most frequent morbid appearances in both diseases, and in both, the changes that these glands are found to have undergone, are more advanced and more extensive in proportion to their nearness to the ileocæcal valve. In both, too, the mesenteric glands are enlarged, swollen, of a more or less deep-red color, and manifestly increased in vascularity; while the softened state of the spleen, the gorged condition of the lungs, and the congestion of the membranes of the brain, are appearances common to both diseases. There is, however, no more relation between the severity of the intestinal lesion, and the intensity of the symptoms in the fever of the child, than in that of the adult; and there is no ground for regarding the disease as the mere effect of the constitution sympathizing with a certain local mischief in the former case, which may not be equally alleged with reference to the latter. The symptoms in both "are the expression of the influence of the disease on the whole economy, of the disorder which it occasions in the principal functions of the body, and are an essential part of the disease itself, rather than the secondary effects of certain lesions of the bowels."[1]

If, however, this be so, it will tend greatly to the avoidance of errors which time has rendered popular, if for the future we altogether discard the term infantile remittent fever from our scientific nomenclature, and speak, as many French writers do, only of *Typhoid Fever* in children.[2]

The different degrees of severity which a disease may present in different cases do not in general form a good basis on which to found any classification of its varieties; but in the case of typhoid fever the differences are so great between its milder and its severer form as to warrant our adopting them as a ground for its subdivision into two classes. In *cases of the first or milder kind*, the disease usually comes on very gradually, often so much so that the parents of a child who is attacked by it are unable to name any fixed time as that at which the illness began. The child loses its cheerfulness, the appearance of health leaves it, the appetite fails, and the thirst becomes troublesome; by daytime it is listless and fretful, and drowsy towards evening; but the nights are often restless, or the slumber broken and unrefreshing; while all these symptoms come on without any evident cause, and are not accompanied by any definite illness. When once the attention of the parents has been excited to the condition of the child, it is soon ascertained that the skin is often hotter, and almost always drier than natural, though now and then rather profuse sweats break out causelessly on the surface, and continuing for an hour or two, leave the patient in no

---

[1] Chomel, Leçons de Clinique Médicale: Fièvre Typhoïde, p. 231, 8vo. Paris, 1834.

[2] Dr. Murchison, whose Treatise on Continued Fevers, 8vo., London, 1862, has appeared since the fourth edition of these Lectures, suggests as most appropriate the name Pythogenic Fever, from its connection with imperfect drainage, and similar causes. No one can consult this work and fail to do homage to the merits of one of the most remarkable monuments of patient investigation, original thinking, and lucid statement with which our medical literature has been enriched in the present generation. by the most [illegible] er of Sir W. Jenner at the Fever Hospital.

respect relieved by their occurrence. The bowels are ... even at the onset of the disease, or if not they are in ... turbed by medicine; a very mild aperient being not ... lowed by three or four actions of the bowels daily for ... three days. In a few instances there is a condition of ... constipation at the onset of the disease, requiring ... overcome it; but this is not often the case, and when ... is, I think, more frequently in the severer than in the ... the disease. The appearance of the evacuations is ... healthy, and they are usually relaxed, very offensive, of ... low-ochrey color, and separate on standing into a supernat... a flaky sediment; appearances which become more marked in ... week of the disease. The tongue is generally rather deficient ... ture, red at the tip and edges, thinly coated on the dorsum ... mucus, through which the papillæ appear of a deep-red ... abdomen is soft, though there is some flatus in the intestines ... sure is usually borne without pain. These characters often ... through the whole course of the affection, though sometimes ... middle of the second week, pressure in either iliac region, ... the right, appears to cause suffering. The pulse is generally ... from the very commencement of the illness; sometimes it is ... so, but there is by no means a constant relation between ... skin and the rapidity of the pulse. Occasionally there is slight ... but this symptom is very frequently absent in the milder ... disease. As the symptoms which constitute this affection come ... gradually, so they often continue for several days with little ... change from day to day, though the patient is far from seeming ... ill at all times of the day; and this periodical exacerbation and ... of the symptoms obtained for the disorder the name of remittent ... In some instances two distinct exacerbations and remissions ... observed in the course of every twenty-four hours, but in the ... cases only one is well marked. The child, who during the ... been listless and poorly, but yet not incapable of being ... has had the appearance of a patient convalescent from illness ... than of one still suffering from disease, becomes flushed and ... and feverish as evening approaches; and sometimes slight ... ushers in the evening exacerbation of fever. He seems drowsy ... begs to be put to bed, where sometimes he sleeps, though seldom ... quilly, till morning. In the second week, the nights generally ... worse than they were at an earlier stage of the disease; the ... is very dry and hot, he sleeps with his eyes half open, talks ... wakes often to ask for drink, and occasionally has ... Early in the morning he wakes pale and unrefreshed, but ... o'clock seems to have recovered something of his cheerful... the succeeding three or four hours appears tolerably ... ing approaches he seems weary and drowsy, again the ... occurs, and the succeeding night closely resembles ... Sometimes, in addition to the evening exacerbation ... one though less severe at about 11 o'clock in ... the child has hardly recovered before the ...

on. As the case advances towards recovery, the morning attack disappears long before the evening paroxysm ceases to recur; and it happens not infrequently that a slight threatening of the evening exacerbation continues to return for some time after the child has seemed in other respects quite well. It is during the second week of the disease that the rose spots characteristic of typhoid fever generally make their appearance if they appear at all; but they are often very few in number, and not infrequently are altogether absent. Towards the end of the second, or the beginning of the third week, the symptoms begin to abate, the bowels act more regularly, the appearance of the evacuations becomes more natural, the tongue grows cleaner and uniformly moist, the thirst diminishes, and the evening exacerbations of fever become shorter and less severe; while the child's cheerfulness by day gradually returns, and his face resumes the aspect of health. Convalescence, however, after even a mild attack of the disease, is rarely established before the end of the third week, while the child is in general left extremely weak, and greatly emaciated; the loss of flesh and strength being quite out of proportion to the severity of the illness, and the progress to complete recovery being usually very slow.

It sometimes happens that, having set in with comparatively mild symptoms, the typhoid fever assumes a serious character in the course of the second week. In the majority of instances, however, the *severer* form of the disease gives some earnest of its severity at a very early period. It commonly sets in with vomiting, accompanied in many cases by headache, or by a remarkable degree of drowsiness and heaviness of the head. Coupled with these symptoms, there are those indications of fever which attend the milder forms of the disease, though in this case with a proportionate increase in their severity; and sometimes distinct rigors may be observed alternating with the heat of the surface, or preceding the evening exacerbations of the fever. In the greater number of instances, the vomiting with which the fever sets in does not return after the second or third day of the patient's illness; but to this there are occasional exceptions; and as the sickness is usually more severe in cases in which constipation is present, there is some risk of mistaking the real nature of the affection, and of regarding the irritability of the stomach as a sign of approaching cerebral disease. Now and then too, the drowsiness at the onset of the disease is so overwhelming that I have known a child fall asleep two or three times during breakfast, while his dizziness and inability to walk steadily still further strengthened the impression that he was suffering from some affection of the brain. Either of these occurrences, however, is unusual; and, though listless and drowsy, the child is in general unwilling to keep his bed, while by night he is commonly very restless, waking often in a state of alarm, or talking much in his sleep. The countenance before long begins to wear the peculiar heavy
earance of a fever patient, and by the end of the first or the begin-
f the second week the child is usually found to have sunk into
from which he seems unwilling to be roused. The
most constantly hot as well as dry; the tem-
n in any other disease, with the excep-

tion of scarlatina, and in a few instances ranging as high [illegible] My own observations with reference to the date of app[illegible] eruption on the surface are neither sufficiently numerous [illegible] accurate for me to rely on their authority. MM. Rillie[illegible] observe that it very seldom appears so early as the fourth, [illegible] sixth to the tenth being the most common date of its appea[illegible] both the period during which it remains visible and the [illegible] are liable to great variation. In by far the greater numb[illegible] the eruption at any one time is extremely scanty; not i[illegible] spite of careful daily examination of my patients in the [illegible] Hospital, two or three spots only have been discovered [illegible] these have remained visible for only two or three days; [illegible] spots not infrequently appear as the others fade, for several [illegible] days. Now and then I have observed an abundant eruption [illegible] or forty spots being scattered at one time over the whole ab[illegible] this is altogether an exceptional occurrence. I have obs[illegible] abundant eruption only in severe cases of the fever, but [illegible] constant relation between the amount of eruption and the [illegible] the fever; and in some of the severest cases, the most careful [illegible] tion has failed to discover the characteristic spots at any stage [illegible] disease. In a few cases profuse sweats take place, but they [illegible] seem to have anything of a critical character. The pulse is [illegible] quent, and I have known it to continue at nearly 140 in the [illegible] for several days together, during the increase of the fever [illegible] eight years old. A frequent short hacking cough often occur[illegible] the first week; and rhonchus sibilus, and occasional large cre[illegible] are heard, in many cases in both lungs. Now and then, too, the [illegible] ration continues much accelerated for several days, without any [illegible] sign of serious pulmonary disease being present, and gradually [illegible] its proper frequency as the febrile symptoms subside. Tender[illegible] the abdomen is generally very evident before the first week [illegible] but frequently there is no complaint of pain, even in severe [illegible] except on pressure; though that seldom or never fails to elicit [illegible] dences of uneasiness, often to excite distinct complaints. Du[illegible] first week, the condition of the abdomen is usually natural [illegible] even though slightly tender; it afterwards becomes somewh[illegible] tended with flatus, and a sense of gurgling is often perceptible [illegible] pressure in one or other iliac region; but it rarely becomes [illegible] tympanitic. Diarrhœa is usually present, though it is not in [illegible] severe, the bowels not acting above four or five times in the [illegible] four hours. The tongue is usually more thickly coated at the [illegible] mencement than in the milder forms of the disease; a dry stre[illegible] appears down the centre, and by degrees the tongue becomes [illegible] dry, red, and glazed; or less often it is partially covered with [illegible] In the course of the second week the patient generally sink[illegible] more profound stupor—a condition which alternates in [illegible] with delirium. Sometimes the mind wanders occasionally [illegible] the commencement of the disease, in other cases deli[illegible] temporary symptom, occurring only at night, or when the [illegible] the daytime wakes from sleep. Now and then, though [illegible] the delirium is of a noisy kind, but the child not infrequently tries to get out of bed; and both the restlessness and delirium, though generally present in bad cases during the daytime, are aggravated in a marked degree at night. Once or twice I have known violent delirium come on towards evening, the child crying and shouting aloud during nearly the whole night, and sinking into a state of stupor by day. The child now seems nearly or quite unconscious of all that goes on around it; its evacuations are passed unconsciously, and it often seems dead to the sensation of thirst, by which, in the earlier stages of the disease, it was so much distressed; but this stupor of fever is so different from the coma which supervenes in affections of the brain, and the insensibility which characterizes it is so much less profound, that one can hardly be mistaken for the other. Once only I have seen convulsions occur in a child between two and three years old, who together with his two brothers suffered from very severe typhoid fever. The convulsions, which recurred on two successive days at the middle of the third week of the fever, were succeeded by paralysis of one side, which continued, though gradually diminishing, for four days. The child was unconscious even before their occurrence, and continued so for several days, though he eventually recovered. Even when the disease is most severe, neither subsultus nor floccitation is frequent, though it often happens that during the tedious and fluctuating convalescence, the child picks its nose till it bleeds, or makes the tips of its fingers, or different parts of its body sore by picking them. The patient is by the end of the second week, sometimes earlier, reduced by the continuance of these symptoms to the most extreme degree of emaciation, and to a condition apparently hopeless; but there is no other disease incidental to childhood from which recovery so often takes place, in spite of even the most unfavorable symptoms. The signs of recovery are, in the main, the same as betoken the recovery of an adult suffering from fever; but the amendment has seemed to me always to be gradual, and in no case the result of any critical occurrence. Moisture begins to reappear upon the edges of the tongue, the pulse loses its frequency, the delirium ceases by degrees, more quiet rest is enjoyed at night. Such signs of improvement may in general be looked for about or before the middle of the third week, but for days after their appearance the child's unconsciousness in many instances continues. He does not speak; he neither knows nor notices any one; and the mother, longing once more for her little one's fond look of recognition, and each day being disappointed of it, mistrusts the assurances that we may have given her, and loses heart and hope at a time when danger is really almost passed. At length it comes—a look, a smile, a gesture—but still no word; and slowly, very slowly, do the intellectual powers return, or does speech come back again. The first signs of amendment, however, may be taken as giving almost certain promise of complete recovery; but it is well to bear in mind that there is no disease of early life in which the mental faculties, though time brings them back at length uninjured, yet remain so long in a state of feebleness and torpor as in typhoid fever. Though the first signs of [illegible]ment, too, are very seldom deceptive, yet the

fever in these severer cases can scarcely be considered
the thirtieth day; sometimes not till even a week
patient's convalescence is almost always very slow, and
many fluctuations.

In the few cases, and according to my experience they
tively few, in which typhoid fever in children termin
death is seldom the result of complications such as
supervene in the course of fever in the adult, but the vital
way under the severity of the constitutional affection, the
which assume more and more of a typhoid character.
the end of the second, or at the beginning of the third
death in these circumstances is most likely to occur;
take place as late as the twenty-ninth day in one instance,
end of the fifth week in another; but in both of these instances
of the mouth came on after the more alarming general sym
begun to subside; and to this the death of the child was
while on another occasion perforation of the intestine
on the thirty-sixth day after the attack, when apparently
favorably towards recovery. Now and then a fatal termination
place after the lapse of little more than a week from the com
of the illness, under signs of cerebral disturbance which
general febrile symptoms into the shade; great restlessness
tion, with loud cries, being succeeded by convulsions,
their turn, being followed by coma, in which the child dies;
examination after death discovers nothing more serious than
what greater vascularity than natural of the brain and its

The *diagnosis* of the disease has been rendered needlessly
by the loose manner in which the name remittent fever has
plied to a variety of affections: still it must be confessed that
several maladies between which and typhoid fever points of
exist in some parts of their course that may easily deceive the
The resemblance is often very close between the milder varieties
fever and some of those cases of gastro-intestinal disorder, by
unusual in young children, which are excited by errors of diet,
either associated with diarrhœa or preceded by it. Something
done, however, towards guarding against error in all doubtful
by bearing in mind that typhoid fever occurs more than twice
in boys as in girls; that it is rare before five years of age,
uncommon before the age of two; and when it does happen,
young subjects, can almost always be traced to contagion. The
forms of gastric disorder attending or following dentition may
most absolute certainty be determined to be local ailments,
more or less constitutional disturbance: and thus essentially
from typhoid fever. But even in cases where the patient's

[1] Of 84 cases of typhoid fever under my care in the Children's Hospital
minated fatally. I believe this to be a far higher death rate than
private practice would in general yield, though MM. Rilliet and
mortality in their private practice to have been one in ten. The mortality
in four in the Hôpital des Enfans, at Paris, is obviously due rather
diseases contracted in the hospital than to the fever itself.

such as to raise a presumption one way or the other, the degree of loss of strength, and the rapidity with which it becomes apparent, the dry heat of the skin, and its intensity at the time of the exacerbations of the fever, the marked disturbance of the sensorium, and the delirium at night, are characters by which typhoid fever may be known, and whose absence would suffice to disprove the existence of that disorder. General tubercular disease, running an acute course, may indeed be taken for typhoid fever; and the distinction between the two affections is sometimes attended by very considerable difficulty;[1] especially if the case is not seen until the symptoms have become severe. Even then, however, something may be gathered for our guidance from the absence of rose spots, from the abdomen being generally flat, often shrunken, and from diarrhœa being absent, or at any rate not having occurred in acute tuberculosis until all the symptoms have assumed an extreme degree of severity. Auscultation, too, will often show good reason for suspecting the real nature of the case, or the previous history of the child will afford some clue with reference to it, though I believe that, with every care, instances will sometimes occur in which doubt will remain until removed by examination of the body after death. There are two other affections, between which and typhoid fever, though their resemblance is far less deceptive than that of acute tuberculosis, it is often far from easy to distinguish, while, unfortunately, the practical evils which follow from a wrong diagnosis are of a very serious nature. When speaking, however, of tubercular meningitis[2] and of pneumonia,[3] I dwelt so fully on the circumstances that might lead you to mistake either of those diseases for typhoid fever, and of the characteristics which belong to the last-named affection, that it can scarcely be necessary to do more than refer you to the observations made on those occasions. I have already said so much of the value of the indications furnished by the thermometer in guarding us from error in diagnosis, that I need now scarcely do more than remind you that the one great unfailing evidence of the existence of typhoid fever, is the invariable increase of temperature; an increase quite out of proportion to the acceleration of breathing, or the increased rapidity of pulse; and further, the law, to which there is no exception, of marked evening increase, and morning diminution of that heightened temperature, which yet continues above the natural degree throughout and is higher in proportion to the danger of the case.

I am anxious, before we pass to the treatment of the disease, to guard against an error which may possibly arise from my having pointed out certain well-marked distinctions between the cerebral symptoms of tubercular meningitis, and those which accompany typhoid fever. Now, although it is perfectly true that the disturbance of the brain in the latter case is the result of mere functional disorder, which, with the abatement of the fever, will, in general, by degrees pass away, still it is not to be forgotten that serious and even fatal

[1] See remarks on this subject in Lecture XXIX, p. 420.

[2] See Lecture VII, p. 85, and especially the remarks at p. 86 on the temperature in typhoid fever.

[3] Lecture XXI, p. 292.

cerebral affection occasionally attends it. It [illegible] at an early stage of the fever that we need be [illegible] for dangerous cerebral complications seldom occur [illegible] the second week, sometimes even later; while [illegible] ceed to a sort of imperfect convalescence, from the [illegible] had already begun to hope that the most anxious [illegible] The indications of their supervention are various, [illegible] kind as, considering the character of the child's [illegible] fail to excite that attention which otherwise they [illegible] more than ordinary excitability of the patient, the [illegible] his delirium, and the ungovernableness of his [illegible] our suspicions even in the case of an ill-managed [illegible] in whom these symptoms may in part be due [illegible] Sometimes, however, the mode of approach of serious [illegible] even more treacherous. The fever has already abated, [illegible] grown somewhat moister, the delirium is less [illegible] less distressing, and the child even has some quiet [illegible] often grinding his teeth, or there is frequent [illegible] twitchings of the facial muscles occur occasionally. [illegible] intolerant of light, and as the child opens them [illegible] please themselves with its fancied improvement, fondly [illegible] looks around and notices again. The pupils, however, [illegible] than natural, and act more sluggishly; the pulse [illegible] irregularity or intermission; sensibility to external [illegible] coma steals on almost imperceptibly, while in other [illegible] toms of tubercular meningitis by degrees develop [illegible]

The unobserved supervention of pneumonia is [illegible] daily careful auscultation; the existence of diarrhœa [illegible] the abdominal complication for that to be overlooked [illegible] much disturbance of the nervous system is part and [illegible] tion, some excess of it may readily pass without due [illegible] attached to it. When, then, you may ask, are we to [illegible] about the head? I should say, whenever delirium [illegible] merely during the night, or on waking from slumber [illegible] but whenever it also continues during the day, or when [illegible] the day an extremely excitable and unmanageable [illegible] not amounting to actual delirium. Or, secondly, [illegible] abatement of the fever, the cerebral symptoms do not [illegible] portion; or some new, even though very slight, [illegible] of the nervous system appears, although the [illegible] the earlier stages of the affection may have almost or [illegible] away. These symptoms may, indeed, speedily subside, [illegible] yield, and probably will, to judicious treatment, but [illegible] source of danger against which you cannot be too [illegible] ceasingly on the watch.

Thus much concerning the disease; now, in [illegible] *treatment.* In the management of typhoid fever in [illegible] of fever in the adult, the grand object to which our [illegible] be turned is to carry the patient through an affection [illegible] cut short, with as small an amount of suffering and [illegible]

"*Medicus curat, natura sanat morbum,*" says an old Latin adage; and in no disease is it of so much importance as in fever, that we should assign to our art its proper position as the handmaid of nature. The gradual approach of the disorder, in the great majority of instances, of itself points out the propriety of that expectant mode of treatment which is generally the most appropriate during the first week of the child's illness. The languid and listless state of the little patient, his headache and drowsiness, often lead him to wish to remain in bed all day long; but there is no reason for confining him to bed, if during the period of remission of the fever he should prefer to sit up. The impaired appetite often renders any other directions about the diet unnecessary, than a caution to the parents or nurse not to coax or tempt the child to take food, which it is and will probably for some days continue to be entirely unable to digest. The heat of skin and the craving thirst are the two most urgent symptoms in the early stages of the affection. The first of these is generally relieved by sponging the surface of the body several times a day with lukewarm water. The desire for cold drinks is often very urgent, and no beverage is half so grateful as cold water to the child. Of this it would, if permitted, take abundant draughts; but it should be explained to the attendants that the thirst is not more effectually relieved by them than by small quantities of fluid, while pain in the abdomen is very likely to be caused by the overdistension of the stomach. The cup given to the child should therefore only have a dessert or tablespoonful of water in it, for it irritates the little patient to remove the vessel from its lips unemptied. In the milder forms of the disease, and during the first week, medicine is little needed; but a simple saline may be given, such as the citrate of potass, in a mixture to which small doses of vinum ipecacuanhæ may be added, if as sometimes happens the cough is troublesome. If the bowels act with due frequency, and the appearance of the evacuations is not extremely unhealthy, it is well to abstain from the employment of any remedy that might act upon them, for fear of occasioning diarrhœa, which is so apt to supervene in the course of this affection. For the same reason, if an aperient is indicated, drastic purgatives are not to be given, but a moderate dose of castor oil should be administered. Now and then, however, cases are met with in which the bowels remain confined during a great part of the affection, and in which such purgatives as senna are not only borne, but are absolutely necessary. They, however, are purely exceptional cases; and it will generally suffice if there exists any tendency to constipation, to give a small dose of the mercury and chalk night and morning, and during the daytime a small quantity of the tartrate of soda or sulphate of magnesia, dissolved in some simple saline mixture, every six or eight hours.

The unhealthy state of the evacuations that exists in a large number of cases is generally associated with a disposition to diarrhœa, which becomes a more prominent symptom in the second than it was in the first week of the disorder. Equal parts of the Hydrargyrum cum Cretâ and Dover's powder are the best means of relieving both these morbid conditions; the remedy being given either once or twice a day, or more frequently, according to the urgency of the symptoms [illegible] of abdominal pain and tenderness must be ascertained [illegible] a few leeches must be applied to either iliac region if [illegible] seems considerable, or if the child appears to suffer much [illegible] the abdomen, or if the diarrhœa is severe. If depletion [illegible] application of but a small number of leeches will generally [illegible] requirements of the case, while copious bleeding is [illegible] well borne. Even in children of ten years old I never [illegible] four or six leeches, and it is very seldom that any occasion [illegible] repetition of the bleeding. The application of poultices [illegible] or scalded bran to the abdomen, and their frequent repetition [illegible] valuable means of relieving the griping pain which [illegible] children; and in most cases it is desirable to make trial [illegible] having recourse to depletion.

There is but one other class of symptoms likely to occur [illegible] first week of the fever, to the management of which I have [illegible] referred; namely, those signs of cerebral disturbance which [illegible] times so serious as to call for treatment. The early [illegible] delirium, though it generally implies that the disease will [illegible] rather serious character, yet does not of itself indicate the [illegible] taking blood from the head; but if the child is quiet [illegible] rational during the daytime, and though dull yet not in [illegible] stupor, while the delirium at night is of a tranquil kind, [illegible] rupted by frequent and tolerably quiet slumber, it will [illegible] the hair quite short, apply cold to the head by means of [illegible] in a bladder or india-rubber bag, as I have already explained [illegible] speaking of the management of acute cerebral disease, and to [illegible] apartment cool and absolutely quiet. The irritability, [illegible] and restlessness at night, accompanied by loud and noisy [illegible] from which the child gets scarcely any respite all night long [illegible] quently arrested at once by an opiate. Unless some abdominal [illegible] plication should forbid its employment, the tartar emetic is [illegible] cases a most valuable adjunct to the opium.[1] A draught [illegible] five minims of laudanum, and a quarter of a grain of tartar [illegible] will be a suitable anodyne for a child of five years old, and [illegible] repeated night after night with almost magical effect. On the [illegible] too, I think the action of opium is more satisfactory than that of [illegible] in the restlessness of fever. When the delirium at night is [illegible] during the daytime by an almost equally distressing condition [illegible] citement, accompanied with a burning skin, and a very [illegible] though feeble pulse, the continuing the tartar emetic in slightly [illegible] seating doses, combined with smaller quantities of laudanum [illegible] hours, will often be of essential service. If, however, there [illegible] injection of the conjunctivæ, or if the head is in a marked degree [illegible] than the surface generally, or if any other indication of disorder [illegible] brain is present besides the delirium and excitement, leeches [illegible]

[1] The remarks of Dr. Graves, in his Lectures on Clinical Medicine, vol. [illegible] on the use of Tartar Emetic and Opium in Fever, are little less applicable [illegible] management in the child than in the adult.

applied to the head—though depletion should in these cases be used sparingly; and after the abstraction of blood by the application of half a dozen leeches, we should return to the tartar emetic and opium, remembering that we have no active inflammation to combat, nor even that intense cerebral congestion which we occasionally meet with in other circumstances, and safety from which is found only in very active depletory measures.

Depletion is also called for in cases, not very commonly met with, in which even at an early period of the disease there is a great degree of stupor and apathy, with a dilated and sluggish pupil, but little complaint of thirst, and none of headache or local suffering. By the cautious abstraction of blood we may here sometimes anticipate the development of the more alarming head-symptoms, which, if we leave the patient alone, lulled into a false security by the absence of any signs of active mischief, will not fail before long to manifest themselves. As a general rule, indeed, it must be our object in the management of this fever to anticipate the head-symptoms as far as possible, to keep down the excitement and quiet the delirium by tartar emetic and opium, or by the local abstraction of blood; a purely expectant course of practice, when the cerebral disturbance is considerable, is neither wise nor safe. The head-symptoms, which come on slowly and almost imperceptibly at a more advanced stage of the disease, are sometimes very unmanageable. Depletion is no longer of service, but blisters may be applied to the occiput and nape of the neck with advantage; they should, however, not be kept on so long as to produce complete vesication; but only for a time sufficient to obtain their counter-irritant effect, and to allow of their reapplication in the same neighborhood, if not upon exactly the same spot, on the next day. The unfavorable termination of the disease in this stage is, I apprehend, due, in the great majority of cases, to the development of some previously latent tendency to tubercular meningitis; while the more active head-symptoms, which are met with at an earlier period, are often merely the result of functional disturbance, and therefore generally yield to well-considered treatment.

In mild cases of the disease, the expectant treatment usually appropriate during its earlier stages, may be continued throughout its course; great caution being exercised as the child begins to improve, to prevent its committing any error in diet. When severe, however, the second week often brings with it a train of symptoms that require many modifications in the plan of treatment. The vital powers need to be supported, and the nervous system requires to be tranquillized; and this is to be attempted by means similar to those which we should employ in the management of fever in the adult. The mere diluents which were given during the previous course of the disease must now be exchanged for beef or veal tea or chicken broth, unless the existence of severe diarrhœa contraindicate their administration; in which case we must substitute arrowroot, milk, and isinglass, for animal broths. In a large proportion of cases nutritious food is all that will be required; but wine is sometimes as essential as in the fevers of the adult; and the indications for giving it are much the same at all ages, while its influence on the patient must be the only measure of the quantity to be administered; and I have on some occasions given as [illegible] ounces of wine and four ounces of brandy daily, to chil[illegible] ten years old, and believe that this copious use of stimu[illegible] served their life. Even though wine be not necessary, [illegible] some form of stimulant during the second and third week [illegible] tion. The prescription[1] that I usually follow is one [illegible] such circumstances by Dr. Stieglitz, of St. Petersburg, [illegible] dients of which are ether and hydrochloric acid, and [illegible] frequently add either the tincture or Battley's concentrated [illegible] bark, or else quinine in moderate doses. I have no exp[illegible] employment of large doses of quinine as recommended by [illegible] physicians, either given by the mouth or in enema. It [illegible] the bowels if they are not much disturbed at the time of [illegible] its administration, while if this is the case, a small do[illegible] powder, as a grain or a grain and a half at bedtime, will [illegible] useful, both in checking the tendency to diarrhœa, and in [illegible] sleep for the child, who, without it, would probably be [illegible] delirious all night long. If diarrhœa is present, I either [illegible] the use of the acid mixture, or add a drop or two of lau[illegible] dose. If purging becomes really severe, aromatics and astr[illegible] be employed, and small doses of mercury and chalk with Dover[illegible] and bismuth may be given with much advantage for two or [illegible] at intervals of four or six hours. An opiate enema, as sm[illegible] as possible, will more effectually quiet the intestines than [illegible] doses given by the mouth.

The only other complication that is apt to be troublesome [illegible] chitis. Usually, however, the cough to which this gives [illegible] annoying rather than a dangerous symptom; and it is in ge[illegible] harassing at the commencement of the affection, and again [illegible] valescence is beginning, than during the time when the gra[illegible] toms are present. A little ipecacuanha wine, nitrous ether, [illegible] pound tincture of camphor, will usually relieve it, to which [illegible] occasionally be expedient to add the application of a mustard [illegible] to the chest.

The convalescence is often extremely tedious; the child is [illegible] the disease not only extremely weak and emaciated, but with [illegible] tive powers greatly impaired. It is often many days be[illegible] stomach is able to digest any solid food; even a piece of [illegible] sometimes irritate the intestines, and bring on a return of [illegible] The appetite seems sometimes quite lost; tonics either do [illegible] are actually injurious by rekindling the fever; or symptoms [illegible] which seem to threaten the development of tubercular disease, [illegible] quence that not very seldom follows severe attacks of remitt[illegible]

---

[1] (No. 39.)

℞. Acid. Hydrochlor. dil., ♏xxxij.
Spt. Æth. co., ʒj ♏xx.
Syr. Rhœados, ʒiv.
Mist. Camph., ℥iijss. M.

A tablespoonful every six hours. For a child five years old.

In such circumstances, change of air and the removal, if possible, to the seaside, are often the only means of restoring the child to health; a means which you may recommend with the more confidence, since it hardly ever fails to be successful.[1]

I know of no better place than the present for making a few remarks to you concerning *intermittent fever* or *ague* as it occurs in early life. In some countries, as you know, this disorder affects persons at all ages, but in healthier regions it is found commonly to spare the two extremes of life, and to attack but seldom either the aged or the very young. Accordingly, in this country, ague is seldom observed in infancy and childhood, and is so uncommon in this metropolis, that in almost all of the instances of it which have come under my observation in early life the disorder was not contracted in London.

Considering its rarity, therefore, I should not occupy your time by speaking of ague, if it were not that it presents certain peculiarities in early life, and those of a kind to render its nature obscure, and to lead you altogether to overlook its existence, or to mistake it for some other disease. These peculiarities consist in the ill-marked character, or even the complete absence of shivering, the place of which is taken by a condition of extreme nervous depression, or sometimes even by a disturbance of the nervous system issuing in convulsions—in the severity and long continuance of the hot stage, and in the absence of any distinct sweating stage, the child recovering by degrees, but without the well-marked crisis which marks the cessation of each fit of ague in the grown person. When to this is added that the child always appears more ailing between the fits than is usual with the adult, that dulness, heaviness, and fretfulness, with some degree of febrile disturbance, continue in the intervals, and that the periodicity of the attacks is not so regular as in the adult, you will at once see that an erroneous diagnosis is very possible, I might almost say very pardonable.

The youngest child whom I have seen suffering from ague was not quite two years old, and in his case the rigors were so slight that they did not attract the mother's notice until her attention was especially called to their occurrence. In proportion to the tender age of the child are the above-named peculiarities distinctly marked, while after the age of five years the few cases of ague which I have seen scarcely differed from the same disease in the adult.

The *treatment* of the affection is the same in the child or infant as in the grown person, and quinine is no less a specific for it in the one case than in the other. The tendency to relapse, however, I believe to be very great in early life, and I have known ague return after several months, on removal to a district which though healthy, and free from ague, was yet somewhat lower and less dry than the child's previous residence. On this account much care is needed, and that continued for a considerable period, in the selection of the dwelling of a child who has to all appearance perfectly recovered from an attack of intermittent fever.

---

[1] I have said nothing, because I know nothing practically, of the hydropathic treatment of typhoid fever. I feel, however, that far too high authorities have been adduced in its favor to warrant its being passed over without mention.

LECTURE XLIII.

SMALL POX.—Checked but not extirpated by vaccination—Its chief mortality among children—Rate of mortality in cases of the disease undiminished during the last fifty years—Its symptoms—Their early differences from those of the other exanthemata—Characters and progress of the eruption—Peculiarities of confluent small-pox—Dangers attending the maturation of the pustules, and the secondary fever—Treatment.

MODIFIED SMALL-POX—Its low rate of mortality—Protective and mitigating power of vaccination—Objections to vaccination—Communication of syphilis by vaccination. Peculiarities of modified small-pox.

CHICKEN-POX.—Its symptoms, and differences from small-pox.

UNTIL the commencement of this century, the disease to which I wish to-day briefly to call your attention, possessed a degree of importance far greater than that which attaches to it at present. Before the introduction of vaccination, the *small-pox* was a disease of almost universal prevalence, causing at the least eight per cent. of the total mortality of this metropolis, and disfiguring for life thousands whom it did not destroy. Its loathsome character, and its formidable symptoms, when it attacked the constitution at unawares, led to the adoption of variolous inoculation, by which the disease was communicated in a mild form, and under favorable conditions; and persons having undergone comparatively little suffering, and having been exposed to still less danger, enjoyed by this means almost complete immunity from subsequent attacks of small-pox. But great as its benefits were, variolous inoculation perpetuated at all times, and in all places, a disease which would otherwise have obeyed the general law of epidemics, and would have had its periods of rare occurrence as well as those of widespread prevalence. Thus, as has been well observed, while the advantages of the practice were great and obvious to the individual, to the community at large they were very doubtful.

No such drawback exists to detract from the benefits of vaccination, though unfortunately our present experience does not altogether justify the sanguine expectations entertained concerning it by its first promoters. Peculiarities of climate oppose a serious barrier to its successful introduction into some countries,[1] and even in our own land individuals are occasionally met with in whom vaccination altogether fails, or over whom it seems to extend but a partial or temporary protective power.

But I will not enter on the question of the merits of vaccination, nor of the circumstances that impair its preservative power, or call for its repetition; for though the subject is one important alike to the phy-

[1] Dr. Duncan Stewart's valuable Report on Small-pox in Calcutta, and Vaccination in Bengal, 8vo., Calcutta, 1844, shows conclusively that the peculiarities of the Indian climate present obstacles to vaccination such as greatly to detract from its value; while it is to be feared that they are of a nature which the greatest care will never wholly overcome.

sician and the philanthropist, I have had no opportunities of forming a judgment concerning it which are not alike open to you all. Probably indeed, I have seen much less of it than many others. Properly enough, small-pox cases are not received into the Children's Hospital; and I do not think that within the past twenty years as many as five cases of the disease have come under my care. In the writings of the late Dr. Gregory, physician to the Small-Pox Hospital, in the treatise on vaccination by Dr. Steinbrenner, to which the Institute of France adjudged a prize in 1835, and in the still more recent Report to the Board of Health, drawn up by Mr. Simon, in 1857,[1] you will find everything that either large experience or unwearied research can bring to its elucidation.

One fact which it behooves us always to bear in mind, is that albeit the prevalence of the disease has been greatly checked by vaccination, small-pox is still one of the most fatal maladies of this country; and further, that it selects its victims, as heretofore, chiefly from among children and young persons—nearly three-fourths of the fatal cases of this affection occurring before the age of five, and more than nine-tenths before the age of fifteen years.

In spite, too, of the increase of medical knowledge during the past fifty years, the proportion of small-pox cases that terminate fatally has been estimated by the best authorities to be as great now as it was half a century ago. To some extent, perhaps, the very diminution in the frequency of the disease may have had an unfavorable influence on its issue in individual cases; for practitioners, meeting with it now less often than medical men in former days were wont to do, are not so familiar with the meaning of those minuter variations in its symptoms, from which important practical conclusions might be drawn by those who knew how to interpret them aright.

Let me therefore urge you to watch every case of this formidable disease that may come under your observation with most minute care, lest you misinterpret the symptoms, or mistake the treatment of some patient affected with it, whose well-being may be dependent on your skill. For my own part, I cannot pretend to give you more than an outline sketch of its characters, and must refer you to the writings of others who have had greater opportunities of watching it than have fallen to my share, to fill up the portrait.

The early *symptoms* of small-pox are those of approaching fever, and if any other febrile disorder be prevalent at the time of their occurrence, they may possibly be taken for the indications of an approaching attack of the prevailing epidemic. There are, however, some peculiarities in the mode of onset of small-pox which are sufficiently charac-

---

[1] Nothing can more conclusively establish the immensity of the boon which vaccination has conferred on society, than the contrast which Mr. Simon's report exhibits between the mortality from small-pox before and after its introduction. "The fatality of small-pox in Copenhagen is but an eleventh of what it was; in Sweden a little over a thirteenth; in Berlin and in large parts of Austria but a twentieth; in Westphalia but a twenty-fifth. In the last-named instance, there now die of small-pox but five persons, where formerly there died a hundred." See p. xxiii of the Report.

teristic of it even in the child, and which generally dis[illegible] any of the other eruptive fevers. The sickness with wh[illegible] in general severe, and the disorder of the stomach [illegible] forty-eight hours, during which time vomiting recur[illegible] measles there is comparatively little gastric disorder; and [illegible] that often ushers in scarlatina, though frequently severe, [illegible] long continuance. In young children we lose those co[illegible] tense pain in the back which in the case of older patients [illegible] our suspicion; but on the other hand, the severity of [illegible] turbance is an important feature in the early stage of th[illegible] the commencement of measles, the brain is in general [illegible] turbed; in scarlatina, delirium often occurs very early; [illegible] pox the condition is one rather of stupor than of deli[illegible] vulsions sometimes take place, and continue alternating [illegible] as long a period as twenty-four or thirty-six hours. [illegible] the skin in small-pox is hot, it is neither so hot nor so [illegible] fever; the tongue does not present the peculiar redness [illegible] nence of its papillæ, which are observable in scarlatina; [illegible] any of the sore throat which forms so characteristic a sym[illegible] disease. The early stages of small-pox are not attend[illegible] catarrhal symptoms which accompany measles; the eruption [illegible] usually appears later, that of scarlet fever always sooner, [illegible] tion of small-pox; while its papular character is in general [illegible] well marked to distinguish it from the rash of either of [illegible] It never appears in less than forty-eight hours from the [illegible] indisposition, often not till after a somewhat longer time, [illegible] itself in the form of small papulæ, which are first disc[illegible] face, forehead, and wrists, whence they extend to the tr[illegible] and lastly to the lower extremities. These papulæ are at [illegible] red, somewhat acuminated elevations, so minute that the[illegible] easily overlooked on a hasty examination, but yet convey[illegible] sense of irregularity to the finger when passed over the sur[illegible] increase in size, and in the course of forty-eight hours assum[illegible] lar character, and contain a whey-like fluid; while, instead of [illegible] form, they now present a central depression. During another [illegible] of forty-eight hours or thereabouts, these vesicles go on enlarg[illegible] central depression grows more and more apparent, and the[illegible] become white and opaque; they are no longer vesicles, but ha[illegible] converted into pustules, each of which, if they are distinc[illegible] areola of a red hue round its base. As the pustules enlarg[illegible] hands, and feet become swollen, and a general redness of [illegible] succeeds to the more circumscribed areola which had previ[illegible] rounded each separate pustule. As the size of the pustules [illegible] they lose that central depression which they had presented [illegible] cles; they assume a spheroidal form, or even become slig[illegible] The next change observable in them is an alteration of the[illegible] a white to a dirty yellow tint, which they continue to re[illegible] desiccation of the eruption commences. This token of [illegible] the disease is first apparent on the face, where, as you [illegible] the eruption is earliest observable; while on the hand[illegible] ably owing to the thickness of the epidermis in those situations, this change is longest delayed, and the pustules there attain a greater size than in any other situation. The *maturation* of the pustules usually occupies from the commencement of the fifth to the commencement of the eighth day of the eruption, or from the eighth to the eleventh day of the disease, when the process of *desiccation* begins. A few of the smaller pustules dry up and become converted into crusts, which afterwards drop off; but the greater number of them burst, and the pus that they discharge, together with a very adhesive matter which they continue to secrete for two or three days, contribute to form the scab, which incrusts more or less extensively the surface of a small-pox patient during the decline of the disease. When the scab falls off, which it does in from three to five or six days, the skin appears stained of a reddish-brown color, which often does not disappear for several weeks; but it is only in cases where the pustule has gone so deep as to destroy a portion of the true skin, that permanent disfigurement, the so-called pitting of the small-pox, is produced.

It is only in cases of *discrete* small-pox, in which the eruption is but moderately abundant, and the pustules consequently run their course without coalescing with each other, that the above-mentioned changes can be distinctly traced. In the *confluent* variety of the disease, in which the pustules are so numerous that they run together as they increase in size, the characteristic alterations in the individual pustules cannot be followed. In those situations where the eruption is confluent, the pustules never attain the size which separate pustules often reach; they do not become so prominent, nor do their contents in general assume the same yellowish color, but several of them coalesce to form a slightly irregular surface of a whitish hue; while, when the stage of desiccation comes on, each of these patches becomes converted into a moist brown scab, which is many days before it is detached. Nor is it merely at those parts, such as the face, where the eruption is actually confluent, that its character is modified, but even where the pustules are distinct, their advance goes on more slowly, and the maturative stage is longer in being completed, than in less severe cases of the disease. It is, moreover, in cases of confluent small-pox that the ulceration of the pustules most commonly invades the true skin, and that serious disfigurement is most likely to take place; while, further, the degree of danger to life is in almost direct proportion, in every case of small-pox, to the amount of confluence of the eruption.

The appearance of the eruption of small-pox is attended with a great abatement, sometimes with the almost complete disappearance, of those signs of constitutional disturbance with which the disease sets in; and in mild cases the child shows few other indications of illness than are furnished by the eruption on the skin. But with the maturation of the pustules, the *secondary fever*, as it is called, is excited, and the period of the greatest danger to the patient now comes on. The skin once more grows hot; the pulse rises in frequency; restlessness, thirst, and all the phenomena of inflammatory fever, develop themselves, and continue with more or less intensity for about three [illegible]s. These symptoms afterwards diminish, and finally disappear as the pustules burst, and the stage of desiccation is accomplished. [illegible] however, only in cases of a favorable kind that the [illegible] runs so mild a course. In confluent small-pox the secondary [illegible] always more severe than in the discrete form of the disease, [illegible] comes on later, in consequence of the more tardy [illegible] pustules. Often, indeed, it assumes a typhoid character; [illegible] becomes extremely frequent and feeble, the tongue dry and [illegible] and the patient dies delirious. In other instances the [illegible] the pustules goes on for a day or two with very slight [illegible] were it not that this extreme mildness of the secondary fever, [illegible] where the eruption has been abundant, is itself a suspicious [illegible] stance, we should be disposed to express, without hesitation, [illegible] favorable opinion as to the patient's condition. Suddenly, [illegible] the pulse begins to falter; the pustules, which before [illegible] collapse; the extremities grow cold, and in a few hours [illegible] dies. This fatal change is sometimes ushered in by a fit of [illegible] sions; at other times it is preceded by a condition of [illegible] lessness, which contrasts remarkably with the quietude of the [illegible] manner for the two or three previous days; and it is well to [illegible] mind that the supervention of either of these two symptoms [illegible] maturative stage of small-pox is the almost certain herald of [illegible] approaching death. One other not infrequent source of danger [illegible] this period arises from the pustules which have formed on the [illegible] membrane of the mouth, fauces, and air-passages. In almost [illegible] case of small-pox, a few spots of the eruption may be seen [illegible] tongue and on the interior of the mouth; while an inspection [illegible] bodies of patients to whom it has proved fatal has shown [illegible] pustules form likewise on the interior of the larynx and [illegible] sometimes in considerable numbers. It is to the presence of [illegible] in these situations that the hoarse or altered voice, and the [illegible] of deglutition, which are observed in most cases of severe [illegible] are due; as well as that short hacking cough which sometimes [illegible] a very troublesome symptom. The ptyalism, too, which [illegible] many instances, is apparently owing to the salivary glands [illegible] ing with the irritated and inflamed state of the mucous [illegible] the mouth. In cases which run a fortunate course, those [illegible] have come on about the third or fourth day of the eruption, [illegible] ing increased in severity until the eighth or ninth, then [illegible] decline. In less favorable circumstances, however, they [illegible] grow worse; the voice becomes perfectly extinct, and deglutition [illegible] impossible, and the patient dies from the obstacle which the [illegible] mation and swelling of the lining membrane of the larynx [illegible] the free access of air to the lungs; though the symptoms are [illegible] never those of active inflammatory croup.

You will find in the writings of those whose opportunities of [illegible] ing small-pox have been considerable, the description of [illegible] modes in which it occasionally proves fatal. Thus, it is [illegible] associated with a great tendency to hemorrhage; petechiæ [illegible] on the surface of the body, and the pustules assuming a [illegible] from the extravasation of blood into them. In other [illegible] grene attacks the feet or some other part of the body. But these are occurrences which it has not been my lot to witness, and I will not therefore take up your time by detailing them at second hand.

Let us now glance for a few minutes at the *treatment* to be pursued in this disease. You know that before the time of Sydenham, physicians adopted a heating regimen in cases of small-pox; excluding fresh air from the chamber, covering the patient with blankets, and administering stimulating medicines and cordial drinks. To this practice the then prevalent theory of fermentation, and of nature's efforts in disease being directed to eliminate the peccant matter from the blood, had given occasion. In accordance with these notions, it was assumed that the more abundant the eruption, the more complete would be the separation of these noxious matters, and consequently the better the chance of the patient's well-doing. The observation of nature, however, taught Sydenham that the very reverse was the case; that the more abundant the eruption, the greater the danger—the fewer the pustules, the more favorable the prospect of the patient's recovery. A cooling regimen, therefore, is now universally adopted in the early stage of the disease, and fresh air is freely admitted into the chamber, in order to prevent, if possible, a copious eruption, while the same end is sought to be still further promoted by keeping the bowels gently open, by a spare diet, and by mild antiphlogistic medicines. Depletion, which even in the adult is not to be practiced merely with the hope of thereby diminishing the quantity of the eruption, is still less to be resorted to in the child, unless evidently called for by symptoms of severe cerebral disturbance; such as convulsions frequently recurring, or ending in coma. Such occurrences as those, however, demand not merely the abstraction of blood, but its removal with an unsparing hand; for as I told you at the commencement of these lectures, the cerebral congestion which attends the onset of the eruptive fevers, if not speedily relieved, may prove very quickly fatal. Cases of an opposite kind are sometimes met with in which the patient, before the appearance of the eruption, is in a state of depression so great as to call for warmth to the surface, or for the hot bath, for diaphoretic medicines, and sometimes even for stimulants. In this, however, there is nothing more than we may occasionally witness in a patient completely prostrated during the first stage of typhus fever, and needing perhaps the free administration of wine and ammonia to preserve him from death.

With the outbreak of the eruption there ensues a lull in the symptoms, and a period now succeeds during which we have nothing else to do than to leave nature to her workings undisturbed. Even in cases of confluent small-pox, there is in many instances not a single symptom just at this time which could either excite solicitude or call for treatment, and you must therefore take care not to allow yourself at this moment to be betrayed into the hasty expression of a very favorable prognosis, which the supervention of the secondary fever may perhaps in a day or two most grievously belie. If, however, the number of pustules should be but small, the secondary fever will be slight: our [fav]orable opinion may, in these circumstances, be expressed with some confidence, and most probably no deviation from [illegible] tant plan of treatment will be required during the [illegible] of the disease. If the eruption is more abundant, [illegible] ing secondary fever consequently severe, an antiphlo[illegible] ment must be carried out more strictly, while in all [illegible] ness which is so common a symptom during the [illegible] small-pox must be controlled by the administration of [illegible] or of some other form of opiate, once or twice a day. [illegible] fluent small-pox, the patient needs to be very closely [illegible] the maturation of the pustules, for on the second or [illegible] process the vital powers sometimes suddenly fail. The [illegible] of any such occurrence, which would be furnished by a [illegible] tion of the previous restlessness, by the subsidence of [illegible] the face and hands, the paleness of the skin in the [illegible] the pustules, and the collapse of the pustules themselves, [illegible] a sinking in the temperature of the surface, and a great [illegible] the power of the pulse, call at once for the energetic [illegible] stimulants, for the administration of wine, and the [illegible] nutritious food for the previous meagre diet. A similar [illegible] also be pursued whenever the secondary fever shows any [illegible] assume a typhoid character, while, irrespective of any [illegible] symptoms, it is not infrequently expedient, if the eruption [illegible] to give beef tea, and to adopt other means for supporting the [illegible] from the fifth or sixth day of the eruption,—a period corres[illegible] I hardly need remind you, with the eighth or ninth day of the [illegible]

Various local means have been recommended to be adopted [illegible] early stage of the disease, with the view of preventing the full [illegible] ment of the pustules, and consequently of preserving the [illegible] the disfigurement produced by the pitting of the eruption. [illegible] terization of each individual pock with the nitrate of silver [illegible] impracticable from its tediousness, while there is some [illegible] the results which different persons allege that they have [illegible] applying mercurial ointment or plaster, or by washing the surface [illegible] it is wished to defend with a solution of corrosive sublimate. [illegible] weight of evidence appears to me, however, to be in favor of [illegible] ceeding of this kind; and that which seems to have been the [illegible] cessful, is the application of the mercurial plaster at a period [illegible] than the third day from the outbreak of the eruption, or the [illegible] the surface with the elastic collodion.

Attention must be paid to the state of the eyes, which [illegible] much during attacks of the small-pox, though Dr. Gregory [illegible] the conjunctiva never becomes the seat of the pustules. From the [illegible] when the swelling of the face begins during the maturation [illegible] eruption, the eyelids are often so much swollen as completely [illegible] the eyes, while their edges are glued together by a tenacious [illegible] from the Meibomian glands. The patient will be much relieved [illegible] bathing the eyes frequently with warm water, and any pustules [illegible] occupy the margins of the palpebræ should be carefully cauterized [illegible] the nitrate of silver.

The condition of the mouth and throat must not be neglected [illegible] old enough, the child may be made to gargle with the infusion of roses, while, should it be too young to do this, the endeavor must be made to keep the mouth and throat free from the secretions which collect there, by washing or syringing them frequently with warm water, and by applying a weak solution of chloride of lime to the fauces. If difficult respiration should come on, in consequence of the affection seriously involving the larynx and trachea, the patient's condition, according to the testimony of almost all writers, is rendered nearly hopeless.

The intense itching of the eruption during the latter part of the period of maturation, and the stage of desiccation, not only distresses the patient exceedingly, but is often the occasion of subsequent disfigurement, in consequence of the desire to scratch being irresistible, and the pustules being converted by abrasion of their heads into troublesome ulcerations.

The application of sweet oil, cold cream, or spermaceti ointment, will do something towards allaying the irritation; but you will often find it necessary to muffle the hands of children, in order to prevent their producing troublesome sores by scratching themselves.

The convalescence from small-pox is often very tedious; the patient's recovery is frequently interrupted by various intercurrent affections, and the latent seeds of scrofulous disorder are in many instances called into activity by its attack. These, however, are occurrences which present nothing of a special character, and it is therefore unnecessary to make any observation with reference to their treatment.

Although previous vaccination usually confers upon the system a complete immunity from subsequent attacks of small-pox, yet to this rule there are occasional exceptions. In many instances, indeed, the occurrence of *small-pox after* alleged successful *vaccination* may be accounted for by the careless performance of that operation, by the use of lymph taken from the arm at too late a period, or by the production in some way of a spurious instead of a genuine vaccine vesicle. It must be confessed, however, that when every allowance has been made for these casualties, the number of cases of small-pox occurring after successful vaccination is proportionably much greater than the number in which a second attack of small-pox is experienced by those who have either had that disease casually, or in whom it has been produced by variolous inoculation. It would occupy far more time than we have at our command, if we were to attempt to enter upon the inquiry as to the causes of the failure in the protective power of vaccination. Different views have been taken by very high authorities upon this subject; but there is one important fact concerning which nearly all are agreed, namely, that the liability to a subsequent attack of small-pox is almost incalculably diminished by revaccination. Considering, then, how simple the operation is, and how nearly painless its performance, while the benefit to be obtained by it is so inestimable, I would strongly urge you to revaccinate all persons turned twelve years old, even though they had been vaccinated with the most complete success in their infancy.[1]

---

[1] For facts showing the preservative influence of revaccination, see Steinbrenner, Traité sur la Vaccine, 8vo., pp. 683–784. Paris, 1846. The report of Mr. Simon,

But although we should take a comparatively low [illegible] value of vaccination, and confess to the fullest extent the [illegible] *complete* preservative virtue, we shall yet find, in the [illegible] mitigating influence which it exerts over small-pox, more [illegible] to make us value it as a priceless boon. Thirty years ago, [illegible] raged epidemically at Marseilles, where it attacked almost [illegible] persons under 30 years of age. M. Favart,[1] who sent an [illegible] this epidemic to the Academy of Medicine at Marseilles, [illegible] number of the inhabitants of that city under 30 years of age at [illegible] Of those, about 30,000 had been vaccinated, 2000 had had [illegible] casually or by inoculation, and 8000 had had neither variola [illegible] pox. Of this last class 4000, or 1 in 2, were attacked by [illegible] and 1000 of them, or 1 in 4, died. Of those who had had [illegible] previously, only 20, or 6 in 1000, were again affected; but 4 [illegible] 1 in 5, died; while of the vaccinated, although 2000, or 1 in [illegible] it, yet it proved fatal only to 20, or 1 per cent. If we come [illegible] the present day, and to our country, the results at which [illegible] but little less striking. During the recent epidemic [illegible] small-pox in London and its vicinity in the years 1870–187[illegible] [illegible] mortality among 3634 unvaccinated patients, at all ages, was [illegible] rate of 44.80 per cent., and among 11,174 vaccinated [illegible] rate of 10.15 per cent. Further, if the patients alleged to [illegible] vaccinated are divided into classes according as the evidence of [illegible] vaccination is more or less conclusive, we find that the number [illegible] attacked diminishes in proportion to the number of vaccination [illegible] and also that the mortality lessens in the same proportion, [illegible] case of those in whom there are five marks or more as [illegible] cessful vaccination, it amounts to only 5.5 per cent., or little [illegible] one-tenth of the mortality among the non-vaccinated.[2]

It may indeed be said that vaccination has recently been [illegible] upon its trial; and the report to the House of Commons in 18[illegible] committee appointed to inquire into the operation of the V[illegible] Act of 1867, contains all that can be reasonably alleged, or I [illegible] may say fondly imagined, to the discredit of vaccination. [illegible] only fact of importance put on record by the committee is [illegible] occasional communication of syphilis by vaccination, to [illegible] Hutchinson, of the London Hospital, had already drawn the [illegible] of the profession at a meeting of the Medico-Chirurgical Society, [illegible] accident which, though very rare, was yet not of that [illegible]

---

to which reference has already been made, contains a mass of most [illegible] dence illustrative both of the value of vaccination, of the share which [illegible] cination has in the production of its apparent failures, and lastly, of [illegible] importance of revaccination as a means by which, if it were but [illegible] practiced, small-pox would be almost or altogether exterminated. [illegible] Mr. Marson and Dr. Balfour, originally published in the Medico-Chir[illegible] actions, but reprinted in the Appendix to the Report, have afforded [illegible] able elucidation of these last two points.

[1] As reported by Steinbrenner, op. cit., p. 166.

[2] See Tables in the Report of a Committee of the Managers of the [illegible] Asylum District, July 13, 1872. Folio.

[3] Transactions of Medico-Chirurgical Society, vol. liv, 1872, and [illegible] 1873, vol. vii, No. III, p. 109.

quency which had been supposed, and not due in all instances, as it appeared to have been in the cases previously related by Continental observers, to grave carelessness on the part of the vaccinator. It is, however, more satisfactory to know that no one could speak more strongly than Mr. Hutchinson did, in spite of these facts, of the importance of vaccination, and next, that the precautions which he suggests for the prevention of the evil are so simple, that nothing can be easier than their observance. He advises first, that the possibility of this disaster be always borne in mind by the vaccinator, next that he never vaccinate from a child whose parents are unknown to him, and as far as possible also not from first-born children, and lastly, that he invariably take care to use only the perfectly transparent lymph, and to avoid bloodstained lymph or any recent exudation from the walls of the vesicle.

The influence of vaccination in rendering attacks of small-pox which may succeed to it so much less severe and so much less dangerous than the unmodified disease, does not in many instances manifest itself in any diminution of the intensity of the primary fever. The symptoms with which modified small-pox sets in are often as severe as those of the unmodified disease, and are also in general of the same duration. So soon as the eruption begins to make its appearance, however, the difference between the two diseases usually becomes apparent. In many instances, notwithstanding the sharp onset of the patient's illness, the eruption is exceedingly scanty, not more than from twenty to a hundred pustules appearing over the whole body. In other instances, the eruption is much more abundant, and in a few exceptional cases the pustules are actually confluent. But even when they are most numerous, the pustules seldom fail to follow a different course from that which they pursue in ordinary variola, and run through their different stages within little more than half the period required by the eruption of unmodified small-pox. The small size of the pocks, the frequent absence of the central depression, their imperfect suppuration, and their speedy desiccation, are the chief local characters of this affection; while the almost complete absence of the secondary fever, is both its grand constitutional peculiarity and the main source of the patient's safety.

Besides the modified small-pox to which reference has just been made, there is another and still milder affection often observed in children, to which, from the extreme lightness of the symptoms that usually attend it, the diminutive appellation of *varicella* or *chicken-pox* has been given. Much difference of opinion has existed with reference to the relations borne by this disease to small-pox; and even at the present day writers are not quite agreed whether to regard it as an extremely mild form of variola, or as an affection altogether distinct from it. The weight of evidence, however, is decidedly in favor of the opinion that varicella is an affection distinct from, and wholly independent of, small-pox, not being produced by any modification of the poison of that disorder, nor affording any kind of protection from its attacks.

Varicella is almost exclusively a disease of childhood, and in the great majority of cases it occurs prior to the completion of the first dentition. Its initiatory fever, which is scarcely ever severe, is sometimes altogether wanting, so that the appearance of the eruption on the surface is the first occurrence that calls attention to the child's condition. Now and then, however, exceptions occur to this mildness in the onset of the disease; and I have occasionally seen children (chiefly those in whom the process of dentition was going on with activity at the time of the attack) suffer for twenty-four or thirty-six hours from febrile symptoms quite as severe as those which precede the outbreak of measles, or as accompany a sharp attack of influenza. The duration of this premonitory stage of chicken-pox is somewhat uncertain; the vesicles which characterize it making their appearance after twenty-four hours in some cases, not for thirty-six or forty-eight hours in others; while, as already mentioned, the eruption is occasionally the first symptom of the existence of the disease.

The eruption usually consists of more or less numerous minute, circular vesicles, containing a transparent serum, irregularly distributed over the face, head, shoulders, and trunk, but rarely appearing on the lower extremities; and, even when present in considerable abundance, being very seldom confluent at any part. These vesicles differ essentially from those of small-pox in the absence of the central depression and of the multilocular structure which characterize the varioloid pustules. The former, composed of a single cell, collapse at once if punctured, but no such effect follows puncture of the small-pox pustule. For two or three days the vesicles of chicken-pox increase somewhat in size, but their contents then become turbid and milky; about the fourth or fifth day they shrivel, and then dry up into a light pulverulent scab, which falls off on the eighth or ninth day of the disease. It very seldom happens that any cicatrix is left after the detachment of the scab of varicella, unless the skin has been irritated by the patient scratching it in order to relieve the itching, which is sometimes very troublesome. Besides these differences between the eruption of chicken-pox and that of variola, another, and still more striking peculiarity of the former disease consists in the appearance of two or three successive crops of vesicles, so that after the third day of the affection vesicles may be observed close to each other in all stages of their progress.

The disease is one so void of danger, that it requires hardly any treatment beyond the adoption of a mild antiphlogistic regimen; and no complications occur during its course, nor sequelæ remain after its disappearance, concerning which anything more need be added.

LECTURE XLIV.

Measles once confounded with scarlatina, though essentially different diseases.—Share of contagion in producing it—Symptoms of measles—Its dangers depend chiefly on its complications—With convulsions, with inflammation of the lungs, which occurs at different stages of the disease—Sequelæ of measles—Treatment.

Scarlatina.—Great differences in its severity in different cases—Its three varieties—Scarlatina simplex—Scarlatina anginosa—Sources of danger in it—Its disposition to assume characters of scarlatina maligna—Occasional rapid course of that variety—Modes in which it proves fatal—Complications and sequelæ of the disease—Diagnosis—Treatment, use of inunction—Treatment of complications.—Prophylaxis, use of belladonna.

When the short-lived prejudices which at first were entertained against vaccination had been removed, men passed, as they not seldom do, to the opposite extreme, and overestimated the worth of that discovery which they had before undervalued. Physicians rejoiced in it, as a means of getting rid forever of a disease which might well be counted among the opprobria of their art—philanthropists exulted in the probable extermination of one of the most terrible scourges of the human race, and statisticians counted the increase brought to the population, and drew up elaborate tables to illustrate their bright anticipations of the future.[1] In these oversanguine calculations, however, they almost entirely lost sight of the fact, that not all who were preserved from small-pox would be added to the useful population of the country, but that the life of many would be prolonged only for a short season, to be cut off soon by some other disease, against which neither science nor fortunate accident has hitherto discovered a talisman. Experience has proved the truth of what calm reflection might have suggested, and with the diminution in the frequency of small-pox there has been an increase, though not to an equal extent, in the prevalence of *measles* and *scarlatina*.

It is not easy to state with exactness the amount of mortality which these two diseases occasion, for though they are never altogether absent from a large city like London, yet their frequency and their fatality vary much in different years. At one time they occur sporadically, and are then in most instances mild in their character and readily amenable to treatment; while at another time they prevail as epidemics, and are attended with alarming symptoms which it is often not in the power of medicine to control. Dr. Gregory, who, in his work on the Eruptive Fevers has collected together with much labor the statistics of these diseases, presents us with a table, from which it appears that, on an average of five years, very nearly six per cent. of the mortality of London is due to measles and scarlatina. This number, indeed, is not

[1] As an instance of which may be mentioned the work of Duvillard, De l'Influence de la Petite-Vérole sur la Mortalité, 4to., Paris, 1806.

so great as at once to impress us with the formidable [illegible] two affections; but it should not be forgotten, that [illegible] Fifth Report of the Registrar-General) 81 per cent. of [illegible] occurs in children under five; and 97 per cent. in children [illegible] years old; while no figures can accurately represent the [illegible] which death is occasioned by their complications or their [illegible]

These two diseases present many points of resemblance [illegible] indeed, that they were long supposed to be but variations [illegible] malady; and the essential differences between them were [illegible] till within the last eighty years. It is, however, [illegible] important to distinguish between them,—for not only [illegible] attended by the same degree of danger, but this danger [illegible] dissimilar causes, the treatment which they require is [illegible] different. We shall presently examine into some of those [illegible] in their symptoms on which we chiefly rely in forming [illegible] between the two affections; but I may even now state [illegible] broad distinctions between them.

Measles is still more eminently than scarlet fever a disease of childhood,—for of 1293 deaths which it occasioned in London [illegible] 93.8 per cent. occurred in children under five years old, [illegible] cent. in those under the age of ten; while of 1224 deaths [illegible] tina, 31 per cent. occurred after five, and 10 per cent. [illegible] of age. Though there are great fluctuation both in its [illegible] in the mortality which it occasions, yet its variations in [illegible] are less considerable than those of scarlet fever; while the [illegible] persons who pass through life without having experienced [illegible] is smaller than of those who die without ever having [illegible] with scarlatina. But though this is the case, and though [illegible] the disease to occur in many instances where we are unable [illegible] the influence of contagion, there yet seems good reason [illegible] that in every case it has been communicated through some [illegible] other. Facts such as the absence of the disease for the period [illegible] years from the Cape of Good Hope,[1] and its development [illegible] arrival there of a vessel from Europe, in which several [illegible] curred during the voyage, substantiate the correctness of [illegible] The strongest proof of it, however, is afforded by the circum[illegible] which measles prevailed in the Feroe Islands in 1846,[2] after [illegible] val of sixty-five years. They were then introduced into [illegible] islands by a workman, who leaving Copenhagen on [illegible] reached the Feroe Islands on the 28th, apparently in [illegible] but fell ill with measles on April 1st. His two most intimate [illegible] were next attacked; and from that time the disease could be [illegible] hamlet to hamlet, and from island to island, until 6000 [illegible] population of 7782 had been attacked by it; age bringing [illegible] immunity from the contagion, though the disease was [illegible] all who in their childhood had suffered from it at the time [illegible]

[1] Mentioned by Dr. Copland, in his Dictionary, art. "Measles [illegible]

[2] Of which an account, by the commissioner from the Danish [illegible] Pannum, is given in the Archives Gén. de Méd., April, [illegible]

vious epidemic. It is probable, then, that the extreme contagiousness of measles is the reason of its greater prevalence, and that it is so peculiarly a disease of early life not so much on account of any special susceptibility to it then, as because the subtle *materies morbi* is so widely diffused as to leave little chance of any escaping it.

Though a more universally prevalent disease, however, than scarlatina, it is fortunately less dangerous, its mortality not exceeding 3 per cent. of the patients attacked by it, while the average rate of mortality from scarlet fever is estimated as at least double that amount. When measles proves fatal, too, it is very seldom the fever itself which occasions the patient's death, but generally its complication with inflammatory disease of the respiratory organs. Scarlet fever, on the contrary, destroys its victims in all stages of the disease; and in many of the worst cases, in which death takes place early, no organic change is left behind which the scrutiny of the anatomist can discover.

Within a period of thirteen or fourteen days (according to the observations made on this subject in the Feroe Islands) from the reception of the contagion, the eruption of measles makes its appearance. But though this period is tolerably constant, the duration of the premonitory *symptoms* is very variable; the fourth day being that on which the rash most frequently appears, but the extremes varying as widely as twenty-four hours, and thirteen days, according to the careful observations of M. Rilliet. In the premonitory symptoms themselves, there is little besides their greater severity to distinguish them from ordinary catarrh. A child, previously in perfect health, becomes suddenly restless, thirsty and feverish, and, if able to talk, generally complains of headache. The eyes grow red, weak, and watery, and are unable to bear the light; the child sneezes very frequently, sometimes almost every five minutes, and is troubled by a constant short dry cough. Usually, on or about the fourth day from the commencement of these symptoms, a rash makes its appearance on the face, whence it extends in the course of about forty-eight hours to the rest of the body and the extremities, travelling in a direction from above downwards. The rash is made up of a number of minute deep-red, circular stigmata not unlike flea-bites, slightly elevated, especially on the face, and though close together, yet usually distinct from each other, the skin in the interspaces between them retaining its natural color. On the cheeks, the spots sometimes become confluent, and then form irregular blotches about a third of an inch long by half that breadth, while the spots elsewhere often present an indistinctly crescentic arrangement. The eruption fades in the same order as that in which it appeared, and after the lapse of forty-eight hours from its appearance, at which time it is at its height on the trunk, it is beginning to disappear from the face. On the seventh day of the disease the rash grows faint on the body generally, and on the eighth, or at latest the ninth day, it has entirely vanished, leaving behind either a little general redness of the surface, or a few yellowish-red spots, corresponding to some of the situations which the eruption itself had ed. In some cases a partial desquamation of the cuticle takes place after the rash has disappeared; but this is by no [illegible] while, when it occurs, the epidermis separates in [illegible] never in large portions, as it often does after [illegible]

Unlike small-pox, in which the appearance of the [illegible] diately followed by the subsidence of all the previous [illegible] constitutional disturbance of measles is often not at all [illegible] the outbreak of the rash. The reverse, indeed, is [illegible] and in many instances, for twenty-four or forty-eight hours [illegible] the fever is aggravated, and the cough more troublesome [illegible] while the voice often becomes hoarser, and the throat [illegible] in consequence of the inflammation of the palate and [illegible] may be seen to be the seat of a punctated redness, resembling [illegible] duced by the eruption on the skin.

The aggravation of the symptoms, however, when [illegible] only temporary; and on the sixth day of the disease, [illegible] amelioration in the patient's condition becomes apparent, [illegible] diminishing, the cough growing looser and less frequent, [illegible] sounds becoming audible in the lungs, where previously [illegible] heard but rhonchus or sibilus. This amelioration goes on [illegible] day to day, and in ten days or a fortnight from the first [illegible] illness, convalescence is, in favorable cases, fully established.

Such as I have described, and sometimes even less [illegible] symptoms of uncomplicated measles; a disease attended by [illegible] rather than danger, and requiring judicious nursing more than [illegible] medical interference. But to this favorable course of the [illegible] are numerous exceptions, and these are more frequent in [illegible] demics than in others. Occasionally, though very rarely, [illegible] break of the eruption is preceded by convulsions, which [illegible] before the rash becomes visible, and are not succeeded by any [illegible] ing symptom of cerebral disorder. Only one instance of this [illegible] has come under my notice; and that was in a child aged two [illegible] ten months, in whom also an attack of chicken-pox a year [illegible] been ushered in by convulsions. The fits in this case [illegible] own accord, though the rash of measles did not come out [illegible] four hours afterwards. There are, however, a few instances [illegible] of the supervention of convulsions after the eruption has [illegible] and of their succeeding each other rapidly till the patient's [illegible] others in which the sudden disappearance of the rash has [illegible] ceeded by violent convulsions.

Dangerous complications of measles, however, but seldom [illegible] themselves on the side of the nervous system, but generally [illegible] form of disorders of the respiratory organs. The cough, [illegible] ness, and suppressed voice which accompany the onset of [illegible] sometimes so marked as to raise the apprehension that croup [illegible] to come on; and now and then this actually occurs, though [illegible] great majority of instances the symptoms apparently so [illegible] subside readily under small doses of antimonial and anodyne [illegible] cines. The risk, indeed, either of real cynanche trachealis [illegible] or of that form of ulcerative laryngitis to which I referred [illegible] ago[1] attacking the patient, is much greater when the eruption is on the decline, or even at a later period, constituting a sequela of the disease more often than an actual complication.

The most serious as well as the most frequent complication of measles is that with bronchitis or pneumonia. This is not equally frequent at all periods of the disease, being much commoner about the third or fourth day of the eruption than at an earlier time; while on the decline of the disease it is likewise that sequela against which we have to watch with the most sedulous care. When pulmonary inflammation comes on early in the disease, the retrocession of the eruption from exposure to cold is its most frequent cause, though sometimes it seems to occur causelessly, its symptoms developing themselves simultaneously with the outbreak of the rash. In that case, however, the rash almost invariably fades earlier than it should do, and disappears in thirty-six or forty-eight hours; no desquamation succeeding to it, nor any roughness of the skin remaining behind; while the pulmonary affection runs its course rapidly to a fatal issue.

In other instances the rash comes out imperfectly, and presents from the first a dark, livid hue, almost like that of the rash in some cases of malignant scarlet fever; while coupled with this there are great oppression and extreme dyspnœa; and subcrepitant râle, more or less abundant, is perceptible in the chest. Cases of this congestive form of measles are, I believe, less common now than they were some forty years ago, when the fevers which our fathers treated seemed to require free venesection, and actually benefited by its employment. I will therefore relate to you a well-marked instance of it, both to point out its general characters, and also to impress upon you the necessity for occasionally adopting a much more active mode of treatment than is applicable to the great majority of the cases of measles which at present come under our notice.

A little girl, ten years of age, had had slight catarrhal symptoms for a few days, when she was attacked, on the evening of June 7th, 1843, by shivering, pain in the head, and a feeling of sickness. Her head pained her much, and she was very drowsy on the two following days, and on the 10th she came under my notice, when, though no eruption had appeared on the surface, yet the child's history, coupled with the severity of her catarrhal and febrile symptoms, left little room for doubting that she was about to have an attack of measles. On the evening of the 11th of June the rash appeared, and twenty-four hours afterwards I visited the child at her mother's request, who told me that though the rash was fully out, yet the respiration was greatly oppressed. The child was lying in bed, her face puffy, covered by an abundant purple-red rash, of an almost livid hue. The rash was in patches of an irregular form and size, running into each other; while a few small, slightly elevated, dark-purple stigmata were scattered here and there, and a few also were collected together into a crescentic arrangement. On the arms and legs the rash had not the patchy appearance, but an immense number of distinct stigmata, very like petechiæ, except that they

[1] See Lecture XXV, p. 366.

were a little larger, and slightly raised, covered
were much swollen, and glued together by a thick
the lips were dry, the teeth covered with sordes,
dry, and glazed in the centre, with a thin coating
edges; and the nares were perfectly dry. The pulse
respiration sixty in the minute, hurried, loud, and
by very frequent hard and short cough. The child was
but sensible when roused, and she then complained of
and of great soreness of all her limbs.

Air did not enter the lungs freely, and on a deep
crepitant râle was heard in both infrascapular regions
the right. The child was at once bled to ℥vj, which
cause faintness, and was ordered ¼ gr. of tartar emetic

The good effect of these measures was not immediately
in the course of some six hours the child felt relief.
lowing morning I saw her, and found that the rash had
lost its patchy character, and was now universal over
while it was of a bright red color, almost as vivid as
fever. The tongue was no longer glazed and dry,
covered with sordes, while the respiration, though still
minute, was neither so hurried nor so oppressed as on the
and the cough had lost much of its hardness. The
toms, however, were not much altered. The antimonial
ment was continued, but as on the following day the cough
and the subcrepitant râle more abundant, ℥iv of blood
cupping from between the scapulæ, and from this period
ble symptom manifested itself.

This case, however, and cases similar to it, may be
ceptional. In most instances, either the slight cough
panied the early stage of measles increases in severity with
of the disease, and the signs of thoracic mischief creep on
till they assume an alarming character about the fifth or
or in other cases the symptoms of affection of the chest do
fest themselves at all till the eruption is already declining,
that the chest complication is generally serious in proportion
on early and sets in severely; though still more hazardous
lapses which sometimes succeed to improvement, even after
sisted for three or four days, and which are peculiarly
and issue with great rapidity in extensive hepatization of
The symptoms to which inflammation of the lungs at the
measles gives rise are sometimes very slight, so slight that
short of careful daily auscultation will in many instances
tect it. Two circumstances which are especially calculated
are the fact that the pneumonia is often unattended by
dyspnœa, while it is frequently associated with considerable
disturbance of the stomach and bowels. The course of the
the lungs in these cases is usually chronic; the child loses
the subject of an irregular hectic fever, and when at length
symptoms become more apparent than at first they had been,
the cough grows more frequent, and is attended by some

the case so closely resembles one of acute tubercular phthisis that it is extremely difficult to avoid an erroneous diagnosis.

That extreme susceptibility of the mucous membranes, to which are due the persistence of the cough, the supervention of bronchitis, or the occurrence of ulcerative inflammation of the fauces and larynx on the decline of the rubeoloid eruption, very frequently extends to the intestinal canal and gives rise to diarrhœa. The character of the attack corresponds in general to those which some days ago I described under the name of catarrhal diarrhœa, and in the greater number of instances its symptoms yield readily to treatment. Among the poor, however, who, in accordance with the notions of humoral pathology current among the vulgar, generally regard looseness of the bowels after fever as a salutary provision of nature, I have not infrequently met with cases of neglected diarrhœa, in which the symptoms have put on a dysenteric character, and have either seriously threatened life, or in some instances have actually destroyed it. Sometimes, too, the acute stage of diarrhœa is succeeded by an habitual chronic relaxation of the bowels, not only serious in itself, but still more so from its persistence, not infrequently issuing in the development of phthisical disease.

This last hazard is one which, though perhaps overrated by the older observers, who had not the means which we now possess of forming a correct diagnosis, is yet a very real one, and one too against which it behooves us to be on our guard, not simply during the decline of the eruption, but also throughout the whole period of convalescence. Phthisis coming on early in the disease often runs an acute course, developing itself apparently out of the fever itself, and being often difficultly distinguished from the inflammatory affection of the lungs, of which I have already spoken. When it comes on later its course is more chronic, its symptoms are more easily recognizable as those of ordinary phthisis, and the child's history is that of an incomplete recovery from measles having been succeeded by progressive failure in health, and by the gradual appearance of consumption, which proves fatal in some months, or a year, or even not till after a longer period from the occurrence of the fever.

The danger of measles, you must have already seen, depends almost exclusively on its complications, and as in their absence there is little to excite alarm, so also there is little to call for *treatment*. In mild cases, indeed, scarcely anything is needed beyond confinement to a warm chamber, a spare diet, and gentle antiphlogistic remedies. The cough, which is the most troublesome symptom—frequently, indeed, the only one that calls for much attention—is often very much relieved by the application for three or four hours of a small blister, no bigger than a shilling, to the trachea, at the point just above the sterum; and this slight counter-irritation, which seldom produces any vesication of the surface, may be repeated during the course of the affection. If more than this is needed, small doses of antimonial and ipecacuanha wine, with laudanum or the compound tincture of camphor, may be given every few hours. The imperfect desquamation that sometimes takes place as the eruption declines, is often attended with very distressing itching of the whole surface; while the cough is sometimes frequent and troublesome at night, and the child is thus ... ing. To relieve these troublesome symptoms, as well ... tendency to diarrhœa which often comes on at the ... it is desirable to follow the plan pursued by Sydenham ... opiate every night,—a small dose of Dover's powder ... form in which it can be administered, while the warm ... ing both soothes the patient and expedites the completion ... quamative process.

But though these simple measures are amply sufficient ... majority of cases, we yet must not allow ourselves to be ... inertness when any indications of mischief in the chest ... appearance. Such symptoms sometimes come on early ... and before the eruption has well appeared, the child ... pressed, and experiencing considerable dyspnœa, although ... tatory evidences of disease in the chest may be but small ... dyspnœa is often relieved by the application of a mustard ... the chest, and by placing the child in a hot bath,—a proceeding ... will very frequently be followed by the appearance of the ... dantly over the whole surface. Should these measures ... to produce relief, or should the symptoms from the first ... the distress and dyspnœa very considerable, and the ... scanty, but of a dark or livid hue wherever it has appeared ... case I just now related to you, the abstraction of blood ... required; and general depletion should, in such circumstances ... ployed in preference to merely local bleeding. If bronchitis ... monia should come on at a later period of the disease, when ... has already fully appeared, or is beginning to decline, the ... bleeding, as well as of the mode in which the depletion should ... ticed, must be determined entirely by the severity of the ... toms, and is little if at all modified by any considerations ... the circumstance of their supervening during the course ... disease. The unfavorable conditions under which infants ... in the Hôpital des Enfans at Paris, have induced, on the part ... physicians, a dread of depletion in the course of measles ... tainly not justified by the characters that the disease ... country. A repetition of depletion is, however, not generally ... necessary or useful, especially if the first abstraction of blood ... up, as it ought to be, by the free employment of tartar ... dyspnœa, which is frequently exacerbated towards evening ... course of the pneumonia and bronchitis that accompany ... generally much relieved by mustard poultices; but the ... blisters in these circumstances is hazardous, since the sores ... produce are often very intractable; and the irritation and ... occasion prove, in many instances, seriously prejudicial to the ... It is important, too, to bear in mind that little reliance can ... on mercurial remedies in the treatment of active rubeolous ... though small doses of the Hydr. c. Cretâ with Dover's ... often exceedingly useful in cases where a hepatized state of ... left behind after the subsidence of the fever, and of the ... flammatory symptoms. I spoke so fully some time ...

croup succeeding to measles, that it cannot be necessary to repeat the remarks which were then made; neither need I add anything to what I said on a former occasion about cancrum oris—which distressing affection occasionally supervenes on its decline, as also does otorrhœa, though with far less frequency than after scarlatina. The period of convalescence, too, and the ailments which I have referred to as sometimes coming on at that time, require no special notice now. I have described the dangers; the general principles of medical treatment must guide your endeavors either to avert or to remove them.

I will now, in conclusion, briefly sketch the most striking features of *scarlet fever*. Like measles, it is a disease chiefly occurring in early childhood, and the highest mortality from it takes place during the third year of life.[1] It differs, however, from measles, as I have already stated, in not being so generally prevalent at all times, but usually assuming an epidemic form for a season, and then for months disappearing altogether. Its characters also are more variable than those of measles, and one epidemic is often marked by certain distinguishing features quite dissimilar from those which characterized a previous, or which may be observed in a succeeding epidemic. Even when it occurs in a sporadic form its characters are very variable. It presents itself in one case as an ailment so trifling as scarcely to interrupt a child's cheerfulness even for a day; in another it is so deadly that medicine is unable to stay its course even for a moment, and that it destroys life in a few days, sometimes even in a few hours.

These remarkable variations in the character and severity of the affection, and in the symptoms which attend it, have given rise to its subdivision into the three varieties of scarlatina simplex, scarlatina anginosa, and scarlatina maligna. In the first of these the patient experiences an attack of fever, often very mild, always of very short duration, and accompanied by the appearance of a bright scarlet rash over the whole surface, and generally by a slight degree of sore throat. In the second the fever is more intense and subsides less speedily, while, as its name implies, the attendant sore throat is very severe; and in the third the fever generally assumes a typhoid character, sloughing of the inflamed tonsils not infrequently occurs, and a variety of complications in many instances supervene, by which the danger is still further aggravated.

The symptoms of scarlatina usually set in within three days after exposure to its contagion: often indeed the incubation period of the disease is much shorter, sometimes even less than twenty-four hours; while, according to Dr. Murchison's experience, the extreme period does not exceed six days. The law, however, which governs the time of its latency is liable to far greater fluctuations than occur in the case of either small-pox or measles. The symptoms with which the mildest form of the disease, or the *scarlatina simplex*, sets in, vary very much in degree, and sometimes are so slight that the appearance of the rash upon the surface, usually with, but sometimes even without

---

[1] See Table by Dr. Tripe, in Med.-Chir. Review, Jan. 1854, p. 288, whose conclusions are in the main identical with those to which Dr. Murchison's independent researches have led him. See his Lectures in the Lancet for June 18, 1864.

slight sore throat and feverishness, may be the first
existence of an affection which sometimes is so
jority of cases, however, it is ushered in by vomiting
accompanied by headache, heaviness of head, great
some measure of sore throat. The amount of cerebral
the onset of the attack usually furnishes some measure
subsequent severity of its course, though in children who
most part is readily disturbed, delirium sometimes
first twenty-four hours of an attack of scarlatina, but
and the fever runs its subsequent course quite mildly.
row, often indeed within twenty-four hours from the
of the patient's illness, the rash of scarlatina makes its
usually shows itself first on the neck, breast, and
extends, in the course of twenty-four hours, to the trunk
ties. Its color is a very bright red, due in part to a
the skin, in part to the presence of innumerable red
which look like minute red papillæ, though often they
no sense of roughness to the hand. To this, however,
sional exceptions: the rash on the chest and body
times, when at its height, a slightly papular character
then minute sudamina are intermingled with the eruption
instances the redness of the surface is universal, but in others
rash appears in patches of uncertain size and irregular
never affect any definite shape, and never present a
scribed margin. For three days the rash usually continues
of a deeper color, and more generally diffused over the
it then slowly declines, but does not wholly disappear until
or sometimes the eighth day of the disease. The appearance
eruption is not in general succeeded by any immediate
the other symptoms; but on the contrary, they often
verity until the eruption has reached its acme, when
decline with the disappearance of the rash. Sometimes
the case is very mild, the fever abates so soon as the rash
and the child regaining its cheerfulness on the third day
further signs of illness, though the rash remains visible
days longer. Now and then, too, as I have mentioned
young infants, the affection throughout consists of little
eruption on the skin, the presence of which is almost
altogether, the only evidence of their having been attacked
ease. Such, however, are exceptional cases; and in
even when the disease is mild, a slight degree of soreness
comes on on the second or third day; the palate and
red, the latter are generally somewhat swollen, and
slightly impeded. The tongue also is preternaturally
papillæ, which are very prominent, project through the
lowish fur which coats it, and thus form an appearance as
istic of scarlatina as the rash itself. The redness fades from
and the fur disappears from the tongue, as the eruption
the prominence of the papillæ often continues for some
and the tongue presents a vivid red color, and appears

the absence of its ordinary mucous coating. As the rash subsides, desquamation of the epidermis generally commences, the cuticle peeling off from the hands and feet in large flakes, though on the face and trunk the desquamation usually takes place in furfuraceous scales. Both its degree and duration vary much in different cases; sometimes it is over in five or six days, while in other cases the cuticle is reproduced, and then desquamates several times in succession, and the process is thus protracted for three or four weeks, or even longer. It is not possible to assign a cause for these differences. Some epidemics of scarlatina are characterized by the abundance of the desquamation, and its almost universal occurrence, while at other times it is scanty, and often wanting.

The danger of this disease is by no means in proportion to the abundance of the rash, but rather to the degree of the affection of the throat, the severity of which is the distinguishing feature of *scarlatina anginosa*. In this form of the affection the premonitory symptoms are usually much more severe than in the scarlatina simplex: they are also often of longer duration, the rash not showing itself until the end of the second, and sometimes even not until the third day. It is, moreover, less generally diffused over the surface than in the milder variety of the disease, but appears in the form of large scarlet patches irregularly distributed over different parts of the body, especially on the back. In some cases, too, of this variety of scarlet fever, though I think more commonly in the adult than in the child, the rash is altogether wanting, fever and sore throat alone characterizing the disease. In such cases its real nature is sometimes not suspected until other members of the same family are seized with similar symptoms, coupled with a well-marked scarlatinal rash; or, until perhaps the occurrence of dropsy during convalescence awakens suspicion as to the nature of the previous illness. Almost from the commencement of the attack, soreness of the throat is experienced, attended with difficulty of deglutition, and often with considerable stiffness of the neck, and pain and difficulty in moving the lower jaw, due in part to the swelling of the submaxillary glands. On examining the throat, it is seen to be intensely red, and the tonsils are both red and swollen. The swelling of the tonsils increases rapidly, until they almost block up the entrance to the pharynx, and thereby render the attempt to swallow so difficult that fluids are often returned by the nose. An adhesive mucus collects about the back of the throat, and often seems to cause great annoyance to the patient, and specks or patches of lymph form upon the tonsils, and look like sloughs covering ulcers, though, on detaching them, it is seldom that any breach of surface appears beneath. In some of the severest cases, a very troublesome coryza comes on, and an adhesive, yellowish matter is secreted in abundance by the mucous membrane of the nares, whence it runs down upon the upper lip, excoriating the skin over which it passes, and causing still more serious suffering by the obstacle that it presents to free respiration. In some epidemics the inflammation extends to the parotid glands, and to the cellular tissue about the neck, the parts thus affected becoming rapidly swollen, and acquiring a great size and a stony hardness. In some cases this affection is confined to one side; in others, both sides [illegible] cession, while sometimes both are involved [illegible] uments under the chin and in front of the [illegible] flamed and tense and swollen; and the lower [illegible] that the attempt to swallow is rendered almost [illegible] the patient is exposed to a new source of danger, [illegible] taking nutriment in quantity sufficient to [illegible] life. Coupled with this severe local affection, [illegible] expected, a corresponding intensity of the constitu[illegible] The heat of the skin is very great, the pulse extreme[illegible] though not small, it is yet from an early period very [illegible] the sensorial disturbance is considerable, and the [illegible] The tongue does not present that appearance which [illegible] being characteristic of scarlatina in its milder form, [illegible] brown fur, though red at its tip and edges, and often [illegible] a very early period of the disease—partly, no doubt, [illegible] the swelling of the tonsils and of the glands compelling [illegible] breathe with his mouth open.

In cases where the throat affection is very severe, [illegible] arising from the difficult entrance of air into the lungs [illegible] times to be the chief cause of the patient's death; [illegible] rarely, even when the pharyngitis is most intense, [illegible] presents any signs of having been seriously involved in [illegible] In the greater number of instances, however, that [illegible] the local symptoms do not seem to be by any means [illegible] death, but the fever assumes more and more of a typh[illegible] and this even though the throat affection should not [illegible] ity, but should even retrograde. On the other hand, [illegible] scarlatina anginosa generally have a favorable issue [illegible] the severe sore throat the constitutional disorder retains [illegible] of active inflammatory fever, and begins to subside in [illegible] days at the latest; abating as the local symptoms themsel[illegible] which they generally do about this time. The sore throat, [illegible] it comes on early, increases rapidly, and soon attains a [illegible] is yet not accompanied in the majority of instances by [illegible] of the submaxillary glands, which do not assume that [illegible] nor do the surrounding integuments acquire that swelling [illegible] which are observed in less favorable cases. Between the [illegible] of scarlatina anginosa, and that still more dangerous var[illegible] disease to which the name of *malignant* has been applied, [illegible] ences are often rather of degree than of kind. In malig[illegible] fever, however, the sore throat, though a general is by no [illegible] stant symptom; death takes place in some instances before [illegible] ifested itself with much severity, whilst in many other cases [illegible] one of several symptoms which threaten the patient's life. [illegible]

Cases of scarlatina anginosa, even when running the [illegible] course, occupy some days before the dangerous character of [illegible] becomes fully developed. The malignant form, however, [illegible] ill-omened symptoms, and these sometimes are so intense as [illegible] the patient in less than forty-eight hours. One such case [illegible] in which, after exposure to the contagion of scarlatina, convulsions succeeded by coma destroyed in a single day a previously healthy boy of two years of age. In other instances, the onset of the disease announces itself by sudden and intense collapse, from which the patient rallies, but sinks under it in one or two days. Dr. Henry Kennedy, in his very excellent account of the epidemic of scarlatina which prevailed at Dublin between 1834 and 1842,[1] relates some instances of this occurrence far more striking in character than any which have come under my own notice. Among others, he narrates the case of a little girl, four years old, who was seized with the usual symptoms of the epidemic; in about eight hours she lost the power of swallowing, and this was followed by a state of coma, alternating with convulsions of one side of the body. When seen, there was no pulse to be felt at the wrist, the hands and feet were cold and perfectly livid, and the patient's condition was very like that of a person in the last stage of Asiatic cholera, except that her body was covered by a dark-colored eruption. Six hours before death, which took place before the end of the second day, diarrhœa made its appearance, and continued up to the moment of dissolution.[2]

Though no instance comparable with this in the suddenness and completeness of the collapse has presented itself to my observation, I have met with several in which it was apparent, almost from the moment of the seizure, that there was scarcely any chance of the child's recovery. The frequency of such cases varies much in different epidemics, as do also the characters of the symptoms by which the malignancy of the disease announces itself. In some instances, as in that just related, the complete collapse is not succeeded by any attempt at rallying the energies of the system; in others convulsions destroy the patient; in another class uncontrollable diarrhœa sets in almost at the commencement, and speedily exhausts the patient's powers; in others petechiæ and vibices appear on the surface, or hemorrhage takes place from the bowels,—the tokens and consequences of the changes in the circulating fluid; while in other instances typhoid symptoms come on on the second or third day; and death takes place long before the termination of the first week, with phenomena such as one would scarcely expect to meet with earlier than the second or third week of severe typhus fever. One or other of these types is that which in each epidemic of severe scarlet fever characterizes the majority of the worst cases, but isolated cases of the disease sometimes occur sporadically, marked by its worst features, or present themselves as exceptions to the generally mild character of some epidemic of the disease. Of this I saw a striking example some years ago in a large public school some miles from London, in which scarlet fever became prevalent. Almost all of the cases, which occurred among lads from fourteen to eighteen years of age, were extremely mild; but one youth more robust than most of the others, sank from the moment he was taken, and died with typhoid symptoms before the end of the third day. His case stood by itself, unlike any of those which preceded or which followed it.

---

[1] Dublin, 1848. 12mo.

[2] Op. cit., p. 62.

Sometimes, too, we meet with instances where [illegible] observed the same fact with diphtheria) appears to [illegible] fatal influence over the members of one family, [illegible] liar idiosyncrasy on their part tended to render [illegible] The two children of a person in a good position [illegible] forty-eight hours of the appearance of the first symptoms [illegible] Five years afterwards two other children were attacked [illegible] the family then residing in a different locality, in a [illegible] hood, and in a perfectly well-ventilated and well-drained [illegible] boy, aged four years, sickened on the 6th of September [illegible] scarlatina appeared on the 7th; fatal convulsions occurred [illegible] His sister, aged five years, vomited on the morning [illegible] vomiting continued at frequent intervals with some [illegible] rhœa. The skin on the trunk was burning hot, but the [illegible] ities was cold, the soft palate and tonsils were greatly [illegible] there was no rash on the surface twelve hours after the [illegible] sickened. In eighteen hours convulsions came on, and [illegible] within twenty-four hours from the first symptom of illness [illegible] remaining child, an infant at the breast, escaped the disease.

Even in the malignant form of scarlatina, however, it is [illegible] death takes place with this extreme rapidity; but the [illegible] commonly survives to the end of the sixth or seventh [illegible] these circumstances the affection of the throat generally [illegible] creasing in severity. The inflammation of the tonsils [illegible] terminates in the formation of excavated, ragged, unhealthy [illegible] tions, which I have occasionally found also in the pharynx [illegible] upper part of the œsophagus; or sometimes a more extensive [illegible] ing involves the parts at the back of the throat. The tongue [illegible] palate are found denuded of their epithelium; the papillæ [illegible] very prominent, and those at its base, as well as the lingual [illegible] that situation, extremely enlarged, and covered by a dirty [illegible] mucus. The coryza, to which reference was made just now [illegible] ally very severe, while the mischief at the back of the throat [illegible] times extends to the air-passages; and I have found the mucous [illegible] brane at the under surface of the epiglottis, and about the [illegible] cartilages, much injected and thickened; a condition which [illegible] was sufficient to occasion intense dyspnœa, and to give [illegible] attempt at deglutition, during the last twenty-four hours of [illegible] life, to a struggle for breath which threatened every [illegible] fatal. Now and then, too, diphtheritic deposit takes place [illegible] of the fauces, and extending into the larynx, destroys [illegible] producing the ordinary symptoms of croup. The swelling [illegible] parotids in some of these cases increases with very great [illegible] forms not unfrequently, by the implication of the integuments [illegible] neck, a sort of collar of brawny hardness, which interferes [illegible] deglutition and respiration. These swellings are remarkable [illegible] slight tendency which they show to suppurate; and even [illegible] have attained a very considerable size, and have been in [illegible] ure instrumental in occasioning the child's death, I have [illegible] parotids much enlarged, of a rose-red color, infiltrated [illegible] serum, and a dirty seropurulent fluid also pervading the cervical cellular tissue, but no true pus either in the substance of the gland itself, or in the surrounding cellular tissue. Now and then, however, suppuration takes place, not in the substance of the glands themselves, but in the surrounding cellular tissue; and the quantity of pus which is formed there is sometimes very considerable. The destruction of tissue, too, is not always the result of mere suppuration, but a process of sloughing sometimes destroys the cellular membrane very extensively; and, by involving the large vessels of the neck, has caused the child's sudden death from hemorrhage—an occurrence, indeed, which I have only twice met with, but which came thrice under the observation of Dr. H. Kennedy, of Dublin, whose excellent account of the epidemic which prevailed in that city will well repay your attentive perusal.

As in other blood diseases, so in scarlatina, we meet now and then with secondary inflammation of the joints, which may even go on to the formation of pus. It is, however, not a common occurrence; but I saw the hand thus affected in a child who died on the sixth day of the disease, and in another child who had recovery from scarlatina, in the course of which inflammation attacked the right shoulder-joint, the humerus remained permanently anchylosed. Several other instances have of late years come under my notice. The wrist and the back of the hands are the parts usually affected. The symptom is always a very ill-omened one, even though it should be but evanescent, and should disappear one day from the part affected the day before, for its reappearance at some other joint in general indicates but too plainly that the system at large is poisoned by the disease. It is not, however, necessarily a fatal sign, and I have met with other cases than the one just mentioned of recovery even after suppuration had occurred in the affected joint. Both the pericardium and endocardium are also sometimes affected, but in this stage of the disease that special tendency to inflammation of the serous membranes which is afterwards observed does not manifest itself. Pneumonia, indeed, is a more frequent affection, running its course without any marked symptom, though a large portion of one or both lungs may be found after death in a state of hepatization.

The other post-mortem appearances observed in scarlatina are to a great degree identical with those observed in malignant fevers generally. The blood is usually semi-coagulated, of the appearance and consistence of gooseberry jelly, or even altogether fluid, and the coats of the vessels are often stained by it. The mucous membrane of the bronchi, stomach, œsophagus, and trachea, is often of an intensely red color, though nothing can be more arbitrary than the extent, degree, and situation of this redness. The texture of the kidneys and heart is also often very much softer than natural, so as to tear very readily; and once I found the heart exceedingly flaccid, its tissue infiltrated with reddish serum; and not merely tearing easily, but even being so soft that the finger could be pushed through its walls with the slightest effort. As in the case of other fevers, and as is especially observable in puerperal fevers, the character of the epidemic constitution of the period often governs the symptoms, and modif[illegible] appearances. There was an epidemic of puerper[illegible] ago in Paris, in which symptoms of disorder[illegible] nated, and in which tumefaction of the mesenteric [illegible] tion of Peyer's patches, were constant morbid appear[illegible] in accordance with the same law that the characters [illegible] approach to those of typhoid fever, as in the cases [illegible] John Harley;[1] cases illustrating affinity between [illegible] no more; or perhaps rather the influence of a common [illegible] ing the characters of both.

Such are the chief modes of death from scarlet fever [illegible] more important appearances discovered afterwards; [illegible] my personal observation extends, though I scarcely [illegible] that there are but few diseases of which the character [illegible] greater variations; so that no account, how minute soever [illegible] as a true portraiture of more than just that one form of [illegible] which its describer may chance to be most familiar.

Unhappily the first few days of the disease do not [illegible] comprise the whole period of danger, but even though [illegible] should survive the peril of the fever, a long catalogue [illegible] mains, some of which may endanger or even destroy life. [illegible] indeed, the patient passes through the first week of the disease [illegible] or no symptoms to excite anxiety, and then when the [illegible] decline, the parotid glands swell, grow hard and intensely [illegible] on one or two occasions I have seen the integuments [illegible] become gangrenous; or sloughing ulcers form on the [illegible] had not seemed to be very much inflamed previously, [illegible] discharge takes place from the nostrils, and death follows [illegible] of four or five days. In the majority of instances, however, [illegible] ular swellings which come on after the lapse of a week [illegible] mencement of the disease, though tedious and painful, [illegible] danger life. Occasionally, indeed, death occurs in consequence [illegible] matter formed by the inflammation of the glands, or of [illegible] tissue around them, burrowing backwards behind the pharynx [illegible] of pointing externally, and constituting retropharyngeal [illegible] affection concerning which I spoke to you a few days ago.[2]

Coupled with the swelling of the parotid glands, or [illegible] ently of it, inflammation of the internal ear is often met with [illegible] sequence of scarlatina. This otitis terminates in abundant [illegible] discharge, which sometimes continues for many weeks; [illegible] ally it completely destroys the organ of hearing, and [illegible] tient hopelessly deaf for the remainder of his life.

I have already spoken, in a previous lecture,[3] of that [illegible] and very serious occurrence, the dropsy which succeeds to [illegible] and need not, therefore, refer to that subject now. But there [illegible] cases in which, without any definite local complication, [illegible]

[1] Med.-Chir. Transactions, vol. lv, p. 102.
[2] See Lecture XXXIII, p. 462. [3] See Lecture XXX[illegible]

cence from scarlet fever is fluctuating and protracted. In such cases the bowels are irregular in their action, alternately relaxed and constipated; the evacuations unhealthy; the tongue red and raw; and aphthous ulcerations sometimes appear on the inside of the mouth; while an irregularly remittent fever harasses and weakens the child. These symptoms, however, which closely resemble those that sometimes come on during convalescence from measles, are of much less frequent occurrence as consequences of scarlatina.

The *diagnosis* of scarlatina is not in general attended with much difficulty; and the points of difference between it and measles are so well marked, that it is not easy to understand how the two diseases should so long have been confounded together. Their period of incubation is different; that of scarlatina not exceeding a week, that of measles extending to two. Their premonitory symptoms are very dissimilar, those of measles closely resembling the signs of a severe catarrh; while the attack of scarlatina is announced by sickness, succeeded by intense heat of skin, by sore throat, great sensorial disturbance, and extreme rapidity of the pulse. There is no other disease of childhood, indeed, in which the two last-named symptoms supervene so speedily after the commencement of illness; and their occurrence will often enable you, even before the appearance of the rash or any complaint of sore throat, to form a correct conclusion with reference to the nature of the affection. The premonitory stage of measles usually continues for three or four days; that of scarlet fever, in its regular form, only for twenty-four hours; while the other symptoms that appear in cases of scarlet fever, in which the rash is delayed, are such as quite to forbid the supposition of the patient being affected with measles. The character of the two eruptions is so dissimilar, that I need not here dwell on their peculiarities, nor do more than remind you that while in measles the great danger to life arises from the supervention of bronchitis or pneumonia, the two great sources of hazard in scarlet fever are the affection of the throat during its progress and the occurrence of dropsy after its decline.

With a few words on the *treatment* of scarlatina, I will bring this subject and the present course of lectures to a close. The milder forms of the disease require, as you know, but little interference; and you fulfil every indication by keeping the child in a cool and well-ventilated chamber, placing him on a spare diet, giving some mild antiphlogistic medicine during the progress of the fever, and sponging the surface occasionally with tepid water if the heat of the skin is considerable.

For the past several years, however, I have been accustomed to substitute for tepid sponging the inunction of suet into the whole surface twice a day; and my experience leads me very strongly to recommend the adoption of this practice. I was led to try it by the strong encomiums which the late Professor Mauthner, of Vienna, bestowed upon the use of inunctions in these cases, as originally advocated by Dr. Schneeman, of Hanover.[1] It seems to relieve the sense of burning

---

[1] In a work published at Hanover, in 1848, and of which an analysis is given in the Journal für Kinderkrankheiten, March, 1848, p. 214. With no previous knowl-

heat, so distressing to the patient, more effectually than tepid or cold sponging, however often repeated; while it has the further advantage of not requiring repetition above twice in the twenty-four hours, by which the patient is spared much otherwise unavoidable fatigue. To the hand of a bystander it seems to have the effect of removing the pungent heat so remarkable in most cases of scarlet fever, and of keeping the skin supple and comparatively cool, though I am not prepared to say whether it exerts any real influence on the temperature of the surface as estimated by the thermometer. It does not prevent the desquamation of the cuticle after the decline of the eruption, nor does its most diligent employment exclude the occurrence of albuminous urine; though I think it considerably lessens the amount of the former, and diminishes the risk of the latter assuming a serious character.

This immunity from bad symptoms, however, is doubtless in great measure due to the circumstance that the cases in which the inunction was employed were those which came earliest under treatment, and in which, consequently, opportunity existed for carrying out a judicious management of the disease through all its stages. I believe it promotes the patient's comfort, and lessens the risks of some of the ordinary sequelæ of the disease; but the extravagant laudations which this proceeding has received from some medical men, induce me to add that I do not consider it as anything more than a useful adjunct to appropriate treatment, and in no sense a substitute for it. During the period of development of the rash, the inunction should be practiced twice a day: when the eruption is on the decline, its employment once in the twenty-four hours is generally sufficient; whilst, if the desquamation is at all abundant, the hot-air bath is of the greatest service in facilitating its completion and maintaining the activity of the skin. How slight soever the attack of scarlet fever may have been, it is prudent to confine the patient to bed for three weeks, since it is not until after the lapse of that time that one can feel absolutely secure from the supervention of albuminuria; and the urine during the whole of this period ought to be tested for albumen twice a day, in order that the first threatening of so serious an evil as scarlatinal dropsy may at once be met by appropriate treatment. During the whole of the stage of convalescence, or so long at least as the skin shows any trace of desquamation, even though the child is allowed to leave his bed, the inunction should be continued every morning, while the child should be placed in a warm bath every evening, and well rubbed with a soft towel on being placed in bed again. During the whole of this time the diet must be mild and unstimulating, and due attention must be paid to the state of the bowels. For some time after, much caution must be exercised in not allowing the child to go out when the air is cool, and in avoiding all errors of diet, while it is also expedient that

edge of the observations of others, Mr. W. Taylor, of London, was accustomed, from the year 1829, as he states in a little work published in 1850, to adopt a very similar course in the treatment of various febrile diseases, for which he regards it as almost a panacea.

flannel should be worn next to the skin for a considerable period after apparent convalescence from scarlet fever. I know that these precautions may appear to you overstrained,—they often do to our patients; but I can only say that every year of added experience leads me to insist upon them more and more, just as each year shows me more of the dangers of scarlatinal dropsy, and of its intractable character.

Even in severer cases of the disease, you must not be in too great a hurry to resort to active measures, for you will remember that a somewhat stormy onset is characteristic of all but the very mildest forms of scarlatina. That disturbance of the sensorium, for instance, which, when the child is sufficiently old, shows itself by the early occurrence of delirium, must not lead you to have recourse hastily to depletion either general or local, in order to quiet the disorder of the brain. The results afforded by depletion in scarlet fever even when the disease occurs in the adult are by no means encouraging; and in the child the loss of blood in these circumstances is even less well borne; so that, unless the patient is robust and plethoric, and the cerebral disturbance very serious, you should content yourselves with the application of cold to the head, perhaps employing cold affusion, if the symptoms are very urgent. These are the cases, too, in which the results of hydropathic treatment are often most remarkable, and I have seen the gravest symptoms of brain disturbance subside, the temperature fall, and the rash appear upon the skin under the use of the wet sheet. It is indeed many years since I employed depletion in the course of scarlet fever, though, as I have already mentioned, the abstraction of blood is frequently needed in the dropsy which constitutes its most formidable sequela. In the malignant forms of the disease there is often very considerable disturbance of the sensorium, great restlessness alternating with a state of stupor; but the frequent and feeble pulse at once forbids depletion in such cases, and points out the necessity for adopting every means to support the feeble powers of life. It is very likely that the low type which a disease such as scarlatina is almost sure to assume in the crowded dwellings of the poor, has rendered my practice in this respect somewhat different from that which might be advantageously pursued in the case of children more favorably situated. To the same circumstance it is also probably due that, in a large proportion of cases, I have found it desirable to give ammonia almost from the outset of the disease; a practice which has been recommended as universally applicable, and which (though the remedy does not deserve the indiscriminate praises that have been lavished on it) you will do well to follow, whenever the pulse presents the characters of frequency and softness combined. The state of the throat must be carefully watched in every case of scarlet fever; and whenever there is much swelling of the tonsils, if the child is too young to gargle, a slightly acidulated lotion should be injected into the throat by means of a syringe every few hours, in order to free it from the mucus which is so apt to collect there, and to be the source of much discomfort; or the solution of chlorate of soda or of permanganate of potash largely diluted, may be used for the same purpose, or the sulphurous acid in the proportion of one part to eight of water may be frequently employed with the spray-producer. [illegible] is much deposit of lymph upon the tonsils, it is generally [illegible] apply strong hydrochloric acid, mixed with honey, in the [illegible] about one part of the former to six of the latter, by means [illegible] hair pencil, or a solution of twenty grains of nitrate of [illegible] ounce of distilled water, once or twice at intervals of twenty [illegible] but I do not think that in scarlatinal sore throat, any more [illegible] of diphtheria, the frequent application of strong caustics [illegible] much good, or yields as much relief, as the frequent gargling or [illegible] ing the throat with milder remedies. The coryza, which is [illegible] and so ill-omened a symptom in cases of severe scarlatina, is [illegible] by throwing a small quantity of a solution of gr. j or gr. ij [illegible] silver in ℥j of distilled water, up the nostrils every four or [illegible] hours. The glandular swellings are very difficult to relieve, though [illegible] development sometimes seems to be retarded by painting the [illegible] them, two or three times a day, with tincture of iodine. When [illegible] erable, they do not seem to be benefited by leeches; the employment [illegible] which is also contraindicated by the feeble state of the patient's [illegible] while they show very little disposition to suppurate, and [illegible] are not relieved by lancing; so that the constant application of a [illegible] poultice is often all that can be done to afford ease to the patient. Children in whom the local affection is severe, or in whom the disease assumes a malignant character, require all those stimulants, and [illegible] nutritious diet, which we are accustomed to give to patients in [illegible] stages of typhus fever; though unfortunately, the best devised [illegible] will in many such cases prove ineffectual.

It may be well to add a few words in conclusion with reference to the alleged virtues of belladonna as a prophylactic against scarlatina. Hahnemann, the founder of the homœopathic system, first introduced it into practice, being induced to try it by certain resemblances which he believed to exist between its effects and the ordinary symptoms of scarlet fever. Other practitioners, without subscribing to homœopathic opinions, have yet adopted this proceeding, and aver that infinitesimal doses of belladonna do in reality exert the marvellous protective power which the drug was said to possess.

The evidence of its virtues, however, is in the last degree unsatisfactory. There are many recorded instances of its failure when tried on a large scale, while the strongest advocates of its use have never put its virtues to the obvious and simple test of administering the remedy to half of a given number of persons placed in similar circumstances as to age, health, and exposure to contagion, and comparing the results thus obtained. In the only instance with which I am personally acquainted where this mode of inquiry was adopted, the results, though the experiment was on too small a scale to justify a positive conclusion, seemed to show that the protective power of belladonna was absolutely null. I cannot do better than relate the experiment which was made at the Royal Military Asylum at Chelsea, by Dr. Balfour, in the words in which he was good enough to communicate it to me. [illegible] fever having broken out in the institution, Dr. Balfour determined to try the virtues of belladonna. "There were," he says, "151 boys of whom I had tolerably satisfactory evidence that they had not had scarlatina; I divided them into two sections, taking them alternately from the list, to prevent the imputation of selection. To the first section (76) I gave belladonna; to the second (75) I gave none; the result was that two in each section were attacked by the disease. The numbers are too small to justify deductions as to the prophylactic power of belladonna, but the observation is good, because it shows how apt we are to be misled by imperfect observation. Had I given the remedy to all the boys, I should probably have attributed to it the cessation of the epidemic."[1]

To these remarks I need add nothing. They convey a most important lesson, but one which I fear we are all too apt to forget in the study and in the practice of medicine.

---

[1] Any one who still feels a lingering faith in the prophylactic powers of belladonna, will do well to read the very careful and candid inquiry into the evidence on both sides of the question, published by Dr. Warburton Begbie, in the British and Foreign Medico-Chirurgical Review for January, 1855.

INDEX.

INDEX.

INDEX TO FORMULÆ.

INDEX TO FORMULÆ.

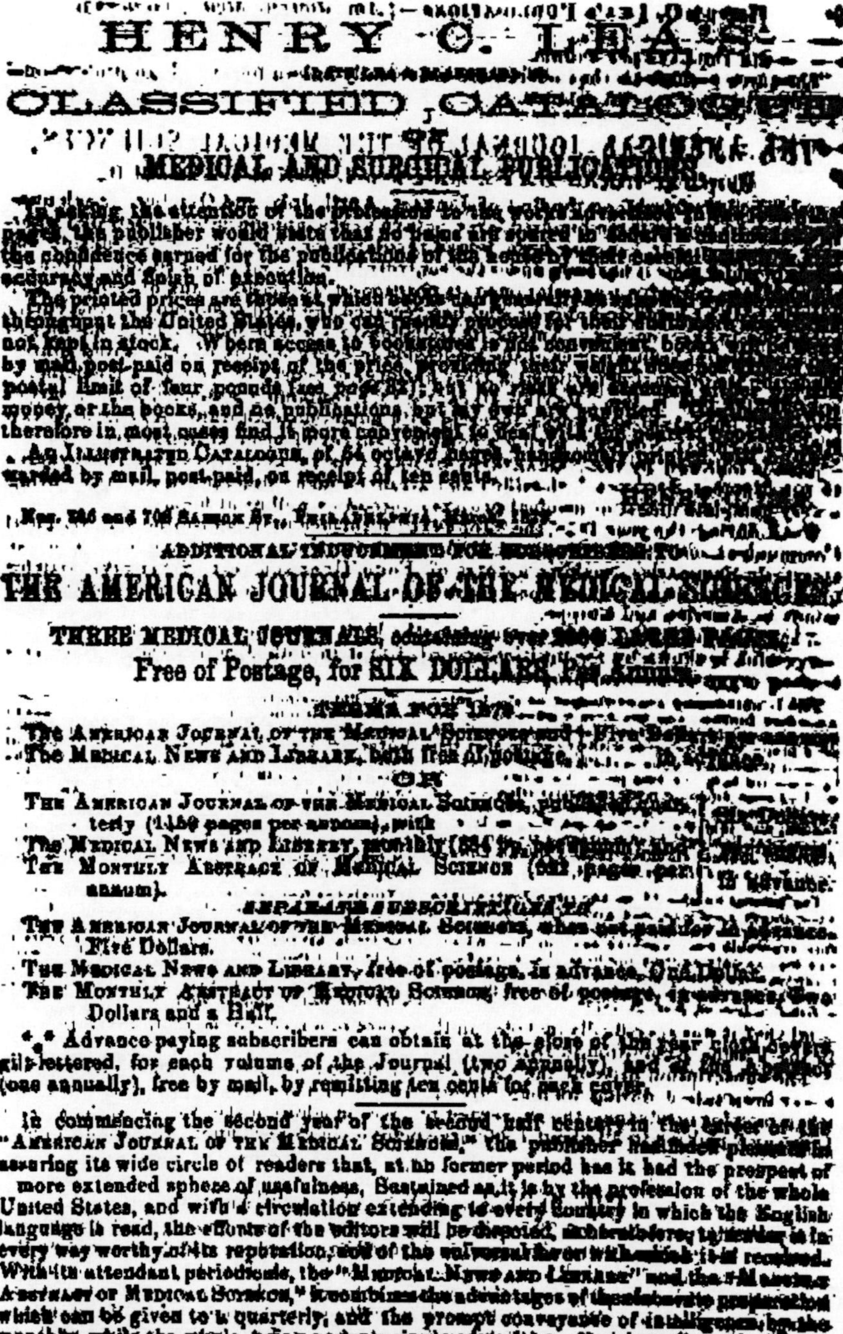

cost of SIX DOLLARS *per annum*.

The three periodicals thus offered are universally known for their high professional standing in their several spheres.

I.

THE AMERICAN JOURNAL OF THE MEDICAL SCIENCES,

EDITED BY ISAAC HAYS, M.D., AND I. MINIS HAYS, M.D.,

is published Quarterly, on the first of January, April, July, and October. Each number contains nearly three hundred large octavo pages, appropriately illustrated wherever necessary. It has now been issued regularly for over FIFTY years, during the whole of which time it has been under the control of the present senior editor. Throughout this long period, it has maintained its position in the highest rank of medical periodicals both at home and abroad, and has received the cordial support of the entire profession in this country. Among its Collaborators will be found a large number of the most distinguished names of the profession in every section of the United States, rendering its original department a truly national exponent of American medicine.*

Following this is the "REVIEW DEPARTMENT," containing extended and impartial reviews of important new works, together with numerous elaborate "ANALYTICAL AND BIBLIOGRAPHICAL NOTICES" giving a complete survey of medical literature.

This is followed by the "QUARTERLY SUMMARY OF IMPROVEMENTS AND DISCOVERIES IN THE MEDICAL SCIENCES," classified and arranged under different heads, presenting a very complete digest of medical progress abroad as well as at home.

Thus, during the year 1878, the "JOURNAL" furnished to its subscribers 77 Original Communications, 133 Reviews and Bibliographical Notices, and 255 articles in the Quarterly Summaries, making a total of FOUR HUNDRED AND SIXTY-FIVE articles illustrated with 48 maps and wood engravings, emanating from the best professional minds in America and Europe.

That the efforts thus made to maintain the high reputation of the "JOURNAL" are successful, is shown by the position accorded to it in both America and Europe as a leading organ of medical progress:—

This is universally acknowledged as the leading American Journal, and has been conducted by Dr Hays alone until 1869, when his son was associated with him. We quite agree with the critic, that this journal is second to none in the language, and cheerfully accord to it the first place, for nowhere shall we find more able and more impartial criticism, and nowhere such a repertory of able original articles. Indeed, now that the "British and Foreign Medico-Chirurgical Review" has terminated its career, the American Journal stands without a rival.—*London Med. Times and Gazette*, Nov 24, 1877.

The present number of the American Journal is an exceedingly good one, and gives every promise of maintaining the well-earned reputation of the review. Our venerable contemporary has our best wishes, and we can only express the hope that it may continue its work with as much vigor and excellence for the next fifty years as it has exhibited in the past.—*London Lancet*, Nov 24, 1877.

The Philadelphia Medical and Physical Journal issued its first number in 1820, and after a brilliant career, was succeeded in 1827 by the American Journal of the Medical Sciences, a periodical of world-wide reputation; the ablest and one of the oldest periodicals in the world—a journal which has an unsullied record.—*Gross's History of American Med. Literature*, 1876.

It is universally acknowledged to be the leading American medical journal, and, in our opinion, is second to none in the language.—*Boston Med. and Surg. Journal*, Oct 1877.

This is the medical journal of our country to which the American physician abroad will point with the greatest satisfaction, as reflecting the state of medical culture in his country. For a great many years it has been the medium through which our ablest writers have made known their discoveries and observations.—*Address of L. P. Yandell, M.D., before International Med. Congress*, Sept 1876.

And that it was specifically included in the award of a medal of merit to the Publisher in the Vienna Exhibition in 1873.

The subscription price of the "AMERICAN JOURNAL OF THE MEDICAL SCIENCES" has never been raised during its long career. It is still FIVE DOLLARS per annum; and when paid for in advance, the subscriber receives in addition the "MEDICAL NEWS AND LIBRARY," making in all about 1500 large octavo pages per annum, free of postage.

II.

THE MEDICAL NEWS AND LIBRARY

is a monthly periodical of Thirty-two large octavo pages, making 384 pages per annum. Its "LIBRARY DEPARTMENT" is devoted to publishing standard works on the various branches of medical science, paged separately, so that they can be detached for binding, when complete. In this manner subscribers have received, without expense, such works as "WATSON'S PRACTICE," "WEST ON CHILDREN," "MALGAIGNE'S SURGERY," "STOKES ON FEVER," GOSSELIN'S "CLINICAL LECTURES ON SURGERY," and many other volumes of the highest reputation and usefulness. With July, 1878, was commenced the publication of "LECTURES ON DISEASES OF THE NERVOUS SYSTEM," by J. M. CHARCOT, Professor in the Faculty of Medicine of Paris, translated from the French by GEORGE SIGERSON, M.D., Lecturer on Biology, etc., Catholic Univ. of

* Communications are invited from gentlemen in all parts of the country. Elaborate articles inserted by the Editor are paid for by the Publisher.

[illegible] (see p. [illegible]), which will be completed [illegible] 1878. New [illegible] commencing with January, 1878 [illegible] [illegible] of 50 cents [illegible]

The "NEWS DEPARTMENT" of the "MEDICAL NEWS" [illegible] current information of the month, with Clinical Lectures [illegible] A new and attractive feature of this will be found in an elaborate [illegible] American Clinical Lectures [illegible] the highest reputation in the profession throughout the United States [illegible] there have appeared Lectures by [illegible]

S. D. GROSS, M.D., Prof. of Surgery, Jefferson Med. Coll., Philada. [illegible]
T. GAILLARD THOMAS, M.D., Prof. Obstetrics, &c., Coll. Phys. and Surg., N. Y. [illegible]
WILLIAM PEPPER, M.D., Prof. Clin. Medicine, Univ. of Penna. [illegible]
LEWIS A. SAYRE, M.D., Prof. Orthopedic Surg., Bellevue Hospital [illegible]
ROBERTS BARTHOLOW, M.D., Prof. Theory and Practice of Medicine [illegible]
T. G. RICHARDSON, M.D., Prof. Genl. and Clin. Surg., Univ. of La. [illegible]
S. W. GROSS, M.D., Surg. to Philada. Hospital [illegible]
[illegible] PEYRE PORCHER, M.D., Prof. of Mat. Med. and Clin. Medicine [illegible]
WILLIAM GOODELL, M.D., Prof. Clin. Gynæcology, Univ. of Penna. [illegible]
N. S. DAVIS, M.D., Prof. Prin. and Prac. of Med., Chicago Med. College [illegible]
W. H. VAN BUREN, M.D., Prof. Surgery, Bellevue Hosp. Med. Coll., N. Y. [illegible]

To be followed by others of similar value, from [illegible]

AUSTIN FLINT, M.D., Prof. Prin. and Pract. of Med., Bellevue Hosp. Med. Coll., N. Y.
FORDYCE BARKER, M.D., Prof. Clin. Midwifery, &c., Bellevue Hosp. Med. Coll., N. Y.
L. A. DUHRING, M.D., Clin. Prof. of Diseases of the Skin, Univ. of Penna.
THEOPHILUS PARVIN, M.D., Prof. Obstetrics, &c., Coll. Phys. and Surg., Indianapolis.
J. P. WHITE, M.D., Prof. of Obstetrics, &c., [illegible]
JOHN ASHHURST, Jr., M.D., Prof. of Clin. Surg., Univ. of Penna.
D. WARREN BRICKELL, M.D., Prof. Obstetrics, &c., [illegible]
J. LEWIS SMITH, M.D., Clin. Lec. on Dis. of Chil., Bellevue [illegible]
WILLIAM E. NORRIS, M.D., Clin. Prof. of Diseases of the Eye [illegible]
P. S. CONNER, M.D., Prof. of Anat. and Clin. Surgery, Med. Coll. of Ohio, Cin.
S. WEIR MITCHELL, M.D., Phys. to the Infirmary for Nervous Diseases, Philada.
J. M. DACOSTA, M.D., Prof. Prin. and Prac. of Med., Jeff. Med. Coll., Philada.
THOMAS G. MORTON, M.D., Surgeon to Penna. Hospital, Philada.
F. J. BUMSTEAD, M.D., late Prof. of Venereal Dis., Coll. Phys. and Surg., N. Y.
J. H. HUTCHINSON, M.D., Physician to Penna. Hospital.
CHRISTOPHER JOHNSON, M.D., Prof. of Surgery, Univ. of Md., Baltimore.
WILLIAM THOMSON, M.D., Lecturer on Ophthalmology, Jeff. Med. Coll., Philada.

With contributors such as these, representing so many [illegible] the publisher feels safe in promising to the subscribers a course of [illegible] unsurpassed in variety, interest, and value.

As stated above, the subscription price of the "MEDICAL NEWS AND LIBRARY" is ONE DOLLAR per annum in advance, and it is furnished [illegible] to all paying subscribers to the "AMERICAN JOURNAL OF THE MEDICAL SCIENCES."

[illegible]

THE MONTHLY ABSTRACT OF MEDICAL SCIENCE

is issued on the first of every month, each number containing forty-eight [illegible] pages, thus furnishing, in the course of the year, [illegible] The [illegible] of the "ABSTRACT" is to present—without duplicating the matter in the "JOURNAL" and "NEWS"—a careful condensation of all that is new and important in the medical journalism of the world, and all the prominent professional periodicals of both hemispheres are at the disposal of the Editors. To show the manner in which this plan has been carried out, it is sufficient to state that during the year 1877 it contained

No. Articles on [illegible]
58 [illegible] Materia Medica and Therapeutics.
230 [illegible] Medicine.
154 [illegible] Surgery.
78 [illegible] Midwifery and Gynæcology.
33 [illegible] Medical Jurisprudence and Toxicology.

making in all 553 articles in a single year.

The subscription to the "MONTHLY ABSTRACT," [illegible] is TWO DOLLARS AND A HALF a year, in advance.

[illegible] above, however, it will be supplied in conjunction with the "American [illegible]

[illegible]

[illegible]

which must be for a new subscriber, will receive [illegible]

[illegible]

well to forward their [illegible]

complete [illegible]

to the order of the undersigned. [illegible]

[illegible]

DUNGLISON (ROBLEY) [illegible]

late Professor of [illegible]

MEDICAL LEXICON. A DICTIONARY [illegible]

taining a concise explanation of the various Subjects [illegible] ... Hygiene, Therapeutics [illegible] ... Jurisprudence, and Dentistry [illegible] ... Officinal, Empirical, and Dietetic Preparations; with the [illegible] ... the Terms, and the French and other Synonymes [illegible] ... English Medical Lexicon. A New Edition. [illegible] ... vised and Augmented. By Richard J. Dunglison, [illegible] ... royal octavo volume of over 1100 pages. [illegible]

(*Just Issued.*)

The object of the author from the outset has not been [illegible] ... of terms, but to afford, under each, a condensed view [illegible] ... to render the work an epitome of the existing condition [illegible] ... the immense demand which has existed [illegible] ... revisions, to augment its completeness and usefulness, [illegible] ... of a recognized and standard authority wherever the language [illegible] ... have been taken in the preparation of the [illegible] ... During the [illegible] years which have elapsed since [illegible] ... to the nomenclature of the medical sciences have been greater [illegible] ... of the past, and up to the time of his death the author labored [illegible] ... thing requiring the attention of the student or practitioner. [illegible] ... equally industrious to add the additions to the vocabulary [illegible] ... vious revision. Especial attention has been bestowed on the accentuation [illegible] ... marked on every word. The typographical arrangement has been [illegible] ... reference more easy, and every care has been taken with the [illegible] ... work has been printed on new type, small but exceedingly clear, [illegible] ... the additions have been incorporated without increase of but little [illegible] ... the volume now contains the matter of at least four ordinary octavo [illegible]

[illegible] well known to our readers, and of which every American ought to be proud. When the learned author of the work passed away, probably all of us feared lest the book should not maintain its place in the advancing science whose terms it defines. Fortunately, Dr. Richard J. Dunglison, having assisted his father in the revision of several editions of the work, and having been, therefore, trained in the methods and imbued with the spirit of the book, has been able to edit it, not in the patchwork manner so dear to the heart of book editors, so repulsive to the taste of intelligent book readers, but to edit it as a work of the kind should be edited—to carry it on steadily, without [illegible] or interruption, along the grooves of thought it has [illegible] during its lifetime. To show the magnitude of the task which Dr. Dunglison has assumed and carried [illegible], it is only necessary to state that more than six thousand new subjects have been added in the present edition.—*Phila. Med. Times*, Jan. 3, 1874.

About the first book purchased by the medical student is the Medical Dictionary. The lexicon explanatory of technical terms is simply a sine qua non. In a

[illegible] ... physician, [illegible] ... became Dunglison's [illegible] ... nothing was needed [illegible] ... former revisions [illegible] ... have been added. [illegible] ... latter, while the [illegible] ... arrangement which [illegible] ... that the work, which [illegible] ... of individual [illegible] ... standard authority.—[illegible]

It has the rare merit that it [illegible] ... in the English language [illegible] ... —London [illegible]

A CENTURY OF AMERICAN MEDICINE, 1776–1876. By Doctors [illegible] Clarke, H. J. Bigelow, S. D. Gross, T. G. Thomas, and J. S. Billings. In one very handsome 12mo. volume of about [illegible] pages [illegible]

This work has appeared in the pages of the American Journal of the Medical Sciences [illegible] year 1876. As a detailed account of the development of medical science in America [illegible] men of the highest authority in their respective departments, [illegible] come in a form adapted for preservation and reference.

HOBLYN (RICHARD D.), M.D.

A DICTIONARY OF THE TERMS USED IN MEDICINE [illegible] THE COLLATERAL SCIENCES. [illegible] M.D., Editor of the "American Journal of the Medical Sciences." [illegible] 12mo. volume of over [illegible] double-columned [illegible]

It is the best book of definitions we have [illegible] *Med. and Surg. Journal.*

RODWELL (G. F.), F.R.A.S.

A DICTIONARY OF SCIENCE: Comprising Astronomy, Chemistry, Dynamics, Electricity, Heat, Hydrodynamics, Hydrostatics, Light, Magnetism, Mechanics, Meteorology, Pneumatics, Sound, and Statics. Preceded by an Essay on the History of the Physical Sciences. In one handsome octavo volume of [illegible] pages, with many illustrations; cloth, $5.

NEILL (JOHN), M.D., and SMITH (FRANCIS G.), M.D.,
Prof. of the Institutes of Medicine in the Univ. of Penna.

AN ANALYTICAL COMPENDIUM OF THE VARIOUS BRANCHES OF MEDICAL SCIENCE; for the Use and Examination of Students. A new edition, revised and improved. In one very large and handsomely printed royal 12mo. volume, of about one thousand pages, with 374 wood-cuts, cloth, $4; strongly bound in leather, with raised bands, $4 75.

HARTSHORNE (HENRY), M.D.,
Professor of Hygiene in the University of Pennsylvania.

A CONSPECTUS OF THE MEDICAL SCIENCES; Containing Handbooks on Anatomy, Physiology, Chemistry, Materia Medica, Practical Medicine, Surgery, and Obstetrics. Second Edition, thoroughly revised and improved. In one large royal 12mo. volume of more than 1000 closely printed pages, with 477 illustrations on wood. Cloth, $4 25; leather, $5 00. (*Lately Issued.*)

We can say with the strictest truth that it is the best work of the kind with which we are acquainted. It embodies in a condensed form all recent contributions to practical medicine, and is therefore useful to every busy practitioner throughout our country, besides being admirably adapted to the use of students of medicine. The book is faithfully and ably executed.—*Charleston Med. Journ.*, April, 1875.

The work is intended as an aid to the medical student, and as such appears to admirably fulfil its object by its excellent arrangement, the full compilation of facts, the perspicuity and terseness of language, and the clear and instructive illustrations in some parts of the work.—*American Journ. of Pharmacy*, Philadelphia, July, 1874.

The volume will be found useful, not only to students, [illegible] who may [illegible] wish to refresh their memories with the smallest possible expenditure of time.—*N. Y. Med. Journal*, [illegible]

The student will find this the most convenient and useful book of the kind on which he can lay his hand.—*Pacific Med. and Surg. Journ.*, Aug. 1874.

This is the best book of its kind that we have ever examined. It is an honest, accurate, and concise compend of medical sciences, [illegible] representing their present condition. The changes and the additions have been so judiciously [illegible] as to render it, so far as it goes, entirely trustworthy. If students must have a compend, [illegible] to procure that of Dr. Hartshorne.—*Detroit Review of Med. and Pharm.*, Aug. 1874.

LUDLOW (J. L.), M.D.

A MANUAL OF EXAMINATIONS upon Anatomy, Physiology, Surgery, Practice of Medicine, Obstetrics, Materia Medica, Chemistry, Pharmacy, and Therapeutics. To which is added a Medical Formulary. Third edition, thoroughly revised and greatly extended and enlarged. With 370 illustrations. In one handsome royal 12mo. volume of 816 large pages, cloth, $3 25; leather, $3 75.

The arrangement of this volume in the form of question and answer renders it especially suitable for the office examination of students, and for those preparing for graduation.

TANNER (THOMAS HAWKES), M.D.

A MANUAL OF CLINICAL MEDICINE AND PHYSICAL DIAGNOSIS. Third American from the Second London Edition. Revised and Enlarged by Tilbury Fox, M.D., Physician to the Skin Department in University College Hospital, &c. In one neat volume small 12mo., of about 375 pages, cloth, $1 50.

*** On page 3, it will be seen that this work is offered as a premium to new subscribers to the "American Journal of the Medical Sciences."

[illegible]

ANATOMY, [illegible]

[illegible], M.A., Surgeon to St. [illegible] enlarged and improved London edition. [illegible] Surgical," by Luther Holden, F.R.C.S., author of [illegible] of Dissections," etc. In one magnificent [illegible] large and elaborate engravings on wood. [illegible]

[illegible] original, and having the names of the various parts printed on [illegible] spaces of reference, with descriptions at the foot. They thus [illegible] which will greatly assist the student in obtaining a clear [illegible] [illegible] pupil of much labor in laying the groundwork of a thorough [illegible]

Since the appearance of the last American Edition, the work [illegible] hands of its accomplished editor, Mr. Holmes, who [illegible] [illegible] work by the distinguished anatomist, Mr. Luther Holden, [illegible] [illegible] complete, the work, it is believed, will furnish [illegible] illustration in anatomical study. No pains have been [illegible] the volume, which will be found in all respects superior to former [illegible] increase of size, amounting to over 100 pages and [illegible] at a price rendering it one of the cheapest works ever [illegible]

The recent work of Mr. Holden, which was [illegible] [illegible] of this volume, has been added [illegible] [illegible] the most [illegible] and complete anatomical treatise [illegible] [illegible] students and physicians. The former [illegible] the necessary guide in [illegible] tions; a very comprehensive chapter on [illegible] [illegible] about all that can be taught him on general and special anatomy; while the latter, in its treatment of each region from a surgical point of view, and in the valuable edition of Mr. Holden, [illegible] all that will be essential to him in his practice.—*New Remedies*, Aug. 1878.

This work is as near perfection as one could possibly or reasonably expect any book intended as a text-book or a general reference book on anatomy to be. The American publishers deserve the thanks of the profession for appending the recent work of Mr. Holden, "Landmarks, Medical and Surgical," which has already been commended as a separate book. The latter work—treating of topographical anatomy—has become an essential to the library of every intelligent practitioner. We know of no book that can take its place, written as it is by a most distinguished anatomist. It would be simply a waste of words to say anything further in praise of Gray's anatomy, the text-book in almost every medical college in this country, and the daily reference book of every practitioner who has occasion to consult [illegible] simply [illegible] [illegible] Aug. 1878.

The [illegible] [illegible] who [illegible] [illegible] Aug. 1878.

It is difficult [illegible] new edition of [illegible] perfect as it is [illegible] any branch of [illegible] eminent men [illegible] eight editions [illegible] seem to leave [illegible] addition of Holden's [illegible] indispensable to the [illegible] surgery as it has [illegible] regards completeness, [illegible] beauty, and cheapness [illegible] dent should [illegible] physician can afford [illegible] library.—*St. Louis* [illegible]

ALSO FOR SALE SEPARATE—

HOLDEN (LUTHER), F.R.C.S.,

Surgeon to St. Bartholomew's and the Foundling Hospitals.

LANDMARKS, MEDICAL AND SURGICAL. [illegible]

Ed. In one handsome volume, royal 12mo., of 128 pages; cloth, [illegible]

The title of this book is very suggestive of its practical value, while the perusal of the work itself realizes the most extravagant expectations. The object of the author has been to collect in compact form the landmarks, or surface-marks of the different parts of the body, and indicate their relation to the deeper-seated parts. The value of this sort of knowledge to the physician, but especially to the surgeon [illegible] with anatomical eye, can make the [illegible] transparent before him [illegible] ping out of the human body [illegible] structive to the [illegible] after considerable [illegible] of his own; but in [illegible] knowledge is [illegible] manner as to place it [illegible] one of the most interesting [illegible] for a long time.—*N. Y.* [illegible]

ALLEN (HARRISON), M.D.
Professor of Physiology in the Univ. of Pa. [illegible]

A SYSTEM OF HUMAN ANATOMY; INCLUDING ITS MEDICAL and Surgical Relations. For the Use of Practitioners and Students [illegible] Introductory Chapter on Histology. By E. O. Shakespeare [illegible] [illegible]. In one large and handsome quarto volume [illegible] illustrations on lithographic plates, and numerous wood-cuts [illegible]

In this elaborate work, which has been in active preparation for [illegible] sought to give, not only the details of descriptive anatomy in a clear and condensed [illegible] the practical applications of the science to medicine and surgery. The [illegible] the attention of the general practitioner, as well as of the student, enabling him [illegible] fresh his recollections of the dissecting room, but also to recognize the [illegible] from normal conditions. The marked ability of the [illegible] self-evident, and his long experience and assiduous devotion to the [illegible] sufficient guarantee of the manner in which his task [illegible] spared with the illustrations. Those of normal anatomy are from original [illegible] stone by Mr. Hermann Faber, with the name of every part [illegible] after the manner of "Holden" and "Gray" [illegible] effort of the publisher to render the volume worthy of the very [illegible] anticipated for it.

ELLIS (GEORGE VINER),
[illegible]

DEMONSTRATIONS IN ANATOMY; Being a Guide to the Knowledge of the Human Body by Dissection. By George Viner Ellis, [illegible] of Anatomy in University College, London. From the [illegible] Edition. In one very handsome octavo volume [illegible] *(Nearly Ready.)*

This work has long been known in England as the leading authority [illegible] and the favorite guide in the dissecting-room, [illegible] which it has passed. In the last edition, which has just [illegible] author has sought to bring it on a level with the most recent [illegible] necessary changes in his account of the microscopic structure of the [illegible] oped by the latest researches in textural anatomy.

WILSON (ERASMUS), F.R.S.

A SYSTEM OF HUMAN ANATOMY, General and Special. Edited by W. H. Gobrecht, M.D., Professor of [illegible] College of Ohio. Illustrated with three hundred and [illegible] one large and handsome octavo volume, of over 600 [illegible]

HEATH (CHRISTOPHER), F.R.C.S.,
Teacher of Operative Surgery in University College, London.

PRACTICAL ANATOMY: A Manual of Dissections. [illegible] Second revised and improved London edition. Edited, with additions, by [illegible] M. D., Lecturer on Pathological Anatomy in the Jefferson Medical College, Philadelphia. In one handsome royal 12mo. volume of 578 pages, with 247 illustrations. Cloth, [illegible] leather, $4 00.

SMITH (HENRY H.), M.D., and **HORNER (WILLIAM E.), M.D.,**
Prof. of Surgery in the Univ. of Penna., &c. — *Late Prof. of Anatomy in the Univ. of Penna.*

AN ANATOMICAL ATLAS, illustrative of the Structure of the Human Body. In one volume, large imperial octavo, cloth, with about six hundred and fifty beautiful figures. $4 50.

BELLAMY (E.), F.R.C.S.

THE STUDENT'S GUIDE TO SURGICAL ANATOMY: A Text-Book for Students preparing for their Pass Examination. With [illegible] one handsome royal 12mo. volume. Cloth, [illegible] (Lately Published.)

CLELAND (JOHN), M.D.,
Professor of Anatomy and Physiology in Queen's College, [illegible]

A DIRECTORY FOR THE DISSECTION OF THE HUMAN BODY. In one small volume, royal 12mo. of 182 pages; cloth, [illegible]

SCHAFER (EDWARD ALBERT), M.D.,
Assistant Professor of Physiology in University College, London.

A COURSE OF PRACTICAL HISTOLOGY: Being an Introduction to the Use of the Microscope. In one handsome royal 12mo. volume of [illegible] pages, with numerous illustrations: cloth, [illegible] (Just Issued.)

HORNER'S SPECIAL ANATOMY AND HISTOLOGY. Eighth edition, extensively revised and modified. In 2 vols. 8vo., of over 1000 pages, with 320 wood-cuts; cloth, [illegible]

[illegible]

[illegible]

English edition. In conclusion, we can give our cordial recommendation to the work as it now appears. The editors have, with their additions to the only work on physiology in our language that, [illegible] [illegible] it will [illegible] maintain the place it has [illegible] to the favor of the medical profession.—*Journ. of Nervous and Mental Disease*, April, 1877.

"Good wine needs no bush" says the proverb, and an old and faithful servant like the "[illegible]" Carpenter, [illegible] [illegible]
[illegible] has been a received and established fact for years. In this encyclopædic way it is unrivalled. Here, as it seems to us, is the great value of the book [illegible] [illegible]

[illegible] *Med. and Surg.* [illegible]

KIRKES (WILLIAM SENHOUSE), M.D.

A MANUAL OF PHYSIOLOGY. Edited by [illegible] M.D., F.R.C.S. A new American from the eighth [illegible] about two hundred and fifty illustrations. In one large [illegible] ume. Cloth, $3 25; leather, $3 75. (*Lately Issued.*)

Kirkes' Physiology has long been known as a concise and exceedingly [illegible] presenting within a narrow compass all that is important for the student [illegible] which successive editions have followed each other in England has enabled [illegible] thoroughly on a level with the changes and new discoveries made in the science [illegible] edition, of which the present is a reprint, has appeared so recently [illegible] the latest accessible exposition of the subject.

On the whole, there is very little in the book which either the student or practitioner will not find of practical value and consistent with our present knowledge of this rapidly changing science; and we have no hesitation in expressing our opinion that this eighth edition is one of the best handbooks on physiology which we have in our language.—*N. Y. Med. Record*, April 15, 1873.

The book is admirably adapted to be placed in the hands of students.—[illegible] *Journ.*, April 15, 1873.

In its enlarged form it is [illegible] best book on physiology [illegible] —*Phila. Med. Times*, [illegible]

This is undoubtedly the [illegible] physiology extant.—[illegible]

HARTSHORNE (HENRY), M.D.,

Professor of Hygiene, etc., in the Univ. of Penna.

HANDBOOK OF ANATOMY AND PHYSIOLOGY. [illegible] tion, revised. In one royal 12mo. volume, with 220 wood-cuts. cloth, $1 [illegible]

DALTON (J. C.), M.D.,
Professor of Physiology in the College of Physicians and Surgeons, New York, &c.

A TREATISE ON HUMAN PHYSIOLOGY [illegible]

[illegible] pages. Cloth [illegible]

From the Preface to the Sixth Edition. [illegible]

In the present edition of this book, while every part has [illegible] original plan of arrangement has been changed only so far as was necessary for the [illegible] new material. [illegible]

The additions and alterations in the text, requisite to present [illegible] physiological knowledge, have resulted, in spite of the author's [illegible] in an increase of fully fifty per cent. in the matter of the work. A change, [illegible] typographical arrangement has accommodated these additions without [illegible] bulk of the volume. [illegible]

The new chemical notation and nomenclature [illegible] introduced into the present edition, [illegible] now so generally taken the place of the old, that [illegible] The centigrade system of measurements for length, volume and weight, [illegible] measurements being at present almost universally employed in original physiological [illegible] tions and their published accounts. Temperatures are given in degrees of the centigrade [illegible] usually accompanied by the corresponding degrees of Fahrenheit's scale, inclosed in brackets.

NEW YORK, September, 1875.

During the past few years several new works on physiology, and new editions of old works, have appeared, competing for the favor of the medical student, but none will rival this new edition of Dalton. It now enlarged, it will be found [illegible] work of reference for the practitioner.—*Chicago Med. Journ. and Examiner*, Jan. 1876.

Prof. Dalton, has discussed conflicting theories and conclusions regarding physiological questions with a fairness, a [illegible] and a conciseness which lend freshness and vigor to the entire book. But his discussions have been so guarded by a [illegible] of admission to those speculative and theoretical explanations, which at best exist in the minds of observers themselves as only probabilities, that none of his readers need be led into grave errors while making them a study.—*The Medical Record*, Feb. 19, 1876.

The revision of this great work has brought it abreast with the physiological advances of the day, and renders it, as it has ever been, the finest work for students extant.—*Nashville Journ. of Med. and Surg.*, Jan. 1876.

For clearness and perspicuity, Dalton's Physiology commended itself to the student years ago, and was a pleasant relief from the verbose productions which it supplanted. Physiology has, however, made many advances since then—and while the style has been preserved intact, the work in the present edition has been brought up fully abreast of the times. The new chemical notation and nomenclature have also been introduced into the present edition. Notwithstanding the multiplicity of text-books on physiology, this will [illegible] none of its old time popularity. The mechanical execution of the work is all that could be desired.—*Peninsular Journal of Medicine*, Dec. 1875.

[illegible]

We heartily welcome this, the [illegible] edition of this [illegible] [illegible] has been appreciated. [illegible] admirably executed illustrations, has been [illegible] revised and very much enlarged, [illegible] not [illegible]—*[illegible] Medical and Surgical Journal*, March, 1876.

The present edition is very much [illegible] other, not only in that it brings the subject up to the times, but [illegible] than any previous edition. [illegible] physiology [illegible] in any land or language.—*[illegible]*

As a whole, we cordially recommend the work as a text-book for the student [illegible]—*The Journal of Nervous and Mental Disease*, [illegible] 1876.

Still holds the position [illegible] of [illegible] written, and is, we believe, on the whole, the best book to place in the hands of the student.—*London Students' Journal.*

DUNGLISON (ROBLEY), M.D.,
Professor of Institutes of Medicine in Jefferson Medical College, Philadelphia.

HUMAN PHYSIOLOGY. Eighth edition. Thoroughly revised and extensively modified and enlarged, with five hundred and thirty-two illustrations. In two large and handsomely printed octavo volumes of [illegible] pages. [illegible]

LEHMANN (C. G.).

PHYSIOLOGICAL CHEMISTRY. Translated from the second edition by GEORGE E. DAY, M.D., F.R.S., &c., edited by R. E. ROGERS, M.D., Professor of Chemistry in the Medical Department of the University of Pennsylvania, with illustrations selected from Funke's Atlas of Physiological Chemistry, and an Appendix of plates. Complete in two large and handsome octavo volumes, containing [illegible] pages, with nearly two hundred illustrations, cloth, $[illegible].

BY THE SAME AUTHOR.

MANUAL OF CHEMICAL PHYSIOLOGY. Translated from the German, with Notes and Additions, by J. CHESTON MORRIS, M.D., with an Introductory Essay on Vital Force, by Professor SAMUEL JACKSON, M.D., of the University of Pennsylvania. With illustrations on wood. In one very handsome octavo volume of [illegible] pages, cloth, $2 25.

FOWNES (GEORGE), Ph.D.

A MANUAL OF ELEMENTARY CHEMI[illegible]

Practical. Revised and corrected by Henry Watts, [illegible] ary of Chemistry," etc. With a colored plate, [illegible] trations. A new American, from the [illegible] and [illegible] Robert Bridges, M.D. In one large royal [illegible] cloth, $2 75; leather, $3 25. (Just Ready.)

Two careful revisions by Mr. Watts, since the [illegible] "Fownes," have so enlarged the work that in England [illegible] reprinting it, by the use of a small and exceedingly clear type, [illegible] found possible to comprise the whole, without omission, in one [illegible] reference. The enlargement of the work has induced the American [illegible] to the narrowest compass, and he has accordingly inserted [illegible] noticed since the very recent appearance of the work in England [illegible] in popular use to the Decimal and Centigrade systems employed in the [illegible]

Among the additions to this edition will be found a very [illegible] a number of spectra in the spectroscope. Every care has been taken [illegible] tion to render the volume worthy in every respect of its high reputation [illegible] though it has been enlarged by more than one hundred and [illegible] will still maintain it as one of the cheapest volumes accessible to the [illegible]

This work, inorganic and organic, is complete in one convenient volume. In its earliest editions it was fully up to the latest advancements and theories of that time. In its present form, it presents, in a remarkably convenient and satisfactory manner, the principles and leading facts of the chemistry of to-day. Concerning the manner in which the various subjects are treated, much deserves to be said, and [illegible], etc. in praise of the book. A review of such a work as Fownes's Chemistry within the limits of a book-notice for a medical weekly is simply out of the question.—*Cincinnati Lancet and Clinic*, Dec. 14, 1878.

When we state that, in our opinion, the present edition sustains in every respect the high reputation which its predecessors have acquired and enjoyed, we express therewith our full belief in its intrinsic value as a text-book and work of reference.—*Am. Journ. of Pharm.*, Aug. 1878.

The conscientious care which has been bestowed upon it by the American and English editors renders it still, perhaps, the best book for the student and the practitioner who would keep alive the acquisitions of his student days. It has, indeed, reached a some[illegible] [illegible] thousand pages, [illegible] reputation of [illegible] type is small [illegible] [illegible] arranged [illegible] and [illegible]

The work is [illegible] in need, any [illegible] the revision by the [illegible] [illegible], and thus [illegible] from the valuable [illegible] [illegible] chemistry. [illegible] volume to [illegible] fail to retain all its [illegible] of Chemistry [illegible]

It will be [illegible] [illegible] Manual, for [illegible] most place as a [illegible] thorough revision [illegible] volume [illegible] step before [illegible]

As a manual of [illegible] in the language [illegible]

ATTFIELD (JOHN), Ph.D.,

Professor of Practical Chemistry to the Pharmaceutical Society of [illegible]

CHEMISTRY, GENERAL, MEDICAL, AND PHA[illegible]

Including the Chemistry of the U. S. Pharmacopœia. A Manual [illegible] of the Science, and their Application to Medicine and Pharma[illegible] tion, revised from the Seventh English edition by the author. [illegible] volume of over 700 pages, with Illustrations. (In press.)

A few notices of the previous edition are subjoined.

It is a valuable work for the busy practitioner, excluding as it does everything that would be of interest only to the scientific chemist, and having a comprehensive index which renders after consultation easy. That portion devoted to urinalysis and practical toxicology, and the tests for impurities in medicinal preparations, is especially valuable to the practising physician. For the student it is desirable, for the reason that it is so arranged that he may, without an instructor, study the science experimentally.—*Am. Practitioner*, March, 1877.

After having used it as a text-book in the laboratory of the Philadelphia College of Pharmacy during the last two years, we can speak from our own experience, and testify to its intrinsic value in the instruction of the student. The more we [illegible] pleased with it, and on the [illegible] and enlarged edition [illegible] [illegible] recommend it [illegible] struction of pharma[illegible] has no superior [illegible] *of Pharm.*, Nov. 18[illegible]

As a compact [illegible] science and their [illegible] macy, it has no rival, [illegible] revision it receives keeps [illegible] times. The American [illegible] States Pharmacopœia, [illegible] supervision.—[illegible]

BOWMAN (JOHN E.), M.D.

INTRODUCTION TO PRACTICAL CHEMIST[illegible]

ANALYSIS. Sixth American, from the sixth and revised London [illegible] ous illustrations. In one neat vol., royal 12mo., cloth, $2 25. [illegible]

BY THE SAME AUTHOR.

PRACTICAL HANDBOOK OF MEDICAL CHE[illegible]

neat volume, royal 12mo., pp. 351, with numerous illustrations. [illegible]

KNAPP'S TECHNOLOGY; or Chemistry Applied to the Arts, and to Manufactures. With American additions by Prof. Walter R. Johnson. In two very handsome [illegible] engravings, cloth, [illegible]

BLOXAM (C. L.).

Professor of Chemistry in King's College, London.

CHEMISTRY, INORGANIC AND ORGANIC. [illegible] Edition. In one very handsome octavo volume, of [illegible]. Cloth, $4 [illegible]; leather, $[illegible]. (*Lately Issued.*)

We have in this work a complete and [illegible] text-book for the use of schools, and can heartily recommend it as such.—*Boston Med. and Surg. Journ.*, May 28, 1874.

[illegible] the title of a work which we can most [illegible] recommend to students of chemistry [illegible] a work on chemistry could be made [illegible] at the same time that it presents a full account of [illegible] work [illegible] it is quite as well suited [illegible] [illegible]

CLASSEN (ALEXANDER).

Professor in the Royal [illegible] School, Aix-la-Chapelle.

ELEMENTARY QUANTITATIVE ANALYSIS. Translated, with notes and additions by Edgar F. Smith, Ph.D., Assist. Prof. of Chemistry in the Towne Scientific School, Univ. of Penna. In one handsome [illegible] pages, with illustrations; cloth, $2 00. (*Just Ready.*)

This little book will supply a want of a condensed and [illegible] laboratory guide [illegible] student in quantitative analysis. Since its appearance in Germany, two or three [illegible] it has been received throughout the continent as a [illegible] into French and Russian shows that the author has [illegible] at which he aimed. The translator has added such [illegible] adapt the volume more thoroughly to the wants [illegible]

A small, practical, comprehensive, and [illegible] guide to practical elementary quantitative analysis, and is particularly adapted to the wants of the beginner with laboratory work.—*N. Y. Med. Record*, Nov. 12, 1878.

It is probably the best manual of an elementary [illegible] is [illegible] by [illegible] determinations [illegible] advancing to the analysis of minerals and such products as are met with in applied chemistry. It is an indispensable book [illegible] *[illegible] Journal of Chemistry* [illegible]

CLOWES (FRANK), D.Sc., London.

Senior Science-Master at the High School, Newcastle-under-Lyme, [illegible].

AN ELEMENTARY TREATISE ON PRACTICAL CHEMISTRY AND QUALITATIVE INORGANIC ANALYSIS. Specially adapted for Use in the Laboratories of Schools and Colleges and by Beginners. From the Second and Revised English Edition, with about fifty illustrations on wood. In one [illegible] 12mo. volume of 372 pages; cloth, $2 50. (*Now Ready.*)

It is short, concise, and eminently practical. We therefore heartily commend it to students, and especially to those who are obliged to dispense with a master. Of course a teacher is in every way desirable, but a good degree of technical skill and practical knowledge can be attained with no other instructor than the very valuable handbook now under consideration.—*St. Louis Clin. Record*, Oct. 1877.

The work is so written and arranged that it can be comprehended by the student without a teacher, and the descriptions and directions for the various work are so simple, and yet [illegible] theoretical [illegible] practical matter, which [illegible] text-book [illegible] analytical methods [illegible] author and the [illegible] printed text. We can heartily commend the work to the student of chemistry as being a reliable and comprehensive one.—*[illegible]*, [illegible] 20, 1877.

GALLOWAY (ROBERT), F.C.S.,

Prof. of Applied Chemistry in the Royal College of Science for Ireland, etc.

A MANUAL OF QUALITATIVE ANALYSIS. From the [illegible] London Edition. In one neat royal 12mo. volume, with illustrations; cloth, $2 [illegible]. (*Lately Issued.*)

The success which has carried this work through repeated editions in England, and its adoption as a text-book in several of the leading institutions in this country, show that the author has succeeded in the endeavor to produce a sound practical manual and book of reference for the chemical student.

We regard this volume as a valuable addition to the chemical text-books, and as particularly calculated to instruct the student in analytical [illegible] of the inorganic compounds, the important vegetable [illegible] and [illegible]—*Am. Journ. of [illegible]*, Sept. 1872.

REMSEN (IRA), M.D., Ph.D.,

Professor of Chemistry in the Johns Hopkins University, Baltimore.

PRINCIPLES OF THEORETICAL CHEMISTRY, with special reference to the Constitution of Chemical Compounds. In one handsome royal 12mo. volume of 232 pages; cloth, $1 50. (*Just Issued.*)

WÖHLER AND FITTIG.

OUTLINES OF ORGANIC CHEMISTRY. Translated, with Additions from the Eighth German Ed. By Ira Remsen, M.D., Ph.D., Prof. of Chem. and Physics in Williams College, Mass. In one volume, royal 12mo. of 550 pp., cloth, $3.

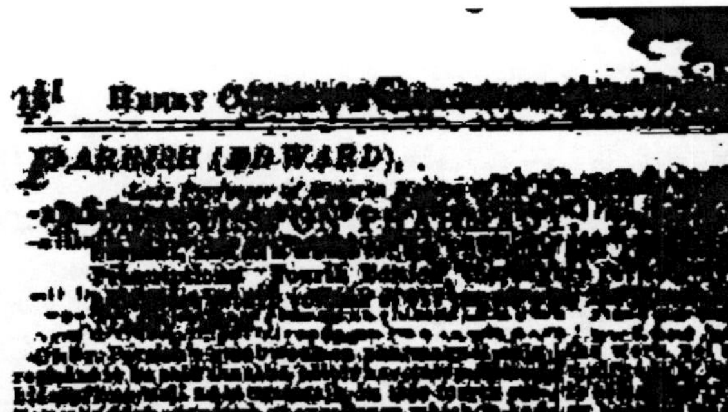

Parrish (Edward).

[illegible] accomplished author. This has not been accomplished without much labor, and many additions and improvements, involving changes in the arrangement of the several parts of the work, and the addition of much new matter. With the [illegible] the pharmaceutical preparation of the [illegible] [illegible]—*Chicago Med. Journ.* [illegible]

[illegible] lisher it will convey some idea [illegible] have been bestowed upon its production [illegible] illustrations. In conclusion, we heartily recommend [illegible]

Stillé (Alfred), M.D.,

Professor of Theory and Practice of Medicine [illegible]

THERAPEUTICS AND MATERIA MEDICA [illegible]

on the Action and Uses of Medicinal Agents [illegible] Fourth edition, revised and enlarged. In two [illegible] pages. Cloth, $10; leather, $12. (*Lately Issued.*)

It is unnecessary to do much more than to announce the appearance of this fourth edition of this well known and excellent work.—*Cin. and [illegible] Med. Chir. Review*, Oct. 1874.

To all who desire a complete work on therapeutics and materia medica for reference, in cases involving medico-legal questions, as well as for information concerning remedial agents, Dr. Stillé's is "[illegible] of the work." The work being out of print, by the exhaustion of former editions the author has laid the profession under renewed obligations, by the careful revision, important additions, and timely re[illegible] issuing a work not scarcely supplemented by any other in the English language, if in any language. The mechanical execution handsomely sustains the well-known skill and good taste of the publisher.—*St. Louis Med. and Surg. Journal*, Dec. 1874.

From the publication of the first edition "Stillé's Therapeutics" has been one of the classics; its absence from our libraries would create a vacuum which could be filled by no other work in the language, and its predominant place, in the two volumes [illegible]

of the [illegible] [illegible]

[illegible] a place in the physician's [illegible] fully representing the [illegible] pharmacopœia [illegible] treatise upon the [illegible] question.—*Boston Med. and Surg. [illegible]* 1874.

Griffith (Robert E.), M.D.

A UNIVERSAL FORMULARY, Containing the Methods of [illegible]

ing and Administering Officinal and other Medicines. The whole adapted [illegible] Pharmaceutists. Third edition, thoroughly revised, with numerous [illegible] Maisch, Professor of Materia Medica in the Philadelphia College of [illegible] and handsome octavo volume of about 800 pp. cloth, $4 50; leather, $5 [illegible]

To the druggist a good formulary is simply indispensable, and perhaps no formulary has been more extensively used than the well-known work before us. Many physicians have to officiate, also, as druggists. This is true especially of the country physician, and a work which shall teach him the means by which to administer or combine his remedies in the most efficacious and pleasant manner, will always hold its place upon his shelf. A formulary of this kind is of benefit also to the city physician in larger practice.—*Cincinnati Clinic*, Feb. 21, 1874.

A more complete formulary [illegible] cal form the pharmacist or physician [illegible] desire. To the first some such [illegible] ble, and it is hardly less [illegible] who compounds his own medicines [illegible] is contained in the introduction [illegible] mitted to memory by [illegible] As a help to physicians it will [illegible] and doubtless will make [illegible] already supplied with a standard [illegible] —*The American Practitioner*, [illegible]

STILLE (ALFRED), M.D., LL.D., and MAISCH (JOHN M.), [illegible]

Prof. of Theory and Practice of Medicine [illegible] [illegible]

THE NATIONAL DISPENSATORY: [illegible] and Chemistry, Pharmacy, [illegible] the Pharmacopoeias of the United States and Great Britain [illegible] octavo volume of 1628 pages, with over 200 illustrations. [illegible] raised bands [illegible]

[illegible] this work exceeds [illegible] copies have been done up in two parts [illegible] desire to procure the work by mail. [illegible]

EXTRACT FROM THE PREFACE.

"In the rapid progress of modern [illegible] sions of facts than the group of sciences connected with materia medica and [illegible] new resources thus placed at the command of the pharmaceutist and physician have [illegible] authors to justify an attempt to make, from the advanced stand-point of the present day, a concise but complete statement of all that is of practical importance [illegible] that which is old and that which is new shall be brought together [illegible] the most moderate practicable compass, all the [illegible] pensing, which he is likely to need in his daily avocations. [illegible] material, this has required a careful and conscientious [illegible] untrustworthy, or comparatively trivial, without impairing [illegible] work. That they have wholly accomplished their [illegible] they can say that years of constant labor have been [illegible] which the inquirer may refer with the certainty of [illegible] up as worthy of confidence in the [illegible]

"To this end there have been [illegible] drugs and [illegible] preparations official in the Pharmacopoeias of the United States and Great Britain, together with the more important medicines of the French Codex and German Pharmacopoeia, which are to some extent prescribed here, or which may serve for comparison with similar articles in the English and American standards. Besides these, a large number of drugs [illegible] Pharmacopoeia, are often kept in the shops because they are prescribed by physicians or used in domestic practice. Some of these give promise of future importance, and [illegible] among this class of remedies it was deemed best [illegible] on the [illegible]

"The alphabetical order of arrangement has been adopted throughout [illegible] the whole the most convenient for reference. In this the non-official medicines have been included with the official, the latter being distinguished by an affix showing the Pharmacopoeia in which they have been admitted. The title of each article is followed by [illegible] and German, together with Latin [illegible] prescriptions and standard works, [illegible] have thus their appropriate place in the body of the work [illegible] for the Appendix, in which may be found the leading reagents, tables of weights and measures, [illegible] scales of different hydrometers, alcoholometers, and thermometers, [illegible]

"With regard to Pharmacodynamics, there is presented, for the [illegible] succinct account of the physiological action of medicines. The results of [illegible] as clearly as possible, and occasionally in the theoretical language of the day; but as a rule, terms have been employed whose meaning is not likely to become obsolete [illegible]

"In treating of Therapeutics, the most trustworthy results of clinical experience [illegible] set forth, without discussing the grounds on which they rest. [illegible]

"Another feature, novel in a Dispensatory, is the Therapeutical Index. Care has been taken to render it as complete as possible, in order that the inquirer may be enabled to [illegible] all of the more important medicines that have been employed in the treatment of each disease. Such an Index thus becomes, to some extent, a therapeutical classification of medicines, and it is believed must greatly enhance, by its suggestiveness, the working value of the book to the practitioner."

The very thorough manner in which the authors have carried out their [illegible] from the extent of the Indexes. Thus the "Index of Materia Medica" covers [illegible] columned pages, and contains [illegible] references. The "Therapeutical Index" [illegible] under the head of each disease the principal remedies recommended for its treatment, [illegible] double-columned pages, and contains [illegible] references.

FARQUHARSON (ROBERT), M.D.,

Lecturer on Materia Medica [illegible] Hospital Medical School.

A GUIDE TO THERAPEUTICS. Edited, with Additions, [illegible] the U. S. Pharmacopoeia. By FRANK WOODBURY, M.D. [illegible] volume of over [illegible] pages. [illegible]

Many persons who [illegible] the physiological action of remedies [illegible] students find it difficult to discover [illegible] physiological action [illegible] from ordinary text-books. Dr. Farquharson [illegible] ingeniously shown [illegible] the two in parallel columns [illegible] running the eye down the left-hand side [illegible] get the physiological action of a drug, and on the right-hand the therapeutical [illegible]

[illegible] the work is likely to be useful, [illegible] between the [illegible]

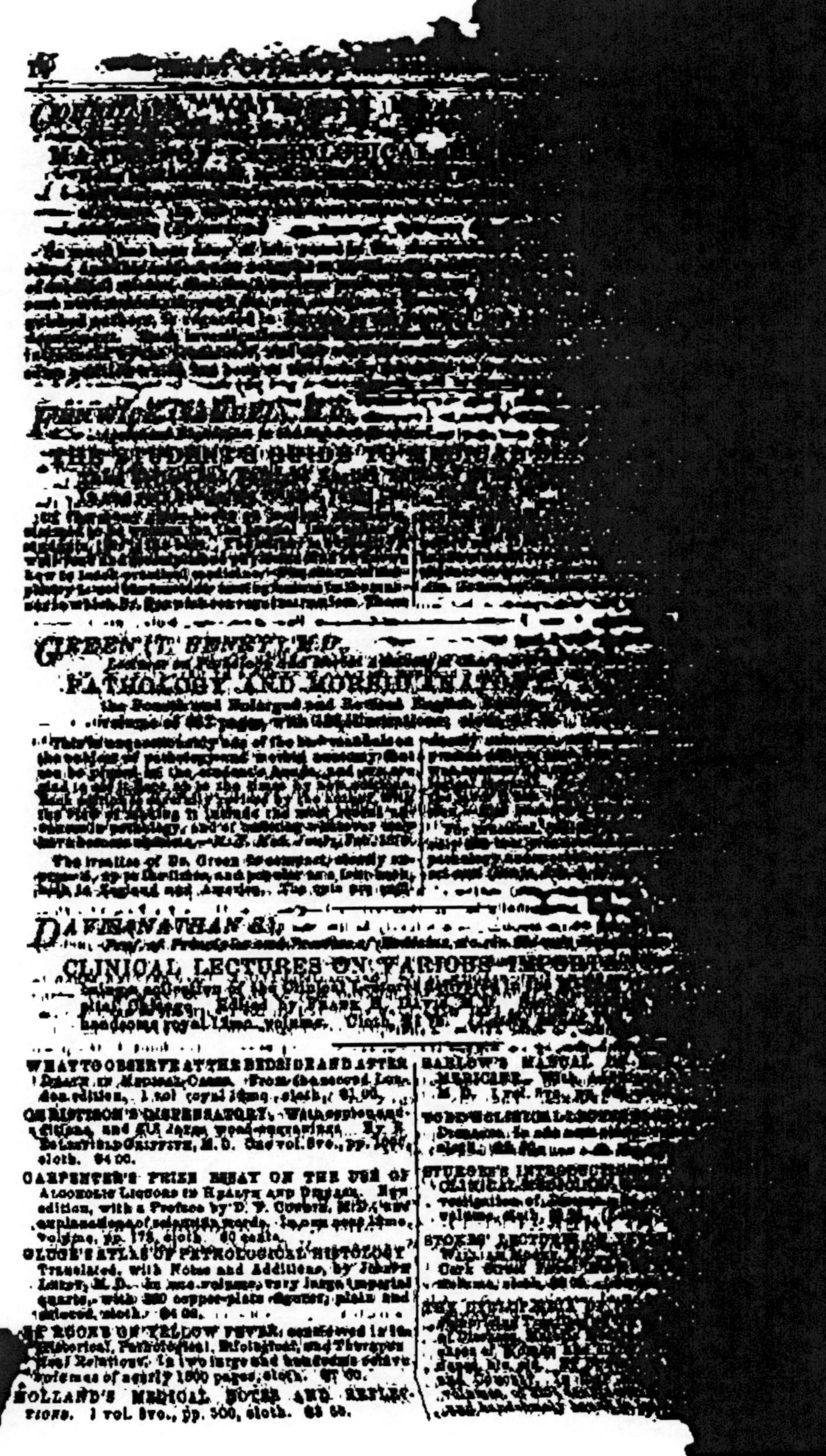

GREEN (T. HENRY), M.D.

PATHOLOGY AND MORBID ANATOMY.

The treatise of Dr. Green is compact, clearly ... England and America.

DA ... NATHAN S.,

CLINICAL LECTURES ON VARIOUS IMPORTANT ...

... Edited by FRANK H. DAVIS ... handsome royal 12mo. volume. Cloth, ...

WHAT TO OBSERVE AT THE BEDSIDE AND AFTER DEATH IN MEDICAL CASES. From the second London edition. 1 vol. royal 12mo., cloth. $1.00.

CHRISTISON'S DISPENSATORY. With copious additions, and 213 large wood-engravings. By R. EGLESFIELD GRIFFITH, M.D. One vol. 8vo., pp. 1000, cloth. $4.00.

CARPENTER'S PRIZE ESSAY ON THE USE OF ALCOHOLIC LIQUORS IN HEALTH AND DISEASE. New edition, with a Preface by D. F. CONDIE, M.D., and explanations of scientific words. In one neat 12mo. volume, pp. 178, cloth. 60 cents.

GLUGE'S ATLAS OF PATHOLOGICAL HISTOLOGY. Translated, with Notes and Additions, by JOSEPH LEIDY, M.D. In one volume, very large imperial quarto, with 320 copper-plate figures, plain and colored, cloth. $4.00.

LA ROCHE ON YELLOW FEVER, considered in its Historical, Pathological, Etiological, and Therapeutical Relations. In two large and handsome octavo volumes of nearly 1500 pages, cloth. $7.00.

HOLLAND'S MEDICAL NOTES AND REFLECTIONS. 1 vol. 8vo., pp. 500, cloth. $3.00.

BARLOW'S MANUAL ... MEDICINE. With ... M.D. 1 vol. ...

STOKES' LECTURES ...

FLINT (AUSTIN), M.D.

Professor of the [illegible]

A TREATISE ON THE PRINCIPLES AND PRACTICE OF MEDICINE; [illegible] edition, revised and enlarged. [illegible]

By common consent of the English and American [illegible] to the highest position as a complete and comprehensive [illegible] of medical science. [illegible]

[illegible]

[illegible] of Sir Thomas Watson. [illegible]

[illegible] English text-books of [illegible] —*British and Foreign Med.-Chir. Rev.* [illegible]

It is of course unnecessary to introduce or eulogize this new standard treatise [illegible] mend it as a text-book, and there are few libraries in which one of its editions is not to be found. The present edition has been enlarged and revised [illegible] reading. [illegible]

[illegible] Dec. '78.

BY THE SAME AUTHOR.

ESSAYS ON CONSERVATIVE MEDICINE AND KINDRED TOPICS.

In one very handsome royal 12mo. volume. [illegible]

WOODBURY (FRANK), M.D.

Physician to the German Hospital, Philadelphia, late Physician to the Out-patient Department of the Jeff. College Hospital, etc.

A HANDBOOK OF THE PRINCIPLES AND PRACTICE OF Medicine; for the use of Students and Practitioners. [illegible] Handbook of Practice. In one 12mo. volume, royal 12mo. [illegible]

HARTSHORNE (HENRY), M.D.

Professor of Hygiene in the University of Pennsylvania.

ESSENTIALS OF THE PRINCIPLES AND PRACTICE OF MEDICINE. A handy-book for Students and Practitioners. [illegible] edition, revised and improved. With about one hundred illustrations. In one handsome royal 12mo. volume, of about 550 pages, cloth, $2 63; half bound, $2 88. [illegible]

As a handbook, which [illegible] do not know its equal. —*N. Y. Med. Journal.* [illegible]

As a brief, condensed, but comprehensive hand-book, it cannot be improved upon. —*Chicago Med. Examiner*, Nov. 15, 1874.

The work is brought fully up to the [illegible]

WATSON (THOMAS), M.D., etc.

LECTURES ON THE PRINCIPLES AND PRACTICE OF PHYSIC. Delivered at King's College, London. A new American from the fifth revised and enlarged English edition, [illegible] by Henry Hartshorne, M.D., Professor of Hygiene in the University of Pennsylvania. In two large [illegible] 8vo. volumes [illegible]

It is a subject for congratulation [illegible] ance that Sir Thomas Watson, during a period of comparative leisure, after a long, laborious, and most honorable professional career, while retaining full possession of his high mental faculties, should have employed the opportunity to [illegible] a more thorough revision than was possible during the earlier and busier period of his life. [illegible] [illegible] tains of his clear insight and his calm judgment are now recorded for the [illegible] The re- [illegible] done, and [illegible] —*Brit. Med. Journal.* [illegible]

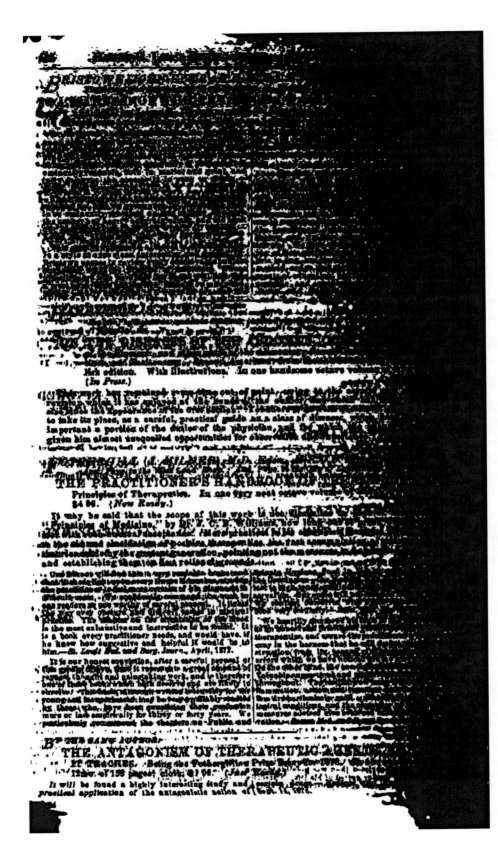

[illegible]

[illegible] edition. With illustrations. In one handsome octavo volume [illegible] (*In Press.*)

This work has remained [illegible] out of print, [illegible] revision which it has enjoyed at the hands of the author [illegible] the appearance of the [illegible] to take its place, as a careful, practical guide in a class of diseases [illegible] important a portion of the duties of the physician, and [illegible] given him almost unequalled opportunities for observation [illegible]

[illegible]

THE PRACTITIONER'S HANDBOOK [illegible]

Principles of Therapeutics. In one very neat octavo volume [illegible] $4 00. (*Now Ready.*)

It may be said that the scope of this work is [illegible] "Principles of Medicine," by Dr. [illegible] Williams, [illegible] [illegible] and establishing them [illegible]

[illegible] is the most exhaustive and instructive to be found. It is a book every practitioner needs, and would have, if he knew how suggestive and helpful it would be to him.—*St. Louis Med. and Surg. Journ.*, April, 1877.

It is our honest conviction, after a careful perusal of [illegible] earnest thought and painstaking work, and is therefore one of those books which [illegible] and are likely to [illegible] more or less empirically for thirty or forty years. We particularly [illegible] the chapters on Public and [illegible]

[illegible] therapeutics, and [illegible] away in the harness that he [illegible] errors which we have [illegible] On the other hand, [illegible] throughout. [illegible] logical conditions, and [illegible] measures [illegible]

BY THE SAME AUTHOR.

THE ANTAGONISM OF THERAPEUTIC AGENTS [illegible]

IT TEACHES. Being the Fothergillian Prize Essay for 1878. [illegible] 12mo. of 156 pages; cloth, $1 00. (*Just Ready.*)

It will be found a highly interesting study and [illegible] practical application of the antagonistic action of [illegible]

FINLAYSON (JAMES), M.D.

Physician and [illegible] in the Glasgow Western Infirmary, &c.

CLINICAL DIAGNOSIS; A Handbook for Students and Practitioners of Medicine. [illegible] Cloth, $2 62. (Just Ready.)

The co-operation of gentlemen specially familiar with [illegible] of Prof. Gairdner, who has contributed the chapter on the [illegible] Stephenson that on Disorders of the Female Organs [illegible] Prof. Simpson [illegible] Chapters on the Fauces, Larynx, [illegible] examinations. Other chapters [illegible] the advantage of [illegible] versed in their several subjects, and the [illegible] the most advanced condition of knowledge in a department which has made such [illegible] of advancement within the last few years.

The book is an excellent one, clear, concise, convenient, practical. It is replete with the very knowledge the student needs when he quits the lecture-room and the laboratory for the wards and [illegible], and does not lack in information that will meet the wants of experienced and older men.—*Phila. Med. Times*, Jan. [illegible]

"The aim of the treatise is to teach a student and practitioner how to [illegible] his knowledge" in arriving at a diagnosis. All the various symptoms of the several systems are grouped together in such a manner as to [illegible] [illegible] diagnosis [illegible]. This work has been done by men of large experience and trained observation, who have been long recognized as authorities upon the subjects which they treat. There is a profusion of illustrations to illustrate subjects under discussion. The application of electricity, and instruments of precision [illegible] is fully discussed. This book is all good. We recommend it to all students and practitioners of medicine as a work worthy of a place in their [illegible].—*N. Y. Med. Recorder*, Dec. 1878.

This is one of the really useful books [illegible] [illegible]

HAMILTON (ALLAN McLANE), M.D.

Attending Physician at the Hospital for Epileptics and Paralytics, Blackwell's Island, N. Y., and at the Out-Patient Department of the New York Hospital.

NERVOUS DISEASES; THEIR DESCRIPTION AND TREATMENT.

In one handsome octavo volume of [illegible] pages, with [illegible] illustrations. [illegible] (Just Ready.)

This is unquestionably the best and most complete text-book of nervous diseases that has yet appeared, and were international jealousy in scientific affairs at all possible, we might be excused for a feeling of chagrin that it should be of American [illegible]. This work, however, has been [illegible] in New York, and has been [illegible] that no room is left for anything but commendation. With great skill, Dr. Hamilton has presented to his readers a succinct and lucid survey of all that is known of the pathology of the nervous system, viewed in the light of the most recent researches. From the preliminary description of the methods of examination and study, and of the instruments of precision employed in the investigation of nervous diseases, up till the final [illegible], the book is eminently practical.—*Brain*, London, Oct. 1878.

The author tells us in his preface that it has been his object to produce a concise, practical book, and we think he has been successful, considering the extent of the subject which he has undertaken. In fact, it is more extensive than the title properly or accurately indicates, embracing—besides what are usually regarded as nervous diseases—inflammatory affections, both acute and chronic, hemorrhages and tumors of the cerebrum and cerebellum, medulla oblongata, spinal cord and meninges, while thrombosis and embolism of the arteries, sinuses and veins. The reader may therefore expect information, more or less full and satisfactory, [illegible] [illegible] connected with the nervous system. We have no hesitation in saying that reliance may be placed on Dr. Hamilton's [illegible] [illegible] [illegible] Oct. 1878.

[illegible] the whole work, we can [illegible] not only clearly and fully treated of diagnosis and treatment, but, unlike most works of this class, is [illegible] in regard to etiology, and [illegible] the pathology of nervous diseases in the light of the very latest experiments and discoveries. The drawings are excellent and well selected. After this careful revision, we can heartily recommend this work to students and general practitioners in particular as being a full [illegible] of the nervous system, their pathology and treatment [illegible].—[illegible] Aug. [illegible]

As stated in the preface, the author's object has been to write a concise and practical book, for which there is certainly a place, and we think he has succeeded admirably in fulfilling his object. The usual plan is adopted in the consideration of [illegible] July, 1878.

CHARCOT (J. M.)

Professor to the Faculty of Med. Paris, Physician to the Salpêtrière, &c.

LECTURES ON DISEASES OF THE NERVOUS SYSTEM. Translated from the Second Edition by George Sigerson, M.D., M.Ch., [illegible] etc., Cath. Univ. of Ireland. With illustrations. (Publishing in the Medical News and Library, commencing with the July No. 1878. See page [illegible].)

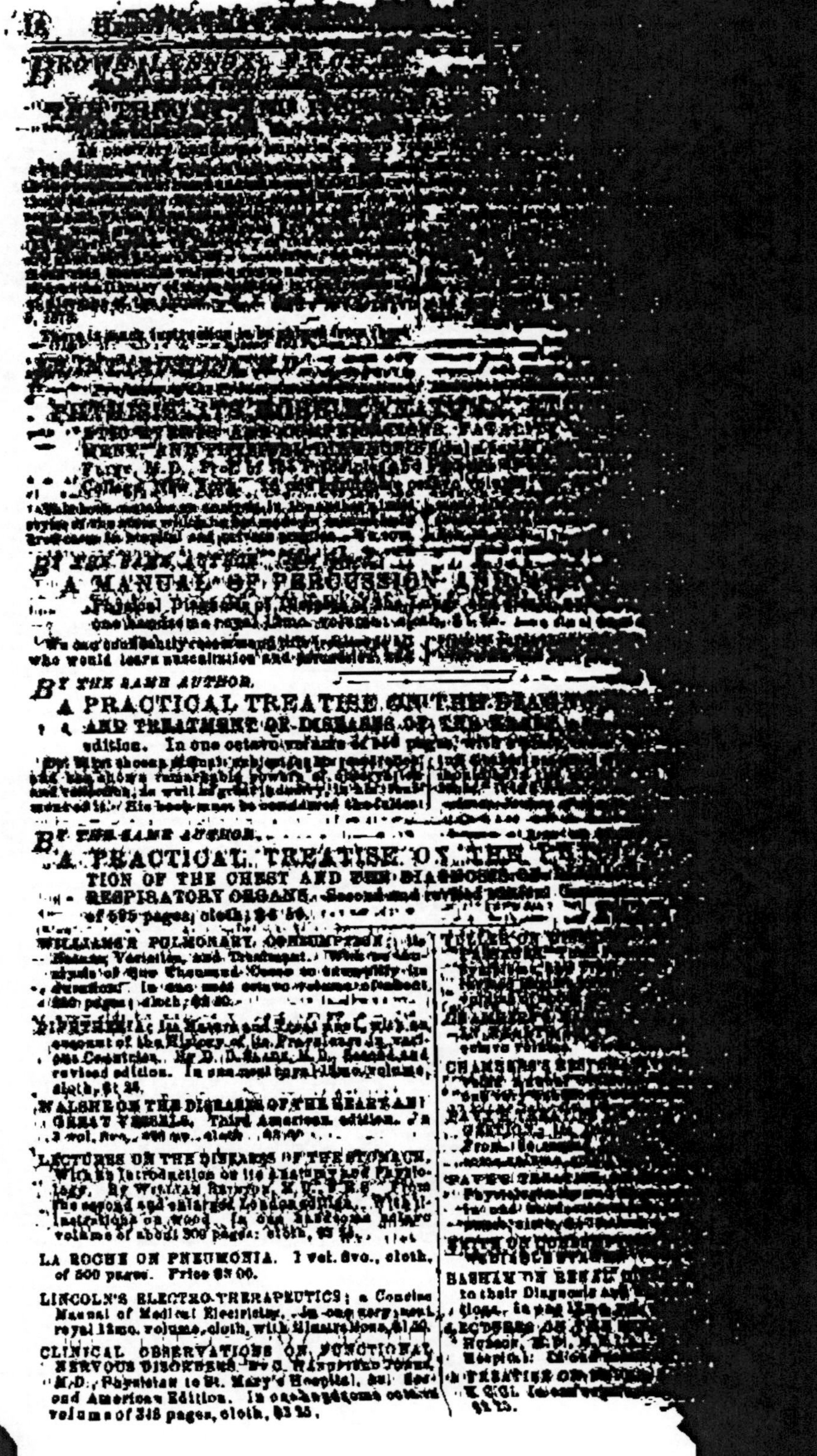

BY THE SAME AUTHOR.

A MANUAL OF PERCUSSION [illegible]

who would learn auscultation and percussion [illegible]

BY THE SAME AUTHOR.

A PRACTICAL TREATISE ON THE [illegible] AND TREATMENT OF DISEASES OF THE [illegible] edition. In one octavo volume of [illegible] pages, [illegible]

[illegible] has shown remarkable powers of [illegible] His book must be considered the fullest [illegible]

BY THE SAME AUTHOR.

A PRACTICAL TREATISE ON THE [illegible] TION OF THE CHEST AND THE DIAGNOSIS [illegible] RESPIRATORY ORGANS. Second and revised edition [illegible] of 595 pages, cloth, $4 50.

WILLIAMS'S PULMONARY CONSUMPTION; its Nature, Variation, and Treatment. With an Analysis of One Thousand Cases to exemplify its duration. In one neat octavo volume of about [illegible] pages, cloth, $2 50.

DIPHTHERIA; its Nature and Treatment, with an account of the History of its Prevalence in various Countries. By D. D. Slade, M.D. Second and revised edition. In one neat royal 12mo. volume, cloth, $1 25.

WALSHE ON THE DISEASES OF THE HEART AND GREAT VESSELS. Third American edition. In 1 vol. 8vo., [illegible] pp., cloth. $3 [illegible]

LECTURES ON THE DISEASES OF THE STOMACH. With an Introduction on its Anatomy and Physiology. By William Brinton, M.D., F.R.S. From the second and enlarged London edition. With illustrations on wood. In one handsome octavo volume of about 300 pages; cloth, $3 [illegible]

LA ROCHE ON PNEUMONIA. 1 vol. 8vo., cloth, of 500 pages. Price $3 00.

LINCOLN'S ELECTRO-THERAPEUTICS; a Concise Manual of Medical Electricity. In one very neat royal 12mo. volume, cloth, with illustrations, $1 50.

CLINICAL OBSERVATIONS ON FUNCTIONAL NERVOUS DISORDERS. By C. Handfield Jones, M.D., Physician to St. Mary's Hospital, &c. Second American Edition. In one handsome octavo volume of 348 pages, cloth, $3 25.

BASHAM ON RENAL [illegible] to their Diagnosis and [illegible]

BUMSTEAD (FREEMAN J.), M.D.,

Professor of Venereal Diseases at the Col. of Phys. and Surgs. New York, etc.

THE PATHOLOGY AND TREATMENT OF VENEREAL DISEASES. Including the results of recent investigations upon the subject. Third edition, revised and enlarged, with illustrations. In one large and handsome octavo volume of over 700 pages, cloth, $5 00; leather, $6 00.

In preparing this standard work again for the press, the author has [illegible] thorough revision. Many portions have been rewritten, and much new matter added [illegible] bring it completely on a level with the most advanced condition of [illegible] ... [illegible] of the text of previous editions, the work has been increased by [illegible] pages. The labor thus bestowed upon it, it is hoped, will insure for it a continuance of the position as a complete and trustworthy guide for the practitioner.

[illegible] work on Venereal Diseases, which has not only been a wide circulation in this country, but been accepted as the standard, but appears to have [illegible], to a large extent, of many of the books and articles which have been written on the same subject and published in England.—*The Glasgow Med. Journ.*, Oct. 1877.

It is the most complete book with which we are acquainted in the language. The latest views of the best authorities are put forward, and the information is well arranged—a great point for the student and still more for the practitioner. The subjects of visceral syphilis, syphilitic affections of the eyes, and the treatment of syphilis by repeated inoculations, are very fully discussed.—*London Lancet*, [illegible], 1877.

Dr. Bumstead's work is already so universally known as the best treatise in the English language on venereal diseases, that it may seem almost superfluous [illegible] ... [illegible] new edition [illegible] much special attention [illegible] ... on a class of diseases which form a large share of nearly every physician's practice [illegible] ... [illegible].

It is safe to say [illegible] ... book which contains all that a practitioner needs to know [illegible] ... [illegible] ... [illegible] or treatment of these affections.—[illegible] *Journal*, March, 1878.

CULLERIER (A.),

Surgeon to the Hôpital du Midi.

BUMSTEAD (FREEMAN J.),

Professor of Venereal Diseases at the Col. of Phys. and Surgs., New York.

AN ATLAS OF VENEREAL DISEASES. Translated and Edited by FREEMAN J. BUMSTEAD. In one large imperial 4to. volume of 328 pages, double columns, with 26 plates, containing about 150 figures, beautifully colored, many of them the size of life; strongly bound in cloth, $17 00; also, in five parts, stout wrappers, at $3 per part.

Anticipating a very large sale for this work, it is offered at the very low price of THREE DOLLARS a Part, thus placing it within the reach of all who are interested in this department of practice. Gentlemen desiring early impressions of the plates would do well to order it without delay.

A specimen of the plates and text sent free by mail, on receipt of 25 cents.

We wish for once that our province was not restricted to [illegible] of [illegible], that we might say something of the exquisite colored plates in this volume.—*London Practitioner*, May, 1869.

As a whole, it teaches all that can be taught by means of plates and print.—*London Lancet*, March 13, 1869.

Superior to anything of the kind ever before issued on [illegible].—*Canada Med. Journal*, March, '69.

The practitioner who desires to understand this branch of medicine thoroughly should obtain this, the most complete and best work ever published.—*Dominion Med. Journal*, May, 1869.

This is a work of master hands on both sides. M. Cullerier is [illegible] ... [illegible] ... [illegible] ... Dr. Bumstead, as an authority, is without a rival. Assuring our readers that these illustrations tell the whole history of venereal disease, from its inception to the end, we do not know a single medical work which for its kind is more necessary for them to have.—*California Med. Gazette*, March, 1869.

The most splendidly illustrated work in the language, and in our opinion far more useful than the French original.—*Am. Journ. Med. Sciences*, Jan. '69.

The [illegible] ... work has reached us, and we have no hesitation in saying that its illustrations surpass those of previous numbers.—*Bost. Med. and Surg. Journ.*, Jan. 14, 1869.

Other writers besides M. Cullerier have given us a good account of the diseases of which he treats, but no one has furnished us with such a complete series of illustrations of the venereal diseases. There is, however, an additional interest and value possessed by the volume before us; for it is an American reprint and translation of M. Cullerier's work, with incidental remarks by one of the most eminent American syphilographers, Mr. Bumstead.—*Brit. and For. Medico-Chir. Review*, July, 1869.

LEE (HENRY),

Prof. of Surgery at the Royal College of Surgeons of England, etc.

LECTURES ON SYPHILIS AND ON SOME FORMS OF LOCAL DISEASE AFFECTING PRINCIPALLY THE ORGANS OF GENERATION. In one handsome octavo volume: cloth, $2 25. (*Lately Published.*)

The work is valuable, as it treats quite fully of subjects which are not dwelt upon in the systematic works of other English authors of the present day, as the transmissibility of syphilitic blood; the conditions under which the discharges of primary and secondary syphilitic manifestations may be inoculated naturally or artificially; the morbid processes produced by such inoculation; the modifications of those [illegible] patients previously syphilitic; primary and secondary syphilitic diseases of the [illegible] ... [illegible] to constitutional syphilis, etc. The book is full of [illegible] ... [illegible].—*Archives of Dermatology*, April, 1875.

HILL (BERKELEY),

Surgeon to the Lock Hospital, London.

ON SYPHILIS AND LOCAL CONTAGIOUS DISORDERS. In one handsome octavo volume; cloth, $3 25.

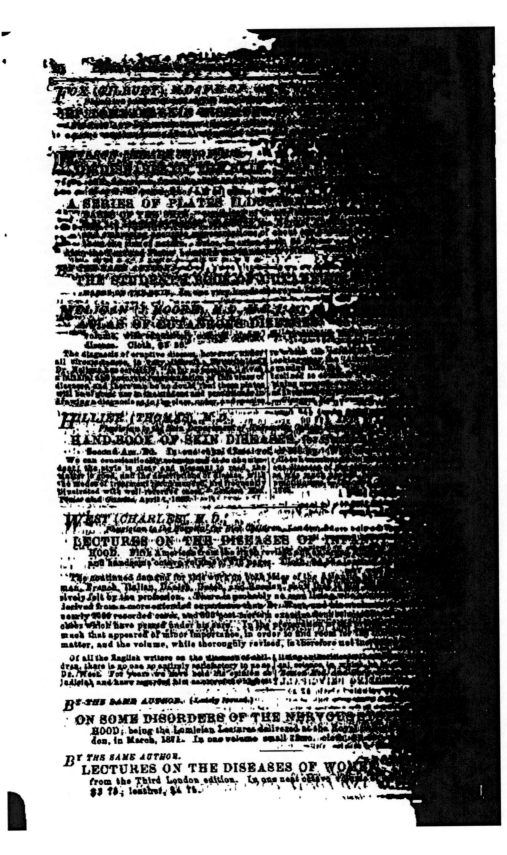

A SERIES OF PLATES ILLUS[illegible]

[illegible]

NELIGAN (J. MOORE), M.D., M.R.I.A.

ATLAS OF CUTANEOUS DISEASES. [illegible] volume, with [illegible] diseases. Cloth, $5 50.

The diagnosis of eruptive disease, however, under all circumstances, is very difficult. [illegible] Dr. Neligan has certainly [illegible] a faithful and accurate representation of this class of diseases, and there can be no doubt that these plates will be of great use to the student and practitioner in drawing a diagnosis as to the class, order, and species [illegible]

HILLIER (THOMAS), M.D.,
Physician to the Skin Department of [illegible]

HAND-BOOK OF SKIN DISEASES, [illegible] Second Am. Ed. In one royal 12mo. vol. [illegible]

We can conscientiously recommend it to the student; the style is clear and pleasant to read, the matter is good, and the descriptions of disease, with the modes of treatment recommended, are frequently illustrated with well-recorded cases.—*London Med. Times and Gazette*, April [illegible]

WEST (CHARLES), M.D.,
Physician to the Hospital for Sick Children, London, [illegible]

LECTURES ON THE DISEASES OF INFAN[illegible]HOOD. Fifth American from the sixth revised [illegible] and handsome octavo volume of [illegible] pages. Cloth, [illegible]

The continued demand for this work on both sides of the Atlantic [illegible] man, French, Italian, Danish, Dutch, and Russian, [illegible] sively felt by the profession. There is probably no man living [illegible] derived from a more extended experience than Dr. West [illegible] nearly 2000 recorded cases, and 600 post-mortem examinations [illegible] cases which have passed under his care. In the preparation [illegible] much that appeared of minor importance, in order to find room for the [illegible] matter, and the volume, while thoroughly revised, is therefore not in[illegible]

Of all the English writers on the diseases of children, there is no one so entirely satisfactory to us as Dr. West. For years we have held his opinion as judicial, and have regarded him as [illegible] highest [illegible]

BY THE SAME AUTHOR. (*Lately Issued.*)

ON SOME DISORDERS OF THE NERVOUS [illegible] HOOD; being the Lumleian Lectures delivered at the Royal [illegible] don, in March, 1871. In one volume small 12mo. cloth, [illegible]

BY THE SAME AUTHOR.

LECTURES ON THE DISEASES OF WOM[illegible] from the Third London edition. In one neat octavo volume [illegible] $3 75; leather, $4 75.

SMITH (J. LEWIS), M.D.,

Clinical Professor of Diseases of Children in the Bellevue Hospital Med. College, N.Y.

A COMPLETE PRACTICAL TREATISE ON THE DISEASES OF CHILDREN. Fourth Edition, revised and enlarged. In one handsome octavo volume of about 750 pages, with illustrations. [illegible]

The very marked favor with which this work has been received [illegible] the author [illegible] no pains in the endeavor to render it [illegible] in every respect [illegible] Many portions of the volume have been rewritten [illegible] but by an earnest effort at condensation the size of the work has not [illegible] increased. It is now passing rapidly through the press, and [illegible]

CONDIE (D. FRANCIS), M.D.

A PRACTICAL TREATISE ON THE DISEASES OF CHILDREN. Sixth edition, revised and augmented. In one large octavo volume of nearly 800 closely printed pages, cloth, $5 25; leather, $6 25.

The present edition, which is the sixth, is fully up to the times in the discussion of all those points in the pathology and treatment of infantile diseases which have been brought forward by the German and French [illegible] As a whole, however, the work is the best American one that we have, and in its special adaptation to American [illegible] — *New York Med. Record*, [illegible]

SMITH (EUSTACE), M.D.,

Physician to the Northwest London Free Dispensary for Sick Children.

A PRACTICAL TREATISE ON THE WASTING DISEASES OF INFANCY AND CHILDHOOD. Second American, from the second revised and enlarged English edition. In one handsome octavo volume, cloth, $2 50. (*Lately Issued.*)

This is in every way an admirable book. The modest title which the author has chosen for it barely conveys an adequate idea of the many subjects upon which it treats. Wasting is so constant an attendant upon the maladies of childhood, that a treatise upon the wasting diseases of children must necessarily embrace the consideration of many affections of which it is a symptom; and this is excellently well done by Dr. Smith. The book might fairly be described as a practical handbook of the common diseases of children, so arranged as [illegible] either collectively or directly. We are acquainted with no safer guide to the treatment of children's diseases, and few books give the insight into the [illegible] and other peculiarities of children that Dr. Smith's book does. — *Brit. Med. Journal*, April 8, 1871.

SWAYNE (JOSEPH GRIFFITHS), M.D.,

Physician-Accoucheur to the British General Hospital, &c.

OBSTETRIC APHORISMS FOR THE USE OF STUDENTS COMMENCING MIDWIFERY PRACTICE. Second American, from the Fifth and Revised London Edition, with Additions by E. R. Hutchins, M.D. With Illustrations. In one neat 12mo. volume. Cloth, $1 25. (*Lately Issued.*)

*** See p. 4 of this Catalogue for the terms on which this work is offered as a premium to subscribers to the "American Journal of the Medical Sciences."

CHURCHILL ON THE PUERPERAL FEVER AND OTHER DISEASES PECULIAR TO WOMEN. 1 vol. 8vo., pp. 450, cloth. $2 50.

DEWEES'S TREATISE ON THE DISEASES OF FEMALES. With illustrations. Eleventh Edition, with the Author's last improvements and corrections. In one octavo volume of 536 pages, with plates, cloth. $3 00.

MEIGS ON THE NATURE, SIGNS, AND TREATMENT OF CHILDBED FEVERS. 1 vol. 8vo., pp. 346, cloth. $2 00.

ASHWELL'S PRACTICAL TREATISE ON THE DISEASES PECULIAR TO WOMEN. Third American from the Third and revised London edition. 1 vol. 8vo., pp. 528, cloth. $3 50.

HODGE (HUGH L.), M.D.,

Emeritus Professor of Obstetrics, &c., in the University of Pennsylvania.

ON DISEASES PECULIAR TO WOMEN; including Displacements of the Uterus. With original illustrations. Second edition, revised and enlarged. In one beautifully printed octavo volume of 531 pages, cloth. $4 50.

Professor Hodge's work is truly an original one from beginning to end, consequently no one can peruse its pages without learning something [illegible] contribution to the literature of [illegible] is of great value, and is abundantly able to stand on its own merits. — *N. Y. Medical Record*, [illegible]

CHURCHILL (FLEETWOOD), M.D., M.R.I.A.

ON THE THEORY AND PRACTICE OF MIDWIFERY. A new American from the fourth revised and enlarged London edition. With notes and additions by D. Francis Condie, M.D., author of a "Practical Treatise on the Diseases of Children," &c. With one hundred and ninety-four illustrations. In one very handsome octavo volume of nearly 700 large pages. Cloth, $4 00; leather, $5 00.

MONTGOMERY'S EXPOSITION OF THE SIGNS AND SYMPTOMS OF PREGNANCY. With two exquisite colored plates, and numerous wood-cuts. In 1 vol. 8vo., of nearly 600 pp., cloth. $3 75.

RIGBY'S SYSTEM OF MIDWIFERY. With notes and Additional Illustrations. Second American edition. One volume octavo, cloth, 422 pages. $2 50.

THOMAS (T. GAILLARD), M.D.

[illegible]

... pages, with [illegible] illustrations [illegible]

[illegible]

A work which [illegible] that too, in the short space of [illegible] years, has attained a reputation which places it almost beyond the reach of criticism, and the favorable opinions which we have already expressed of the former editions [illegible] that [illegible] this new issue. We cannot [illegible] as a practical work, [illegible] lish, or, indeed, in any other language. This arrangement of the contents, the admirable [illegible] in which the subject of the [illegible] of the diseases is handled, [illegible] desired by the practitioner [illegible] clinical work, one to which he can refer in cases of doubtful diagnosis with the certainty of obtaining light and instruction. Dr. Thomas is a man with a very clear head and decided views, and there seems to be nothing which he [illegible] position. The [illegible] who will [illegible] study this book [illegible] certainly [illegible].—*London Lancet*, Feb. 12, 1876.

[illegible] to close this [illegible] notice of so excellent a work, and in conclusion would remark that, as a teacher of gynecology, both didactic and clinical, Prof. Thomas has [illegible] the [illegible] of his [illegible], and as an author he certainly has met with unusual and merited success.—*Am. Journ. of Obstetrics*, Nov. 1876.

This volume of Prof. Thomas in its revised form [illegible]

BARNES (ROBERT), M.D., F.R.C.P.,

Obstetric Physician to St. Thomas's Hospital, [illegible]

A CLINICAL EXPOSITION OF THE [illegible] CAL DISEASES OF WOMEN.

Second American [illegible] from the [illegible] English Edition. In one handsome octavo volume of [illegible] Cloth, \$4.50; leather, \$5.50. (*Just Ready.*)

The call for a new edition of Dr. Barnes' work on the Diseases of [illegible] the author to make it even more worthy of the favor of the profession [illegible] rangement and careful printing space has been found for [illegible] Relations of the Bladder and Bowel Disorders, without [illegible] many new illustrations have been introduced [illegible] is therefore hoped that the volume will be found to [illegible] condition of gynæcological science.

Dr. Barnes stands at the head of his profession in the old country, and it requires but scant scrutiny of his book to show that it has been sketched by a master. It is plain, practical common sense; shows very deep research without being pedantic; is eminently calculated to inspire enthusiasm without inculcating rashness; points out the dangers to be avoided as well as the success to be achieved in the various operations connected with this branch of medicine; and will do much to smooth the rugged path of the young gynæcologist and relieve the perplexity of the man of mature years.—*Canadian Journ. of Med. Science*, Nov. 1876.

We pity the doctor who, having any considerable practice in diseases of women, has no copy of "Barnes" for daily consultation and instruction. It is, at once a work of great learning, research, and individual experience, and at the same time eminently practical. That it has been appreciated by the profession, both in Great Britain and in this country, is shown by the second edition following so soon upon the first.—*Am. Practitioner*, Nov. 1876.

Dr. Barnes's work is one of a practical character, largely illustrated from cases in his own experience, but by no means confined to such, as will be learned from the fact that he quotes from no less than [illegible] medical authors in numerous countries. Coming from such an author, it is not necessary to say that the work is [illegible] consulted by the profession [illegible] *Journ. of British and* [illegible]

No other [illegible] diseases of women [illegible] fully [illegible] of his library, and the [illegible] text-book.—[illegible]

This second [illegible] the American [illegible] additions [illegible] all the additions in our [illegible] have been made [illegible] tion. The American [illegible] work, [illegible] cordially recommend [illegible] are.—*Journal of* [illegible] 1876.

This second [illegible] seems to be [illegible] ments which bring it up [illegible] The excellence of the work [illegible] require [illegible] that they will [illegible] which as a standard [illegible] students and practitioners [illegible] Oct. 1876.

EMMET (THOMAS ADDIS), M.D. [illegible]

Surgeon to the Woman's Hospital, New York, &c. [illegible]

THE PRINCIPLES AND PRACTICE OF GYNÆCOLOGY; for the use of Students and Practitioners of Medicine. [illegible] octavo volume of nearly 900 pages, with numerous illustrations. [illegible]

Dr Emmet is so widely known as among the most eminent of those who have made gynæcology a peculiar American science, that the profession cannot [illegible] condensed the results of his long and extensive experience. [illegible] the whole subject of the diseases peculiar to females in a manner [illegible] not only to the wants of the student as a text-book, but to those of [illegible] the emergencies of daily practice. A special feature of the work will be [illegible] condensed tables, which convey at a glance, and within the narrowest [illegible] to be drawn from the many thousand cases which have passed under the [illegible]. With trifling exceptions, the illustrations are all original, and the volume will be [illegible] point of typographical execution worthy of the distinguished position which is [illegible] cipated for it.

CHADWICK (JAMES R.), A.M., M.D.

A MANUAL OF THE DISEASES PECULIAR TO WOMEN. [illegible] neat volume, royal 12mo., with illustrations. (Preparing.)

America has contributed so largely to the advances which have made [illegible] eases of Women a distinctive department of medical science, that the student [illegible] turn to American Books for the latest and most [illegible] most modern aspect. Yet there has thus far been no attempt [illegible] manual, presenting in a condensed and convenient form the information [illegible] or for the general practitioner. This want it has been the effort of the [illegible] the special attention which he has devoted to the subject is a guarantee of the value of [illegible]. A distinguishing feature of the work will be a number of diagrammatic illustrations [illegible] greatly the comprehension of the text.

WINCKEL (F.).

Professor and Director of the Gynæcological Clinic in the University of [illegible]

A COMPLETE TREATISE ON THE PATHOLOGY AND TREATMENT OF CHILDBED, for Students and Practitioners. Translated, with the consent of the author, from the Second German Edition, by JAMES READ CHADWICK, M.D. [illegible] octavo volume. Cloth, $4 00. (Lately Issued.)

This work was written, as the author tells us in his preface, to supply a want arising from the very brief consideration given to puerperal diseases by writers on Obstetrics, in which respect the state of the profession in his country is not different from ours, and to fill a blank left between the treatises upon the subject already in the field, and the present [illegible]. The work has reached a second edition, and bears evidence [illegible] of careful study and practical experience. As [illegible] rather than [illegible].—*American Journal of* [illegible], April, 1881.

THE OBSTETRICAL JOURNAL. (Free of postage for 1879.)

THE OBSTETRICAL JOURNAL of Great Britain and Ireland; including MIDWIFERY, and the DISEASES OF WOMEN AND INFANTS. With an American Supplement, edited by J. V. INGHAM, M.D. A monthly of about 80 octavo pages, very handsomely printed. Subscription, Five Dollars per annum. Single Numbers, 50 cents each.

Commencing with April, 1873, the Obstetrical Journal consists of Original Papers by British and Foreign Contributors; Transactions of the Obstetrical Societies in England and abroad; Reports of Hospital Practice; Reviews and Bibliographical Notices; Articles and Notes, Editorial, Historical, Forensic, and Miscellaneous; Selections from Journals; Correspondence, &c. Collecting together the vast amount of material daily accumulating in this important and rapidly improving department of medical science, the value of the information which it presents to the subscriber may be estimated from the character of the gentlemen who have already promised their support, including such names as Drs. [illegible], J. HENRY BENNET, NATHAN BOZEMAN, THOMAS CHAMBERS, FLEETWOOD CHURCHILL, CHARLES CLAY, JOHN CLAY, MATTHEWS DUNCAN, ARTHUR FARRE, ROBERT GREENHALGH, GRAILY HEWITT, BRAXTON HICKS, ALFRED MEADOWS, W. LEISHMAN, ALEX. SIMPSON, HEYWOOD SMITH, TYLER SMITH, EDWARD J. TILT, LAWSON TAIT, SPENCER WELLS, &c. &c.; in short, the representative men of British Obstetrics and Gynæcology.

In order to render the OBSTETRICAL JOURNAL fully adequate to the wants of the American profession, each number contains a Supplement devoted to the progress made in Obstetrics and Gynæcology on this side of the Atlantic. This portion of the Journal is under the editorial charge of Dr. J. V. INGHAM, to whom editorial communications, exchanges, books for review, &c., may be addressed, to the care of the publisher.

*** Complete sets from the beginning can no longer be furnished, but subscriptions can commence with Vol. VI., No. 1, April, 1878, or January, 1879.

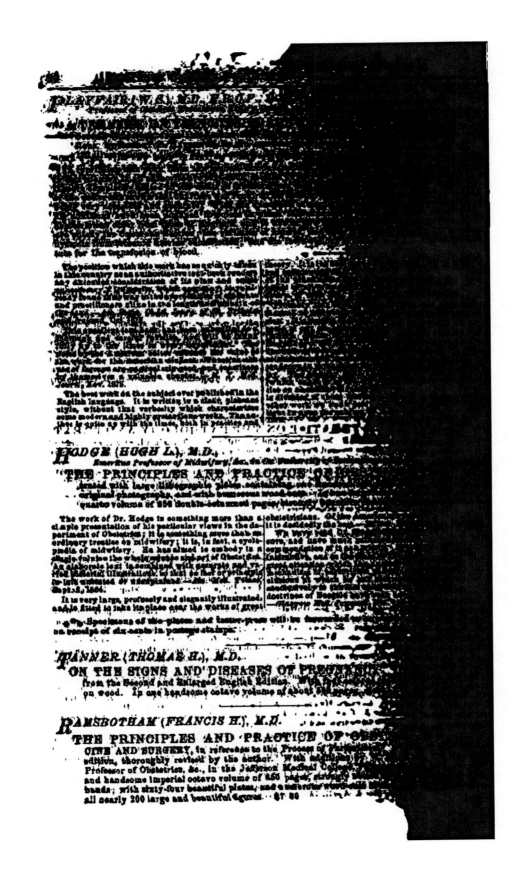

PLAYFAIR (W. S.), M.D., F.R.C.P. [illegible]

[illegible]

tute for the transfusion of blood.

The position which this work has so quickly attained in this country as an authoritative text-book renders any extended consideration of its plan and scope [illegible] ... and practitioners alike in the length and breadth [illegible]

[illegible]

The best work on the subject ever published in the English language. It is written in a clear, pleasant style, without that verbosity which characterizes some modern and highly pretentious works. ... that is quite up with the times, both in practice and [illegible]

[illegible]

HODGE (HUGH L.), M.D.,

Emeritus Professor of Midwifery, &c., in the University of [illegible]

THE PRINCIPLES AND PRACTICE OF [illegible] ...trated with large lithographic plates containing [illegible] original photographs, and with numerous wood-cuts. [illegible] quarto volume of 550 double-columned pages, [illegible]

The work of Dr. Hodge is something more than a simple presentation of his particular views in the department of Obstetrics; it is something more than an ordinary treatise on midwifery; it is, in fact, a cyclopædia of midwifery. He has aimed to embody in a single volume the whole science and art of Obstetrics. An elaborate text is combined with accurate and varied pictorial illustrations, so that no fact or principle is left unstated or unexplained.—*Am. Med. Times*, Sept. 3, 1864.

It is very large, profusely and elegantly illustrated, and is fitted to take its place near the works of great obstetricians. Of the [illegible] it is decidedly the [illegible]

We have read [illegible] care, and have much [illegible] commendation of [illegible] [illegible] doctrines of [illegible] —*Glasgow Med. Journal*. [illegible]

☞ Specimens of the plates and letter-press will be forwarded [illegible] on receipt of six cents in postage stamps.

TANNER (THOMAS H.), M.D.

ON THE SIGNS AND DISEASES OF PREG[illegible] from the Second and Enlarged English Edition. [illegible] on wood. In one handsome octavo volume of about [illegible]

RAMSBOTHAM (FRANCIS H.), M.D.

THE PRINCIPLES AND PRACTICE OF OBS[illegible]**CINE AND SURGERY**, in reference to the Process of [illegible] edition, thoroughly revised by the author. With [illegible] Professor of Obstetrics, &c., in the Jefferson Medical College, [illegible] and handsome imperial octavo volume of 650 pages, strongly [illegible] bands; with sixty-four beautiful plates, and numerous wood-cuts [illegible] all nearly 200 large and beautiful figures. $7 00

LEISHMAN (WILLIAM), M.D.,

Regius Professor of [illegible]

A SYSTEM OF MIDWIFERY, INCLUDING THE DISEASES OF PREGNANCY AND THE PUERPERAL STATE. [illegible] and Revised English Edition, with additions by John S. Parry, M.D., Obstetrician to the Philadelphia Hospital, &c. In one large and very handsome octavo volume [illegible] pages, with about two hundred illustrations; cloth, [illegible]

[illegible] many of the leading scholars of medicine [illegible] in a work, we know of no [illegible] our language, [illegible] The value of the book [illegible] edition, which contains [illegible] —*Chicago Med. Journ. and Examiner*, [illegible]

But the most valuable additions to the volume are those made by the American editor. One of the best tests of a man's ability is for him to take a standard work in our profession, like this of Dr. Leishman, and materially improve it. Many a one, with more [illegible] than wisdom, has attempted it with other books and failed. But Dr. Parry has succeeded most admirably. We know no obstetrical work that has anything better [illegible] than that which Dr. Parry has given in this, and no work that has the rational and intelligent views upon lactation with which he has enriched this. Having used "Leishman" for two years as a text-book for students, we can cordially commend it and are quite satisfied to continue such use now.—*Am. Practitioner*, May, 1876.

This new edition decidedly confirms the opinion which we expressed of the first edition of the work, in the May, 1874, number of this Journal, that this is "the best modern work on the subject in the English language." The excellent practical notes contributed by Dr. Parry refer principally to the use of the forceps, [illegible] the puerperal diseases, and are intended to increase the usefulness of the work in this country. An entirely new chapter on diphtheria of puerperal wounds has been [illegible]

[illegible] —*[illegible] Surg. Journal*, Nov. 1876.

PARRY (JOHN S.), M.D.,

Obstetrician to the Philadelphia Hospital, Vice-President of the Obstet. Society of Philadelphia, etc.

EXTRA-UTERINE PREGNANCY; ITS CLINICAL HISTORY, DIAGNOSIS, PROGNOSIS, AND TREATMENT. In one handsome octavo volume. Cloth, $2 50. (*Lately Issued.*)

In this work Dr. Parry has added a most valuable contribution to obstetric literature, and one which meets a want long felt by those of the profession who have ever been called upon to deal with this class of cases.—*Boston Med. and Surg. Journ.*, March 2, 1876.

This work, being as near as possible a collection of the experiences of many persons, will afford a [illegible] guide, both in diagnosis and treatment, for this [illegible] interesting and fatal malady. We think it should be in the hands of all physicians practising midwifery.—*Cincinnati Clinic*, Feb. [illegible], 1876.

STIMSON (LEWIS A.), A.M., M.D.,

Surgeon to the Presbyterian Hospital.

A MANUAL OF OPERATIVE SURGERY. In one very handsome royal 12mo. volume of about 500 pages, with [illegible] illustrations; cloth, $2 50. (*New Ready.*)

The work before us is a well printed, profusely illustrated manual of over four hundred and seventy pages. The novice, by a perusal of the work, will gain a good idea of the general domain of operative surgery, while the practical surgeon has presented to him within a very concise and intelligible form the latest and most approved selections of operative procedure. The precision and conciseness with which the different operations are described enable the author to compress an immense amount of practical information in a very small compass.—*N. Y. Medical Record*, Aug. 3, 1878.

This volume is devoted entirely to operative surgery, and is intended to familiarize the student with the details of operations and the different modes of performing them. The work is handsomely illustrated, and the descriptions are clear and well drawn. It is a [illegible] should possess [illegible] —*Md. Med. Journal*, Aug. 1878.

The author's [illegible] the work [illegible] surgery, and as one of reference to the practitioner. —*Cincinnati Lancet and Clinic*, July [illegible], 1878.

SKEY'S OPERATIVE SURGERY. In 1 vol. 8vo. cl., of 650 pages; with about 100 wood-cuts. [illegible]

COOPER'S LECTURES ON THE PRINCIPLES AND PRACTICE OF SURGERY. In 1 vol. 8vo. cl. 750 p. [illegible]

GIBSON'S INSTITUTES AND PRACTICE OF SURGERY. Eighth edition, improved and altered. With thirty-four plates. In two handsome octavo volumes, about 1000 pp. [illegible]

THE PRINCIPLES AND PRACTICE OF SURGERY. By WILLIAM PIRRIE, F.R.S.E., Professor of Surgery in the University of Aberdeen. Edited by JOHN NEILL, M.D., Professor of Surgery in the Penn. [illegible]

[illegible] Medical College, [illegible] Hospital, [illegible] [illegible] 500 pages, with [illegible] illustrations.

[illegible] PRINCIPLES OF SURGERY. Fourth American, from the Third Edinburgh Edition. In one large 8vo. vol. [illegible] pages, with [illegible] illustrations. [illegible]

[illegible] PRACTICE OF SURGERY. Fourth American, from the [illegible] Edition, [illegible] the American editor. [illegible]

GROSS (SAMUEL D.), M.D.

[illegible]

greater, both in size and worth, in its new edition. The difference in actual number of pages is not more than 130, but the size of the page having been increased to what we believe is technically termed "elephant," there has been [illegible] with the alterations, [illegible]

[illegible] a text-book and work of reference. We think this last edition of Gross's "Surgery," will confirm his title of [illegible]

BY THE SAME AUTHOR.

A PRACTICAL TREATISE ON THE [illegible]

and Malformations of the Urinary Bladder, the Prostate [illegible] Edition, thoroughly Revised and Condensed, by Samuel W. [illegible] the Philadelphia Hospital. In one handsome [illegible] trations: cloth, $4 50. (*Just Issued.*)

[illegible]

BY THE SAME AUTHOR.

A PRACTICAL TREATISE ON FOREIGN [illegible]

AIR-PASSAGES. In 1 vol. 8vo., with illustrations, pp. [illegible]

DRUITT (ROBERT), M.R.C.S., &c.

THE PRINCIPLES AND PRACTICE OF MOD[illegible]

A new and revised American, from the eighth enlarged and [illegible] trated with four hundred and thirty-two wood-engravings [illegible] volume, of nearly 700 large and closely printed pages [illegible]

All that the surgical student or practitioner could desire.—*Dublin Quarterly Journal.*

It is a most admirable book. We do not know when we have examined one with more pleasure.—*Boston Med. and Surg. Journal.*

In Mr. Druitt's book, though containing only some seven hundred pages, both the principles and the [illegible]

ASHHURST (JOHN, Jr.), M.D.,

Prof. of Clinical Surgery, Univ. of Pa., [illegible]

THE PRINCIPLES AND PRACTICE OF SURGERY. [illegible]

edition, enlarged and revised. In one [illegible] 1000 pages, with [illegible] illustrations. Cloth, [illegible]

Conscientiousness and thoroughness are two very marked traits of character in the author of this book. One of these traits largely has given the [illegible] [illegible] [illegible] before. The general arrangement of the edition is the same as in the first edition, but every part has been carefully revised, and much new matter added.—*Phila. Med. Times*, Feb. 1, 1879.

We have previously spoken of Dr. Ashhurst's work in terms of praise. We wish to [illegible] those terms here, and to add that no more satisfactory representation of modern surgery has yet fallen from the press. In point of judicial fairness, of power of condensation, of accuracy and conciseness of expression and thoroughly good English, Prof. Ashhurst has no superior among the surgical writers in America.—*Am. Practitioner*, Jan. 1879.

The attempt to compress in a volume of 1000 pages the whole field of surgery, general and special, would be a hopeless task, unless [illegible] the most [illegible] industry in collating and arranging, and the wisest judgment in condensing and excluding. These qualities have been abundantly employed by the author, and he has given us a most excellent treatise, brought up by the revision for the second edition to the latest date. Of course this book is not designed for specialists, but as a source of general surgical knowledge and for general practitioners and as a text-book for students it is not surpassed by any that has yet appeared, whether of home or foreign authorship.—*N. Carolina Med. Journal*, Jan. 1879.

[illegible] in this country is [illegible] [illegible] numerous additions [illegible] work is not [illegible] of text books of surgery [illegible] [illegible] the [illegible] past.—*Nashville Journ. of Med. and Surg.* [illegible]

The favorable reception of the first edition is [illegible] guarantee of the popularity of this edition, which is fresh from the author's [illegible] and improved. [illegible] [illegible] [illegible] [illegible] [illegible] practical surgery and [illegible] [illegible] practice.—*N. Y. Med. Journal*, Jan. 1879.

The fact that this work has reached a second edition so very soon after the publication of the first one, speaks more highly of its merits than anything we might say in the way of commendation. [illegible] [illegible] [illegible]

HOLMES (TIMOTHY), M.D.,

Surgeon to St. George's Hospital, London.

SURGERY, ITS PRINCIPLES AND PRACTICE. In one hand-

some octavo volume of nearly 1000 pages, with 411 illustrations. Cloth, $6; leather, $7. (*Just Issued.*)

This is a work which has been looked for on both sides of the Atlantic with much interest. Mr. Holmes is a surgeon of large and varied experience, and one of the best known, and perhaps the most brilliant writer upon surgical subjects in England. It is a book for students—and an admirable one—and for the busy general practitioner. It will give a student all the knowledge needed to pass a rigid examination. The book fairly justifies the high expectations that were formed of it. Its style is clear and forcible, even brilliant at times, and the conciseness needed to bring it within its proper limits has not impaired its [illegible].—*N. Y. Med. Record*, April 15, 1876.

It will be found a most excellent volume of surgery by the general practitioner [illegible] [illegible] and to the medical student. In fact, [illegible] one we can more cordially recommend. The author has succeeded well in giving a plain and practical account of each surgical injury and disease, and of the treatment which is most commonly [illegible]. It will no doubt become a popular work in the profession, and especially as a text-book.—*Cincinnati Med. News*, April, 1876.

HAMILTON (FRANK H.), M.D.,

Professor of Fractures and Dislocations, &c., in Bellevue Hosp. Med. College, New York.

A PRACTICAL TREATISE ON FRACTURES AND DISLOCATIONS.

Fifth edition, revised and improved. In one large and handsome octavo volume of nearly 800 pages, with 344 illustrations. Cloth, $5 75; leather, $6 75. (*Lately Issued.*)

This work is well known, abroad as well as at home, as the highest authority on its important subject—an authority recognized in the courts as well as in the schools and in practice—and again manifested, not only by the demand for a fifth edition, but by arrangements now in progress for the speedy appearance of a translation in Germany. The repeated revisions which the author has thus had the opportunity of making have enabled him to give the most careful consideration to every portion of the volume, and he has sedulously endeavored in the present issue, to perfect the work by the aid of his own enlarged experience and to incorporate in it whatever of value has been added in this department since the issue of the fourth edition. It will therefore be found considerably improved in matter, while the most careful attention has been paid to the typographical execution, and the volume is presented to the profession in the confident hope that it will more than maintain its very distinguished reputation.

There is no better work on the subject in existence than that of Dr. Hamilton. It should be in the possession of every general practitioner and surgeon.—*Am. Journ. of Obstetrics*, Feb. 1876.

The value of a work like this to the practical physician and surgeon can hardly be over-estimated, and the necessity of having such a book revised to the latest date, not merely on account of the practical importance of its teachings, but [illegible] [illegible] the [illegible] of which [illegible] and which have recently been the subject of useful papers by Dr. Hamilton and [illegible] [illegible] The present volume seems to supply all [illegible] We can safely recommend it as the best of its kind in the English language, and not equalled in any other.—*Journ. of Nervous and Mental Disease*, Jan. 1876.

ERICHSEN (JOHN E.),

[illegible]

[illegible] tioner, April, 1873.

[illegible] edition Mr. Erichsen has ever produced of his [illegible] book. Besides inheriting the [illegible] of its predecessors, it possesses excellences quite [illegible]. Having stated that Mr. Erichsen has [illegible] into this edition every [illegible] improvement in the science and art of surgery, it would be a [illegible] tion to give a detailed criticism. In short, we un-hesitatingly aver that we know of no other single work where the student and practitioner can gain at once so clear an insight into the principles of surgery, and so complete a knowledge of the [illegible] of surgical practice.—*London Lancet*, Feb. [illegible], 1873.

For the past twenty years Erichsen's Surgery has maintained its place as the leading text-book, not only in this country, but in Great Britain. That it [illegible] to hold its ground, is abundantly proven by the [illegible] with which the present edition has been revised, and by the large amount of valuable material that has been added. Aside from this, two hundred and fifty new illustrations have been inserted, including quite a number of microscopical appearances of pathological processes. So marked is this change for the better, that the work almost appears as an entirely new one.—*Med. Record*, Feb. 15, 1873.

[illegible] Journal, March, 1873.

GOSSELIN (L.),

Professor of Clinical Surgery in the Faculty of Medicine, Paris, [illegible]

CLINICAL LECTURES ON SURGERY, [illegible] La Charité. Translated from the French by Lewis A. [illegible] Presbyterian Hospital, New York. With Illustrations. [illegible] 350 pages; cloth, $3 50. *(Now Ready.)* From the [illegible]

SUMMARY OF CONTENTS.

PART I. SURGICAL DISEASES OF YOUTH. 5 LECT.
" II. FRACTURES OF THE LIMBS. 18 "
" III. TRAUMATIC OSTEITIS AND NECROSIS. 3 "
PART IV. [illegible]
PART V. [illegible]
" VI. [illegible]

It will be seen from this brief abstract of the contents that these [illegible] which are of daily interest to the practitioner, while some of [illegible] books the attention which their importance deserves.

ASHTON ON THE DISEASES, INJURIES, AND MALFORMATIONS OF THE RECTUM AND ANUS; with remarks on Habitual Constipation. Second American, from the fourth and enlarged London Edition. With illustrations. In one 8vo. vol. of 287 pages. [illegible]

SARGENT ON [illegible] TIONS OF MINOR SURGERY [illegible] An additional [illegible] 12mo. vol. [illegible] $1 75.

BRYANT (THOMAS), F.R.C.S.,

Surgeon to Guy's Hospital.

THE PRACTICE OF SURGERY. Second American, from the Second and Revised English Edition. [illegible] Wood. In one large and very handsome imperial octavo volume of [illegible] closely printed pages. Cloth, $6; leather, $7. (*Just Ready.*)

This work has enjoyed the advantage of two thorough revisions [illegible] the appearance of the first American edition, [illegible] improvement of matter. [illegible] which are here [illegible] a condensed but clear [illegible] be found correspondingly improved.

The marked success of the work on both sides of the Atlantic shows that the author has succeeded in the effort to place [illegible] practice of Surgery; while the simultaneous appearance of [illegible] in this country affords to the American reader the [illegible] advance in surgical science.

BROWNE (EDGAR A.),

[illegible]

HOW TO USE THE OPHTHALMOSCOPE. Being [illegible] Instructions in Ophthalmoscopy, arranged for the Use of Students. With [illegible] tions. In one small volume royal 12mo. of [illegible] pages. Cloth, [illegible] (*Now Ready.*)

This capital little work should be in the hands of every medical student, and would [illegible] every general practitioner. Its explanation of the optical principles on which the ophthalmoscope is [illegible] is so clear and simple that the most stupid reader could scarcely fail of understanding them. [illegible] satisfactory are the directions for the use of [illegible] what is seen.—[illegible]

[illegible]

CARTER (R. BRUDENELL), F.R.C.S.,

Ophthalmic Surgeon to St. George's Hospital, &c.

A PRACTICAL TREATISE ON DISEASES OF THE EYE. Edited, with test-types and Additions, by John Green, M.D. (of St. Louis, Mo.) [illegible] handsome octavo volume of about [illegible] pages, and [illegible] illustrations. Cloth, [illegible] (*Just Issued.*)

Dr. Green, whose reputation and experience in this department are well known, has given this work a very careful revision, and has introduced much matter which will be found of importance to the practitioner. As his system of test-types is the one recommended by the author, they have been inserted in the volume in a shape which will admit of their being [illegible] and mounted for convenient office use.

These test-types, on a sheet for mounting, can be had separate, price [illegible] cents.

It would be difficult for Mr. Carter to write an uninstructive book, and impossible for him to write an uninteresting one. Even on subjects with which he is most bound to be familiar, he can discourse with a rare degree of elegance and effect. Our readers will therefore not be surprised to learn that a work by him on the Diseases of the Eye makes a very valuable addition to ophthalmic literature. . . . The book will remain one useful alike to the general and the special practitioner. Not the least valuable result which we expect from it is that it will to some considerable extent despecialize this brilliant department of medicine.—*London Lancet*, Oct. 30, 1875.

It is with great pleasure that we can endorse the work as a most valuable contribution to practical ophthalmology. Mr. Carter never deviates from the end he has in view, and presents the subject in [illegible] manner, easy of comprehension, and hence [illegible] valuable. We would especially commend [illegible] worthy of high praise, the manner in which [illegible] of diseases of the eye is [illegible] the author is particularly clear and [illegible] writers are [illegible] The final chapter is devoted to a discussion of the uses and selection of spectacles, and is admirably compact, plain, and useful, especially the paragraphs on the treatment of presbyopia and myopia. In conclusion, our thanks are due the author for many useful hints in the great subject of ophthalmic surgery and therapeutics, [illegible] of late years, [illegible] from a [illegible]—*New York Medical Record*, Oct. [illegible], 1876.

WELLS (J. SOELBERG),

Professor of Ophthalmology in King's College Hospital, &c.

A TREATISE ON DISEASES OF THE EYE. Third American, from the Fourth and Revised London Edition, with additions; illustrated with numerous engravings on wood, and six colored plates. Together with selections from the Test-types of Jaeger and Snellen. In one large and very handsome octavo volume. (*Preparing.*)

LAURENCE (JOHN Z.), F.R.C.S.,

Editor of the Ophthalmic Review, &c.

A HANDY-BOOK OF OPHTHALMIC SURGERY, for the use of Practitioners. Second Edition, revised and enlarged. With numerous illustrations. In one very handsome octavo volume, cloth, $2 75.

LAWSON (GEORGE), F.R.C.S., Engl.,

Assistant Surgeon to the Royal London Ophthalmic Hospital, Moorfields, &c.

INJURIES OF THE EYE, ORBIT, AND EYELIDS: their Immediate and Remote Effects. With about one hundred illustrations. In one very handsome octavo volume, cloth, $3 50.

THOMPSON (SIR HENRY),
Surgeon and Professor of Clinical Surgery to University College Hospital.

LECTURES ON DISEASES OF THE URINARY ORGANS. With illustrations on wood. Second American from the Third English Edition. In one neat octavo volume. Cloth, $2 25. (*Just Issued.*)

BY THE SAME AUTHOR.

ON THE PATHOLOGY AND TREATMENT OF STRICTURE OF THE URETHRA AND URINARY FISTULÆ. With plates and wood-cuts. From the third and revised English edition. In one very handsome octavo volume, cloth, $3 50. (*Lately Published.*)

ROBERTS (WILLIAM), M.D.,
Lecturer on Medicine in the Manchester School of Medicine, etc.

A PRACTICAL TREATISE ON URINARY AND RENAL DISEASES, including Urinary Deposits. Illustrated by numerous cases and engravings. Second American, from the Second Revised and Enlarged London Edition. In one large and handsome octavo volume of 616 pages, with a colored plate; cloth, $4 50. (*Lately Published.*)

TUKE (DANIEL HACK), M.D.,
Joint author of "The Manual of Psychological Medicine," &c.

ILLUSTRATIONS OF THE INFLUENCE OF THE MIND UPON THE BODY IN HEALTH AND DISEASE. Designed to illustrate the Action of the Imagination. In one handsome octavo volume of 416 pages; cloth, $3 25. (*Lately Issued.*)

BLANDFORD (G. FIELDING), M.D., F.R.C.P.,
Lecturer on Psychological Medicine at the School of St George's Hospital, &c.

INSANITY AND ITS TREATMENT: Lectures on the Treatment, Medical and Legal, of Insane Patients. With a Summary of the Laws in force in the United States on the Confinement of the Insane. By ISAAC RAY, M. D. In one very handsome octavo volume of 471 pages; cloth, $3 25.

It satisfies a want which must have been sorely felt by the busy general practitioners of this country. It takes the form of a manual of clinical description of the various forms of insanity, with a description of the mode of examining persons suspected of insanity. We call particular attention to this feature of the book, as giving it a unique value to the general practitioner. If we pass from theoretical considerations to descriptions of the varieties of insanity as actually seen in practice and the appropriate treatment for them, we find in Dr. Blandford's work a considerable advance over previous writings on the subject. His pictures of the various forms of mental disease are so clear and good that no reader can fail to be struck with their superiority to those given in ordinary manuals in the English language or (so far as our own reading extends) in any other.—*London Practitioner*, Feb. 1871.

LEA (HENRY C.).

SUPERSTITION AND FORCE: ESSAYS ON THE WAGER OF LAW, THE WAGER OF BATTLE, THE ORDEAL, AND TORTURE. Third Revised and Enlarged Edition. In one handsome royal 12mo. volume of 552 pages. Cloth, $2 50. (*Just Ready.*)

The appearance of a new edition of Mr. Henry C. Lea's "Superstition and Force" is a sign that our highest scholarship is not without honor in its native country. Mr. Lea has met every fresh demand for his work with a careful revision of it, and the present edition is not only fuller and, if possible, more accurate than either of the preceding, but, from the thorough elaboration is more like a harmonious concert and less like a baton of studies.—*The Nation*, Aug. 1, 1878.

Many will be tempted to say that this, like the "Decline and Fall," is one of the uncriticizable books. Its facts are innumerable, its deductions simple and inevitable, and its *chevaux-de-frise* of references bristling and dense enough to make the keenest, stoutest, and best equipped assailant think twice before advancing. Nor is there anything controversial in it to provoke assault. The author is no polemic. Though he obviously feels and thinks strongly, he succeeds in attaining impartiality. Whether looked on as a picture or a mirror, a work such as this has a lasting value.—*Lippincott's Magazine*, Oct. 1878.

Mr. Lea's curious historical monographs, of which one of the most important is here reproduced in an enlarged form, have given him an unique position among English and American scholars. He is distinguished for his recondite and affluent learning, his power of exhaustive historical analysis, the breadth and accuracy of his researches among the rarer sources of knowledge, the gravity and temperance of his statements, combined with singular earnestness of conviction, and his warm attachment to the cause of human freedom and intellectual progress.—*N. Y. Tribune*, Aug. 9, 1878.

BY THE SAME AUTHOR. (*Lately Published.*)

STUDIES IN CHURCH HISTORY—THE RISE OF THE TEMPORAL POWER—BENEFIT OF CLERGY—EXCOMMUNICATION. In one large royal 12mo. volume of 516 pp.; cloth, $2 75.

The story was never told more calmly or with greater learning or wiser thought. We doubt, indeed, if any other study of this field can be compared with this for clearness, accuracy, and power.—*Chicago Examiner*, Dec. 1870.

Mr. Lea's latest work, "Studies in Church History," fully sustains the promise of the first. It deals with three subjects—the Temporal Power, Benefit of Clergy, and Excommunication, the record of which has a peculiar importance for the English student, and is a chapter on Ancient Law likely to be regarded as final. We can hardly pass from our mention of such works as these—with which that on "Sacerdotal Celibacy" should be included—without noting the literary phenomenon that the head of one of the first American houses is also the writer of some of its most original books.—*London Athenæum*, Jan 7, 1871.

[illegible] Books marked with * exceed the limit of Four Pounds [illegible] and therefore not mailable. [illegible] forwarding.

Lightning Source UK Ltd.
Milton Keynes UK
UKOW021953181012

200821UK00009B/150/P